5th Edition

Professional Issues
in Nursing

CHALLENGES AND OPPORTUNITIES

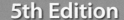
5th Edition

Professional Issues
in Nursing

CHALLENGES AND OPPORTUNITIES

Carol J. Huston, RN, MSN, MPA, DPA, FAAN
Professor Emerita, School of Nursing
California State University
Chico, California

 Wolters Kluwer

Philadelphia • Baltimore • New York • London
Buenos Aires • Hong Kong • Sydney • Tokyo

Vice President and Publisher: Julie K. Stegman
Senior Acquisitions Editor: Christina Burns
Director of Product Development: Jennifer K. Forestieri
Senior Development Editor: Michael Kerns
Editorial Coordinator: Tim Rinehart
Marketing Manager: Brittany Clements
Editorial Assistant: Kaitlin Campbell
Art Director: Elaine Kasmer
Art Director, Illustration: Jennifer Clements
Production Coordinator: Sadie Buckallew
Manufacturing Coordinator: Karin Duffield
Prepress Vendor: S4Carlisle Publishing Services

5th edition

9 8 7 6 5 4 3 2

Printed in China

Library of Congress Cataloging-in-Publication Data

Names: Huston, Carol Jorgensen, author.
Title: Professional issues in nursing: challenges and opportunities / Carol
  J. Huston.
Description: 5th edition. | Philadelphia, PA: Wolters Kluwer, [2020] |
  Includes bibliographical references and index.
Identifiers: LCCN 2018049595 | ISBN 9781496398185
Subjects: | MESH: Nursing—trends | Nurse's Role | Professional Competence |
  Nursing—manpower | Ethics, Nursing | United States
Classification: LCC RT82 | NLM WY 16 AA1 | DDC 610.73—dc23 LC record available at
  https://lccn.loc.gov/2018049595

CCS0719

I dedicate this book to my grandson Jackson. Your determination, courage, and love inspires all of us.

Carol J. Huston

Contributors

Sheila A. Burke, DNP, MBA, MSN, RN, BC-NEA
Vice President of Nursing
Nursing Division
Education Affiliates, Inc.
Baltimore, Maryland
(CHAPTER 24)

Jennifer Dine, PhD, RN
Adjunct Assistant Professor
Nursing PhD Program
The Graduate Center, City University of New York
New York, New York
(CHAPTER 24)

Cassandra D. Ford, PhD, RN, FAHA, FGSA
Associate Professor
Capstone College of Nursing
The University of Alabama
Tuscaloosa, Alabama
(CHAPTER 5)

Ryan M. Fuller, MSN, RN, CNML
Strategy Integration Program Director
Kaiser Permanente Nurse Scholars Academy
Kaiser Permanente–Northern California
Oakland, California
(CHAPTER 2)

Lynn Gallagher-Ford, PhD, RN, NE-BC, DPFNAP, FAAN
Senior Director
Helene Fuld Health Trust National Institute for Evidence-based Practice in Nursing and Healthcare
Director
Clinical Core, Helene Fuld Health Trust National Institute for Evidence-based Practice in Nursing and Healthcare
The Ohio State University–College of Nursing
Columbus, Ohio
(CHAPTER 3)

Perry M. Gee, PhD, RN
Adjunct Assistant Professor
College of Nursing
University of Utah
Salt Lake City, Utah
Nurse Scientist
Nursing Research and Analytics
Dignity Health
Phoenix, Arizona
(CHAPTER 13)

Charmaine Hockley, PhD, MEd Admin, LLB, RN, FACN, JP
Adjunct Senior Lecturer
College of Nursing and Health Sciences
Flinders University
Bedford Park, South Australia
(CHAPTER 12)

Carol J. Huston, RN, MSN, MPA, DPA, FAAN
Professor Emerita
School of Nursing
California State University
Chico, California
(CHAPTERS 1, 6, 7, 8, 9, 10, 11, 14, 15, 16, 19, 20, 21, 22, 23)

Holly T. Kralj, DNP, CNM, PHN, IBCLC
Associate Professor
School of Nursing
California State University
Chico, California
Certified Nurse Midwife
Enloe Women's Services
Chico, California
(CHAPTER 4)

Jennifer Lillibridge, PhD, RN
Professor Emerita
School of Nursing
California State University
Chico, California
(CHAPTER 17)

Michelle L. Litchman, PhD, FNP-BC, FAANP
Assistant Professor
College of Nursing
University of Utah
Salt Lake City, Utah
(CHAPTER 13)

Kathy Malloch, PhD, MBA, RN, FAAN
President, KMLS, LLC
Professor of Practice
Arizona State University
College of Nursing and Health Innovation
Phoenix, Arizona
Clinical Professor
Ohio State University, College of Nursing
Columbus, Ohio
Clinical Consultant
API Healthcare Inc
Hartford, Wisconsin
(CHAPTER 3)

Bernadette Mazurek Melnyk, PhD, RN, APRN-CNP
Vice President for Health Promotion
University Chief Wellness Officer
Dean and Professor, College of Nursing
Professor of Pediatrics and Psychiatry, College of Medicine
Executive Director, The Helene Fuld Health Trust National Institute for EBP
The Ohio State University
Columbus, Ohio
(CHAPTER 13)

Donna M. Nickitas, PhD, RN, NEA-BC, FNAP, FAAN
Dean and Professor
Rutgers School of Nursing-Camden–Rutgers University
Camden, New Jersey
Editor
Nursing Economics
The Journal for Health Care Leaders
Pitman, New Jersey
(CHAPTER 24)

George C. Pittman, RN, CCRN, MSN
Associate Professor
School of Nursing
California State University
Chico, California
(CHAPTER 18)

Suzanne S. Prevost, PhD, RN,
    FAAN
Professor and Dean
Capstone College of Nursing
The University of Alabama
Tuscaloosa, Alabama
(CHAPTER 5)

Margaret J. Rowberg, DNP, APRN
Professor Emerita
School of Nursing
California State University
Chico, California
(CHAPTER 4)

Patricia E. Thompson, RN, EdD
CEO, Retired
Sigma Theta Tau International
Indianapolis, Indiana
(CHAPTER 25)

Cynthia Vlasich, MBA, BSN, RN,
    FAAN
Director
Global Initiatives
Sigma Theta Tau International
Indianapolis, Indiana
(CHAPTER 25)

Jonalyn Wallace, DNP, MSN,
    RN-BC, CENP
Academic Relations Director
Kaiser Permanente–Northern
    California
Oakland, California
(CHAPTER 2)

Nikki West, MPH
Director
Health Care Education
    Management
Northern California Patient Care
    Services
Kaiser Permanente
Oakland, California
(CHAPTER 2)

Reviewers

Jill Bass, DNP, MSN, RN, GCNS-BC
Virginia Western Community College
Roanoke, Virginia

Dawn R. Bunting, EdD, MSN, RN, CNE
Capital Community College
Hartford, Connecticut

Karen Cooper, MSN, RN
Clinical Assistant Professor
Towson University
Towson, Maryland

Betty Daniels, PhD, RN
Brenau University
Gainesville, Georgia

Beena Davis, RN, MSN
LA County College of Nursing and Allied Health
Los Angeles, California

Drew Ellen Gogian, EdD, MSN, RN
Mary Baldwin University
Staunton, Virginia

Karla Haug, MS, RN
North Dakota State University
Fargo, North Dakota

Kathleen M. Kennedy, PhD, RN, PHN
Concordia University Irvine
Irvine, California

J. Mari Beth Linder, PhD, RN, BC
Missouri Southern State University
Joplin, Missouri

Dr. Ladonna Michelle McClave, EdD, MSN, RN
Morehead State University
Morehead, Kentucky

Janet Tompkins McMahon, DNP, MSN, RN, ANEF
Towson University
Towson, Maryland

Dolores Minchhoff, DNP, CRNP
Pennsylvania College of Health Sciences
Lancaster, Pennsylvania

Sharvette Law Philmon, MSN, RN, NEA-BC, CNE
Lincoln University
Lincoln, New Zealand

Kimberly Sharp, RN, PhD
Mississippi College
Clinton, Mississippi

Danielle White, MSN, RN
Austin Peay State University
Clarksville, Tennessee

Mary B. Williams, MS, RN
Associate Professor of Nursing
Gordon State College
Barnesville, Georgia

Karen A. Zapko, PhD, MSN, RN
Kent State University
Kent, Ohio

Preface

As a nursing educator for almost 38 years, I have taught many courses dealing with the significant issues that impact the nursing profession. I often felt frustrated that textbooks that were supposed to be devoted to professional issues in the field instead deviated significantly into other areas, including nursing research and theory. In addition, while many of the existing professional issues books dealt with the enduring issues of the profession, it was difficult to find a book for my students that incorporated those with the "hot topics" of the time. The first four editions of *Professional Issues in Nursing: Challenges and Opportunities* were efforts to address both needs. The fifth edition maintains this precedent with significant content updates, the deletion of three chapters, and the addition of two new chapters.

This book continues, however, to be first and foremost a professional issues book. Although an effort has been made to integrate research and theory into chapters where it seemed appropriate, these topics in and of themselves are too broad to be fully addressed in a professional issues book. This book is also directed at what my expert nursing colleagues and I have identified as both enduring professional issues and the most pressing contemporary issues facing the profession. It is my hope, then, that this book fills an unmet need in the current professional issues text market. It has an undiluted focus on professional issues in nursing and includes many timely issues not addressed in other professional issues texts. This is an edited book, with 15 chapters contributed by the primary author and the remaining 10 chapters by guest contributors with expertise in the specific subject material.

This book has been designed primarily for use at both the baccalaureate and the graduate levels. It is envisioned that it will be used as a primary textbook or as a supplement for a typical two- to three-unit professional issues course. It would also be appropriate for most RN–BSN bridge courses and may be considered by some faculty as a supplemental reader to a leadership/management course that includes professional issues.

The book can be used in both the traditional classroom and online courses because the discussion question format works well for both small and large groups onsite as well as in bulletin board and chat room venues.

ORGANIZATION AND FEATURES

The book is divided into five units, representing contemporary and enduring issues in professional nursing including Furthering the Profession, Workforce Issues, Workplace Issues, Legal and Ethical Issues, and Professional Power. Each unit has four to six chapters.

FEATURES

Each chapter begins with **Learning Objectives** and an overview of the professional issue being discussed. Multiple perspectives on each issue are then identified in an effort to reflect the diversity of thought found in the literature as well as espoused by experts in the field and varied professional nursing and health care organizations. **Discussion Points** encourage readers to pause and reflect on specific questions (individually or in groups), and **Consider This** features encourage active learning, critical thinking, and values clarification by the users. In addition, at least one research study is profiled in every chapter in **Research Fuels the Controversy**, an effort to promote evidence-based analysis of the issue. Each chapter ends with **Conclusions** about the issues discussed, questions **For Additional Discussion**, and a comprehensive and current reference list. Also included in each chapter are multiple displays, boxes, and tables to help the user visualize important concepts.

NEW TO THIS EDITION

- A new chapter on the opportunities, limitations, and challenges of emerging technologies in health care has been added.

- A new chapter on health care reform and the dismantling of the Affordable Care Act has been added.

- New or updated content has been added throughout the book to reflect cutting-edge trends in health care, including the ongoing demand for quality and safety in the workplace for patients as well as workers; workforce projections and changing population demographics; the recommendations of the Institute of Medicine (IOM) put forth in *The Future of Nursing: Leading Change, Advancing Health*; and the challenges and opportunities that accompany the provision of nursing care in an increasingly global, rapidly changing, technology-driven world.

TEACHING/LEARNING RESOURCES

Professional Issues in Nursing: Challenges and Opportunities, fifth edition, includes additional resources for both instructors and students that are available on the book's companion website at http://thePoint.lww.com/Huston3e.

Instructor Resources

Approved adopting instructors will be given access to the following additional resources:

- Test Generator containing NCLEX-style questions
- PowerPoint Presentations
- Journal Articles
- Answers to Journal Articles Critical Thinking Questions

- Lab Activities with Answers
- Teaching/Learning Activities

Student Resources

Students who have purchased *Professional Issues in Nursing: Challenges and Opportunities*, fifth edition, have access to the following additional resources:

- Journal Articles
- Journal Articles Critical Thinking Questions
- Spanish–English Audio Glossary
- Learning Objectives

In addition, purchasers of the text can access the searchable full text online by going to the *Professional Issues in Nursing: Challenges and Opportunities*, fourth edition, website at http://thePoint.lww.com/Huston3e. See inside the front cover of this text for more details, including the passcode you will need to gain access to the website.

Carol J. Huston

Contents

UNIT 5   PROFESSIONAL POWER

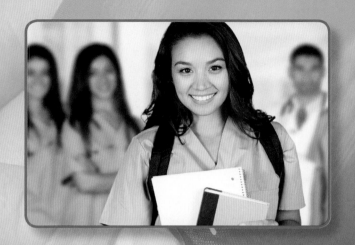

1

FURTHERING THE PROFESSION

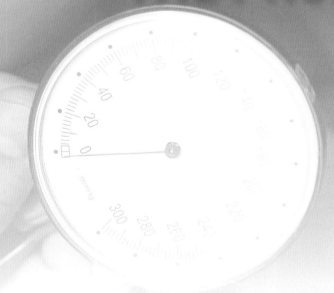

Entry Into Practice
The Debate Rages On
Carol J. Huston

LEARNING OBJECTIVES

The learner will be able to:

1. Differentiate between technical and professional nurses as outlined in Esther Lucille Brown's classic *Nursing for the Future*.

2. Identify what, if any, progress has been made on increasing the educational entry level for professional registered nursing since publication of the 1965 position paper of the American Nurses Association on entry into practice.

3. Identify similarities and differences between contemporary associate and baccalaureate degree nursing programs.

4. Describe basic components of associate degree educational programs as outlined by Mildred Montag and compare those with typical associate degree programs in the 21st century.

5. Analyze how having one NCLEX for entry into practice, regardless of educational entry level, impacts the entry-into-practice dilemma.

6. Identify key driving and restraining forces for increasing the educational entry level for professional nursing.

7. Analyze the potential impacts of raising the educational entry level on the current nursing shortage, workforce diversity, and intraprofessional conflict.

8. Examine current research that explores the impact of registered nurse educational level on patient outcomes.

9. Explore how shifting health care delivery sites and increasing registered nursing competency

requirements are impacting employer preferences for hiring a more educated nursing workforce.

10. Compare the nursing profession's educational entry standards with that of the other health care professions.

11. Identify positions taken by specific professional organizations, certifying bodies, and employers

regarding the appropriate educational level for entry into practice for professional nursing.

12. Explore personal values, beliefs, and feelings regarding whether the educational entry level in nursing should be increased to a baccalaureate or higher degree.

INTRODUCTION

Few issues have been as long-standing or as contentious in nursing as the entry-into-practice debate. Although the entry-into-practice debate dates back to the 1940s with the publication of Esther Lucille Brown's classic *Nursing for the Future*, the debate came to the forefront with a 1965 position paper by the American Nurses Association (ANA, 1965a, 1965b). This position paper suggested an orderly transition from hospital-based diploma nursing preparation to nursing education in colleges or universities based on the following premises:

- The education of all those who are licensed to practice nursing should take place in institutions of higher education.
- Minimum preparation for beginning professional nursing practice should be baccalaureate education in nursing.
- Minimum preparation for beginning technical practice should be associate degree education in nursing.
- Education for assistants in the health care occupations should be short, intensive, preservice programs in vocational education institutions rather than on-the-job training programs.

In essence, two levels of preparation were suggested for registered nurses (RNs): *technical* and *professional*. Persons interested in technical practice would enroll in junior or community colleges and earn associate degrees in 2-year programs. Those interested in professional nursing would enroll in 4-year programs in colleges or universities. Hospital-based diploma programs were to be phased out.

The curricula for the two programs were to be very different, as were each program's foci. The 2-year technical degree was to result in an associate degree in nursing (ADN). This degree, as proposed by Mildred Montag (Fig. 1.1) in her dissertation in 1952, with direction and support from R. Louise McManus, would prepare a beginning, technical practitioner who would provide care in acute-care settings, under the supervision of a professional nurse.

In a typical associate degree program, approximately half of the credits would be fulfilled by general education courses such as English, anatomy, physiology, speech, psychology, and sociology and the other half were fulfilled by nursing courses. The 4-year degree would result in a Bachelor of Science in nursing (BSN) and would encompass coursework taught in ADN programs as well as more in-depth treatment of the physical and social sciences, nursing research, public and community health, nursing management, and the humanities. The additional course work in the BSN was intended to enhance the students' professional development, prepare them for a broader scope of

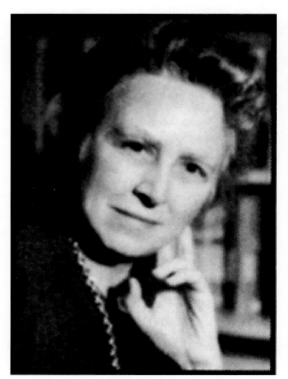

Figure 1.1 Mildred Montag.

practice, and provide a better understanding of the cultural, political, economic, and social issues affecting patients and health care delivery.

The ANA 1965 position statement was reaffirmed by a resolution at the ANA House of Delegates in 1978, which set forth the requirement that the baccalaureate degree would be the entry level into professional nursing practice by 1985. Associate degree and diploma programs responded strongly to what they viewed as inflammatory terminology and clearly stated that not being considered "professional" was unacceptable. In the end, both ADN and diploma programs refused to compromise title or licensure. Dissension ensued both within and among nursing groups, but little movement occurred to make the position statement a reality.

> **Consider This** Titling (professional vs. technical) was and will be an important consideration before consensus can be reached on the entry-into-practice debate.

Finally, in 2008, 30 years later, the ANA House of Delegates stepped forth once again to pass a resolution supporting initiatives to require diploma- and associate-degree-educated nurses to obtain a BSN within 10 years of license. The responsibility for mandating and implementing this new resolution was passed on to individual states.

Just one state, however, North Dakota, became successful in changing the Nurse Practice Act so that baccalaureate education was necessary for initial RN licensure. For 15 years, it was the only state to recognize baccalaureate education as the minimal education for professional nursing, despite challenges from opposing groups. Unfortunately, however, North Dakota repealed this act in 2003, bowing to pressure from nurses and some health care organizations, to once again allowing nonbaccalaureate entry into practice.

Other states, however, continue to consider increasing educational entry levels. California, for example, requires a BSN for certification as a public health nurse in that state, and multiple states require a BSN to be a school nurse because it is part of public health nursing. New York signed a "BSN in 10" bill into law on December 19, 2017, making it a leader in recognizing the significance of baccalaureate preparation for RNs (Newland, 2018). The purpose of the law was to increase the level of education for professional RNs, requiring that newly licensed nurses already have a BSN at the time of entry into practice or achieve a BSN within 10 years after initial licensure.

In addition, state nursing associations or other nursing coalitions in California, Rhode Island, and New Jersey have, over the past few years, called for initiatives to establish the BSN as the entry level for nursing in their respective state. Other states are pursuing some type of initiative requiring newly graduated RNs to obtain a BSN within a certain time frame to maintain their licensure.

The end result, however, is that almost 55 years after the initial ANA resolution, entry into practice at the baccalaureate level has not been accomplished. Even the strongest supporters of the BSN for entry into practice cannot deny that, despite almost six decades of efforts, RN entry at the baccalaureate level continues to be an elusive goal.

PROLIFERATION OF ADN EDUCATION

It is doubtful that Mildred Montag had any idea in 1952 that ADN programs would someday become the predominant entry level for nursing practice or that this education model would proliferate like it did in the 1960s—just one decade after she completed her doctoral work. While the overwhelming majority of nurses in the early 1960s were educated in diploma schools of nursing, enrollment in baccalaureate programs was increasing and associate degree programs were just beginning. By the year 2000, diploma education had virtually disappeared, and although BSN education had increased significantly, it was ADN education, that represented nearly two thirds of all nursing school graduates.

Indeed, ADN education continues to be the primary model for initial nursing education in the United States today. According to a 2013 HRSA report, titled *The U.S. Nursing Workforce: Trends in Supply and Education*, only 55% of the RN workforce currently holds a baccalaureate or higher degree. Further, only 43% of first-time NCLEX test takers were graduates of baccalaureate nursing programs (American Association of Colleges of Nursing [AACN], 2015b). Yet, enrollment in baccalaureate nursing programs is on the rise with 15 consecutive years of enrollment growth. Indeed, Clarke (2017) notes that although the majority of new nursing graduates seeking RN licensure still come from associate degree programs, with each passing year, the proportion of entry-level NCLEX test takers moves closer to a 50-50 split.

LICENSURE AND ENTRY INTO PRACTICE

Critics of BSN as a requirement for entry into practice argue that there is no need to raise entry levels because passing rates for the National Council Licensure Examination (NCLEX) show only small differences between ADN, diploma, and BSN graduates (Table 1.1). Although some might argue that this suggests similar competencies across the educational spectrum, the more common precept is

TABLE 1.1	2017 NCLEX-RN Passage Rate per Educational Program Type	
Program Type	**Number of Graduates**	**NCLEX-RN Passage Rate (%)**
Diploma	2,222	90.23
Associate degree	79,511	84.24
Baccalaureate degree	75,944	90.04

Source: National Council of State Boards of Nursing. (2018, January 19). *2017: Number of candidates taking NCLEX examination and percent passing, by type of candidate.* Retrieved April 12, 2018, from https://www.ncsbn.org/Table_of_Pass_Rates_2017.pdf

that the NCLEX is a test that measures minimum technical competencies for safe entry into basic nursing practice and, as such, may not measure performance over time or test for all of the knowledge and skills developed through a BSN program.

One must also ask why the nursing profession has not differentiated RN licensure testing based on educational preparation for RNs, just as has been done for practical nurses and advanced practice nurses. Hewitt (2016) suggests that at some point, conversations about how to lessen the confusion between levels of nursing should include the possibility of two levels of NCLEX-RN licensing. This would celebrate each level of nursing education and help to clarify differentiated levels of practice. Complicating the picture, however, is that both ADN and BSN schools preparing graduates for RN licensure meet similar criteria for state board approval and have roughly the same number of nursing coursework units. These factors contribute to confusion about differentiations between ADN- and BSN-prepared nurses and result in an inability to move forward on implementing the BSN as the entry level for professional nursing.

Discussion Point

Should separate licensing examinations be developed for ADN-, diploma-, and BSN-educated nurses?

Consider This Critics of BSN entry into practice argue that ADN-, diploma-, and BSN-educated nurses all take the same licensing examination and therefore have earned the title of RN. In addition, nurses prepared at all three levels have successfully worked side by side, under the same scope of practice, for more than 55 years.

In addition, many employers state that they are unable to differentiate roles for nurses based on education because both ADN- and BSN-prepared nurses hold the same license. Ironically, state boards of nursing have asserted their inability to develop a different licensure system given the fact that employers have not developed different roles.

Discussion Point

Should licensure be equated with professional status?

EDUCATIONAL LEVELS AND PATIENT OUTCOMES

Perhaps the most common argument against raising the entry level in nursing is an emotional one, with ADN-prepared nurses arguing that "caring does not require a baccalaureate degree." Many ADN-educated nurses argue passionately that patients do not know or care what educational degree is held by their nurse as long as they receive high-quality care by the nurse at their bedside. ADN nurses also frequently claim that BSN-prepared nurses are too theoretically oriented and thus are not in touch with real practice. In addition, many ADN nurses suggest that baccalaureate-prepared nurses are deficient in basic skills mastery and conclude that care provided by ADN nurses is at least as good as, if not better than, that provided by their BSN counterparts.

Consider This Most ADN-prepared nurses argue that significant differences exist between their practice and that of a licensed vocational/practical nurse (LVN/LPN), despite there typically being only 12 months' difference in length of educational preparation. Yet, many ADN-educated nurses argue that the additional education that BSN-educated nurses have makes little difference in their practice over that of their ADN counterparts. How can this argument be justified?

An increasing number of studies, however, report differences between the performance levels of ADN- and BSN-prepared nurses. In a landmark study, Aiken, Clarke, Cheung, Sloane, and Silber (2003) at the University of Pennsylvania identified a clear link between higher levels of nursing education and better patient outcomes (AACN, 2018c). This study found that surgical patients have a "substantial survival advantage" if treated in hospitals with higher proportions of nurses educated at the baccalaureate or higher degree level and that a 10% increase in the proportion of nurses holding BSN degrees decreased the risk of patient death and failure to rescue by 5% (AACN, 2018c).

Research by Aiken and colleagues also showed that hospitals with better care environments, the best nurse staffing levels, and the most highly educated nurses had the lowest surgical mortality rates. In fact, the researchers found that every 10% increase in the proportion of BSN nurses on the hospital staff was associated with a 4% decrease in the risk of death (Aiken, Clarke, Sloane, Lake, & Cheney, 2008).

A more recent study by Yakusheva, Lindrooth, and Weiss (2014) of 8,526 adult medical-surgical patients found similar results with BSN education being associated with lower mortality ($p < 0.01$), lower odds of readmission ($p = 0.04$), and 1.9% shorter length of stay ($p = 0.03$). Economic simulations supported a strong business case for increasing the proportion of BSN-educated nurses in the workforce.

Another study by Kutney-Lee and colleagues found that a 10-point increase in the percentage of nurses holding a BSN within a hospital was associated with an average reduction of 2.12 deaths for every 1,000 patients—and for a subset of patients with complications, an average reduction of 7.47 deaths per 1,000 patients (AACN, 2018c). In a cross-sectional study of 21 University Health System Consortium hospitals, Blegen, Goode, Park, Vaughn, and Spetz (2013) analyzed the association between RN education and patient outcomes. The researchers found that hospitals with a higher percentage of RNs with baccalaureate or higher degrees had lower congestive heart failure mortality, decubitus ulcers, failure to rescue, and postoperative deep vein thrombosis or pulmonary embolism and shorter length of stay (AACN, 2018c).

As more outcome research becomes available suggesting an empirical link between educational entry level of nurses and patient outcomes, nursing leaders, professional associations, and employers are increasingly speaking out on the need to raise the profession's entry level as a means of improving quality patient care and patient safety. Yet, Clarke (2017) raises at least some doubt about concluding that these outcomes are clearly due to baccalaureate-educated nurses providing a higher quality of care. He notes it is possible that conditions favoring better patient outcomes, such as an attractive labor market, a range of higher education opportunities, and a better professional practice environment, may simply be more common in hospitals where there are more baccalaureate-prepared nurses.

EMPLOYERS' VIEWS AND PREFERENCES

Nursing employers are still somewhat divided on the issue of entry into practice. The academic requirements of associate degree, diploma, and baccalaureate programs vary widely, yet health care settings that employ nursing graduates often make no distinction in the scope of practice among nurses with different levels of preparation. Furthermore, many employers provide no incentives for BSN education in terms of pay, recognition, or career mobility and are afraid to do so, fearing they may be unable to fill vacant nursing positions. The starting rate of pay for ADN- and BSN-prepared nurses historically has not been significantly different, although this appears to be changing.

Employers, however, appear to be increasingly aware of purported differences between BSN and ADN graduates, and this is increasingly being reflected in their hiring preferences. A 2014 survey by the AACN found that 45.1% of hospitals across the country required new hires to have a bachelor's degree ("The Ultimate Guide," 2017). Similarly, AACN reported that 59% of new BSN graduates had jobs at the time of graduation, compared to the national average across all professions of 29.3% and that 89% of new BSN graduates had secured employment in nursing within 4 to 6 months after graduation (New AACN Data, 2014). One reason is the Magnet Recognition Program's requirement that nurse managers and leaders have at least a baccalaureate in nursing. Magnet hospitals are also required to have a higher percentage of nurses educated at the baccalaureate level.

In addition, some employers are now giving preference for clinical placements to students in baccalaureate and higher degree programs over those enrolled in associate degree programs.

Indeed, LaRocco (2014) suggests that

. . .while state boards of nursing and legislatures fail to act to change the entry requirements for professional nursing, in many areas of the country the baccalaureate is becoming the de facto requirement. Major medical centers in the Boston area no longer hire nurses with associate's degrees. At least one large, for-profit hospital chain has decreed that their nurses must obtain a baccalaureate within a stipulated period of time, typically 3 to 5 years. Nurses with associate's degrees are limited in both their initial employment and their long-term options. (p. 11)

Discussion Point

If indeed employers prefer hiring BSN-prepared RNs, why don't more employers offer pay differentials for nurses with BSN degrees?

The Veterans Administration (VA), with its 35,000 nurses on staff, is leading the nation in raising the bar for a higher educational entry hire level in nursing. The VA established the BSN as the minimum education level for new hires and as the minimum preparation its nurses must have for promotion beyond the entry level (AACN, 2018c).

SHIFTING HEALTH CARE DELIVERY SITES AND REQUIRED COMPETENCIES

Although hospitals continue to be the main site of employment for nurses, there is an ongoing shift in health care from acute-care settings to the community and integrated health care settings. This shift will clearly require more highly educated nurses who can function autonomously as caregivers, leaders, managers, and change agents. These are all skills that are emphasized in a baccalaureate nursing curriculum.

In addition, in response to changes in health care as the result of the Affordable Care Act, RNs must now be skilled in population health, case management, and quality metrics, which are competencies obtained through baccalaureate education (Auerbach, Buerhaus, & Staiger, 2015). In addition, a 2014 study by Kumm, Godfrey, Martin, Tucci, Muenks, and Spaeth, of curriculum in 17 ADN programs found that two thirds were missing identified competencies considered essential for nurses including population health, evidence-based practice, and leadership (Baur, Moore, & Wendler, 2017).

> *Consider This* Baccalaureate and graduate-level skills in research, leadership, management, and community health are increasingly needed in nursing as health care extends beyond the acute-care hospital.

In May 2010, the Tri-Council for Nursing, a coalition of four steering organizations for the nursing profession (AACN, ANA, the American Organization of Nurse Executives [AONE], and the National League for Nursing [NLN]), issued a consensus statement calling for all RNs to advance their education in the interest of enhancing quality and safety across health care settings. The statement suggested that a more highly educated nursing workforce will be critical to meeting the nation's nursing needs and delivering safe, effective patient care and that failure to do so will place the nation's health at further risk (AACN, 2015a).

The recommendations of the IOM (2010) report, *The Future of Nursing*, were even stronger. This landmark report called for increasing the number of baccalaureate-prepared nurses in the workforce from 50% to 80% over the next 10 years and doubling the population of nurses with doctorates to meet the demands of an evolving health care system and changing patient needs.

In addition, in December 2009, Patricia Benner and her team at the Carnegie Foundation for the Advancement of Teaching released a new study titled *Educating*

Nurses: A Call for Radical Transformation, which recommended preparing all entry-level RNs at the baccalaureate level and requiring all RNs to earn a master's degree within 10 years of initial licensure (Benner, Sutphen, Leonard, & Day, 2010). The authors found that many of today's new nurses are "undereducated" to meet practice demands across settings. Their strong support for high-quality baccalaureate degree programs as the appropriate pathway for RNs entering the profession is consistent with the views of many leading nursing organizations, including AACN (AACN, 2015b).

Similarly, the National Advisory Council on Nurse Education and Practice (NACNEP) suggests that nursing's role for the future calls for RNs to manage care along a continuum, to work as peers in interdisciplinary teams, and to integrate clinical expertise with knowledge of community resources. This increased complexity of scope of practice will require the capacity to adapt to change; critical thinking and problem-solving skills; a social foundation in a broad range of basic sciences; knowledge of behavioral, social, and management sciences; and the ability to analyze and communicate data (AACN, 2015b). All these are integral components of BSN education. As a result, the NACNEP has recommended to Congress that at least two thirds of the nurse workforce hold baccalaureate or higher degrees in nursing (AACN, 2015a, 2015b).

The Council on Physician and Nurse Supply also released a statement in 2007 calling for a national effort to substantially expand baccalaureate nursing programs, citing the growing body of evidence that nursing education impacts both the quality and safety of patient care. Consequently, the group is calling on policy makers to shift federal funding priorities in favor of supporting more baccalaureate-level nursing programs (AACN, 2018c). Some nurse leaders have even suggested that a BSN degree may not be an adequate preparation for these expanded roles and that, instead, master's or doctoral degrees should be required for entry into practice for registered nursing.

Discussion Point

Would raising the entry level to the master's or doctoral degree eliminate the tension between supporters of ADN and BSN as entry levels into nursing, since both educational preparations would be considered inadequate? Is a graduate degree currently feasible as the entry level for professional nursing? If not, what would it take to make it happen?

ENTRY LEVEL AND PROFESSIONAL STATUS

Nurses, consumers, and allied health care professionals are currently questioning why the entry level into professional nursing is so much lower than other health care professions. Does nursing require less skill? Is the knowledge base needed to provide nursing care skill based instead of knowledge based? Should nursing be reclassified as a vocational trade and not a profession? The answer to these questions, of course, is no. Yet clearly, nurses have resisted the normal course of occupational development that other health care professions have pursued. As a result, nurses are now the least educated of the health care professionals, with most health care professions now requiring graduate degrees for entry. Indeed, one must question whether nursing is at risk for losing its designation as a profession because of its failure to maintain educational equity.

Discussion Point

Is nursing in danger of losing its designation as a "profession" if it fails to maintain educational entry levels comparable to those of the other health professions?

The primary identity of any professional group is based on the established education entry level. Attorneys, physicians, social workers, engineers, clergy, and physical therapists, to list a few examples, have in common an essential education at the bachelor's level. Nursing is unique among the health care professions in having multiple educational pathways lead to the same entry-level license to practice. In fact, advanced degrees are required in many professions for entry positions at the professional level. Only nursing continues the hypocrisy of pretending that education is unimportant and does not make a difference. Only nursing allows individuals with no college course work, or with limited college study that lacks a well-rounded global college education, to lay claim to the same licensure and identity as that held by nurses having a baccalaureate education.

Indeed, the educational gap between nursing and other health professions continues to grow (Table 1.2). Disciplines such as occupational therapy, physical therapy, speech therapy, and social work all require master's or doctoral degrees. Pharmacy has also raised its educational entry level standards to that of a doctoral degree.

Consider This   Unlike the other health care professions which now require master's and doctoral degrees, nursing continues to put forth an argument that educational degree does not matter or that requiring a BSN for entry into practice is elitist.

TABLE 1.2	Entry-Level Degrees for the Health Professions
Health Profession	**Entry-Level Degree**
Medicine	Doctorate
Pharmacy	Doctorate
Social work	Master's
Speech pathology	Master's
Physical therapy	Master's transitioning to doctorate
Occupational therapy	Master's
Nursing	Associate

Failure to maintain educational parity with other health care professions also contributes to nursing being viewed as a "second-class citizen" in the health care arena. It is difficult to justify the profession's argument that nursing should be an equal partner in health care decision making when other professions are so much better educated, suggesting that nurses are either undereducated for the roles they assume or that the nursing role lacks complexity.

Consider This   Nursing is the only health care "profession" that does not require at least a bachelor's or higher degree for entry into practice.

THE 2-YEAR ADN PROGRAM?

Many ADN-prepared nurses also express frustration when discussing the need to raise the entry level in professional nursing because they feel the ADN degree does not appropriately represent the scope of their education or the time they had to put in to earn what is typically considered to be a 2-year degree. ADN nurses argue that the "2-year" ADN program is a myth. Many ADN students follow nontraditional education paths, and almost all ADN programs currently require three or more years of education, not two, with a minimum of 12 to 24 months of prerequisites and a full 2 years of nursing education. Most associate degrees require approximately 60 semester units or 90 quarter units of coursework, although there is a great deal of variance with some programs now requiring more than 70 semester units and over 100 quarter units.

Consider This   The 2-year ADN program is a myth.

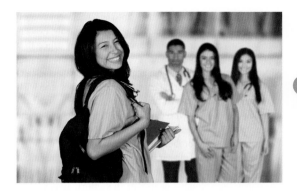

Indeed, it is almost impossible to graduate from an ADN program in less than 3 years and often four or more years are required to complete the general education, prerequisite, and nursing requirements. Given that most BSN programs require approximately 120 semester units for graduation, the question must be asked whether requiring so many units at the associate degree level, without granting the upper division credit that could lead to a BSN degree, is an injustice to ADN graduates.

This addition of units and extension of educational time in ADN programs has generally been attributed to the need to respond to a changing job market; that is, the need to prepare ADNs to work in more diverse environments (nonhospital) and to increasingly assume positions requiring management skills. While Montag clearly intended a differentiation between level of education and level of practice between ADN- and BSN-prepared nurses, many ADN programs have added leadership, management, research, and home health and community health courses to their curricula in the past two decades.

One must ask then what part of the associate degree curriculum should be cut to add these new experiences. What should the balance be between community and acute-care experiences in ADN programs? How much management content do ADN nurses need and what roles will they be expected to assume? If no content is deleted from the ADN programs to accommodate the new content, how can ADN education reasonably be completed within a 2-year framework?

Montag expressed concern that when ADN programs add content inappropriate for technical practice, appropriate content may have to be deleted to maintain the estimated time for completion. The question that follows then is, If ADN education now incorporates much of what was meant to be BSN content, and if the time needed to complete this education is near that of a bachelor's degree, why are ADN graduates being given associate degrees,

which reflect expertise in technical practice, rather than BSN degrees, which reflect achievement of these higher-level competencies?

SHORTAGES AND ENTRY-LEVEL REQUIREMENTS

Whenever there are shortages, legislators and workforce experts suggest a need to reexamine or reduce educational requirements. Indeed, Montag's original project to create ADN education was directed at reducing the workforce shortage of nurses that existed at that time, by reducing the length of the education process to 2 years. Clearly, the immediate short-term threat of raising the entry level to the bachelor's degree may be to exacerbate predicted nursing shortages.

In addition, raising the entry level may, in the long run, elevate the public image of nursing and increase recruitment to the field since the best and the brightest may seek professions with greater academic prestige. Raising the entry level may also impact retention rates in nursing. Having more BSN nurses may actually then stabilize the nursing workforce as a result of their higher levels of job satisfaction, a key to nurse retention.

> **Consider This**   The impact of raising the entry level in nursing to the baccalaureate level on the current nursing shortage is not known.

The other reality is that a chronic shortage of nursing personnel has persisted despite the proliferation of ADN programs. This negates the argument that the current nursing shortage should be used as an excuse for postponing action to raise educational standards. A nursing shortage existed at the time of the 1965 ANA proposal and has occurred intermittently since that time. Clearly, nursing has been swept along by a host of social, economic, and educational circumstances that have little to do with nursing or the clients we serve. Perhaps, then, the decision to raise the entry-to-practice level in nursing should be made because it is the right and necessary thing to do and not as a result of the influence of external communities of interest.

> **Consider This**   Nurses, professional health care and nursing organizations, credentialing programs, and employers are divided on the entry-into-practice issue.

Debate over entry into practice is as varied among professional health care and nursing organizations, credentialing programs, and employers as it is among individual nurses. Getting support for the BSN as the entry-level requirement for nursing will be difficult because the overwhelming majority of nurses are currently ADN prepared and there are inadequate workplace incentives to increase entry requirements to the BSN degree.

PROFESSIONAL ORGANIZATIONS, UNIONS, AND ADVISORY BODIES SPEAK OUT

Not surprisingly, a 2006 position statement issued by the National Organization for Associate Degree Nursing (NOADN) on entry into practice reaffirmed the role and value of associate degree nursing education and practice. The position statement suggested that ADN graduates were essential members of the interdisciplinary health care team, that these nurses were prepared to function in diverse health care settings, and that associate degree education provided a dynamic pathway for entry into professional RN practice. A follow-up position statement issued by the NOADN in 2008 suggested that a BSN should not be required for continued practice beyond initial licensure as an RN and that the choice to pursue further education should remain the choice of each ADN graduate based on his or her personal preferences and professional career goals.

Similarly, the position of the NLN, the national voice for nurse educators in all types of nursing education programs, historically was that the nursing profession should have multiple entry points. As such, the NLN suggested that instead of investing energy debating entry into the profession, the focus should turn toward opportunities for lifelong learning and progression for those who enter the nursing profession through diploma and associate degree programs.

More recently, however, the NOADN partnered with the American Association of Community Colleges, the Association of Community College Trustees, AACN, and NLN to author a joint statement acknowledging their full support for the academic progression of every nursing student and nurse. This statement was endorsed by the ANA in January 2014 (Joint Statement, 2018). The joint statement suggests that it is only through the collaboration and partnering of organizations that a seamless academic progression of students and nurses will occur.

In addition, the Nurse Alliance of the Service Employees International Union (SEIU, 2014) Health care, an organization of more than 85,000 RNs, has firmly rejected any bill that would limit entry into, or maintenance of, practice to the BSN, arguing that this would only exacerbate the current nursing shortage. Instead, they argue that more resources must be made available to support nursing education at all levels, to give academic credit for work experience, to provide workplace support for nurses who wish to return to school, and to develop more online and hybrid programs for nurses who cannot attend traditional on-site classes to advance their education.

An increasing number of professional nursing organizations, however, are now supporting the BSN requirement for entry into professional nursing. The ANA, however, is no longer the standard bearer in this effort. Instead, organizations such as the AACN, the National Association of Neonatal Nurses (NANN), the American Nephrology Nurses' Association, the Association of peri-Operative Registered Nurses (AORN), and the AONE have published position statements supporting BSN entry.

For example, the AACN suggests that the primary pathway for entry into professional-level nursing, as compared to technical-level practice, is a 4-year BSN. NANN issued its position statement in 2009, arguing that "the increasing acuity of patients and their more complex needs for care in community and home settings demand a higher level of educational preparation for nurses than was necessary in the past" (National Association of Neonatal Nurses, 2009, para. 1).

The AORN has also supported the baccalaureate degree for entry into nursing since 1979. The AORN's current position statement on entry into practice reaffirms its belief that there should be one level for entry into nursing practice and that the minimal preparation for future entry into the practice of nursing should be the baccalaureate degree (Association of peri-Operative Registered Nurses, 2015). In 2004, the AONE also published guiding principles suggesting that "the educational preparation of the nurse of the future should be at the baccalaureate level."

The NACNEP, which advises the Secretary of the U.S. Department of Health and Human Services and the U.S. Congress on policy issues related to nurse workforce supply, education, and practice improvement, also urged in 2007 that a minimum of two thirds of working nurses hold baccalaureate or higher degrees in nursing by 2010 (AACN, 2015a). Yet, federal and state regulation of entry into practice has, for the most part, not occurred. In addition, the Tri-Council for Nursing (ANA, AONE, NLN, and AACN) issued a consensus statement in 2010 calling for all RNs to advance their education in the interest of patient safety and enhanced quality of care across all settings.

Consider This The Tri-Council organizations argue that a more highly educated nursing profession is no longer a preferred future; it is a necessary future in order to meet the nursing needs of the nation and to deliver effective and safe care (AACN, 2018d).

GRANDFATHERING ENTRY LEVELS

Traditionally, when a state licensure law is enacted, or when a current law is repealed and a new law enacted, a process called "grandfathering" occurs. Grandfathering allows individuals to continue to practice his or her profession or occupation despite new qualifications having been enacted into law. Should the entry-level requirement for nursing be raised to a bachelor's or higher degree, debate will undoubtedly occur as to how and when grandfathering should be applied.

Consider This "Grandfathering" current ADN nurses as professional nurses would smooth political tensions between current educational entry levels but threaten the essence of the goal.

Several professional organizations have actively advocated that all RNs should be grandfathered if the entry level is raised. Other professional organizations have argued that it should not occur at all. Still others believe that grandfathering should be conditional. For example, all RNs licensed at the time of the law would be allowed to retain their current title for a certain time, but would be required to return to school to increase their educational preparation if it did not meet the new entry level.

LINKING ADN AND BSN PROGRAMS

Returning to school, unfortunately, is not part of the career path for many nurses, which makes the entry level even more important. Intimidation, cost, impact on family, and lack of clarity about the possible gains from additional education deter many nurses from returning to school. Still, only 25% of respondents in a recent study of nurses with less than a baccalaureate degree felt they were already adequately educated (Byrne, Mayo, & Rosner, 2014). Most felt that furthering their education would provide more career opportunities but that returning to school would not be a pleasant experience.

Indeed, there are many internal and external motivators that encourage or discourage RNs from pursuing higher

degrees. Perceived benefits include expanded knowledge and job opportunities while barriers include time commitment and expenses for books/supplies (Sarver, Cichra, & Kline, 2015). The average time to complete RN-to-BSN education is 2.63 years (Sarver et al., 2015), although fast-track baccalaureate programs may take as little as 11 to 18 months to complete, including prerequisites (AACN, 2018a). RNs also identify a desire to achieve personal and job satisfaction and professional achievement as important motivators.

Yet, research by Byrne et al. (2014) revealed that while 50% of the respondents in their study intended to return to school in the next 12 months, many had a fear of failure. Respondents suggested that more nurses would return to school if their colleagues did and that having the support of a significant person was important in both their decision to return to school and their retention. In addition, positive talk by nurse leaders and educators regarding the importance and value of advancing their education by earning a BSN is often critical to a nurse's decision to return to school.

This was the case in a pilot study by Baur et al. (2017) that examined how motivational interviewing (MI) could positively influence RNs considering a return to school (see Research Fuels the Controversy 1.1). Tuition reimbursement, flexible work hours, and pay for attending classes are also powerful employer-based motivators.

Currently, 747 RN-to-BSN programs nationally build on the education provided in diploma and ADN programs including more than 400 programs that are offered at least partially online (AACN, 2018b). There are also 230 programs available nationwide to transition RNs with diplomas and associate degrees to the master's degree level (MSN, MS, or Master of Science in Nursing degree; AACN, 2018b). The number of RN to MSN programs has more than tripled in the past 20 years, from 70 programs in 1994 to 230 programs as of 2017; 36 new RN to MSN programs are in the planning stages (AACN, 2018b).

In addition, statewide articulation agreements exist in many states, including Florida, California, Connecticut, Arkansas, Texas, Iowa, Maryland, North Carolina, South Carolina, Idaho, Alabama, and Nevada, to facilitate credit transfer from community colleges to universities with BSN programs. Indeed, Knowlton and Angel (2017) argue that creative RN-to-BSN completion pathways will be essential to raising the educational preparation of our nursing workforce with the aim of improving patient outcomes.

Indeed, the growth in RN pathways to baccalaureate and graduate degrees has been so rapid in the past decade that some nurse leaders have suggested that this has resulted in a lack of educational standardization and significant variability in expectations and requirements among

Research Fuels the Controversy 1.1

The focus of this pilot project was to identify and remove perceived barriers to returning to school through motivational interviewing (MI). MI is a framework providing interactions designed to help interviewees move through the change process with specific behaviors within a supportive and caring context. MI in this study focused on identifying the individual, specific barriers that prevented commitment to Bachelor of Science in Nursing (BSN) completion and determining if the interviewer could provide additional information, such as educational assistance information for a financial barrier. Thus, MI served as the unfreezing trigger. Eight registered nurses without BSN degrees volunteered to participate in the study.

Source: Baur, K., Moore, B., & Wendler, M. C. (2017, March). Influencing commitment to BSN completion: A pilot project using motivational interviewing. *Journal of Nursing Administration, 47*(3), 172–178.

Study Findings

The project facilitated the identification of many attitudes/barriers/motivators with the unique opportunity for the interviewer to provide additional information, clarify misconceptions, and possibly validate assumptions in real time as the conversation progressed. Ten overarching categories were isolated regarding BSN completion including:

1. Fear of failure
2. I could be a better nurse
3. Influence of others
4. Family stressors/obligations
5. Facilitators for return to school/BSN completion
6. I don't know what I don't know
7. Late starter
8. Career impact
9. Barriers to return to school/BSN education
10. My educational journey.

Facts regarding the IOM report, the impact of higher percentages of BSNs on patient outcomes, availability of financial assistance from the organization/costs of programs, differences in associate degree in nursing (ADN) and BSN curricula, and BSN completion opportunities were woven into each MI session. This open discussion of the participants' current attitudes and feelings and the counter discussion of facts, in a context of caring and support, were foundational to the results. The richness of the dialogue, which produced the overarching qualitative theme of "I know more now . . . I could be a better nurse," was a very powerful message to all ADN and diploma nurses not yet considering BSN completion. These results encourage purposeful communications with all ADN and diploma nurses regarding attitudes toward BSN education.

RN-to-BSN programs. In addition, sometimes there is little integration, standardization, or cooperation between public systems of education. Such integration, standardization, and cooperation will be essential for transition to BSN entry levels. This is why one of the key recommendations in *The Future of Nursing* was that all nursing schools should offer defined academic pathways that promote seamless access for nurses to higher levels of education (Institute of Medicine, 2010). Transition programs or services for non-baccalaureate-prepared nurses must be designed, which facilitate entry into baccalaureate and advanced education and practice programs. In addition, funding must continue to be increased for colleges and universities sponsoring baccalaureate and advanced practice nursing education programs.

Research also suggests that there are differences in the demographics of BSN and ADN graduates with BSN nurses being younger as a cohort than their ADN counterparts. It is also generally believed that ADN graduates represent greater diversity in race, gender, age, and educational experiences than BSN-prepared nurses. Critics of the BSN requirement for entry into professional nursing suggest that greater diversity is needed in nursing, and this may be lost if entry levels are raised. Indeed, recent research by Sabio (2014) supports this concern, suggesting that 37% of ADN students would not have enrolled in a BSN program if the BSN had been the only option for professional nursing practice and up to 89% would not have enrolled in the ADN program. Situational barriers such as the costs of BSN education and home and job responsibilities were of most concern among respondents.

> **Consider This** A broad new system, composed of direct transfer, linkage, and partnership programs, is needed between community college and baccalaureate institutions to ensure a smooth transition from ADN to BSN as the entry-level requirement for professional nursing practice. This transition will be costly.

Finally, raising the entry level in professional nursing practice will be costly. University education simply costs more than education at community colleges and significant increases in federal and state funding for baccalaureate and graduate nursing education will need to occur. Given the significant budget deficit currently faced by almost all states, the likelihood of funding increases for nursing education is directly related to the public and legislative understanding of the complexity of roles nurses assume each and every day and the educational level they perceive is needed to accomplish these tasks.

In addition, Krugman and Goode (2017) ask why federal money is still being directed to more than 35 diploma schools (embedded as part of graduate medical resident funding) when most state boards of nursing closed these schools 30 years ago and there is no such funding for BSN students. They argue that closure of the remaining diploma schools is overdue and that associated government funds should be reallocated to professional nursing education and nurse residency programs.

Clearly, barriers for educational reentry must be removed if the educational entry level in nursing is to be raised to a bachelor's or higher degree. Alternative pathways for RN education must be developed to create opportunities for learners who might not otherwise be able to pursue additional nursing education.

ENTRY INTO PRACTICE AS AN INTERNATIONAL ISSUE

The entry-into-practice debate in nursing is not limited to the United States, although several countries have already established the baccalaureate degree as the minimum entry level and grandfathered all those with a license before that date. For example, since 1982, all the provincial and territorial nurses associations in Canada have advocated the baccalaureate degree as the education entry-to-practice standard and most provincial and territorial regulatory bodies have achieved this goal (all but Quebec). The Canadian Nurses Association (CNA, 2018) believes that the knowledge, skills, and personal attributes that today's health system demands of its RNs can be gained only through broad-based bachelor's nursing programs.

Similarly, Australia moved toward the adoption of a BSN for entry into nursing during the 1980s, initially encountering resistance by both physicians and by nurses themselves, who feared university education would minimize needed hands-on training. Registered nursing as a university degree, however, was mandated in the 1990s. *Enrolled nurses* (scope of practice similar to LPNs/LVNs in the United States) continue to be educated in diploma programs and work under the supervision of the RN. Postgraduate diplomas provide further vocational training for specialist areas.

Similarly, in South Africa, nurses who complete a 2-year course of study are called *enrolled nurses* or *staff nurses*, whereas those who complete 4 years of study attain *professional nurse* or *sister* status. Enrolled nurses can later complete a 2-year bridging program and become *registered general nurses*.

Wales, Scotland, and Northern Ireland also offer only one entry point for nursing entry and that is a 3-year university degree. Other one entry-point countries include Italy, Norway, and Spain (3-year university degree); Ireland (4-year university degree); and Denmark (3.5-year degree at nursing school in university college sector). Many countries, such as Sweden, Portugal, Brazil, Iceland, Korea, Greece, and the Philippines, already require a 4-year undergraduate degree to practice nursing. All new nurses in England were required to hold a degree-level qualification to enter the profession after 2013. The aim was to increase skills and train a medical workforce capable of operating in a more analytical and independent manner.

> ***Consider This*** A growing list of countries, states, and provinces now require baccalaureate education in nursing.

Thus, international efforts to advance nursing education appear to be gaining momentum. The (2009) World Health Organization's Global Standards for the Initial Education of Professional Nurses and Midwives, written between 2005 and 2007, with participation from Sigma Theta Tau International, called for all nurses to be educated with a bachelor's degree, recognizing that country-specific standards would be necessary due to differing resources, history, and environments.

CONCLUSIONS

The entry-into-practice debate in the United States continues to be one of the oldest professional issues nurses face as we enter the second decade of the 21st century. Indeed, Krugman and Goode (2018) suggest the issue of educational entry into professional nursing practice is an "old" issue and that nurse leaders must act now to eliminate the multiple educational levels and require a minimum BSN degree for professional nurse practice. Yet limited progress has been made since 1965 in creating a consensus to raise the entry level into professional nursing practice.

Achieving the BSN as the entry degree for professional nursing practice will take the best thinking of our nursing leaders. It will also require courage, as well as a respect for persons not seen in the entry debate, and collaboration of the highest order. It will also require nurses to depersonalize the issue and look at what is best for both the clients they serve and the profession, rather than for them individually.

LaRocco (2014) suggests:

While the leaders of 1965 were visionary in their proposal of baccalaureate education as the entry to professional nursing, they were less effective in creating the change

that they proposed. Will our current nursing leaders be successful in completing this unfinished business? (p. 11)

Even the most patient planned-change advocate would agree that more than 50 years is a long time for implementation of a position. Clearly, the driving forces for such a change have not yet overcome the restraining forces, although movement is apparent. The question seems to come down to whether the nursing profession wants to spend another 50 years debating the issue or whether it wants to proactively take the steps necessary to make the goal a reality.

For Additional Discussion

1. What are the greatest driving and restraining forces for increasing entry into practice to a bachelor's or higher level?

2. Are the terms *professional* and *technical* unnecessarily inflammatory in the entry-into-practice debate? Why do these terms elicit such a "personal" response?

3. Is calling the associate degree in nursing a 2-year vocational degree an injustice to its graduates?

4. What is the legitimacy of requiring so many units at the community college level for an ADN degree? Should the current movement by community colleges to award baccalaureate degrees in nursing be encouraged?

5. How does the complexity of nursing roles and responsibilities compare to that of other health professions with higher entry levels?

6. What is the likelihood that nurses and the organizations that represent them will be able to achieve consensus on the entry-into-practice issue?

7. If the entry level is raised, should grandfathering be used? If so, should this grandfathering be conditional?

8. Is the goal of BSN entry a realistic one by 2020? If not, when?

References

Aiken, L. H., Clarke, S. P., Cheung, R. B., Sloane, D. M., & Silber, J. H. (2003). Educational levels of hospital nurses and surgical patient mortality. *JAMA, 290*(12), 1617–1623.

Aiken, L. H., Clarke, S. P., Sloane, D. M., Lake, E. T., & Cheney, T. (2008). Effects of hospital care environment on patient mortality and nurse outcomes. *The Journal of Nursing Administration, 38*(5), 223–229.

American Association of Colleges of Nursing. (2015a). *Fact sheet: Creating a more highly qualified nursing workforce.* Retrieved April 12, 2018, from http://www.aacnnursing.org/News-Information/Fact-Sheets/Nursing-Workforce

American Association of Colleges of Nursing. (2015b). *Talking points. HRSA report on nursing workforce projections through 2025.* Retrieved April 12, 2018, from http://www.njccn.org/wp-content/uploads/2015/07/HRSA-Nursing-Workforce-Projections.pdf

American Association of Colleges of Nursing. (2018a). *Accelerated baccalaureate and master's degrees in nursing.* Retrieved April 12, 2018, from http://www.aacnnursing.org/Nursing-Education-Programs/Accelerated-Programs

American Association of Colleges of Nursing. (2018b). *Degree completion programs for registered nurses: RN to master's degree and RN to baccalaureate programs.* Retrieved April 12, 2018, from http://www.aacnnursing.org/News-Information/Fact-Sheets/Degree-Completion-Programs

American Association of Colleges of Nursing. (2018c). *Fact sheet: The impact of education on nursing practice.* Retrieved August 31, 2017, from http://www.aacnnursing.org/News-Information/Fact-Sheets/Impact-of-Education

American Association of Colleges of Nursing. (2018d). *Joint statement from the tri-council for nursing on recent registered nurse supply and demand projections.* Retrieved

April 12, 2018, from http://www.aacn.nche.edu/news/articles/2010/tricouncil

American Nurses Association. (1965a). *A position paper.* New York, NY: Author.

American Nurses Association. (1965b). *Educational preparation for nurse practitioners and assistants to nurses: A position paper.* New York, NY: Author.

Association of peri-Operative Registered Nurses. (2015, February). *AORN position statement on entry into practice. First drafted House of Delegates 1979, St. Louis.* Retrieved from https://www.aorn.org/guidelines/clinical-resources/position-statements

Auerbach, D. I., Buerhaus, P. I., & Staiger D. O. (2015). Do associate degree registered nurses fare differently in the nurse labor market compared to baccalaureate-prepared RNs? *Nursing Economic$, 33,* 8–12, 35.

Baur, K., Moore, B., & Wendler, M. C. (2017, March). Influencing commitment to BSN completion: A pilot project using motivational interviewing. *Journal of Nursing Administration, 47*(3), 172–178.

Benner, P., Sutphen, M., Leonard, V., & Day, L. (2010). *Educating nurses: A call for radical transformation: Preparation for the professions.* San Francisco, CA: Jossey-Bass/The Carnegie Foundation for the Advancement of Teaching.

Blegen, M. A., Goode, C. J., Park, S. H., Vaughn, T., & Spetz, J. (2013, February). Baccalaureate education in nursing and patient outcomes. *Journal of Nursing Administration, 43*(2), 89–94. doi:10.1097/NNA.0b013e31827f2028

Byrne, D., Mayo, R., & Rosner, C. (2014). What internal motivators drive RNs to pursue a BSN? *Nursing, 44*(10), 22–24. doi:10.1097/01.NURSE.0000453707.43199.ea

Canadian Nurses Association. (2018). *Education.* Retrieved April 12, 2018, from https://www.cna-aiic.ca/en/becoming-an-rn/education

Clarke, S. P. (2017). The BSN entry into practice debate. *Nursing Made Incredibly Easy! 15*(1), 6–8.

Hewitt, P. (2016, January-February). The call for 80% BSNs by 2020: Where are we now? *Nurse Educator, 41*(1), 29–32.

Institute of Medicine. (2010, October). *The future of nursing: Leading change, advancing health.* Retrieved January 31, 2015, from http://thefutureofnursing.org/IOM-Report

Joint statement on academic progression for nursing students and graduates. (2018). AACC, ACCT, AACN, NLN, NOADN. Retrieved June 28, 2017, from http://www.aacnnursing.org/News-Information/Position-Statements-White-Papers/Academic-Progression

Knowlton, M. C., & Angel, L. (2017, May-June). Lessons learned: Answering the call to increase the BSN workforce. *Journal of Professional Nursing, 33*(3), 184–193.

Krugman, M., & Goode, C. J. (2018, February). BSN preparation for RNs: The time is now! *Journal of Nursing Administration, 48*(2), 57–60.

Kumm S, Godfrey N, Martin D, Tucci M, Muenks M, & Spaeth T. (2014, Sept.-Oct.). Baccalaureate outcomes met by associate degree nursing programs. *Nurse Educator, 39*(5), 216–220.

LaRocco, S. (2014). Where are the visionary nursing leaders of 1965? *American Journal of Nursing, 114*(4), 11. doi:10.1097/01.NAJ.0000445661.74531.b8

National Association of Neonatal Nurses. (2009). *Educational preparation for nursing practice roles [Position statement No. 3048, NANN Board of Directors].* Retrieved June 29, 2017, from http://nann.org/uploads/About/PositionPDFS/1.4.11_Education%20Preparation%20for%20Nursing%20Practice%20Roles.pdf

New AACN data on BSN-prepared hiring. (2014). *American Nurse, 46*(1), 5.

Newland, J. A. (2018). BSN in 10: It's the law! *Nurse Practitioner, 43*(2), 6.

Sabio, C. C. (2014). *Would you have enrolled? Decision factors in baccalaureate-only nursing among associate degree nursing students.* Capella University. CINAHL Plus with Full Text, EBSCO host. Retrieved November 23, 2014.

Sarver, W., Cichra, N., & Kline, M. (2015, May/June). Perceived benefits, motivators, and barriers to advancing nurse education: Removing barriers to improve success. *Nursing Education Perspectives, 36*(3), 153–156.

Service Employees International Union. (2014). *Position statement on BSN requirement for RN practice.* Retrieved November 24, 2014, from http://www.seiu.org/a/healthcare/position-statement-on-bsn-requirement-for-rn-practice.php

The ultimate guide to online RN-to-BSN programs. (2017, May 10). Post University Insights. Retrieved May 14, 2017, from http://blog.post.edu/2017/05/ultimate-guide-online-rn-to-bsn-programs/

World Health Organization. (2009). *Global standards for the initial education of professional nurses and midwives.* Retrieved June 29, 2017, from http://www.who.int/hrh/nursing_midwifery/hrh_global_standards_education.pdf

Yakusheva, O., Lindrooth, R., & Weiss, M. (2014). Economic evaluation of the 80% baccalaureate nurse workforce recommendation: A patient-level analysis. *Medical Care, 52*(10), 864–869. doi:10.1097/MLR.0000000000000189

Bridging the Academic–Practice Gap in Nursing

Nikki West, Jonalyn Wallace, and Ryan M. Fuller

ADDITIONAL RESOURCES

Visit thePoint° for additional helpful resources

- eBook
- Journal Articles
- WebLinks

CHAPTER OUTLINE

LEARNING OBJECTIVES

The learner will be able to:

1. Define the academic–practice gap in prelicensure nursing.

2. Describe the academic–practice gap's impact on the current and future nursing workforce.

3. Describe changes in the U.S. health care landscape that widen the academic–practice gap.

4. Define nursing practice specialties and care settings that are at risk due to the widening academic–practice gap.

5. Discuss the national spotlight on the academic–practice gap, including findings of the Institute of Medicine (IOM) of the National Academies report *The Future of Nursing: Leading Change, Advancing Health.*

6. Describe strategic and innovative programs and approaches to address the academic–practice gap.

INTRODUCTION

There is an identified gap between completion of academic programs and entry into employment (also referred to as service or practice) as a registered nurse (RN). This chapter explores how the changing U.S. health care landscape, projected workforce needs, and the evolving role of the RN are impacting this gap and potentially making it more challenging to bridge. Transition-to-Practice Programs (TPPs) are outlined as one solution. Additional effective and innovative strategies are described, including those led by academia, practice, and through collaborative efforts. National attention to the academic–practice gap is presented, including reports and updates from the Institute of Medicine (IOM) on *The Future of Nursing*. The chapter concludes with considerations and risks if the gap is not bridged.

THE ACADEMIC–PRACTICE GAP

Negotiating the transition from student to professional nurse can be daunting. New graduate nurses report feeling overwhelmed, unprepared, and shocked by the level of responsibility required (Casey et al., 2011; Huston et al., 2017; Kramer, et al 2013; Spector et al., 2015). These perceptions can lead new nurses to feelings of distress, often resulting in job dissatisfaction and the potential for clinical errors and high turnover in the first year of practice (Casey, Fink, Krugman, & Propst, 2004; Duchscher, 2009; Fink, Krugman, Casey, & Goode, 2008; Goode, Lynn, McElroy, Bednash, & Murray, 2013; Hickerson, Taylor, & Terhaar, 2016; Huston et al., 2017; Robert Wood Johnson Foundation, 2014; Spector et al., 2015; Ulrich et al., 2010).

Complicating the situation is the difference in perceptions of new graduates' readiness for practice upon entering the workforce. Nurse researchers have discovered a significant discrepancy between how deans and chief nurse executives view newly licensed RNs. Among 400 nursing school deans surveyed, 90% reported that newly licensed RNs were fully prepared to practice. In sharp contrast, only 10% of the 5,700 nurse executives responded that new nurses were fully prepared to provide safe and effective care (Berkow, Virkstis, Stewart, & Conway, 2008). In another study, novice nurses expressed a similar viewpoint. More than 50% stated their programs prepared them to pass the National Council Licensure Examination (NCLEX), but did not prepare them for "real-world" practice. In addition, more than 76% believed they did not have enough clinical hours in their nursing program (Candela & Bowles, 2008).

> **Consider This** Evidence of an academic–practice gap is well documented. Academic institutions are criticized for not providing curriculum and training experiences that fully prepare nurses to practice in the current health care environment, while practice settings are criticized for having unrealistic expectations of schools of nursing as well as the abilities of newly licensed nurses to practice safely (Huston et al., 2017; Kellehear, 2014).

Similarly, Kavanagh and Szweda (2017) examined the disconnect between newly licensed RN entry-level competency and NCLEX pass rates. All participants in the study passed the NCLEX. However, the competency assessment tool found that only 23% of new graduates scored in the "safe to practice independently" range. The other 77% were rated as unsafe to practice independently (see Research Fuels the Controversy 2.1).

These challenges are the result of several interconnected issues and are linked to discussions regarding accountability for "fixing" the academic–practice gap. Some researchers suggest that the focus on preparing students to pass the NCLEX limits the scope of education and clinical training that can be accomplished during nursing school. Others suggest that full-time faculty have difficulty staying clinically current and may not present the most relevant or up-to-date material. One survey of nursing students indicated that the students perceived most of their clinical faculty as lacking the expertise to work in the clinical setting. In addition, poor communication between theory based and clinical faculty made it hard for them to link what they were learning in class with direct patient care (Huston et al., 2017; Numminen, Leino-Kilpi, Isoaho, & Mertoja, 2015; Saifan, AbuRauz, & Masa'deh, 2015).

Employers report the existence of the academic–practice gap as well, and note a difference between their expectations and those of academia. Nurse researchers conducted assessments of newly licensed RNs prior to employment and determined that competency gaps spanned the domains of critical thinking, communication, clinical knowledge, time management, professionalism, acquisition of psychomotor skills, physical assessments, and teamwork. Significantly, they identified these skills as critical for providing safe nursing care. Ultimately, these competency gaps put patients, the newly licensed RN, and health systems at risk (Berman et al., 2014; Huston et al., 2017).

Research Fuels the Controversy 2.1

NCLEX Success Versus Real-World Competency

Kavanagh and Szweda examined the disconnect between newly licensed RN entry-level competency and National Council Licensure Examination (NCLEX) pass rates. In their 2017 study, the nurse researchers explored the relationship between successful completion of the NCLEX and the level of clinical competency of recent graduates to work in the complexity of real-world practice. The study administered a nationally recognized competency assessment tool to more than 5,000 newly licensed RNs over a period of 5 years. Nurses in the study came from more than 140 U.S. nursing programs across 21 states. The assessment tool examines critical thinking learning needs, ability to differentiate urgency and justification for actions, provides insight into the thought processes of the nurse, and assists in the development of an individualized orientation action plan to prepare each nurse for safe clinical practice.

Source: Kavanagh, J., & Szweda, C. (2017). A crisis in competency: The strategic and ethical imperative to assessing new graduate nurses' clinical reasoning. *Nursing Education Perspectives, 38*(2), 57–62.

Study Findings

All participants in the study passed the NCLEX. However, the competency assessment tool found that only 23% of new graduates scored in the "safe to practice independently" range. The other 77% were rated as unsafe to practice independently. To note, there was no significant difference in ratings between baccalaureate and associate degree graduates.

These findings demonstrate the gap between the skills and knowledge required to pass the NCLEX, and the competency needed to practice safely as an independent RN. The study authors suggest that the issue belongs to academia and practice alike. Hospital educators must be competent in coaching, guided facilitation, and adult learning theories. Prelicensure academic faculty must respond to the changing landscape of health care as well as the changing learner. This must be achieved while both sides face mounting challenges such as budget cutbacks, aging faculty, lack of trained preceptors, and competition for clinical sites.

Together, undergraduate education and practice partners must prepare nurses beyond the ability to simply pass the NCLEX. Instead, nursing leaders need to look toward knowledge acquisition, clinical application, and critical thinking as desired outcomes for the education of new RNs. The NCLEX is a crucial step in the journey to become a RN. However, many steps must follow initial licensure to obtain the clinical competency necessary for safe and independent RN practice.

Discussion Point

This study was conducted between 2011 and 2015. If the academic–practice gap was evident then, what are the implications for the gap as our population and health care landscape continue to change? Conducted at an acute care medical center, this is only one type of setting where nurses practice. How do you think newly licensed nurses would score on competence in an ambulatory or community-based setting?

Discussion Point

Until the 1960s, nurses were trained primarily using the diploma model (Carter, 2006). This model immersed student RNs in their actual practice environment for 3 years before they were able to work independently. What can we learn from the diploma model of nursing—could clinical and academic settings work together more collaboratively to bridge the academic–practice gap?

UNDERSTANDING THE ACADEMIC–PRACTICE GAP

Discussed for decades, the need to bridge the academic–practice gap gained momentum in the mid-1970s with the release of Kramer's groundbreaking book *Reality Shock: Why Nurses Leave Nursing.* Kramer argued that idealized versions of nursing promoted by academic faculty contrasted significantly with new nurses' experiences upon entering the workforce. This often led to a shock-like reaction, putting the new graduate nurse at risk for job dissatisfaction and disillusionment with the profession of nursing (Kramer, 1974). The book stimulated the development and implementation of programs designed to support newly licensed RNs as they entered into professional practice.

Benner's Novice to Expert theory broadened understanding of how newly licensed nurses acquire the skills necessary to expertly care for patients. According to Benner's research, nurses acquire skill over time by engaging in focused educational opportunities and a multitude of clinically relevant experiences. Through these activities, nurses move along a continuum from novice to advanced beginner; competent; proficient; and finally, expert nurse (Benner, 1984).

TRANSITION-TO-PRACTICE PROGRAM DEFINED

TPPs were developed as one solution to bridge the gap by supporting newly licensed RNs as they progress from their nursing school experience to their first professional nursing role. The National Council for State Boards of Nursing (NCSBN) and the American Association of Colleges of Nursing (AACN, 2007) defined TPPs as a formal program of active learning that includes a series of facilitated educational sessions and precepted work experiences for newly licensed PNs (Spector, et al., 2015). TPP is designated as the period between being a student nurse and an independent professional nurse. TPPs have been given various names including "nurse residencies," "nurse fellowships," "externships," and "work-study internships" (Jones & West, 2017; Wallace, 2016).

Although multiple types of TPPs exist, all are focused on bridging the transition from school into employment. There are programs that begin the final year of nursing school and continue through licensure. Others are structured as employer-based "new graduate classes," typically within a hospital. Some of these programs take up to a year to complete, whereas others are only 12 to 16 weeks in length. Still other programs are for new graduates who have yet to be hired, so they may gain skills to become more employable.

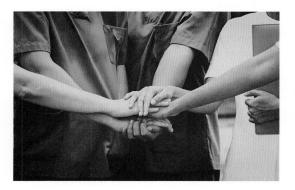

TPPs bridge the gap by providing the newly licensed nurse with opportunities to master the clinical skills that they learned in nursing school and apply them in an expanded, intensive, and integrated clinical learning environment while providing direct patient care under the guidance of a nurse preceptor (Benner, Sutphen, Leonard & Day, 2010; Jones & West, 2017; Spector & Echternacht, 2009).

CHANGING HEALTH CARE LANDSCAPE

Several factors are influencing how nurses should be prepared to meet health needs. The U.S. population is changing, significant workforce shifts are anticipated, and new nursing roles are developing as care moves away from acute care settings toward population health. These factors will impact the transition to practice for newly licensed nurses, and could potentially widen the academic–practice gap.

Changing Health Care Landscape: Population Aging and Sicker

Americans are growing older and living longer than ever before. At the same time, the prevalence of chronic disease and the complexity of patients also continue to increase. Baby boomers (born between 1946 and 1964) number 76 million, and make up the largest generation in history (Colby & Ortman, 2015). It is estimated that the U.S. population of people 85 years and older will double from 6.3 million in 2015 to nearly 13 million by 2035. In addition, the number of U.S. citizens aged 100 years or more will triple between 2017 and 2045 (Buerhaus, Skinner, Auerbach, and Staiger 2017a; Colby & Ortman, 2015).

Despite medical and technologic advances, lower rates of smoking, decreased incidence of emphysema, and access to healthier lifestyles, the prevalence of chronic disease is increasing among aging U.S. adults. Adding burden to an already taxed system, the need for Medicare, the health insurance plan available to U.S. citizens aged 65 years and older, people with specific disabilities, and/or people with end-stage renal failure, is anticipated to rise to 92.5 million people by 2050 (Cubanski et al., 2015). The growth in Medicare is directly related to the surge in U.S. population from the early 1940s through the early 1960s—the baby boomer generation—however, we do not have to wait until 2050 to see the health care implications of an aging generation. By 2030, 40% of baby boomers are expected to be diagnosed with diabetes, 43% will have heart disease, and 25% will have received a diagnosis of cancer. The aging population, coupled with an increasing prevalence of chronic disease, increases the complexity of patient care exponentially for the newly licensed and experienced RN

(Buerhaus, Auerbach, and Staiger 2017b; Gaudette, Tys-inger, Cassil & Goldman 2015; Goldman & Gaudette, 2015).

Academia and practice will both play an important role in developing competent nurses who are able to care for the growing and aging population in the United States. Focusing education on gerontologic and public health nursing will become of increasing importance as these trends continue to climb (Buerhaus, Skinner, Auerbach, & Staiger, 2017; Mullen, 2015; Sherman, Patterson, Avitable, & Dahle, 2014).

Changing Health Care Landscape: Health Care Reform

In 2020, the United States is estimated to spend one-fifth of its economy on health care—five times more than the annual spending on military (Bradley, Sipsma, & Taylor, 2016). Despite this investment, the United States is ranked well below other developed nations in relation to quality outcomes (Davis, Stremikis, Schoen, & Squires, 2014). The passage of the Patient Protection and Affordable Care Act (ACA) in 2010 fundamentally reshaped U.S. health care by driving increased efficiencies, providing broader insurance coverage, promoting preventive care measures, subsidizing provider training, and replacing the fee-for-service model with value-based delivery systems. Yakusheva, O., Lindroth, R. C., Weiner, J., Spetz, J., & Pauly, M. V. (2015). By 2017, more than 20 million people had access to health care through the ACA (Sommers, Maylone, Blendon, Orav, & Epstein, 2017).

> **Consider This** Health care reform presents an important opportunity for both academia and practice to evaluate and imagine how to prepare nurses to deliver high-quality care, while also being stewards for affordability. Under the ACA, nurses have an opportunity to assume new roles that address the growing population health disparities in our country.

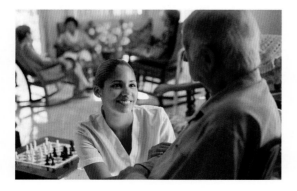

Changing Health Care Landscape: Workforce Changes

Demands upon the health care workforce are shifting. The number of nurses and other health professionals needed, as well as the skills and competencies they require, is changing and will continue to evolve.

Nurses

It is estimated that nurses from the baby boomer generation, born between 1946 and 1964, are leaving practice at a rate of more than 70,000 annually with a million nurses anticipated to retire between 2015 and 2030 (Auerbach, Buerhaus, & Staiger, 2015; Buerhaus et al., 2017; Staiger, Auerbach, & Buerhaus, 2012; U.S. Department of Labor, Bureau of Labor Statistics, 2014). As baby boomer nurses retire, current shortages of nurses in specialty areas including perioperative, behavioral health, and perinatal nursing will increase. Both the limited exposure students get to these specialties during nursing school and the need for lengthy training result in a wider academic–practice gap (Ball, Doyle, & Oocumma, 2015; Bell, Bossier-Bearden, Henry, & Kirksey, 2015; Jansen & Venter, 2015; Monahan, 2015).

The impact of nurse retirements on the health care system is significant and multifaceted. Not only must nurse leaders fill vacant positions in hard-to-fill clinical specialties, they must also account for the loss of accumulated nursing knowledge, expertise, and wisdom as experienced nurses leave practice. Buerhaus quantified the impact of this loss by multiplying the number of retiring RNs in 2015 by their years of experience. This calculation shows that in 2015 alone, the workforce lost 1.7 million "experience years" impacting nurse leaders as they address health system challenges with a less experienced team (Buerhaus et al., 2017).

Physicians

Anticipated changes in the physician workforce will impact nursing practice as well. Over the next two decades, significant numbers of physicians will retire or leave their medical practices. Total numbers vary, as do estimates of anticipated shortages that could result. The American Association of Medical Colleges (AAMC) predicts a shortage of 40,800 to 104,900 physicians by 2030. Professional associations and accrediting bodies disagree on the impact that loss of physicians will have on fulfilling patient care needs. Leaders do agree that the current uneven distribution of physicians across the country will worsen in the future. Currently, rural America has fewer physicians, averaging 60 primary care physicians per 100,000 residents than urban areas with 80 primary care providers per 100,000 residents. People seeking care may notice significant wait times and difficulty accessing necessary care (Buerhaus et al., 2017; Gudbranson, Glickman, & Emanuel, 2017; Kirch & Petelle, 2017).

Nurses can help address the growing physician gap in innovative ways, including broadening the use of nurse practitioners to meet primary care needs, and RNs extending providers by working under standardized protocols within the interprofessional team (Berg & Dickow, 2013; Bodenheimer & Smith, 2013). Both academia and practice will need to consider the implications of the future role of RNs in filling the physician shortage gap when designing prelicensure curriculum and TPPs.

Discussion Point

Upon completion of medical school, newly licensed physicians typically attend a 1-year internship followed by a multiyear residency in a designated specialty. How does this compare to the pathway of a newly licensed nurse?

Changing Health Care Landscape: New Roles for Nurses

The changing health care landscape will result in the development of new care delivery models that address quality and cost containment concerns as providers manage care for a growing population that is older and sicker. Historically, patients have been cared for in hospital environments. In the future, only the sickest of patients will be cared for in hospitals. This trend has been in effect for the last decade; patient stays are shorter in length, resulting in patients transitioning home for convalescence and rehabilitation. In addition to routine preventive health services, patients will receive chronic condition care, behavioral health services, and palliative care in new and innovative ways. Wider use of interventions like telehealth, allowing providers to "visit" patients in their own home, and technologic devices that measure patients' heart rate, blood glucose and other findings will fundamentally change how care is delivered. These shifts from hospital to community-based care are opening new options for the nursing role. Other changes including accountable care organizations (ACOs), medical homes, broadening accountability for home health and hospice teams, and roles in clinical settings for reducing readmissions and improving care quality (care coordination, transition care services, and health education) will add to the opportunities. Nurses can play a pivotal role in the health care system through cost savings and improved quality outcomes (Pittman & Forrest, 2015).

Caring for patients in these new settings will necessitate a mastery of sophisticated nursing competencies, typically not taught in nursing schools, where clinical skills are emphasized (Huston et al., 2017). Sometimes dismissed as "soft skills," research shows that teams can improve outcomes significantly through interprofessional communication, collaboration, delegation, and the ability to apply systems thinking. These competencies are learned over time. Nurses need transition experiences that prepare them to meet the distinct needs of patients in this environment (Spector et al., 2015).

Discussion Point

Nurses of the future will need to be prepared for new roles that address chronic population health outside of the acute care hospital system.

Roles of the future may include (Berg & Dickow, 2013):
- Care coordinator
- Faculty team leader
- Informatics specialist
- Community nurse
- Primary care partner

How could newly licensed RNs help fill these roles?

NATIONAL ATTENTION ON THE ACADEMIC–PRACTICE GAP

The need to bridge the academic–practice gap has received national attention. The release of the landmark IOM (2011) report, *The Future of Nursing: Leading Change, Advancing Health*, stimulated a call to action for the profession of nursing and provided recommendations for the future of the profession, given the numerous factors in the health care landscape. For several years, it has been the IOM's most downloaded report in the history of their organization (Campaign for Action, 2016).

The report identifies barriers that prevent nurses from being effective in a rapidly changing health care system as well as strategies to overcome them. Authored by a prestigious committee of national experts appointed by the IOM, the committee reviewed current issues in nursing, discussed strategies, and then made recommendations. The report provided four key messages:

1. Nurses should practice to the full extent of their education and training.

2. Nurses should achieve higher levels of education and training through an improved education system that promotes seamless academic progression.

3. Nurses should be full partners, with physicians and other health care professionals, in redesigning health care in the United States.

4. Effective workforce planning and policy making require better data collection and an improved information infrastructure (IOM, 2011).

To align education with evolving roles for nurses, the report called for transformation such that nurses become "competent in several disciplines, such as leadership, system improvement, research, teamwork and collaboration, and

public health" (National Academies of Sciences, Engineering, Medicine, 2017; see Fig. 2.1).

The IOM's challenge to bridge the academic–practice gap spanned public and private bodies, academia, practice and policy, urging all to act. Specifically, relative to residency programs, the IOM committee called for:

• State boards of nursing, in collaboration with accrediting bodies such as the Joint Commission and the Community Health Accreditation Program, should support nurses' completion of a residency program after they

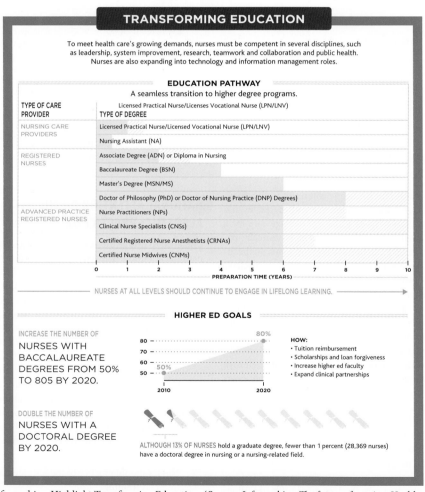

Figure 2.1 Infographic—Highlight Transforming Education. (***Source:*** *Infographic—The future of nursing: Health and medicine division.* Retrieved June 4, 2018, from http://nationalacademies.org/hmd/Reports/2010/The-Future-of-Nursing-Leading-Change-Advancing-Health/Infographic.aspx, with permission.)

have completed a prelicensure or advanced practice degree program or when they are transitioning into new clinical practice areas.

- The Secretary of Health and Human Services should redirect all graduate medical education funding from diploma nursing programs to support the implementation of nurse residency programs in rural and critical access areas.

- Health care organizations, the Health Resources and Services Administration and Centers for Medicare and Medicaid Services, and philanthropic organizations should fund the development and implementation of nurse residency programs across all practice settings.

- Health care organizations that offer nurse residency programs and foundations should evaluate the effectiveness of the residency programs in improving the retention of nurses, expanding competencies, and improving patient outcomes (IOM, 2011).

Implementation of *The Future of Nursing* report's recommendations was taken on by each state in the form of action coalitions. In 2014, the IOM assembled a new national committee, tasked with reviewing the work of the action coalitions, assessing progress on report recommendations, and identifying areas that should be emphasized over the next 5 years. After evaluating progress and incorporating the impact of changes in delivery and payment models, this new committee concluded in the 2015 *Assessing progress on the Institute of Medicine report: The future of nursing*:

No single profession, working alone, can meet the complex needs of patients and communities. Nurses should continue to develop skills and competencies in leadership and innovation and collaborate with other professionals in healthcare delivery and health system redesign. To continue progress on the implementation of report recommendations and to effect change in an evolving healthcare landscape, the nursing community. . .must build and strengthen coalitions with stakeholders both within and outside of nursing. (National Academies of Sciences, Engineering, and Medicine, 2016)

The 2016 report determined:

- As the RN population shifts to becoming increasingly baccalaureate-prepared, unintended consequences (employment, earning power, skills, and roles and responsibilities) for those nurses who do not achieve higher education may occur.

- Further evaluation of transition-to-practice residencies is needed to prove their value with measurable outcomes;

specifically, more attention is needed to determine the effect of these programs on patient outcomes.

- Additional efforts are needed to clarify the roles of PhD and DNP nurses, especially in regard to teaching and research.

- The current health care context makes interprofessional continuing education more important than ever. Current efforts by health care delivery organizations, accreditors, and state regulatory boards to promote these programs need to be expanded and promoted (National Academies of Sciences, Engineering, and Medicine, 2016).

These findings seem to pose as many questions as they answer related to progress. What seems clear, though, is the importance of evaluating the impact of changes in education and continuing to monitor the health care landscape to better educate the current and future nurse. Building closer ties between academia and practice is critical now and for the future.

STRATEGIES AND INNOVATIONS TO BRIDGE THE GAP

Many organizations have implemented programs that help assimilate newly licensed nurses into the profession by providing experiences to develop improved clinical skills and increase the newly licensed nurse's clinical confidence. Programs are of value to health systems, mitigating concerns for patient safety, recruitment, retention, and turnover costs during the initial year of their career (Blegen, Spector, Lynn, Barnsteiner, & Ulrich, 2017; Friday, Zoller, Hollerbach, Jones, & Knofczynski, 2015; Wallace, J. et al 2014).

Huston and colleagues (2017) surveyed the literature to identify programs and strategies that bridge the gap; the researchers organized them into three categories: educational strategies, practice strategies, and collaborative strategies. These strategies and tactics provide guidance for academic and practice partners who want to work together to better manage this critical issue.

Educational Strategies

Simulation

A recent study conducted by the NCSBN considered the impact on student outcomes when simulation was substituted for clinical practicum hours. Positive results were reported in both the control group (students who received 25% of their clinical practicum hours in the simulation lab) and the research group (students who received 50% of their clinical practicum hours via simulation). These findings suggest that learning is enhanced when simulation and debriefing are conducted in a safe, nonthreatening manner. Additionally, simulation is customizable, thus, specific gaps in knowledge can be addressed in "real time" with a student rather than waiting until the next patient interaction. Finally, simulation can be a solution for solving challenges with securing clinical practicum hours for students (Huston et al., 2017).

Active Learning/Flipped Classroom

With active learning, faculty are encouraged to decrease use of lecture and PowerPoint decks, replacing them with activities that facilitate critical thinking and development of clinical judgment. This can be accomplished through use of scenarios and experiences that give students an opportunity to reason through a patient care problem and work together to solve it. The flipped classroom is another methodology where students are assigned to read and learn content prior to attending class with the expectation that they will apply the learning during the classroom session. This strategy requires that students use higher-level skills as opposed to rote memorization and improves problem solving and critical thinking skills and the transfer of knowledge (Hessler, 2017; Huston et al., 2017).

Competency-Based Education

In this learner-centric solution, educators structure learning and provide students with specific ways to demonstrate competency for both "soft" and technical skills necessary for safe nursing practice (Huston et al., 2017).

Practice Strategies

Practice partners typically provide transition experiences to address workforce needs, giving newly licensed and hired RNs an opportunity to prepare for their new role.

Nurse Residency Programs

These are formal TTPs for newly licensed RNs. Length typically ranges from 3 to 12 months with a curriculum that is aligned with national standards and practice needs. Programs are structured to provide a multitude of experiences to participants including online modules, didactic sessions, simulation, and direct patient care orientation under the supervision of an experienced nurse preceptor.

Programs may be either commercially developed and owned or "homegrown" by a health system. Two widely used commercial programs include Vizient (formally known as University Health Consortium/American Association of Colleges of Nursing [UHC/ANCC]) and Versant. These programs provide content, data analysis, and proprietary tools to health systems interested in implementing a TTP.

TPPs may also be developed within an organization. Homegrown refers to the fact that the health system created its own program, instead of purchasing a commercial program. Nurse researchers recently examined 10 years of data on a "homegrown" TTP. The results of a review of more than 1,000 newly licensed RNs demonstrated that it may be equally effective in supporting the growth, development, and retention of newly licensed RNs. Tailored to the specific needs of a health system, "homegrown" programs may become increasingly popular as additional data are available to validate the quality of their outcomes (Cline, La Frentz, Fellman, Summers, & Brassil, 2017).

Clinical Judgment and Competency Assessment

New graduate RNs often lack sufficient experience in applying clinical judgment to patient care situations. As a result, Dorothy Del Bueno (2001) developed the Performance Based Development System (PBDS) in 1985. PBDS is an assessment exam that evaluates the clinical judgment competency of an individual nurse. The exam provides video vignettes, and then asks the examinee to assess, diagnose, plan, intervene, and evaluate a plan of care for the simulated patient. The results of the exam are aggregated and provide insight into the strengths and weaknesses of the individual nurse. Since the introduction of the PBDS, the assessment has been used in more than 450 health systems across the country (Del Bueno, 2005).

Recently, HealthStream purchased the PBDS product and rebranded it under the name Assess. Assess leverages IBM Watson artificial intelligence to provide an interactive clinical judgment assessment experience. Using emerging technologies such as Assess, practice settings will be able to evaluate competency and clinical judgment in ways that were previously not possible. As a result, future clinical orientation programs might be better tailored to the individual new graduate nurse, which may help reduce the time it takes to safely transition the new graduate into clinical practice.

Collaborative Strategies

Academia and practice have come together in effective, creative ways to prepare RNs and bridge the gap. There are multiple examples of collaborative solutions and strategies.

Student Work-Study Internships/Externships

These programs provide senior level nursing students with a paid clinical immersion experience, exposing interns to the realities of clinical practice and allowing them to hone skills they've learned in nursing school. Students work in a variety of settings including hospital units, procedural suites, clinical education, quality and risk, and infection prevention departments. Programs are structured as a clinical course, with a syllabus, faculty of record, and malpractice coverage by the academic partner. Programs may include both clinical and didactic sessions depending on the setting and usually take place in the summer semester when students have fewer school-related obligations. Interns show increased confidence and competence because of the program (Ramirez, Zimmerman, & Judson, 2013; Wallace, 2016).

Specialty-Specific Clinical Immersion

Academic practice partnerships that provide structured clinical immersion experiences for nursing students in specialty areas anticipating critical workforce shortages (e.g., perioperative nursing and maternal child health) provide another example of collaboration. The immersion experience is structured as a clinical practicum course where the school and clinical site collaborate to develop curriculum, select students, and create evaluation tools. In this model, tuition may be paid by the student, covered by the practice partner, or covered through other means, such as grant funding. Examples include a 2-week clinical immersion in the operating room conducted by Kaiser Permanente Northern California (KP NCAL) in partnership with California State University, East Bay (CSUEB) and an operating room immersion offered during the summer session after both junior and senior years for California State University, Los Angeles (CSULA) students in partnership with Cedars-Sinai Heath System.

Dedicated Education Unit

Dedicated education units (DEUs) are student-centered units where nursing students learn theory and direct patient care. In this model, staff nurses are key partners in the student's education and professional role development. An added benefit to DEUs is that they require sharing of resources, and a willingness to work collaboratively to solve operational issues—the foundation of a true partnership (Huston et al., 2017).

Formal Academic–Practice Partnerships

More than arranging clinical practicum and related issues, a formal partnership is bound by clearly defined expectations, the sharing of knowledge, and a commitment to lifelong learning. In this model, partners move out of traditional roles and ways of thinking to rethink nursing education, nursing research, and professional development in ways that support more effective ways to transition into practice (Slaikeu, 2011).

Academic–Practice-Based TPP

A 12-week TPP was developed in the San Francisco Bay Area to address new graduate RNs unable to find work due to the recession of 2008. This standardized curriculum showed positive outcomes in terms of improved competence, confidence, and employment, and was adopted for use in acute care, home health, hospice and public health settings (Jones & West, 2017).

> ### Discussion Point
>
> What additional ideas do you have for better alignment of academia to emerging practice needs?

THINKING BIGGER: CURRICULUM REDESIGN

The academic and practice strategies shared above are built on traditional models of nursing education. The changing health care landscape provides the nursing profession with an opportunity to disrupt current thinking and fundamentally rethink how to prepare a future nursing workforce. Through partnership, academia and practice can redesign curricula that prepare students to pass their board exam *and* safely and effectively provide patient care. What might a new model look like? How might education and practice partners collaborate to create an innovative approach to nursing education? It can be difficult to envision innovative approaches that bridge the academic–practice gap. Fortunately, examples do exist and can be used to illustrate this idea.

Redesign Example From Nursing's Past: Kaiser Foundation School of Nursing

Established in the 1940s, the Kaiser Foundation School of Nursing (KFSN) fundamentally disrupted traditional approaches to the preparation of nurses, breaching norms of the time by providing an experiential curriculum that advocated health promotion, preventive health measures, and wellness over sick care. Nursing courses included clinical experiences that spanned the continuum of care; occupational health and rural nursing were early rotations as were rehabilitation nursing, outpatient/ambulatory care, and home care clinical experiences. The school was led by a doctorally prepared nurse leader and learning was delivered to a diverse student body by nursing and physician educators—including clinical and operational specialists from Kaiser Permanente. The program fostered mutual respect, expansion of nursing roles, and interprofessional collaboration. Many of the graduates went on to achieve leadership positions in the state of California and elsewhere, their legacy still present within nursing.

At that time, the Kaiser Permanente health care model primarily focused on serving employees with an emphasis on worker safety, and the prevention of industrial injuries in the Kaiser Industries shipyards and civil engineering sites. The training environment of KFSN presented an opportunity to align nursing education with the needs of Kaiser workers by providing access to comprehensive care close to their work sites and by providing a robust education to the nursing students that accelerated learning and the acquisition of clinical nursing skills (Moss, D'Alfonso, & Jones, 2018).

Modern Redesign Example: Jefferson College of Nursing

Jefferson College of Nursing in Pennsylvania provides a current example of innovative redesigns in nursing education. The college used a collaborative effort to design and implement a curriculum focused on nurses' expanding roles and the need for preparing a workforce able to function as leaders beyond the traditional acute care environment. The curriculum was developed over 1 year by stakeholders including faculty from prelicensure and graduate programs, students, alumni, practice, and community-based partners.

Jefferson's faculty were asked to explore, "How do employers, the public, professional colleagues, faculty, and the community identify the university's professional RNs from other new graduates and RNs? What characteristics, behaviors, and/or competencies would that product possess after completing the university's program?" (Bouchard, Brown, & Swan, 2017). Senior nursing students, alumni, and practice partners were asked to provide input for improving the disparity of access to health care that many populations experience and the role nursing can play.

Program outcomes and a concept-based curriculum were built around four themes: practice excellence,

interprofessional collaboration, population health, and innovation (Bouchard et al., 2017). Students enrolled in the program are exposed to a range of care settings including the acute environment, continuing care facilities, outpatient rehabilitation centers, pediatric offices, homeless shelters, and ACOs to better understand how health care data are analyzed and applied to keep populations and communities well (Bouchard et al., 2017).

In the words of a professor co-lead for the effort at Jefferson, "We have to prepare a different professional registered nurse today" (Bouchard et al., 2017).

Discussion Point

Have your prelicensure clinical experiences prepared you to work in settings outside of the the hospital? How much experience are you gaining outside the hospital?

WHAT CAN WE DO TO BRIDGE THE GAP? WHAT IS HOLDING US BACK?

Despite data validating the risks of not addressing the academic–practice gap, many organizations continue to resist change. Change can be complex. Schools and clinical sites may be open to new ways of thinking and working, yet they might lack the understanding of, or experience with, how to successfully manage organizational change and the inevitable disruptions that accompany innovation. Strategies such as redesigning relationships between academic and practice partners, providing opportunities for employees to work as clinical faculty, or creating DEUs require collaboration, clear communication, patience, persistence, and resources to conceive and adopt. It is a challenge and a skill to address nursing workforce competencies for evolving health care trends while simultaneously addressing the current demand to graduate nurses and treat a population with chronic disease and illness. In other words, the need and finite resources with which to address immediate issues and challenges can compete with the longer-term investment of time, effort, and funds to create the type of nurse anticipated to be in increasing demand.

Academia faces pressure to meet current educational and regulatory requirements established by accrediting agencies and state boards of nursing. Universities and colleges may be steeped in tradition and committed to adhere to long-established policies, procedures, and approaches to academic learning. The school's business model may be reliant on traditional ways of providing nursing education.

Recommendations for fundamentally redesigning curricula and shifting how knowledge is transferred may challenge both the academic and business sides of universities and colleges. Moving beyond the traditional prelicensure models focused on inpatient medical-surgical nursing represents a dramatic change in paradigm, which may be challenging to overcome.

CONCLUSION

Although the IOM report was released in 2010, schools and practice settings have yet to uniformly incorporate key messages and recommendations. The U.S. population is growing older, and the need to manage chronic health conditions continues to expand. This is occurring concurrently with health care reform as well as significant changes in the clinical workforce. With the right education, nursing can support changing care needs through the emergence of new roles and care delivery models. If academia and practice do not address the apparent trends in American health care, then the academic–practice gap is likely to grow wider.

Much of prelicensure nursing education continues to focus on tasks and memorization. This curriculum was designed for a role that does not match expectations of a contemporary RN. As the authors have established, focusing on NCLEX pass rates does not adequately measure a newly licensed RN's ability to meet the demands of real-world clinical practice. Unlike the physician education model, nursing lacks a standardized postlicensure approach to role acquisition through robust TPPs. This places both newly licensed RNs and the health systems they work for at risk.

Physician residency is not required following initial licensure as a medical doctor. However, it is the standard of practice in most communities across the country. Newly licensed physicians seek placements in competitive multiyear residency programs that help bridge the gap between medical school and safe independent practice. As RN roles and the overall health care system become more complex, standardization of RN TPPs becomes more of a consideration. Facing a multitude of conflicting priorities, health systems have yet to recognize the importance of providing the same rigor of education for newly licensed RNs. Lack of adequate preparation for practice may result in clinical errors, reality shock, job dissatisfaction, and ultimately nurse attrition.

Regulatory and accrediting bodies, such as boards of nursing and the NCSBN, must critically evaluate pre- and postlicensure standards. Revisions to state-mandated prelicensure curriculum outlines may be necessary. Further, TPPs should become the standard of practice to ensure quality and consistency across health systems. Federal regulatory bodies such as the Centers for Medicare and Medicaid should also take an interest in supporting TPPs for newly licensed RNs. Improving initial RN competency could help close the quality and affordability gap that is draining the national economy.

In the current environment, there are opportunities for academia and practice to find creative ways to create the nurse of the future. Examples exist of how academia and practice have aligned to prepare nurses for the modern needs of clinical practice. These examples of schools and practice sites working collaboratively have been possible through an openness to innovation. Stronger collaborative relationships need to be developed between regulatory bodies, academia, and practice partners to advance new models of pre- and postlicensure nursing education.

Risks are high if nursing maintains the status quo—the health of our population and the value of the profession are on the line. Can we afford not to change?

For Additional Discussion

1. In the future, should practice settings be required to offer TPPs to all newly licensed RNs? What role might academia play in these programs? What role might the Centers for Medicare and Medicaid or other public funders play?

2. Do you feel your nursing program has prepared you to fill nursing roles in the community? Have you learned about primary care?

3. Which specialty areas have you been exposed to (emergency department, operating room, catheterization lab, labor and delivery)? Did the exposure provide enough experience for you to work as a competent nurse in that field?

4. How many of your faculty members are still active in clinical practice? Do you think this makes a difference in your education as a future RN?

5. What learning experiences should be offered in the future to help better prepare prelicensure RNs for real-world nursing practice? What gaps do you see?

References

American Association of Colleges of Nursing. (2007, February). *White paper on the education and role of the clinical nurse leader.* Retrieved from https://nursing.uiowa.edu/sites/default/files/documents/academic-programs/graduate/msn-cnl/CNL_White_Paper.pdf

Auerbach, D. I., Buerhaus, P. I., & Staiger, D. O. (2015). Will the RN workforce weather the retirement of the baby boomers? *Medical Care, 53*(10), 840–856. doi:10.1097/MLR.0000000000000415

Ball, K., Doyle, D., & Oocumma, N. I. (2015). Nursing shortages in the OR: Solutions for new models of education. *AORN Journal, 101*(1), 115–136. doi:10.1016/j.aorn.2014.03.015

Bell, R., Bossier-Bearden, M., Henry, A. A, & Kirksey, K. M. (2015). Transitioning experienced registered nurses into an obstetrics specialty. *The Journal of Continuing Education in Nursing, 46*(4), 187–192. doi:10.3928/00220124-20150320-04

Benner, P. (1984). *From novice to expert: Excellence and power in clinical nursing practice.* Menlo Park, CA: Addison-Wesley Publishing Company.

Benner, P., Sutphen, M., Leonard, V., & Day, L. (2010). *Educating nurses: A call for radical transformation.* San Francisco, CA: Jossey-Bass.

Berg, J., & Dickow, M. (2013). *Nurse role exploration project: The affordable care act and new roles for nurses.* California Institute for Nursing & Health Care (CINHC). Retrieved from CINHC Website: http://healthimpact.org/wp-content/uploads/2015/08/NurseRoles-100920131.pdf

Berkow, S., Virkstis, K., Stewart, J., & Conway, L. (2008). Assessing new graduate nurse performance. *Journal of Nursing Administration, 38*(11), 468–474. doi:10.1097/01.NNA.0000339477.50219.06

Berman, A., Beazley, B., Karshmer, J., Prion, S., Van, P., Wallace, J., & West, N. (2014). Competence gaps among unemployed new nursing graduates entering a community-based transition-to-practice program. *Nurse Educator, 39*(2), 56–61. doi:10.1097/NNE.0000000000000018

Blegan, M. A., Spector, N., Lynn, M. R., Barnsteiner, J., & Ulrich, B. (2017, October). Newly licensed RN retention: Hospital and nurse characteristics. *Journal of Nursing Administration, 47*(10), 508–514.

Bodenheimer, T. S., & Smith, M. D. (2013). Primary care: Proposed solutions to the physician shortage without training more physicians. *Health Affairs, 32*(11), 1881–1886.

Bouchard, M., Brown, D., & Swan, B. A. (2017). Creating a new education paradigm to prepare nurses for the 21st century. *Journal of Nursing Education and Practice, 7*(10), 27–35.

Bradley, E. H., Sipsma, H., & Taylor, L. A. (2016). American health care paradox—High spending on health care and poor health. *QJM: An International Journal of Medicine, 110*(2), 61–65.

Buerhaus, P. (2015). *Dr. Peter Buerhaus' perspective on the short- and long-term outlook for registered nurses in the US.* Retrieved from the New Jersey State Nurses Association Website: http://www.njsna.org/?639

Buerhaus, P., Auerbach, D., & Staiger, D. (2017). How should we prepare for the wave of retiring baby boomer nurses? *HealthAffairs Blog.* Retrieved May 31, 2017, from https://www.healthaffairs.org/do/10.1377/hblog20170503.059894/full/

Buerhaus, P., Skinner, L. E., Auerbach, D. I., & Staiger, D. O. (2017). Four challenges facing the nursing workforce in the United States. *Journal of Nursing Regulation, 8*(2), 40–46.

Campaign for Action. (2016, January). *Huge interest in IOM's future of nursing report shows in record number of downloads.* Retrieved from https://campaignforaction.org/huge-interest-ioms-future-nursing-report-shows-record-number-downloads

Candela, L., & Bowles, C. (2008). Recent RN graduate perceptions of educational preparation. *Nursing Education Perspectives, 29*(5), 266–271.

Carter, M. (2006). The evolution of doctoral education in nursing. In C. Bridges, A. Lowenstein, L. Andrist, P. Nicholas, & K. Wolf. (Eds.), *History of nursing ideas* (p. 38). New York, NY: Jones & Bartlett.

Casey, K., Fink, R., Jaynes, C., Campbell, L., Cook, P., & Wilson, V. (2011). Readiness for practice: The senior practicum experience. *Journal of Nursing Education, 50*(11), 646–652. doi:10.3928/01484834-20110817-03

Casey, K., Fink, R., Krugman, M., & Propst, J. (2004). The graduate nurse experience. *Journal of Nursing Administration, 34*(6), 303–311. doi:10.1097/00005110-200406000-00010

Cline, D., La Frentz, K., Fellman, B., Summers, B., & Brassil, K. (2017). Longitudinal outcomes of an institutionally developed nurse residency program. *Journal of Nursing Administration, 47*(7/8), 384–390.

Colby, S. L., & Ortman, J. M. (2015). *Projections of the size and composition of the US population: 2014 to 2060.* Washington, DC: U.S. Census Bureau.

Cubanski, J., Lyons, B., Neuman, T., Snyder, L., Jankiewicz, A., & Rousseau, D. (2015). Medicaid and Medicare trends and challenges. *JAMA, 314*(4), 329–329.

Davis, K., Stremikis, K., Schoen, C., & Squires, D. (2014). Mirror, mirror on the wall, 2014 update: How the US health care system compares internationally. *The Commonwealth Fund, 16*, 1–31.

Del Bueno, D. (2001). Buyer beware: The cost of competence. *Nursing Economic$, 19*(6), 250–255.

Del Bueno, D. (2005). A crisis in critical thinking. *Nursing Education Perspectives,* (5), 278–282.

Duchscher, J. E. (2009). Transition shock: The initial stage of role adaptation for newly graduated registered nurses. *Journal of Advanced Nursing, 65*(5), 1103–1113. doi:10.1111/j.1365-2648.2008.04898.x

Fink, R., Krugman, M., Casey, K., & Goode, C. (2008). The graduate nurse experience: Qualitative residency program outcomes. *Journal of Nursing Administration, 38*(7/8), 341–348. doi:10.1097/01.NNA.0000323943.82016.48

Friday, L., Zoller, J. S., Hollerbach, A. D., Jones, K., & Knofczynski, G. (2015). The effects of a prelicensure extern program and nurse residency program on new graduate outcomes and retention. *Journal for Nurses in Professional Development, 31*(3), 151–157. doi:10.1097/NND.0000000000000158

Gaudette, É., Tysinger, B., Cassil, A., & Goldman, D. P. (2015). Health and health care of Medicare beneficiaries in 2030. *Forum for Health Economics and Policy, 18*(2), 75–96.

Goldman, D., & Gaudette, É. (2015). *Strengthening Medicare for 2030.* Retrieved from Brookings Institute: https://www.brookings.edu/wp-content/uploads/2016/07/Medicare2030_Chartbook.pdf

Goode, C. J., Lynn, M. R., McElroy, D., Bednash, G. D., & Murray, B. (2013). Lessons learned from 10 years of research on a post-baccalaureate nurse residency program. *Journal of Nursing Administration, 43*(2), 73–79. doi:10.1097/nna.0b013e31827f205c

Gudbranson, E., Glickman, A., & Emanuel, E. J. (2017). Reassessing the data on whether a physician shortage exists. *JAMA, 317*(19), 1945–1946.

Hessler, K. (2017). *Flipping the nursing classroom.* Burlington, MA: Jones & Bartlett Learning.

Hickerson, K. A., Taylor, L. A., & Terhaar, M. F. (2016). The preparation-practice gap: An integrative literature review. *The Journal of Continuing Education in Nursing, 47*(1), 17–23.

Huston, C. L., Phillips, B., Jeffries, P., Todero, C., Rich, J., Knecht, P., . . . Lewis, M. P. (2017, August). The academic-practice gap: Strategies for an enduring problem. *Nursing Forum, 53*(1), 27–34. doi:10.1111/nuf.12216

Institute of Medicine. (2011). *The future of nursing: Leading change, advancing health.* Washington, DC: The National Academies Press.

Jansen, R., & Venter, I. (2015). Psychiatric nursing: An unpopular choice. *Journal of Psychiatric and Mental Health Nursing, 22*(2), 142–148.

Jones, D., & West, N. (2017). Chapter 16. New graduate RN transition to practice programs. In C. J. Huston (Ed.), *Professional issues in nursing: Challenges and opportunities* (4th ed, pp. 233–249). Philadelphia, PA: Wolters Kluwer.

Kavanagh, J. M., & Szweda, C. (2017). A crisis in competency: The strategic and ethical imperative to assessing new graduate nurses' clinical reasoning. *Nursing Education Perspectives, 38*(2), 57–62.

Kellehear, K. J. (2014). The theory-practice gap: Well and truly alive in mental health nursing. *Nursing Health Science, 16*(2), 141–142. doi:10.1111/nhs.12156

Kirch, D. G., & Petelle, K. (2017). Addressing the physician shortage: The peril of ignoring demography. *JAMA, 317*(19), 1947–1948.

Kramer, M. (1974). *Reality shock: Why nurses leave nursing.* Saint Louis, MO: CV Mosby.

Kramer, M., Brewer, B. B., & Maguire, P. (2013). Impact of healthy work environments on new graduate nurses' environmental reality shock. *Western Journal of Nursing Research, 35*(3), 348–383. doi:10.1177/0193945911403939

Monahan, J. C. (2015). A student nurse experience of an intervention that addresses the perioperative nursing shortage. *Journal of Perioperative Practice, 25*(11), 230–234.

Moss, T., D'Alfonso J, & Jones, D. (2018). Kaiser's school of nursing: A 70-year legacy of disruptive innovation. *Nursing Administration Quarterly, 42*(1), 35–42.

Mullen, J. (2015). Living longer better: A call to action to promote the health of older adults and their communities. *Journal of Public Health Management and Practice, 21*(4), 410–412.

National Academies of Sciences, Engineering, and Medicine. (2016). *Assessing progress on the Institute of Medicine report The Future of Nursing.* Washington, DC: The National Academies Press.

National Academies of Sciences, Engineering, and Medicine. (2017). *Infographic—The future of nursing.* Retrieved from http://nationalacademies.org/hmd/Reports/2010/The-Future-of-Nursing-Leading-Change-Advancing-Health/Infographic.aspx

Numminen, O., Leino-Kilpi, H., Isoaho, H., & Mertoja, R. (2015). Newly graduated nurses' competence and individual and organizational factors: A multivariate analysis. *Journal of Nursing Scholarship, 47*(5):446–457. doi:10.1111/jnu.12153

Patient Protection and Affordable Care Act, 42 U.S.C. § 18001 (2010).

Pittman, P., & Forrest, W. (2015). The changing roles of registered nurses in pioneer accountable care organizations. *Nursing Outlook, 63*(5), 554–565. doi:10.1016/joutlook.2015.05.008

Ramirez, Y. I., Zimmerman, R., & Judson, L. H. (2013). A student nurse externship program: Academia and service collaboration. *Journal of Nursing Regulation, 4*(1), 39–44. doi:10.1016/S2155-8256(15)30162-9

Robert Wood Johnson Foundation. (2014). *Nearly one in five nurses leaves first job within a year, according to survey of newly-licensed registered nurses.* Retrieved from http://www.rwjf.org/en/library/articles-and-news/2014/09/nearly-one-in-five-new-nurses-leave-first-job-within-a-year--acc.html

Saifan, A., AbuRauz, M. E., & Masa'deh, R. (2015). Theory practice gaps in nursing education: A qualitative perspective. *Journal of Social Sciences, 11*(1), 20–29. Retrieved from http://thescipub.com/PDF/jssp.2015.20.29.pdf

Sherman, R. O., Patterson, P., Avitable, T., & Dahle, J. (2014). Perioperative nurse leader perspectives on succession planning: A call to action. *Nursing Economic$, 32*(4), 186–195.

Slaikeu, K. (2011). Addressing the preparation/practice gap: A new era, new approach. *Nursing Leadership, 9*(2), 46–49.

Sommers, B. D., Maylone, B., Blendon, R. J., Orav, E. J., & Epstein, A. M. (2017). Three-year impacts of the Affordable Care Act: Improved medical care and health among low-income adults. *Health Affairs, 6*(36), 1119–1128. doi:10.1377/hlthaff.2017.0293

Spector, N., Blegen, M. A., Silvestre, J., Barnsteiner, J., Lynn, M. R., Ulrich, B., . . . & Alexander, M. (2015). Transition to practice study in hospital settings. *Journal of Nursing Regulation, 5*(4), 24–38.

Spector, N., & Echternacht, M. (2010). A regulatory model for transitioning newly licensed nurses to practice. *Journal of Nursing Regulation, 1*(2), 18–25.

Staiger, D. O., Auerbach, D. L., & Buerhaus, P. (2012). Registered nurse labor supply and the recession—Are we in a bubble? *New England Journal of Medicine, 366*(16), 1463–1465. doi:10.1056/NEJMp1200641

U.S. Department of Labor, Bureau of Labor Statistics. (2014). *Economic news release. Table 8. Occupations with the largest projected number of job openings due to growth and replacement needs, 2012 and projected 2022*. Retrieved from http://www.bls.gov/news.release/ecopro.t08.htm

Ulrich, B., Krozek, C., Early, S., Ashlock, C. H., Africa, L. M., & Carman, M. L. (2010). Improving retention, confidence, and competence of new graduate nurses: Results from a 10-year longitudinal database. *Nursing Economic$, 28*(6), 363–375. Retrieved from http://www.ndcenterfornursing .org/linked/versant_10_year_article_nec_2010.pdf

Wallace, J. (2016). Nursing student work-study internship program: An academic partnership. *Journal of Nursing Education, 55*(6), 357–359. doi:10.3928/01484834-20160516-11

Wallace, J., Berman, A., Karshmer, J., Prion, S., Van P., & West, N. (2014). Economic aspects of community-based academic-practice transition programs for unemployed new nursing graduates. *Journal of Nurses in Professional Development, 30*(5), 237–241. doi:10.1097/NND.0000000000000094

Yakusheva, O., Lindrooth, R. C., Weiner, J., Spetz, J., & Pauly, M. V. (2015). How nursing affects Medicare's outcome-based hospital payments. Interdisciplinary Nursing Quality Research Initiative. Retrieved from University of Penn Leonard Davis Institute of Health Economics Website: http://ldi.upenn.edu/brief/how-nursing-affectsmedicare%E2%80%99s-outcome-based-hospital-payments

Developing Effective Leaders to Meet 21st-Century Health Care Challenges

Bernadette Mazurek Melnyk, Kathy Malloch, and Lynn Gallagher-Ford

CHAPTER OUTLINE

LEARNING OBJECTIVES

The learner will be able to:

1. Describe factors that are driving the need for in-novative and transformational leaders in health care for the 21st century.

2. Identify nine health care leadership challenges of the 21st century.

3. Delineate three effective strategies to promote and sustain an evidence-based practice organizational culture.

4. Explain why effective leaders in the 21st century must engage in mentoring young leaders and suc-cession planning.

5. Describe the characteristics required of leaders in order to effectively promote innovation and change.

6. Discuss the importance of teamwork, effective com-munication, and transdisciplinary/de-siloed work as they relate to health care outcomes.

7. List 13 essential characteristics of effective leaders.

8. Recognize the areas of change that have occurred as a result of the "electronic world."

9. Discuss the strengths and weaknesses of three lead-ership models: transactional, transformational, and complexity.

10. Distinguish the unique leadership components re-quired in the complexity leadership model.

TODAY'S HEALTH CARE: IN CRITICAL CONDITION

The American health care system is in critical condi-tion, with a tripling of costs over the past two decades, poor-quality services, wasteful spending, and a rise in medical errors (Hader, 2010). Half of the hospitals in the United States are functioning in deficit. There are up to 400,000 unintended patient deaths every year (James, 2013) with medical errors being the third leading cause of death in America (Mackary & Daniel, 2016). Further-more, we are living in an era in which patients receive only approximately 55% of the care they should receive when they enter the health care system (Resar, 2006) and Americans' health care needs are increasing with a higher prevalence of overweight/obesity, chronic diseases, and mental health disorders. The health care system also is facing the most severe shortage of health professionals, including physicians and nurses, it has ever encountered. The changing nature of morbidities in the United States, the current condition of the health care system, and the severe shortage of health care professionals call for trans-formational and innovative leaders who will develop new models of transdisciplinary care and interprofessional education. Such changes will hopefully lead to high qual-ity, evidence-based care and best patient outcomes and, at the same time, decrease health care costs (i.e., high-value health care) as well as limit the number of errors to attain high reliability (Melnyk, 2012).

This chapter presents nine critical leadership challenges for nurse leaders in the 21st century as well as 13 compe-tencies needed to overcome these challenges. The chapter

concludes with a discussion of leadership models for the 21st century and suggests that the complexity leadership model offers a new perspective for leadership and potential to support improved organizational performance.

TWENTY-FIRST-CENTURY LEADERSHIP CHALLENGES

The foregoing health care issues provide challenges or "character-builders" specific to nursing and health care leaders in the 21st century. These challenges are listed in Box 3.1. Each individual nurse leader will have the op-portunity to leverage the challenges of these times or be overwhelmed by them. Old models of autocratic, hierar-chic leadership will be inadequate to handle the fast-paced, complex health care environment of the future. Leaders of today and in the future will need to be evidence based, in-novative, creative, flexible, engaging, courageous, relation-ship based, and dynamic.

Leadership is not a "solo act"; it is imbedded in rela-tionships, effective communication, shared ownership, and coaching and motivating others. Leadership must move from an autocratic, transactional model to innovative com-plexity leadership. Leaders who are steeped in traditional leadership styles and unwilling to grow and change their own practices will be particularly challenged by the dynam-ics of the health care environment that lies ahead. Leaders who are proactive and embrace new approaches, who are better suited for chaotic times, will be in the best position for dealing with the following challenges.

BOX 3.1   Nine 21st-Century Leadership Challenges

* Meeting expectations for increased productivity within budgetary constraints
* Advancing evidence-based practice
* Planning for succession and mentoring young nurse leaders
* Facilitating and enhancing teamwork and effective communication
* Embracing and supporting transdisciplinary health care
* Positioning nursing to influence decision-making in organizational and health policy
* Promoting workplace wellness
* Striking a balance between technology and interpersonal relationships to deliver best care
* Creating cultures of innovation and change

Meeting Expectations for Increased Productivity Within Rigorous Budgetary Constraints

Even in an era of major federal, state, and organizational budget reductions, leaders are expected to be highly productive with a scarcity of resources and a plethora of financial constraints. In the theater of nursing, what exactly does "productive" encompass? Productivity includes both resource stewardship and delivery of the nursing "product" of safe, evidence-based, quality care. A major challenge for nurse leaders is to advocate for, attain, and maintain a balance between these two key factors of nursing productivity. Nurse leaders need to use strategies where "caring management and financial constraints can coexist while promoting quality patient care" (Cara, Nyberg, & Brousseau, 2011).

Nurse leaders also need to understand and clearly articulate the inextricable connectedness of nurse engagement, productivity, and retention with caring and quality outcomes, which ultimately drive satisfaction and the financial well-being of the organization. Therefore, nurse leaders must be evidence based, creative, innovative, entrepreneurial, and resourceful in garnering new resources and strategizing to maintain the core nursing value of caring to increase efficiency and to drive quality outcomes.

Advancing Evidence-Based Practice When Care in Many Health Care Institutions Remains Steeped and Mired in Tradition

Consider This A large number of medical errors occur because clinicians do not practice evidence-based health care.

The Institute of Medicine (IOM) named evidence-based practice (EBP) as a core competency for health care professionals (Greiner & Knebel, 2003). Shortly thereafter, the National Institutes of Health Roadmap initiative prioritized the acceleration of the transfer of knowledge from research into practice (Zerhouni, 2005; Research Fuels the Controversy 3.1). Specific, research-derived

Research Fuels the Controversy 3.1

The Establishment of Evidence-Based Practice Competencies for Practicing Registered Nurses and Advanced Practice Nurses in Real-World Clinical Settings: Proficiencies to Improve Health Care Quality, Reliability, Patient Outcomes, and Costs

In 2014, the first set of evidence-based practice (EBP) competencies for practicing nurses and advanced practice nurses was created. Consensus among a national panel of seven EBP experts was the first step in establishing the competencies followed by two rounds of a Delphi survey with 80 EBP mentors across the United States who validated them.

Source: Melnyk, B. M., Gallagher-Ford, L., Long, L. E., & Fineout-Overholt, E. (2014). The establishment of evidence-based practice competencies for practicing registered nurses and advanced practice nurses in real-world clinical settings: Proficiencies to improve health care quality, reliability, patient outcomes, and costs. *Worldviews on Evidence-Based Nursing, 11*(1), 5–15.

Study Findings

Two rounds of a Delphi survey with the 80 mentors resulted in a final set of 13 EBP competencies for practicing registered nurses and 11 additional competencies for advanced practice nurses. Leaders must create cultures and environments that support the implementation and sustainability of EBP. Integration of these competencies into health care system expectations, orientations, job descriptions, performance appraisals, and clinical ladder promotion processes will enhance health care quality, safety, and consistency of health care interventions as well as reduce costs.

competencies for EBP have been described and disseminated and can easily be integrated into clinical and academic organizations (Melnyk, Gallagher-Ford, & Fineout-Overholt, 2015; Melnyk, Gallagher-Ford, Long, & Fineout-Overholt, 2014). Furthermore, studies have supported that EBP enhances quality of care, improves patient outcomes, and decreases health care costs. Yet, EBP is not the standard of practice in many health care organizations throughout the country (Harding, Porter, Horne-Thompson, Donley, & Taylor, 2014; Melnyk & Fineout-Overholt, 2015; Melnyk, et al., 2018).

Findings from a survey of over 1,000 nurses randomly sampled from the American Nurses Association indicated that only one third of the nurses reported that their colleagues consistently implement EBP and only one third said they had EBP mentors. Further, the older the nurse, the less they were interested in gaining more knowledge and skills in EBP (Melnyk, Fineout-Overholt, Gallagher-Ford, & Kaplan, 2012). Top barriers to EBP included time, organizational culture and politics, lack of EBP knowledge/education, lack of access to evidence/information, and leader/manager resistance.

Identification that leaders were a major barrier to EBP in this survey prompted yet another survey funded by Elsevier to further explore this finding. The survey with over 270 chief nurse executives across the United States revealed that although they believed in EBP, their own implementation of EBP was low. Further, although the chief nurses reported that their top priorities were health care quality and safety, EBP was rated as a low priority. These findings revealed a major disconnect in that many chief nurses do not see EBP as a direct pathway to quality and safety.

Therefore, leaders must have the knowledge and skills to create cultures of EBP that ignite a spirit of inquiry throughout the organization and cultivate an environment where EBP is the standard of care, not the exception. Unfortunately, although leaders report that they believe in the value of EBP, their own implementation of it is low (Melnyk et al., 2012; Sredl et al., 2011). It will be critical for nurse leaders to integrate evidence into their individual professional practices to deliver best leadership practice as well as to serve as EBP role models, which will influence their staff's EBP beliefs and implementation of evidence-based care. Recently developed tools, such as the new EBP competencies for practicing nurses, and advanced practice nurses (Melnyk et al., 2014; Melnyk et al., 2015) will assist leaders in creating an infrastructure that supports EBP.

Discussion Point

As a new nurse leader, you are faced with an organization of nurses who in large part do not believe in or have the skills to deliver evidence-based care. What strategies would you embark upon early in your new role to begin to change that paradigm?

Planning for Leadership Succession and Mentoring Young Nurse Leaders

Continuity is a vital aspect of effective organizations; it is critical to strategic and operational goals. Disruption in an organization's continuity can have dire consequences. Disruption is particularly challenging in health care organizations because of the potential damage to confidence from the community and employees, the cost of unfinished business and negative impact on financing, and the harm to the organization's image and history (Bowen, 2014; Witt/Kieffer, 2004). Succession planning is the cure for this condition as the process is intended to create an internal leadership pipeline that identifies internal candidates to be promoted. These internal candidates require less time and effort to be oriented and are likely to be successful in their new position. This, in turn, allows organizations to accomplish at least two major goals during times of transition and turnover: (1) effective resource stewardship and (2) ongoing focus on accomplishing their strategic mission.

Succession planning also can be a very positive experience for the "up and coming" leaders in the organization. As individuals in the organization are given expanded opportunities, planned support, intentional mentorship, and effective and meaningful rewards and recognition, they develop their leadership portfolio and are less likely to be a "flight risk" (Blouin, McDonagh, Neistadt, & Helfand, 2006) to the organization.

Consider This Succession planning requires . . . planning! Have you thought about who will follow you and how you can influence their success?

One of the critical aspects of effective succession planning is mentoring. Studies have supported that nurses and physicians who have mentors tend to be more successful in and satisfied with their own careers (Beecroft, Santner, Lacy, Kunzman, & Dorey, 2006; Sambunjak,

Straus, & Marusić, 2006). Mentoring can run the gamut from informal "in the moment" coaching to formal, planned meetings. "Giving talented future leaders the time, energy, advice, and experiences to gain new competencies and learn how to begin to prepare for future roles and responsibilities becomes the 'gift' a current leader can bestow upon a future leader" (Blouin et al., 2006, p. 328). Evidence has supported that mentoring programs decrease nursing turnover rates (Zucker et al., 2006). Both mentors and mentees benefit from the process of mentoring as professional and personal growth occurs.

Yet, despite all of its associated positive benefits, there has not been enough mentoring and empowering of young nurse leaders by more seasoned leaders in the nursing profession (Huston, 2017; Titzer & Shirey, 2013). As a result, the profession is highly vulnerable as large numbers of established nurse leaders will be retiring in the next decade and the resulting talent gap may cause nursing to lose much of the ground gained in health care in recent years. Intentional as well as informal mentoring of young leaders and strategic succession planning is an imperative for current nurse leaders in order to sustain the positive changes and significant outcomes cultivated during their tenures.

Facilitating and Enhancing Teamwork and Effective Communication

Communication has always been an important skill for all clinicians and teams with studies demonstrating the relationship between communication and patient safety. Effective communication among team members has been identified by the IOM as one of the markers of safe and highly reliable care (Kohn, Corrigan, & Donaldson, 2000).

Communication is not simply an exchange of information; it is a complex social process in which each party involved in the process brings history, assumptions, and expectations to the interaction (Lyndon, Zlatnik, & Wachter, 2011). "Effective (clinical) communication is clear, direct, explicit, and respectful" and "requires excellent listening skills, superb administrative support, and a collective commitment to move past traditional hierarchy and professional stereotyping" (p. 93). Communication, whether effective or ineffective, is jointly owned by all members of a team and each member is equally capable of engaging in good or bad communication tactics. Each member of the team enters the communication with different worldviews, values, fears, confidence level, and assumed place within the hierarchy. Effective communication requires conscious effort, shared commitment, and hard work.

> **Consider This** Communication is a personal attribute and a learned skill. Do you have an understanding of your personal communication style? (How you communicate/how do you like to be communicated with?) There are many tools available that you can use to gain a better understanding of your style and how you interact with other individuals and teams and how you can modify your style to be more effective.

Leaders can significantly impact the success of teams and communication efforts in their organizations in a wide variety of ways. First, leaders must be effective communicators themselves and role model excellent communication skills in all settings. In addition, leaders are responsible to establish and uphold administrative structures to require and support effective teamwork and communication in their organizations. Finally, leaders must have the skills to effectively confront/manage conflicts that arise out of poor communications.

Embracing and Supporting Transdisciplinary Health Care

The complexity and multidimensional nature of health care and health problems require a different approach than the traditional, segregated, discipline-siloed approach to patient care that has often been the standard in health care organizations for decades. Transdisciplinary care has received a great deal of attention lately and is emerging as an essential requirement for health care. This approach includes true interprofessional decision-making and trust among a variety of health care providers (Clark & Greenwald, 2013; Légaré, Ratté, Gravel, & Graham, 2008; Regan, Laschinger, & Wong, 2015). Transdisciplinary care assumes that merging the specialized knowledge from different health care disciplines together to act upon the same situation results in better and faster results for the recipient of that care (Vyt, 2008). Interprofessional collaboration, a key component of transdisciplinary care, has been demonstrated to improve patient care effectiveness for patients with chronic disease and a higher degree of work satisfaction in health care workers.

The challenge for leaders is to see the dynamics of health care through a contemporary lens, realize its complexities, and acknowledge that care must be evidence based and patient centered, both of which require a transdisciplinary,

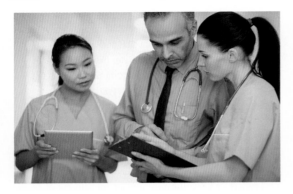

de-siloed approach. Leaders need to be well versed in the tenets of this approach, able to model this approach in their leadership roles, and diligent in creating organizational settings and cultural milieus where this approach can thrive.

Positioning Nursing to Influence Decision-Making in Organizational and Health Policy

Nurse leaders must not only be present in all health care and health policy venues but they must also be active contributors to key discussions and decision-making forums that influence the science and delivery of health care. They must also be proactive in assuring that nurses who are the best in representing certain topics are positioned at the organizational and health policy tables where those topics are being addressed. With an active presence at the "right tables," nurses are able to influence major decisions that positively influence health care quality, safety, and patient outcomes.

Discussion Point

Nurses are the largest sector of health care professionals, yet nurses rarely participate in health care policy decisions. Why does this dilemma persist? What can nurses (individually and as a united group) do to change this?

Promoting Workplace Wellness

Stress, burnout, and turnover continue to plague the nursing profession. This is particularly true for new graduates within the first year of employment (Cho, Laschinger, & Wong, 2006). In a study of new graduate nurses, Melnyk, Hrabe, and Szalacha (2013) found that higher levels of

workplace stress in new graduate nurses were associated with higher levels of depression and anxiety as well as lower levels of resiliency, job satisfaction, and healthy lifestyle beliefs. Furthermore, although nurses are typically great caregivers of others, their own health and wellness often suffer. In a Gallup (2012) survey, it was found that nurses have higher rates of smoking, obesity, hypertension, diabetes, and depression than physicians. Findings from another study by Spence Laschinger, Grau, Finegan, and Wilk (2011) found that, in addition to workload and bullying, psychological capital (i.e., self-efficacy, optimism, hope, and resilience) was an important predictor of burnout in new nurses. Depression also has been found to be associated with prolonged absences from work (Franche et al., 2011). Therefore, it is critical to build supportive workplace cultures of wellness for nurses and other health care professionals.

Wellness includes physical, intellectual, mental, emotional, social, occupational, financial, environmental, and spiritual dimensions. Therefore, promoting workplace wellness in nurses is critical, whether they are new hires or long-term employees, not only to promote the health of nurses directly but also to enhance productivity and decrease absences and high turnover rates, which are very costly to the health care system. A recent study found that new graduate nurses who participated in a 2-day energy management workshop entitled *Nurse Athlete*, which included healthy nutrition, physical activity, and stress reduction, decreased their weight, body mass index, and depressive symptoms at 6 months following completion of the workshop (Hrabe, Melnyk, Buck, & Sinnott, 2017). Workplace wellness requires a culture of respect and support, including definitive programs that address workplace abuse from patients as well as coworkers (Franche et al., 2011). Workplaces also must make healthy choices the easy choice to make.

Discussion Point

How healthy is your workplace culture, physically and emotionally? How healthy are you personally? Are you role modeling and supporting healthy behaviors as a leader?

What single action could you take to make your workplace healthier? When can you initiate that action? How healthy are you? What are you doing to promote *your* physical and emotional well-being? What single action could you take to make yourself healthier? When can you initiate that action?

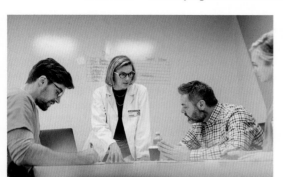

To create a culture of innovation and change, leaders must acknowledge, embrace, and demonstrate engagement in innovation and change in their own leadership practices first. Only then are leaders able to help others to learn, embrace, and imbed the requirements of innovation and change into their individual practices. Creating a culture of innovation and change is not a passive process; it requires active participation, role modeling, and mentorship by the leaders involved. Leaders of organizations who do not model innovation are a barrier in creating and sustaining an innovative environment where positive change and outcomes continually occur (Melnyk & Davidson, 2009).

> **Consider This**   Many people find change stressful. In addition, many people inherently resist change. Embracing change/innovation is a challenge for many traditional managers and leaders.

Striking a Balance Between Technology and Interpersonal Relationships to Deliver Best Care

The impact of technology on health care in the past few decades has been startling, and this trend will surely continue into the future. The challenge for leaders as the next decades unfold will be in shifting from the current trend of technology driving our work to value-based health care quality and relationships as the drivers of our work, with technology supporting those drivers. Effective technology will need to be developed and designed with the "end users" (patients and providers) engaged, valued, and heard throughout the process.

Transformational and innovative leaders well versed in the concepts and language of technology development will be critical in forging the role and place of technology as an integrated component of health care in the future. They will need to understand and articulate the nonlinear and team-based nature of health care work, the innate complexity of the nature of life, and the essential requirement to deliver safe, timely, efficient, effective, equitable, patient-centered care through human interactions and relationships (Berwick, 2002).

Creating Cultures of Innovation and Change

An innovation is more than an idea—it is an idea that comes to fruition and sustains. Although leaders may say that innovation is important, they often do not model it themselves nor provide opportunities that foster innovation in others. For a change to be sustainable, it is not enough to simply create awareness about the change needed. To render a sustainable change, leaders must have the skills and capacity to manage the dynamics and processes associated with innovation as a lived experience (Porter-O'Grady & Malloch, 2010a).

ESSENTIAL CHARACTERISTICS OF EFFECTIVE LEADERS

There are many characteristics that are essential for transformational and innovative leaders, of which 13 are detailed in Box 3.2. It is important to remember that titles do not produce effective leaders; leadership is derived from the combination of an individual's personal characteristics and how they mindfully act and interact with others. Informal leaders without titles who possess these characteristics are often far more respected than formal leaders with titles who do not possess these qualities.

> **BOX 3.2   Thirteen Characteristics of Transformational and Innovative Leaders**
>
> - Vision and the ability to inspire a team vision/dream
> - Passion for patient care and making a difference
> - Transparency, honesty, integrity, and trust
> - Effective communication skills
> - The ability to lead/not micromanage
> - Team, not "I," oriented
> - Risk-taking
> - High level of execution
> - Positive future orientation
> - Innovative and entrepreneurial spirit
> - Dedicated to coaching/mentoring
> - Committed to motivating and empowering others to act/encouraging the heart
> - Passion and persistence through the "character-building" experiences

Vision and the Ability to Inspire a Team Vision/Dream

There is nothing more important to achieving success than a potent dream/vision and an ability to inspire that vision in the team. The change efforts of many leaders fail because they focus too much on process and not enough on an exciting vision, although it does need to be recognized that vision without execution will also deter success. A motivational vision/dream will keep the energy of the leader and the team going when barriers, challenges, or fears are slowing or preventing outcomes from being achieved. Without an inspirational vision and a team who also buys into that vision, the likelihood of new initiatives being successfully attained is doubtful. In the health care environment of the future, characterized by constant change, switching directions, and continuous realignment of resources and priorities, the ability to set and achieve goals will be critical for a leader's success. Effective leaders in the 21st century will be those who can set a vision, guide others toward it, acknowledge progress along the way, and celebrate success relentlessly!

> **Consider This** Nothing happens unless first a dream.
>
> —Carl Sandburg

Passion for Patient Care and Making a Difference

Historically, nurses have been perceived as *the* person on the health care team that "represents the patient" and "advocates for the patient." Placing the patient at the center of our work is not a stretch for nurses . . . it is part of nursing practice and it feels quite right to nurses. However, in the chaos and hustle-bustle of modern health care, it seems that this basic core value is lost at times. This simple idea must be reprioritized and be at the core of nursing, from the bedside to the leadership suite. It must remain an integral part of not only what defines us as clinicians but it must also be translated effectively to represent the value we bring to patients as well as to the health care delivery milieu.

> **Consider This** The main thing is to keep the main thing the main thing.
>
> —Stephen Covey

When patient care and experience are the focus of the leader's efforts, all of the trials and tribulations of the day take on a new perspective. As long as the first question to be answered is "what is the best thing to do for this patient?" a plan can be constructed to get there. With the patient as the focus, it is possible to connect staff with their passion for serving others and define a shared commitment to a set of beliefs about the way patients will be cared for, how families will be treated, how leadership will support that vision, and how staff will help each other. As health care becomes more complex, consumers become more educated, and expectations continue to escalate, having a clear and simple focus that drives the work being done will help nurse leaders to be effective and valued.

Transparency, Honesty, Integrity, and Trust

Transparency, honesty, and integrity are all critical elements for establishing trust. Over the past several decades and across many disciplines, much has been written about the importance of trust. It is considered by many to be the foundation or the basic building block for healthy relationships and effective functional teams. Leaders who are wise know that trust is critical to their success and they work every day to attain and to sustain it. Trust is a "two-way street" and to reap the full benefits of trust, a leader must develop relationships where he/she is trusted by team members *and* where team members are trusted by him/her as well. When words and actions match, when one is perceived as authentic, and when humility and reflection are common actions, trust will flourish. The benefits and rewards of relationships forged from trust are immeasurable, and it is in every nurse leaders' best interest to cultivate this attribute.

> **Consider This** Few things help an individual more than to place responsibility upon him and to let him know that you trust him.
>
> —Booker T. Washington

Discussion Point

As a nurse leader, you have a few nurse managers who hold things "tight to the vest" from their staff; they are not transparent. As a result, there is pervasive mistrust among the staff. How would you handle the situation?

Effective Communication Skills

Effective communication is critical to the safety of patients and the wellness of the workforce. By being effective communicators themselves and role modeling excellent communication skills at all times, leaders can significantly influence the success of teams and organizations. One of the earliest lessons presented in most nursing curriculums is to be attentive to verbal and nonverbal communication and to assess whether they are congruent in all interactions. This is a lesson that resonates whether one is taking care of a patient or presenting a strategic proposal at an executive board meeting. Words, tone, and nonverbal cues, including body language, are all critically meaningful parts of communication. Effective leaders say what they mean, share as much information as they possibly can, and fully engage in their interpersonal interactions.

Within the scope of effective communication skills, the ability to listen cannot be emphasized enough. True listening to others is an incredibly powerful process. The effective listener not only obtains a tremendous amount of valuable information in the interaction but also begins, builds, or enhances their relationship with the other person.

However, it is not enough to simply have these skills and use them in the day-to-day operational context. Leaders must have the additional capacity and courage to use these skills effectively in the challenging times ahead in health care, to confront and manage the conflicts, dilemmas, and conundrums of the coming decades. Finally, in addition to being good communicators, leaders must fulfill their responsibility to establish and uphold administrative structures that assure effective teamwork and communication in their organizations.

The Ability to Lead/Not Micromanage

As a leader, it is critical to lead and sometimes to manage, but never micromanage. When you hire qualified people, you have to give them the freedom to carry out their jobs. Micromanagement is destructive at all levels and in every direction: vertical (manager/subordinate) as well as horizontal (peer/peer). When employees are micromanaged, they believe that their manager does not trust their work or judgment, which can often lead to employees disengaging from their work and simply investing their time, but not their effort or creativity. The resulting dysfunctional work environment is characterized by employees feeling suffocated, which breeds contempt and distrust, both of which are extremely dangerous to teams, organizations, leaders, and, in the health care environment, patients! This cycle is a leader's nightmare.

> **Consider This** If you tell people where to go, but not how to get there, you'll be amazed at the results.
>
> —General Patton

Effective leaders understand and recognize the differences between managing and leading, and they choose to lead whenever possible. Managing people is a skill, whereas leading people is an art and it is an investment. It requires commitment, relationships, emotional intelligence, critical thinking, finesse, and time. The rewards and joys of effective leading compared to the dangers and drain of micromanaging make the effort to lead worthwhile every time.

> **Consider This** Informal leaders without a title can be more effective than leaders with a formal title.

Team, Not "I," Oriented

Teamwork is characterized by a set of interrelated activities accomplished by more than one person to achieve a common objective. Teamwork allows for engagement of many and the distribution of workload that enables each person to be more focused and efficient. Being on a team builds bonds among team members (being part of the team = being part of the solution), spawns creativity, and often generates a more robust outcome than could be achieved by a single individual. With all of this in mind, it would behoove any leaders to embrace the opportunity to work with and build effective teams.

Successful leaders understand the nature of teams and their role on a particular team. The effective leader, when working on a team, understands that the leader's goal is for the *team* to be successful. The effective leader knows that to be successful, each person must relinquish his or her own agenda for personal success and embrace the opportunity to share success with the team. Effective leaders understand that teams need different things from the leader at different stages of their development. A young team needs more direction and hand-holding, whereas a mature team needs more autonomy and freedom. The effective leader guides, motivates, listens to, critiques, and cheerleads the team, and in the end, earns the unique opportunity to celebrate successes as part of the team.

Risk-Taking

Many of the most successful people in life are the greatest risk takers. A definition of a risk taker is "a visionary change leader who can cope with the uncertainty that comes with change at the same time promoting innovation" (McGowan, 2007, p. 106). Risk-taking is often related to "challenging the status quo." It requires a rigorous spirit of inquiry, relentless curiosity about the possibilities, and the courage to engage in both.

Risk-taking is a complex undertaking that includes weighing risks against rewards and moving into a process/project with a clear vision of the benefits overshadowing the doubts. At the same time, successful risk takers proactively recognize the vulnerabilities of moving forward and develop "back up" plans to address unexpected problems.

> **Consider This**   Progress always involves risk; you can't steal second base and keep your foot on first.
>
> —Frederick Wilcox

Leaders of the future will necessarily have to be comfortable with taking risks because the health care environment in the coming decades is bound to be chaotic, unpredictable, messy, and frenetic. Every day in health care will be peppered with opportunities to be risk aversive or risk engaging, and those leaders who embrace and leverage risk effectively will be the success stories, looking at the others in their "rearview mirrors."

High Level of Execution

Effective leaders understand that vision without execution will not lead to success, and so they begin their work with end point(s) in their mind and in their plan. They continuously think about outcomes, the bottom line, and/or the product to be delivered, but the critical difference of this attribute in great leaders is that they do this thinking/planning with finesse. They do not *only* focus on the outcome but also pay attention to the process and the people involved, but they never ever work without the end in mind.

> **Consider This**   We are judged by what we finish, not by what we start.
>
> —Unknown

Positive Future Orientation

Transformational leaders aim high, have a positive future orientation, and "live comfortably in the gap between reality and the organization's vision" (Balik & Gilbert, 2010, p. 14). They are never satisfied, and they are energized by dissatisfaction as opposed to being distressed by it. They convey a positive spirit in their organization as they look to the challenges ahead of them as opportunities, not obstacles (Balik & Gilbert, 2010). Leaders in the chaotic health care environment of the future who address their work with this type of spirit and energy will be more likely to survive and thrive. The key to this attribute is that every individual gets to choose how they will face their day, and those leaders who choose a positive future orientation in their work will be more effective and more likely to *have* a positive future.

Innovative and Entrepreneurial Spirit

The current health care climate calls for leaders who are innovative and entrepreneurial. Resources are dwindling in most health care organizations, which require leaders to be more resourceful and creative in launching innovative and entrepreneurial initiatives that will lead to enhanced efficiency, revenue generation, and reduced costs. Leaders who create cultures of innovation and entrepreneurship will reap the benefits of an organization that thrives through uncertain times and budget constraints. According to Balik and Gilbert (2010), highly successful leaders in health care should "embrace a spirit of innovation, lead bold change, and find ways to lead from inside and outside health care—not only techniques, but changes in mind-set" and "learn to be prepared to lead an interdependent, agile organization with a non-hierarchical mentality that works as a team, with leaders defined by their actions, not by their title" (p. 256).

Dedication to Coaching/Mentoring

Coaching and mentoring young leaders is an imperative for nurse leaders in order to sustain the positive changes and significant outcomes cultivated during their tenure. The ability and desire to find and grow what is good in others is a hallmark of an effective leader. When you ask people . . . "have you ever been mentored by someone?" they are immediately able to tell you who their mentor was and what that mentor did for them that was so life changing. Mentoring is a deep and powerful experience that enriches both the mentee and the mentor. Effective leaders understand the potential power to help others grow and engage in mentoring relationships in order to build effective young leaders and, ultimately, better organizations.

> **Discussion Point**
>
> What were the characteristics of individuals who have mentored you in your career? How did you know you were being mentored? Is there someone in your work environment who you could/should be mentoring now? What can you do to begin that process?

Committed to Motivating and Empowering Others to Act/Encouraging the Heart

The ability to truly motivate and empower others is a skill that effective leaders must possess. People are keenly aware of imposters when it comes to motivation and empowerment. The wise and effective leader knows that this aspect of leadership should only be fulfilled with pure and real intention or the results will be disastrous. Strategies and approaches to connecting with others to motivate them, grow them, and empower them, such as Kouzes and Posner's "encourage the heart," can serve leaders well in developing these attributes (Kouzes & Posner, 2007). These authors stress that leaders must make sure that people feel that what they do matters in their hearts. The practice of encouraging the heart is aligned with two commitments: (1) recognizing contributions by showing appreciation for individual excellence and (2) celebrating the values and victories by creating a spirit of community.

The sharing of stories can be an incredibly powerful tool for motivating and empowering others. Hearing about and relating to what others have lived, learned, or survived has served to help others for decades. Parents who have suffered the loss of a child who share their stories with other parents or with clinicians in training have demonstrated the power of storytelling. This type of exchange is emerging as a powerful tool for leaders to add to their toolkits (Melnyk & Fineout-Overholt, 2015).

Passion and Persistence Through the "Character-Building" Experiences

Passion is so critical, especially to avoid burnout and to keep you going when things get tough. Leaders need to know what their passion is and be able to access it and center on it when the environment intensifies. Persistence, described in the dictionary as an "enduring tenaciously," can be expressed quietly or loudly, but either way it is a key characteristic for effective health care leadership. Persistence is deeply connected to passion in that what you are passionate about you are likely to be persistent about. Nurse leaders must learn the power of passion and persistence and leverage both wisely to attain vision and goals.

> **Consider This**   Many of life's failures are people who had not realized how close they were to success when they gave up.
>
> —Thomas A. Edison

> **Discussion Point**
>
> How many of these 13 essential characteristics have you mastered? Which of these characteristics do your coworkers, peers, direct reports, and supervisors attribute to you? What characteristics can you improve upon?

MODELS OF LEADERSHIP FOR THE 21ST CENTURY

Over the last 30 years, different types and styles of leadership have been used by nurse leaders. Both transactional and transformational models are commonplace in varying degrees in health care organizations. Despite many successes with these models, nurse leaders continue to struggle with patient quality, financial limitations, time management, knowledge access, information sharing, and effective communication. Not surprisingly, leaders are continually searching for the holy grail of leadership, that ultimate, ideal model that effectively guides success in their respective organizations.

The work in today's health care organizations is increasingly complex and filled with digital tools and resources. Specifically, the digital world has changed when we work, where work takes place, and the media for information transfer. This digital revolution results in changes in clinical work processes, including relationships between and among employees, patients, and the community; and the speed at which information is processed, available, and shared. These changes challenge the best of traditional leadership models and render them ineffectual in many situations and settings. Understanding the dynamics of these changes is the first step in determining optimal leadership models that will be effective moving forward.

Scharmer and Käufer (2000) identified four areas of change as a result of the electronic world: media, time, space, and structure. *Media* is the first and refers to the form in which information is documented, shared, and transmitted. In the information age, the Internet has revolutionized how information is transmitted. Flash drives and disks are the norm for data storage. The digitization of information has dramatically reduced the size and format of information. Less physical space is required for papers and files. In many cases, the information is virtual, requiring only electronic storage space. It is now possible for information to be sent to nearly anyone, at anytime, anywhere in the world. The majority of documents can be digitized and thus provide for increased consistency and quality of information. For leaders, the written or typed modality is no longer the most reliable; digitized documentation of information is now the more effective and efficient media for information.

With the nearly open access to the Internet, *time* for work is now wide open as well. The open access to individuals at any time of the day or night increases the emphasis on speed and efficiency. Lag times are decreased allowing for almost instantaneous responses and actions. Given the emphasis on speed and efficiency, this new reality of time as an open concept requires leaders think differently about when work is done. Furthermore, the new reality blurs the work–personal time boundaries creating more challenges. Leaders are now required to shift the emphasis on specific times for work based on a traditional 5-day, 8-hour day in which an individual is present in the workplace to different models. Now, the leader is required to recognize and value work products wherever they are done rather than time present in the workplace. In health care, different models for work time necessarily exist for those providing patient care. The blurring of boundaries for work time necessarily creates two significant challenges: (a) being physically present when there is value in presence and (b) in assuring separation of work and personal time for healthy work–life balance.

As time and media conceptualizations have evolved, the *space* required for work has also changed. While single offices are still commonplace, the actual time spent by individuals in offices is decreasing. The portability of media and ready access to the Internet allows for work to be completed in many locations rather than in the traditional office. It is now possible to perform work wherever the information is accessible. Conference calls and electronic communication have decreased the need for physical gatherings. Individuals gathering at common physical sites are less and less the norm. The trend is to increase flexible spaces for individual and group meetings while decreasing individual office spaces.

The final major change is organizational *structure*. Given the new realities of information and communication exchange, the underlying structure for how work is organized is now open and free flowing. These changes impact organizational structure in numerous ways. The traditional levels of authority diagrams, communication pathways, and span of control are now secondary guides for the organization rather than the primary expectations for communication and permissions. In the digital age, any employee or patient or community members can now communicate with anyone in the organization using electronic mail. Documents or pictures can be shared with anyone in the organization at any time without seeking multiple layers of permissions. For these reasons, it is no wonder that leaders are struggling to be effective and efficient. The rules and principles under which transactional and transformational leadership emerged originally are quite different in the digital age. In the next section, an overview of the strengths and weaknesses of transactional and transformational leadership models followed by the emerging complexity leadership model is presented. Table 3.1 presents a comparison of the three model characteristics. This information is designed to assist leaders in understanding leadership models from a historical perspective and also to determine the role of leaders and leadership for the future.

Transactional/Instrumental Leadership

Transactional or *instrumental* leadership is the most common and well-known leadership style used in health care. In this model, the focus is on task orientation, leader direction, follower participation with the expectation of rewards,

TABLE 3.1 *Characteristics of Three Leadership Models*

	Transactional	Transformational	Complexity
Focus	Planned work	Planned work	Emerging and transitional work
Locus of power	Individual leader-centric/ position; formal	Individual leader-centric/ position; formal	Team/group/relationship-centric network focus; informal
Work	Defined/prescribed; rule driven	Defined/prescribed; rule and principle driven	Emergent; principle driven
Communication direction	Top-down; authoritarian	Top-down; authoritarian	Multiple directions
Competencies	Plan, organize, direct, reward, punish	Plan, organize, direct, reward, punish, empower, collaborate	Facilitate, coach, collaborate
Organizational boundaries	Defined	Defined	Overlapping, informal

threats, or disciplinary action from the leader (Bass & Bass, 2008; see Table 3.1). Research specific to transactional leadership supports the belief that personality traits are consistently correlated with the emergence and effectiveness of leaders. In a transactional model, leaders expect followers to support their goals; a job for the follower is exchanged for support of the leader's vision. In a transactional model, leaders have traditionally relied on traits believed to support and facilitate the role of the leader. Examples of trait theories that focus on the behaviors of the leader include the following:

- Great man theory: Throughout history, great men such as Abraham Lincoln, John Kennedy, and Bill Gates emerged as leaders. The assumption is that strong men emerge as leaders in certain situations.

- Biological-genetic theories: Some individuals were born to lead, a natural leader. The assumption is that leadership cannot be learned; rather one is born a leader.

- Traits of individuals specific to qualities: Intelligence, scholarship, gender, dependability, situation, age, emotional competence, physique, fluency of speech, self-sufficiency, socioeconomic status, social activity, tact, popularity, and so on are common to leaders. The assumption is that certain individuals possess attributes that support their ability to lead; those without these attributes cannot be leaders.

The limitations of transactional leadership include focus on a single individual as the source of knowledge and power; the role of the follower is to follow directions and support the vision of the leader. Creativity, self-actualization, and empowerment of followers are perceived as inappropriate in this model.

Inspirational/Transformational Leadership

The second most common leadership model is *inspirational* or *transformational* and emphasizes the emotional and ideologic appeals using exemplary behavior, confidence, symbolism, and intrinsic motivation (Bass & Bass, 2008). More recently, leaders have embraced the notion of transformational leadership, a style in which the leader forms a relationship of mutual stimulation and elevation that converts followers into leaders (Bryman, Collinson, Grint, Jackson, & Uhl-Bien, 2011). In a transformational leadership model, the work of managing meaning, infusing ideologic values, and co-creation of goals is recognized as processes of empowerment for both the leader and the follower. The exchange between the leader and the follower is elevated to include the value of personal growth for the follower.

Transformational leadership begins to engage followers to self-actualize and contribute to the organization and offers significant advantage over transactional leadership. The limitation of transformational leadership is the locus of power that remains with the leader; the leader is expected to begin the empowerment processes to engage employees rather than employees being expected to lead from their position in the organization. Formal leaders, those designated with an official leadership position, are the norm while informal leadership is not recognized.

Most recently, the concepts of leader authenticity and mindfulness have gained attention (Table 3.2). Models and descriptions of these concepts focus on leadership traits and their relationships to engagement with others in the organization and community as well as a deeper sense of the positive aspects of leadership engagement. The trait of mindfulness from a transactional perspective and authenticity as a transformational approach to self-actualization further defines these basic leadership theories.

These leadership characteristics reflect the complexity of interactions and the limitless potential of other characteristics yet to be identified to guide leaders in recognizing the most contemporary strategies to lead effectively.

Despite the advancements in the transformational leadership model, the ability for the organization to optimize the knowledge and competencies of all members of the organization in a fluid and timely manner is still limited. Continuing to rely on bureaucratic, top-down processes is counterproductive in the presence of the critical dynamics of the digital media, time, space, and structure advancements. Considerations for the changes resulting from the digital advancements are needed to support the uncertain, emergent, and highly interconnected nature of the environment as well as the organizational culture. The addition of appreciative leadership behaviors and strategies may indeed mediate these challenges of transformational leadership.

Complexity Leadership

Congruency between the leadership model, namely, how work occurs, and the underlying assumptions, values, and artifacts of the organization are positively correlated and impact organizational efficiency and effectiveness (Casida & Pinto-Zipp, 2008). Thus, a new leadership model must necessarily integrate the organization culture and local environment. Advancing our current leadership models to address the identified challenges of overwhelming work volumes, fewer financial resources, and increases in complexity of providing patient care will provide an improved framework for leaders. The *complexity leadership model*

TABLE 3.2 **Appreciative Leadership and Mindfulness**	
Appreciative Leadership	**Mindfulness**
Description	
• A process that mobilizes creative potential and unleashes positive power. Five relational strategies—inquiry, inclusion, inspiration, integrity and illumination—are the focus on appreciative leadership (Whitney, Trosten-Bloom, & Rader, 2010).	• Mindfulness is the basic human ability to be fully present, aware of where we are and what we're doing, and not overly reactive or overwhelmed by what's going on around us. Retrieved from https://www.mindful.org/what-is-mindfulness/
Key points	
• A leadership strategy to identify and mobilize creative potential for the individual and the organization. Positive power means bringing your best forward	• The goal is to observe what you are thinking, feeling, and sensing
• Recognizing creative potential	• Develop a spirit of openness and kindness to yourself and others
• Enhancing individual and collective capacity	• Move from automatic processing of information to a high level of presence and engagement in the moment to gain a greater understanding of events
• Opportunities rather than problems are the focus	
Selected References	
• Dewar and Cook (2014)	• Black (2011)
• Keefe and Pesut (2004)	• Boyatzis and McKee (2005)
• Whitney, Trosten-Bloom, and Rader (2010)	• Cullen (2011)
	• Pipe (2008)

offers a futuristic perspective for leadership and potential to support improved organizational performance.

Complexity leadership models are based on complexity leadership theory (CLT) and provide a new lens for leadership to increase effectiveness and efficiency (Uhl-Bien & Marion, 2008). This model recognizes health care organizations as networks of people, resources, knowledge, and other entities composed of overlapping, informal boundaries; leadership is both positional and informal, incorporating the full potential of human and social capital (Hanson & Ford, 2010, p. 6588).

The assumptions in a complexity leadership model are as follows:

• Positional and informal leaders fulfill diverse functions in the organization.
  – Positional leaders carry authority focused on managing organizational dynamics and enabling informal initiatives rather than directing or mandating behaviors.
  – Informal leaders emerge based on relationships and do not require a formal title to lead.

• Control is difficult if not impossible; uncertainty is the norm.

• System boundaries cannot be defined as all interactions are human and interconnected. Boundaries are artificial at best and used to focus on specific projects. Principles increase the effectiveness of the organization and policies are decreased to allow for application of principles by those accountable for the work.

• Leadership is the accountability of every individual in the organization specific to the assigned role. Rather than one great man, everyone has the potential to lead.

• Power does not rest solely with an individual(s); power is distributed among the members of the organization and is located within relationships.

• High degrees of individual interactions are the norm. Communication is critical; transparency as to both positive and negative events is essential.

Within the CLT model, three types of leadership functions are identified—*administrative, adaptive*, and *enabling*.

Interestingly, CLT embraces some aspects of transactional and transformational leadership. The CLT model provides a more robust and congruent model for leadership. The *administrative* leadership component is somewhat similar to the transactional model. This work is about coordinating and planning organizational activities with less hierarchy and formality, thereby sustaining the framework of the organization. The goal is to minimize excessive control and bureaucracy and reinforce the adaptive work of others. The *adaptive* aspect of the model is about the emergence of optimal outcomes from interrelationships and interactions. Collaboration among individuals to produce collective best outcomes is the overall goal of the adaptive leadership role. Some similarities to the transformation model can be gleaned from the adaptive role. The *enabling* role is the new dimension and serves to foster and optimize adaptive work processes and mediate the tensions that occur between administrative and adaptive functions. Enabling leadership works to minimize bureaucratic controls, support the emergence of collective wisdom, and recognize the value of the multiple interactions of individuals as the way work occurs. This brief description of the CLT serves as the foundation for reframing the contemporary leadership model into a trimodal model to better meet the needs of today's challenges (Malloch, 2010).

Trimodal Model

The current work to meet the paradoxical nature of health care in which both stability and creativity are expected encompasses innovation and transition or transformation between operations and innovation. The organizational culture in a trimodal organization reinforces evidence-driven processes. It is also consistent with the work of innovation in which new ideas are encouraged, tested, validated, and implemented when evidence for improvement is available. The organizational culture also strongly supports the transition phase between innovation and operations. Oftentimes, new ideas are embraced and moved from innovation to operations without the necessary time to change to become embedded into the culture. Such changes are often discarded or at best modified. In the trimodal model, transition work is as important as operations and innovation work (Fig. 3.1).

The trimodal model reframes and identifies three vital work processes for leaders: operational stability, innovative leadership, and transformation from innovation to operations. These three categories are designed to manage the present, look to the future, and support the processes in between. A brief explanation of the three components excerpted from Porter-O'Grady and Malloch (2010b) follows.

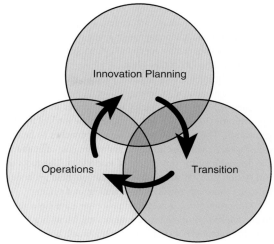

Figure 3.1 Trimodal leadership.

Operations or the work of providing evidence-based patient care within a defined structure with supportive staff and resources comprises the majority of traditional health care work. This work is typically planned, funded, and evaluated within an operations model. Given the predictive nature of this work, it can be thought of as the technical work of an organization, provided by highly skilled professionals. Health care leaders balance and support multiple operational entities and initiatives, medical-surgical services, ambulatory services, pharmacy services, medical imaging, and others.

The new work, with greater variability and complexity, requires leaders to shift from an emphasis on operations to a model that values and integrates the work of change, innovation, and the transition between operations and innovation. The exact proportion of effort needed for each of these modes is unclear; however, it is clear that less time will be spent in operations, with increasing attention to innovation and transition to new levels of operational work.

Traditional operations change in several ways. The emphasis by operations on standardization shifts to one of accountability for work assignments and roles. There is a shift from an emphasis on rules to a focus on principles. Knowing that procedures will change, standardization and consistency must be continually challenged as new information and technologies are introduced. This approach recognizes the temporary nature of most work processes. The emphasis now shifts to the appropriateness of the work performed rather than the completion of checklists.

The second aspect of work in the trimodal model is innovation planning. In this model, innovation work is considered essential rather than optional. Innovation work includes those new ideas, challenges, and product consideration as the means to improve current work. Innovation planning focuses on the continual introduction, modification, and evaluation of new ideas.

Challenging assumptions and asking what if this could happen are normative in innovation work. Innovation work considers all new technologies and processes as potential opportunities to advance and strengthen the work of the organization. The development of new approaches to health care that are safer, less invasive, and more cost-effective is the desired goal for this aspect of leadership. The tools of innovation provide structure and rigor for these processes to assure thorough consideration, testing, and pricing.

Numerous tools, spaces, and processes have been used to accomplish comprehensive evaluations. Many organizations have created physical space for this work; however, the emphasis is more on thinking differently, researching available technologies and the needs of clients. This thinking work does not require a specific physical space, but rather a physical or virtual space that supports creative, safe, and respectful dialogue. Necessarily, the structure for this work is loose to allow for creativity and openness.

The work of innovation planning is not only about looking at new ideas and products but also includes improving or eliminating current ineffective or poorly functioning processes. Furthermore, when organizations are faced with fewer resources, negative outcomes, or shortages of workers, the innovation planning team can begin to assist with creative dialogue to seek greater efficiencies without compromising on quality.

The third aspect of the trimodal model is the transition work that is needed to sustain change and transform work processes. The significance and complexity of facilitating and assuring an effective transition between innovation and operations is too often overlooked or underestimated. Once new ideas are identified and determined to be suitable for future work, sustainable pathways to modify roles, competencies, infrastructure, technology, funding, and the cultural norms must also evolve. Changing the culture requires much more than a single educational program; it requires persistence and focus. When innovations are introduced into a traditional culture without adequate transition support and modification of the existing work, the innovations are most likely to be considered fads and dismissed quickly. New ideas are considered burdens rather than opportunities to remain competitive and achieve the highest-quality outcomes. Participants are more likely to engage in new work at higher levels when they know the rationale for change, are able to test the knowledge in practice, and can support the ethic expectations for professional practice.

Transition is about cultural transformation and requires time, reinforcement, and frequent course corrections to successfully embed new practices into the evolving culture at the point of service level.

Multiple Leadership Perspectives

Given that the needed leadership model necessarily emerges from the time, place, and circumstances in which the organization exists, the leader often relies on multiple leadership perspectives to achieve desired goals. For example, a transactional approach is appropriate when there are regulations to enforce; discussion about whether or not to comply is not appropriate or helpful unless the intent is to propose new regulation. Transformational behaviors—within a complexity leadership model—are appropriate when the focus is on individuals (Malloch, 2014). A complexity approach is most appropriate for the realities of today's health care world. For example, health care reform requirements, namely the emphasis on population health, coordination of care across the life span, and the delivery of value to health care users, are ideally supported by an open and networked approach that aligns the leadership behaviors and beliefs with the nature of this complex and uncertain work.

Understanding one's approach to decision-making, conflict-utilization style, comfort with change, uncertainty, errors, and challenging assumptions are essential for the innovation leader. In addition, basic knowledge of innovation principles, collaboration at the highest and most uncommon levels to foster diversity, and comfort with coaching others to fully engage in the work of the organization are selected competencies that all members of the organization are likely to pursue. The following four principles provide guidance in assuring the alignment of work to be done with supportive leadership behaviors to achieve desired outcomes:

- Self-knowledge: Knowledge of personal ability to manage one's ego, to facilitate others to be fully engaged in the work, and courage to lead in all situations is necessary.

- Value: Value is created through full engagement of all individuals involved in the work of achieving improved health.

- Teamwork: Working in teams is a dynamic process and often requires specific direction from a leader rather than consensus building to achieve timely and value-based outcomes (Coutu, 2009; Frisch, 2008; Hansen, 2009).

- Evidence: When addressing challenges, consideration of available evidence and the need for innovation when evidence is lacking is important in determining the approach that is needed for success—a traditional change process or an innovation strategy.

CONCLUSIONS

To be successful, leaders must possess important characteristics to overcome the major challenges that plague health care in the 21st century. Major challenges facing today's leaders include dwindling resources, organizations, and practices steeped in tradition, and intense pressures to achieve high-value, high-reliability organizations. Leaders must possess numerous essential characteristics, such as an ability to inspire a team vision, effective communication skills, integrity, and an ability to mentor and encourage their team to excel among others, in order to be effective. Although many leadership models exist, the complexity model combined with innovation leadership holds the most promise for best outcomes in dealing with 21st-century leadership challenges.

For Additional Discussion

1. How do traditional attributes associated with the nursing profession (caring, advocacy, service, etc.) promote effective leadership in the 21st century? How might these traditional attributes hinder effective leadership in the 21st century?

2. How could traditional nursing attributes be proactively and thoughtfully leveraged to influence health care decisions in the 21st century?

3. Are health care leaders "walking the talk"/role modeling EBP by integrating evidence into their daily management decision-making? How can this leadership paradigm shift be enhanced?

4. How could formal leadership training for nurse managers and leaders impact hospitals in terms of saving money related to recruitment, nursing satisfaction, nurse wellness, and retention?

5. Compare and contrast the three leadership models identified in Table 3.1. How does each model facilitate patient safety? Also, how can each model be a barrier to patient safety?

6. Is there a model of leadership that better supports leadership at the point of service? Why? Why not?

References

American Hospital Association. (2018). *TrendWatch Chartbook* 2018. Retrieved from https://www.aha.org/guidesreports/2018-05-22-trendwatch-chartbook-2018

Balik, M. B., & Gilbert, J. A. (2010). *The heart of leadership: Inspiration and practical guidance for transforming your health care organization.* Chicago, IL: AHA Press.

Bass, B. M., & Bass, R. (2008). *Handbook of leadership: Theory, research, and management* (4th ed.). New York, NY: Free Press.

Beecroft, P. C., Santner, S., Lacy, M. L., Kunzman, L., & Dorey, F. (2006). New graduate nurses' perceptions of mentoring: Six-year program evaluation. *Journal of Advanced Nursing, 55*(6), 736–747.

Berwick, D. M. (2002). A user's manual for the IOM's "quality chasm" report. *Health Affairs, 21*(3), 80–90.

Black, D. S. (2011). *A brief definition of mindfulness.* Mindfulness Research Guide. Retrieved from http://citeseerx.ist.psu.edu/viewdoc/download?doi=10.1.1.362.6829&rep=rep1&type=pdf

Blouin, A. S., McDonagh, K. J., Neistadt, A. M., & Helfand, B. (2006). Leading tomorrow's healthcare organizations: Strategies and tactics for effective succession planning. *The Journal of Nursing Administration, 36*(6), 325–330.

Bowen, D. J. (2014). The growing importance of succession planning. *Healthcare Executive, 29*(4), 8.

Boyatzis, R. & McKee, A. (2005). *Resonant leadership: Renewing yourself and connecting with others through mindfulness, hope and compassion.* Boston, MA: Harvard Business Press.

Bryman, A., Collinson, D., Grint, K., Jackson, B., & Uhl-Bien, M. (Eds.). (2011). *The SAGE handbook of leadership.* London, England: Sage.

Cara, C. M., Nyberg, J. J., & Brousseau, S. (2011). Fostering the coexistence of caring philosophy and economics in today's health care system. *Nursing Administration Quarterly, 35*(1), 6–14.

Casida, J., & Pinto-Zipp, G. (2008). Leadership–organizational culture relationships in nursing units of acute care hospitals. *Nursing Economic$, 26*(1), 7–15.

Cho, J., Laschinger, H. K., & Wong, C. (2006). Workplace empowerment, work engagement and organizational commitment of new graduate nurses. *Nursing Leadership, 19*(3), 43–60.

Clark, R. C., & Greenwald, M. (2013). Nurse–physician leadership: Insights into interprofessional collaboration. *The Journal of Nursing Administration, 43*(12), 653–659.

Coutu, D. (2009). Why teams don't work. *Harvard Business Review, 87*(5), 99–103, 105.

Cullen, M. (2011). Mindfulness-based interventions: An emerging phenomenon. *Mindfulness, 2*(3), 186–193.

Dewar, B. & Cook, F. (2014). Developing compassion through a relationship centered appreciative leadership programme. *Nurse Education Today, 34*(9), 1258–1264.

Franche, R. L., Murray, E., Ibrahim, S., Smith, P., Carnide, N., Cote, P., . . . Koehoorn, M. (2011). Examining the impact of worker and workplace factors on prolonged work absences among Canadian nurses. *Journal of Occupational and Environmental Medicine, 53*(8), 919–927.

Frisch, B. (2008). When teams can't decide. *Harvard Business Review, 86*(10), 121–126.

Gallup. (2012). *U.S. physicians set good health example.* Retrieved from http://www.gallup.com/poll/157859/physicians-set-good-health-example.aspx

Greiner, A. C., & Knebel, E. (Eds.). (2003). *Health professions education: A bridge to quality.* Washington, DC: The National Academies Press.

Hader, R. (2010). The evidence that isn't. . . Interpreting research. *Nursing Management, 41*(9), 22–26. doi:10.1097/01.NUMA.0000387083.21113.09

Hansen, M. T. (2009). When internal collaboration is bad for your company. *Harvard Business Review, 87*(4), 83–88.

Hanson, W. R., & Ford, R. (2010). Complexity leadership in healthcare: Leader network awareness. *Procedia—Social and Behavioral Sciences, 2*(4), 6587–6596.

Harding, K. E., Porter, J., Horne-Thompson, A., Donley, E., & Taylor, N. F. (2014). Not enough time or a low priority? Barriers to evidence-based practice for allied health clinicians. *The Journal of Continuing Education in the Health Professions, 34*(4), 224–231.

Hrabe, D. P., Melnyk, B. M., Buck, J., & Sinnott, L. (2017). Effects of the nurse athlete program on the healthy lifestyle behaviors, physical health, and mental well-being of new graduate nurses. *Nursing Administration Quarterly, 41*(4), 353–359.

Huston, C. J. (2017). *Professional issues in nursing: Challenges and opportunities* (4th ed.). Philadelphia, PA: Wolters Kluwer.

James, J. (2013). A new, evidence-based estimate of patient harms associated with hospital care. *Journal of Patient Safety, 9*(3), 122–128.

Keefe, M. R., & Pesut, D. (2004). Appreciative inquiry and leadership transitions. *Journal of Professional Nursing, 20*(2), 103–109.

Kohn, L. T., Corrigan, J. M., & Donaldson, M. (Eds.). (2000). *To err is human: Building a safer health system.* Washington, DC: Institute of Medicine.

Kouzes, J. M., & Posner, B. Z. (2007). *The leadership challenge* (4th ed.). San Francisco, CA: Jossey-Bass.

Légaré, F., Ratté, S., Gravel, K., & Graham, I. D. (2008). Barriers and facilitators to implementing shared decision-making in clinical practice: Update of a systematic review of health professionals' perceptions. *Patient Education and Counseling, 73*(3), 526–535.

Lyndon, A., Zlatnik, M. G., & Wachter, R. M. (2011). Effective physician–nurse communication: A patient safety essential for labor and delivery. *American Journal of Obstetrics & Gynecology, 205*(2), 91–96.

Malloch, K. (2010). Innovation leadership: New perspectives for new work. *The Nursing Clinics of North America, 45*(1), 1–10.

Malloch, K. (2014). Beyond transformational leadership to greater engagement: Inspiring innovation in complex organizations. *Nurse Leader, 12*(2), 60–63.

Mackary, M.A. & Daniel, M. (2016). Medical error-the third leading cause of death in the U.S. BJM, 353, i2139. Retrived from https://www.bmj.com/content/353/bmj.i2139/

McGowan, J. J. (2007). Swimming with the sharks: Perspectives on professional risk taking. *Journal of the Medical Library Association, 95*(1), 104–113.

Melnyk, B. M. (2012). Achieving a high reliability organization through implementation of the ARCC model for system-wide sustainability of evidence-based practice. *Nursing Administration Quarterly, 36*(2), 127–135.

Melnyk, B. M., & Davidson, S. (2009). Creating a culture of innovation in nursing education through shared vision, leadership, interdisciplinary partnerships and positive deviance. *Nursing Administration Quarterly, 33*(4), 1–8.

Melnyk, B. M., & Fineout-Overholt, E. (2015). *Evidence-based practice in nursing & healthcare: A guide to best practice* (3rd ed.). Philadelphia, PA: Wolters Kluwer.

Melnyk, B. M., Fineout-Overholt, E., Gallagher-Ford, L., & Kaplan, L. (2012). The state of evidence-based practice in US nurses: Critical implications for nurse leaders and educators. *The Journal of Nursing Administration, 42*(9), 410–417.

Melnyk, B. M., Gallagher-Ford, L., & Fineout-Overholt, E. (2015). *Implementing the evidence-based practice competencies; A practical guide for improving quality, safety and outcomes.* Indianapolis, IN: Sigma Theta Tau International.

Melnyk, B. M., Gallagher-Ford, L., Long, L. E., & Fineout-Overholt, E. (2014). The establishment of evidence-based practice competencies for practicing registered nurses and advanced practice nurses in real-world clinical settings: Proficiencies to improve healthcare quality, reliability, patient outcomes, and costs. *Worldviews on Evidence-Based Nursing, 11*(1), 5–15.

Melnyk, B. M., Hrabe, D. P., & Szalacha, L. A. (2013). Relationships among work stress, job satisfaction, mental health, and healthy lifestyle behaviors in new graduate nurses attending the Nurse Athlete program: A call to action for nursing leaders. *Nursing Administration Quarterly, 37*(4), 278–285.

Melnyk, B.M., Gallagher-Ford, L., Zellefrow, C., Tucker, S., Thomas, B., Sinnott, L.T. & Tan, A. (2018). The first U.S. study on nurses' evidence-based practice competencies indicates major deficits that threaten healthcare quality, safety, and patient outcomes. *Worldviews on Evidence-Based Nursing, 15*(1), 16–25.

Pipe, T. B. (2008). Illuminating the inner leadership journey by engaging intention and mindfulness as guided by caring theory. *Nursing Administration Quarterly, 32*(2), 117–125.

Porter-O'Grady, T., & Malloch, K. (2010a). Innovation: Driving the green culture in healthcare. *Nursing Administration Quarterly, 34*(4), E1–E5.

Porter-O'Grady, T., & Malloch, K. (2010b). *Innovation leadership: Creating the landscape of health care.* Sudbury, MA: Jones & Bartlett.

Regan, S., Laschinger, H. K., & Wong, C. A. (2015). The influence of empowerment, authentic leadership, and professional practice environments on nurses' perceived interprofessional collaboration. *Journal of Nursing Management.* doi:10.1111/jonm.12288

Resar, R. K. (2006). Making noncatastrophic health care processes reliable: Learning to walk before running in creating high reliability organizations. *Health Services Research, 41*(4, Pt. 2), 1677–1689.

Sambunjak, D., Straus, S. E., & Marusić, A. (2006). Mentoring in academic medicine: A systematic review. *The Journal of the American Medical Association, 296*(9), 1103–1115.

Scharmer, C. O., & Käufer, K. (2000). *Universities as the birthplace for the entrepreneuring human being.* Retrieved August 14, 2011, from http://www.ottoscharmer.com/docs/articles/2000_Uni21us.pdf

Spence Laschinger, H. K., Grau, A. L., Finegan, J., & Wilk, P. (2011). Predictors of new graduate nurses' well-being: Testing the job demands-resources model. *Health Care Management Review, 37*(2), 175–186.

Sredl, D., Melnyk, B. M., Hsueh, K. H., Jenkins, R., Ding, C. D., & Durham, J. (2011). Health care in crisis: Can nurse executives' beliefs about and implementation of evidence-based practice be key solutions in health care reform? *Teaching and Learning in Nursing, 6,* 73–79.

Titzer, J. L., & Shirey, M. R. (2013). Nurse manager succession planning: A concept analysis. *Nursing Forum, 48*(3), 155–164. doi:10.1111/nuf.12024

Uhl-Bien, M., & Marion, R. (Eds.). (2008). *Complexity leadership, Part I: Conceptual foundations.* Charlotte, NC: Information Age.

Vyt, A. (2008). Interprofessional and transdisciplinary teamwork in healthcare. *Diabetes/Metabolism Research and Reviews, 24*(Suppl. 1), S106–S109.

What is mindfulness? (2014). Retrieved from https://www.mindful.org/what-is-mindfulness

Whitney, D., Trosten-Bloom, A., & Rader, K. (2010). *Appreciative leadership: Focus on what works to drive winning performance and build a thriving organization (Business Skills and Development).* New York, NY: McGraw Hill.

Witt/Kieffer. (2004). *Putting succession planning in play: Identifying and developing the healthcare organization's successors.* Oak Brook, IL: Author.

Zerhouni, E. (2005). US biomedical research: Basic, translational, and clinical sciences. *JAMA, 294*(11), 1352–1358.

Zucker, B., Goss, C., Williams, D., Bloodworth, L., Lynn, M., Denker, A., & Gibbs, J. D. (2006). Nursing retention in the era of a nursing shortage: Norton Navigators. *Journal for Nurses in Staff Development, 22*(6), 302–306.

Advanced Practice Nursing
Evolving Roles and Striving for Autonomy

Holly T. Kralj and Margaret J. Rowberg

ADDITIONAL RESOURCES

Visit thePoint° for additional helpful resources
- eBook
- Journal Articles
- WebLinks

CHAPTER OUTLINE

LEARNING OBJECTIVES

The learner will be able to:

1. Understand the historical and current roles and impact of advanced practice nursing (APRN).

2. Describe the challenges of variations in practice and autonomy across the United States.

3. Discuss the rationale for the National Council of State Boards of Nursing's APRN Campaign for Consensus.

4. Describe the driving and restraining forces for increasing the entry educational level for APRN to that of a practice doctorate.

5. Discuss the impetus for and controversies associated with the Doctor of Nursing Practice (DNP) degree.

ADVANCED PRACTICE NURSING (APRN)

APRN Roles

In the past three to four decades, the U.S. health care system has experienced an increased focus on cost efficiency and allocation of resources. Primary and preventative care play an increasingly important role in the overall goal of maintaining health of the U.S. populace (Schober, Gerrish, & McDonnell, 2016). With the passage of the Affordable Care Act in 2010, coverage was expanded to millions of previously uninsured Americans, which stressed an already insufficient network of primary care physicians. As a result, many health care policy researchers including the Roberts Wood Johnson Foundation, the Pew Health Commission, and the Institute of Medicine (IOM) recommended the increased utilization of advanced practice registered nurses (APRNs) and other nonphysician primary care providers to fill the gap (Auerbach, 2012; Institute of Medicine of the National Academies [IOM], 2010a).

Although there are many advanced roles and skills in nursing, only four categories are considered APRNs. Those four categories are nurse practitioners (NPs), clinical nurse specialists (CNSs), certified nurse-midwives (CNMs), and certified registered nurse anesthetists (CRNAs). Each of these designated roles requires graduation from a nationally accredited APRN program, licensure and regulation by State Boards of Registered Nursing (BRN), and competency certification from specific national governing bodies (National Council of State Boards of Nursing [NCSBN], 2017). All advanced practice roles require additional education and training in advanced pathophysiology, advanced pharmacology, and advanced health assessment; however, APRN roles typically have a specific population-based focus.

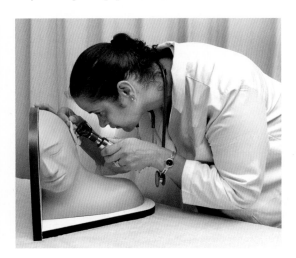

While CRNAs provide anesthesia services across all age ranges, NP and CNS programs focus on specific population-based competencies, including family, neonatal, pediatric (both acute and primary care), adult/gerontology (both acute and primary care), women's health/gender-related, and psychiatric/mental health (NCSBN, 2017). CNMs focus on the primary care and reproductive health care of women from puberty past menopause, with a special focus on pregnancy and childbirth. CNMs also can care for newborns in the first 30 days of life as well as treat sexually transmitted infections in the partners of their patients (American College of Nurse-Midwives [ACNM], 2016).

The APRN Joint Dialogue Group (2008, pp. 3–4) offered the following definition of an APRN as a nurse:

1. *who has completed an accredited graduate-level education program preparing him/her for one of the four recognized APRN roles;*

2. *who has passed a national certification examination that measures APRN role and population-focused competencies and who maintains continued competence as evidenced by recertification in the role and population through the national certification program;*

3. *who has acquired advanced clinical knowledge and skills preparing him/her to provide direct care to patients, as well as a component of indirect care; however, the defining factor for **all** APRNs is that a significant component of the education and practice focuses on direct care of individuals;*

4. *whose practice builds on the competencies of registered nurses (RNs) by demonstrating a greater depth and breadth of knowledge, a greater synthesis of data, increased complexity of skills and interventions, and greater role autonomy;*

5. *who is educationally prepared to assume responsibility and accountability for health promotion and/or maintenance as well as the assessment, diagnosis, and management of patient problems, which includes the use and prescription of pharmacologic and non-pharmacologic interventions;*

6. *who has clinical experience of sufficient depth and breadth to reflect the intended license; and*

7. *who has obtained a license to practice as an APRN in one of the four APRN roles: certified registered nurse anesthetist (CRNA), certified nurse-midwife (CNM), clinical nurse specialist (CNS), or certified nurse practitioner (CNP).*

Certification for each APRN role is managed by different certifying organizations, with differing educational and competency requirements. For CNMs, certification is governed by the American Midwifery Certification Board (AMCB), while CRNAs are governed by the National Board of Certification and Recertification for Nurse Anesthetists (NBCRNA). Certification for a CNS can occur either through the American Nurses Credentialing Center (ANCC) or through the Clinical Nurse Specialist American Association of Critical-Care Nurses (AACN) Certification Corporation. For NPs, there are five different certifying bodies to choose from, depending on area of specialization and provider preference. The four APRN roles, their respective certifying organizations, and specific certifications offered within each category are detailed in Table 4.1.

According to the National Nursing Data Base, there are over three million registered nurses working in the United States, and of those, more than 350,000 are APRNs (NCSBN, 2017). According to the American Association of Nurse Practitioners (AANP, 2018a), more than 248,000 of the APRNs in the United States are NPs. The National Association of Clinical Nurse Specialists (NACNS, 2014)

TABLE 4.1   APRN Role, Certifying Organizations, and Type of Certification

APRN Role	Certifying Organizations	Type of Certification
Certified Nurse-Midwife	American Midwifery Certification Board (AMCB)	• Certified Nurse Midwife (CNM)
Certified Registered Nurse Anesthetist	National Board of Certification and Recertification for Nurse Anesthetists (NBCRNA)	• Certified Registered Nurse Anesthetist (CRNA)
Clinical Nurse Specialist	Clinical Nurse Specialist American Association of Critical-Care Nurses (AACN) Certification Corporation	• Adult-Gerontology CNS (ACCNSAG) • Pediatric CNS (ACCNS-P) • Neonatal CNS (ACCNS-N)
	American Nurses Credentialing Center (ANCC)	• Adult-Gerontology CNS (AGCNS-BC)
Nurse Practitioner	American Academy of Nurse Practitioners Certification Board (AANPCB)	• Family NP (FNP) • Adult-Gerontology Primary Care NP (AGPCNP) • Emergency Care NP (FNP with ED focus)
	American Nurses Credentialing Center (ANCC)	• Adult-Gerontology Acute Care NP (AGACNP-BC) • Adult-Gerontology Primary Care NP (AGPCNP-BC) • Family NP (FNP-BC) • Pediatric Primary Care NP (PPCNP-BC) • Psychiatric Mental Health NP (PMHNP-BC) • Emergency Nurse Practitioner (ENP-BC)
	American Association of Critical-Care Nurses (AACN) Certification Corporation	• Acute Care Nurse Practitioner: Adult-Gerontology (ACNPC-AG)
	Pediatric Nursing Certification Board (PNCB)	• Pediatric Nurse Practitioner Primary Care (CPNP-PC) • Pediatric Nurse Practitioner Acute Care (CPNP-AC)
	National Certification Corporation (NCC)	• Neonatal NP (NNP-BC) • Women's Health Care Nurse Practitioner (WHNP-BC)

Source: ACCN, 2017; American Midwifery Certification Board. (2018). *AMCB Certification Exam Candidate Handbook.* Retrieved from https://www.amcbmidwife.org/docs/board-of-directors-committees/candidate-handbook---updated-april-1-2018.pdf?sfvrsn=0; American Nurses Credentialing Center. (2017). *ANCC Certification Center.* Retrieved from http://www.nursecredentialing.org/Certification; NCC, 2017; Pediatric Nursing Certification Board. (2017). *Steps to CPNP-PC Certification.* Retrieved from https://www.pncb.org/cpnp-pc-certification-steps

reports that there are more than 72,000 CNSs. Additionally, the American College of Nurse-Midwives (ACNM, 2016) suggests there are over 11,000 CNMs, with the American Association of Nurse Anesthetists (AANA, 2015) confirming more than 48,000 CRNAs in the United States. APRNs constitute about 5.5% of the RN workforce in this country (US Department of Labor, 2018), and numbers are expected to continue to grow (Weinberg, Kallerman, & Spetz, 2014).

As the national populace ages and health care reform continues to evolve, there is a call to provide better care at less cost. To achieve this goal, APRNs likely will take an integral role. According to the hallmark IOM (2010) report, "The Future of Nursing: Leading Change, Advancing Health,"

> The nursing profession has the potential capacity to implement wide-reaching changes in the health care system. By virtue of their regular, close proximity to patients and their scientific understandings of care processes across the continuum of care, nurses have a considerable opportunity to act as full partners with other health care professionals and to lead in the improvement and redesign of the health care system and its practice environment. (p. 23)

Yet challenges persist for APRNs regarding acceptance and the ability "to practice to the full extent of their education and training" (IOM, 2010, p. 29).

Brief History of Advanced Practice Nursing

Historically, nurses have stepped in and filled advanced roles as needed. Nurses administered chloroform to soldiers on the front lines of the Civil War (American Association of Nurse Anesthetists [AANA], 2018), and they cared for the poor and vulnerable when few would. Some of the first recognized nurse "specialists" were psychiatric nurses who tended to the mentally ill in the late 1800s hoping to create more humane treatments. The first psychiatric nurse specialty program dates back to 1882 in McLean Hospital, MA (McLean Hospital, 2018). Many other advanced nursing roles can be traced to public health nursing at the turn of the 20th century when care was typically delivered in the home or community clinics, especially to poor pregnant and postpartum women and children. Lillian Wald founded the Henry Street Settlement in New York in 1895 and is credited with starting the U.S. public health movement. Mary Breckinridge founded the first U.S. nurse-midwifery service in the Appalachian Mountains of Kentucky in the 1920s, servicing the rural poor with exceptional results (Hawkins & Bellig, 2000).

The formal development and recognition of APRNs in the United States is often attributed to Loretta Ford and Henry Silva who started the first NP program at the University of Rochester Hospital in 1965 (Parker & Hill, 2017). Initially, it was a hospital-based training program, but it soon expanded to include master's and post-master's degrees and preparation for national certification. The program expanded upon preexisting public health competencies of disease prevention and health promotion and focused heavily on primary preventative care. In addition, APRN programs flourished in the 1970s and 1980s, and along with increased numbers came increased recognition of the need for professional consistency, regulation, and advocacy (Rounds, Zych, & Mallary, 2013).

> **Consider This** How might increasing popularity of the APRN degree strain the profession? What benefits might there be to increasing the number of APRNs?

Variations in APRN Education, Role Recognition, and Licensing

One challenge faced by APRNs is the lack of consistency within states regarding APRN education, role recognition, and licensing agencies. Currently, all states require a graduate degree or postgraduate certification for APRNs except South Dakota and Indiana (which require only a certificate and board certification), but recognition and regulation of specific APRN roles can vary widely. For example, In Indiana and Mississippi, CNSs are not recognized as APRNs, and in New York and Pennsylvania, only NPs and CNSs are recognized as APRNs (while CNMs are licensed by the Board of Medicine, not Nursing). In Virginia, CNSs are not recognized, and the other three APRN roles are recognized but are jointly regulated by both the Boards of Nursing and Medicine (NCSBN, 2017). Obviously, the lack of consistency across state lines can make it difficult for APRNs to practice in states other than their home state of licensure. Additionally, this irregularity in role recognition can decrease access to care for underserved populations by creating additional barriers to practice for APRNs who traditionally serve vulnerable populations (Beaver & Cahill, 2013).

Levels of Independence in Practice

Across the United States, there is a wide variety of APRN practice environments regarding required physician involvement, prescriptive authority, and the ability to bill third-party payors for services rendered. Not only are there discrepancies in the level of physician involvement in APRN practice across state lines, there are also differing levels of independent practice even between APRN roles within individual states. The IOM, the Robert Wood Johnson Foundation, and the National Council of State Boards of Nursing all recommend Independent Practice for APRNs as numerous studies have shown positive patient outcomes, reduced cost, and no compromise of patient safety when APRNs are allowed to practice to the full extent of their education and training (AANP, 2018b). Collaborative care has been held up as a best practice for patient outcomes (IOM, 2010). Interestingly, a study done on primary care NPs in New York showed that APRN and physician teamwork was statistically increased in practice models with the least restrictive practice regulations for the APRNs (Poghosyn, Boyd, & Knutson, 2014). Less restriction increased collaboration between medical and nursing team members. Currently, 24 states grant NPs full independent practice with prescriptive authority (states shown in blue), 17 states require a collaborative agreement with a physician (states with reduced

practice shown in gray), and 12 states require "Physician Supervision" (the most restrictive practice model—states shown in orange; AANP, 2018b; Fig. 4.1).

CRNAs practice almost entirely in inpatient or outpatient surgical suites. In 23 states, CRNAs have independent practice, closely mirroring the pattern of autonomy seen in the NP practice map. In 15 states, CRNAs must practice under "Physician Supervision," and in 10 states, there is no provision for prescriptive authority for CRNAs. Currently, CRNAs are not recognized as APRNs in the states of New York or Pennsylvania (NCSBN, 2017).

As of 2017, CNMs had independent practice in 27 states, some level of collaborative agreement required in 18 states, and "Physician Supervision" (the most restrictive practice type) in five states—California, Nebraska, North Carolina, South Carolina, and Florida (ACNM, 2017). Yet in California, Certified Midwives, who lack the nursing education and background of their CNM counterparts, were granted independent practice in 2013 with the passage of

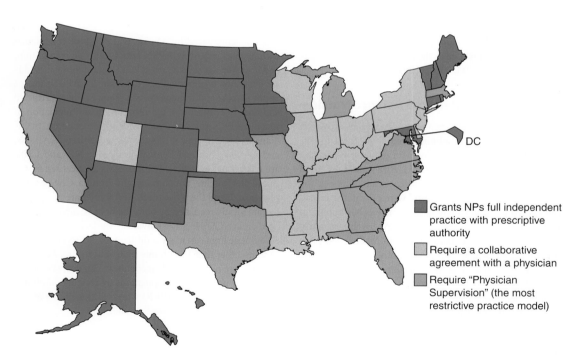

DC

- Grants NPs full independent practice with prescriptive authority
- Require a collaborative agreement with a physician
- Require "Physician Supervision" (the most restrictive practice model)

Figure 4.1 Prescriptive Authority for NPs: Variance by State. (*Source:* Adapted from American Association of Nurse Practitioners. (2018b). *APRN practice authority continues to evolve, and statutes vary based on legislative activity.* An interactive map with up-to-date state-specific details is available at: https://www.aanp.org/legislation-regulation/state-legislation/state-practice-environment.)

Assembly Bill 1308, no longer requiring physician supervision for non-nurse–certified midwives (California Assembly, 2013). In essence, the legislators deemed a hospital or homebirth with a CNM in greater need of physician supervision than a homebirth with a non-nurse-midwife. This decision speaks to a lack of understanding of key health care issues by many legislators as well as the power of successful lobbying groups in shaping health policy. It also reinforces the importance or political competence and engagement on the part of APRN practice (see Research Fuels the Controversy 4.1).

Of the four APRN roles, the CNSs have perhaps the greatest variation of practice recognition and requirements. In some states, the role is not recognized at all, or is recognized as a non-APRN as a nurse role, like that of a nurse educator. In other states, CNSs are allowed independent practice to diagnose, treat, and manage patient care in specific patient populations (NACNS, 2014). In 17 states, CNSs are granted independent practice with prescriptive authority. In 19 other states, CNSs must have a supervising physician agreement for prescriptive authority. In 10 states, there is no prescriptive authority granted to CNSs, and in the remaining states, there are no data available or no recognition of the role as an APRN (NCSBN, 2017).

A MOVEMENT TOWARD AUTONOMY

The IOM's landmark report, *The Future of Nursing* (2010), called for APRNs to be allowed to practice to "the full extent of their education and training" (p. 29). Removing arbitrary, restrictive practice barriers was seen as a key intervention to expand quality, cost-effective care to the additional 30 million individuals who received expanded health coverage under the Affordable Care Act (AANP, 2018b). Decreasing restrictive practice requirements for NPs has been shown to increase access to quality health care for patients (Kuo, Loresto, Rounds, & Goodwin, 2013). Of the recommendations laid out by the IOM, those most impacting APRN practice included: "removing scope of practice barriers, expanding opportunities for nurses to lead and diffuse collaborative improvement efforts, doubling the number of nurses with a doctorate by 2020, and preparing and enabling nurses to lead change to advance health" (IOM, 2010b, pp. 1–7).

Removing Scope of Practice Restrictions

The scope of practice restrictions for APRNs varies widely across the United States. According to Mary Chesney,

---

Research Fuels the Controversy 4.1

Advanced Practice Nursing: Shaping Health Through Policy

Source: Kostas-Polston, E. A., Thanavaro, J., Arividson, C., & Morritt Taub, L. (2015). Advanced practice nursing: Shaping health through policy. *Journal of the American Association of Nurse Practitioners, 27*, 11–20.

On behalf of the Fellows of the American Academy of Nurse Practitioners (FAANP) Health Policy Work Group, the authors put forth a "call to action" for NPs to "become politically engaged to help craft and shape the changes needed to highlight the contributions of NPs in the delivery of quality, safe, and cost-effective services" (p. 11). The authors state that the scope of practice restrictions impedes the ability of NPs to provide needed care in medically underserved areas and it ultimately harms patients.

The authors put forth a tool kit to assist APRNs to engage in legislative advocacy with policy makers. Suggestions included understanding political interests of targeted legislators, having a clear agenda which speaks to the personal interests of the legislator, and arranging face-to-face visits as well as letter writing and social media campaigns. The authors also recommend that NPs join professional organizations, serve on advisory boards, seek out health policy fellowships, write Op-Ed pieces for local papers, and participate in larger lobbying events. The article also stresses the importance of "building partnerships and working with strong coalitions" (p. 18). Utilizing like-minded stakeholder groups brings numbers and credibility to issues of importance and helps leverage important strength and momentum to affect change. The authors conclude:

The overall goal of political engagement is to develop a longstanding relationship with policymakers and their legislative staff. Over time, this relationship grows as a result of the NP expert becoming recognized as a trusted source of nonpartisan, objective information and analysis. . .Whatever the chosen role, NPs need to become politically engaged for the purpose of protecting clinical practice and the healthcare interests of patients and communities (p. 19).

former president and current fellow of the National Association of Pediatric Nurse Practitioners:

> *The national environmental landscape for APRN practice is at best disparate and fragmented and at worst illogical and highly restrictive. Practice laws vary significantly from state to state without evidence-based explanation.* (Chesney, 2015, p. 219)

It has even been suggested that restrictive scope of practice legislation without evidence-based justification is a restriction of trade, based on economic and political factors, not on best practice or the well-being of the U.S. people (Health Policy Briefs: Nurse Practitioners and Primary Care, 2013). Some studies have shown requiring physician supervision of NPs increases cost of care and physician wages, decreases NP wages, and has no benefit to patient outcomes (Kleiner, Marier, Park, & Wing, 2014; Perloff, DesRoches, & Buerhaus, 2016; Weinberg et al., 2014). The IOM report (2010) went so far as to call for an investigation by the Federal Trade Commission (FTC) regarding state policies which restrict APRN practice, since they reduce the well-being of the public through anticompetitive barriers to fair trade health care practices (Health Policy Briefs: Nurse Practitioners and Primary Care, 2013).

According to the Robert Wood Johnson Foundation (RWJF, 2017), restrictive practice legislation for APRNs unnecessarily decreases access to high-quality, affordable care for some of the most vulnerable Americans. APRNs historically have cared for more underserved patients, such as those in rural areas, those with disabilities, or those living in poverty (Weinberg et al., 2014). States which require supervising physicians for APRNs or restrict the ability of APRNs to prescribe medications, order tests or medical equipment, or admit patients to hospitals delay crucial care for patients. Some APRNs have to pay collaborating physicians, and some insurance companies are unwilling to reimburse APRNs or pay them at lower rates than their physician counterparts for the same services rendered (RWJF, 2017). Also, supervisory requirements can take time away from patient care; for unnecessary administrative task, or even more concerning, can keep APRNs from providing needed care in rural areas where a supervising physician is unavailable (Kleiner et al., 2014; Kurtzman et al., 2017; Martsolf, Auerback & Afikhanova, 2015; RWJF, 2017; Weinberg et al., 2014). Restrictive practice legislation then poses economic barriers to practice for APRNs, but more importantly, decreases access to care for citizens in need.

Discussion Point

What role could insurance companies play in increasing access to APRNs?

A number of studies have examined the theoretical impact of removing restrictive scope of practice barriers for APRNs and standardizing independent practice legislation across the United States. Perloff et al. (2016) conducted a study looking at cost of primary care for Medicare recipients delivered by NPs versus physicians. After controlling for variables, their results showed no decrease in quality measures but significant cost savings in the NP group. Weinberg et al. (2014) found that states with restrictive scope of practice legislation have fewer NPs per capita than states with full-practice authority legislation. Their study estimated a 22% increase in primary care providers in restrictive states if APRNs were granted full-practice authority (Weinberg et al., 2014, p. 8). Additionally, they found that that the average price of a preventative care visit in states where NPs lacked prescriptive authority and needed physician supervision was 15% higher than those where NPs had independent practice (p. 18). These findings reinforce other research which suggests that independent practice for APRNs increases access to care for patients and decreases health care costs with no compromise of patient safety or health outcomes (Kleiner et al., 2014; Kurtzman, et al., 2017; Martsolf et al., 2015; Perloff et al., 2016; RWJF, 2017).

NCSBN'S APRN Campaign for Consensus

Inconsistencies in state requirements regarding APRN education and regulation pose barriers for APRNs to work in states other than their home licensure. It may also undermine the credibility of the APRN profession among other health care professionals (APRN Joint Dialogue, 2008). After extensive research, collaboration, and compromise, the APRN Consensus Work Group and the National Council of State Boards of Nursing APRN Advisory Committee issued a document intended to unify nursing regulations for APN across the nation in the areas of licensing, accreditation, credentialing, and education (LACE; APRN Joint Dialogue Group Report, 2008). The document, *Consensus Model for APRN Regulation: Licensure, Accreditation, Certification & Education* (2008), put forth a uniform model of regulation intended to protect the public and create consistency within the APRN recognition nationally.

The Consensus Model stated APRNs would be "licensed as independent practitioners for practice at the level of one of the four APRN roles within at least one of the six identified population foci" (APRN Joint Dialogue Group, 2008, p. 6). Licensure would only be granted to graduates of accredited or pre-accredited programs, ensuring the content and core competencies of the program met the national standards in both broad and population-based foci. Professional certification would still be conducted by the national certifying organizations.

> Advanced practice registered nurses are licensed independent practitioners who are expected to practice within standards established or recognized by a licensing body. Each APRN is accountable to patients, the nursing profession, and the licensing board to comply with the requirements of the state nurse practice act and the quality of advanced nursing care rendered; for recognizing limits of knowledge and experience, planning for the management of situations beyond the APRN's expertise; and for consulting with or referring patients to other health care providers as appropriate. (APRN Joint Dialogue Group, 2008, p. 7)

The NCBN's APRN Campaign for Consensus was overwhelmingly endorsed by the vast majority of major nursing organizations, including the American Academy of Nurse Practitioners (AANP), the American Association of Colleges of Nursing (AACN), the American Association of Nurse Anesthetists (AANA), the American College of Nurse-Midwives (ACNM), the American College of Nurse Practitioners (ACNP), the American Nurses Association (ANA), and the National Council of State Boards of Nursing (NCSBN; for a complete list of nursing organizations endorsing the Campaign for Consensus, see Box 4.1). State Boards of Nursing would still have the responsibility for licensing APRNs, but the consistency in education and regulation would give APRNs the ability to practice in all states adopting the APRN Consensus Model. This would increase access to care for underserved populations. The goal for adoption in all states was 2015 (APRN Joint Dialogue Group, 2008). Unfortunately, legislative issues, and lobbying against independent practice for APRNs in certain states have prevented full adoption moving forward nationally. As of 2018, only 15 states had fully adopted all the elements of the NCSBN Consensus Model (Phillips, 2018).

Discussion Point

How might states work together to achieve consensus regarding licensing, accreditation, certification, and education? What stakeholders might pose the greatest roadblocks?

BOX 4.1   **Organizations Endorsing the APRN Consensus Model**

- Academy of Medical-Surgical Nurses (AMSN)
- Accreditation Commission for Midwifery Education (ACME)
- American Academy of Nurse Practitioners (AANP)
- American Academy of Nurse Practitioners Certification Program
- American Association of Colleges of Nursing (AACN)
- American Association of Critical-Care Nurses (AACN)
- American Association of Critical-Care Nurses Certification Corporation
- American Association of Legal Nurse Consultants (AALNC)
- American Association of Nurse Anesthetists (AANA)
- American Board of Nursing Specialties (ABNS)
- American College of Nurse-Midwives (ACNM)
- American College of Nurse Practitioners (ACNP)
- American Holistic Nurses Association (AHNA)
- American Midwifery Certification Board (AMCB)
- American Nurses Association (ANA)
- American Nurses Credentialing Center (ANCC)
- American Psychiatric Nurses Association (APNA)
- Arkansas State Board of Nursing
- Association of Faculties of Pediatric Nurse Practitioners (AFPNP)
- Association of Women's Health, Obstetric, and Neonatal Nurses (AWHONN)

(continued)

BOX 4.1   **Organizations Endorsing the APRN Consensus Model (*continued*)**

- Commission on Collegiate Nursing Education (CCNE)
- Council on Accreditation of Nurse Anesthesia Educational Programs (COA)
- Dermatology Nurses Association (DNA)
- Dermatology Nursing Certification Board (DNCB)
- Emergency Nurses Association (ENA)
- Gerontological Advanced Practice Nurses Association (GAPNA)
- Hospice and Palliative Nurses Association (HPNA)
- The International Society of Psychiatric Nurses (ISPN)
- National Association of Clinical Nurse Specialists (NACNS)
- National Association of Neonatal Nurses (NANN)
- National Association of Orthopedic Nurses (NAON)
- National Association of Pediatric Nurse Practitioners (NAPNAP)
- National Board for Certification of Hospice and Palliative Nurses (NBCHPN)
- National Board on Certification & Recertification of Nurse Anesthetists (NBCRNA)
- National Certification Corporation (NCC)
- National Council of State Boards of Nursing (NCSBN)
- National Gerontological Nursing Association (NGNA)
- National League for Nursing (NLN)
- National League for Nursing Accrediting Commission, Inc. (NLNAC)
- National Organization of Nurse Practitioner Faculties (NONPF)
- Nurse Practitioners in Women's Health (NPWH)
- Nurses Organization of Veterans Affairs (NOVA)
- Oncology Nursing Certification Corporation (ONCC)
- Oncology Nursing Society (ONS)
- Orthopedic Nurses Certification Board (ONCB)
- Pediatric Nursing Certification Board (PNCB)
- Wound, Ostomy and Continence Nurses Society (WOCN)
- Wound, Ostomy and Continence Nursing Certification Board (WOCNCB)

Source: APRN Consensus Work Group & National Council of State Boards of Nursing APRN Advisory Committee. (2008). *Consensus model for APRN regulation: Licensure, accreditation, certification and education.* pp. 3–4. Retrieved from https://www.ncsbn.org/Consensus_Model_for_APRN_Regulation_July_2008.pdf

---

CONTROVERSIES AND ISSUES IN ADVANCED PRACTICE NURSING

The Doctor of Nursing Practice (DNP) as the Standard for APRNs?

A lack of doctorally prepared nurses reduces the likelihood of achieving the goal of a patient-centered, cost-effective, and safe health care system. Although APRNs are skilled clinical practitioners, many lack the training and expertise needed to address the persistent professional issues that arise in the health care system. In 2004, the AACN initiated several task forces to assess these issues comparing various educational models, and making future recommendations as to the type of leadership needed to move nursing forward. Ultimately, the Board of the AACN proposed that the DNP degree be developed to bring APRN to the doctoral level on a par with other clinical health care professionals, such as physical therapists and pharmacists (American Association of Colleges of Nursing [AACN], 2004).

In addition, *The Future of Nursing* report (IOM, 2010) recognized the need for more nurses who have advanced degrees and recommended that the number of nurses who hold doctorates be doubled by 2020. According to the most recent data available from the Robert Woods Johnson Foundation, of the over 3 million registered nurses in the United States, fewer than 30,000 hold a doctoral degree (RWJF, 2013).

Based on the work of the 2004 task force, the AACN endorsed the *Position Statement on the Practice Doctorate in Nursing* recommending that all APRN education change from graduating APRNs with master's degrees to doctoral degrees by 2015. In 2006, AACN continued its work in this area and approved a document titled "*The Essentials of Doctoral Education for Advanced Practice Nursing*." These *Essentials* are similar in focus to the *Essentials of Baccalaureate Education for Professional Nursing Practice* (AACN, 2008). This *DNP Essentials* document provided schools of nursing with the key content areas that should be included in the DNP curriculum. These essentials are shown in Box 4.2, as well as on the AACN website.

Some of the APRN organizations were quick to respond to the recommendation to adopt the DNP degree as the entry into practice for APRNs by 2015. The National Organization of Nurse Practitioner Faculties (NONPF) began work on the practice doctorate in 2001. In April 2011 and amended in 2012, it released its final document on the core competencies for NP education and practice at the doctoral level. In the end, the NONPF decided that it could not support the 2015 deadline for NP programs to prepare graduates at the doctoral level (National Organization of Nurse Practitioner Faculties [NONPF], 2012) but acknowledged that the DNP is a worthwhile goal for NP programs to attain and recommended that programs transition at a pace that would continue to ensure quality.

The other three advanced practice specialties (CNS, CNM, and CRNA) have been slower to adopt the DNP recommendation. Their representative associations have published position statements that offer different views on the topic. In 2009, the NACNS decided to remain neutral about the recommendation and has requested ongoing dialogue in an effort to tackle lingering concerns. The association stated that:

> NACNS supports CNS education at the master's or the doctoral level, including programs that offer the practice doctorate, providing that established, validated CNS

competencies and education program standards are met. NACNS does not support eliminating MSN programs and moving to practice doctorate programs as the exclusive point-of-entry into CNS practice. (para. 2).

However, in May of 2018, the NACNS issued an updated position statement endorsing the DNP as the entry to practice for clinical nurse specialists by the year 2030. The organization stated:

> While NACNS has consistently supported both masters and DNP preparation for entry into the CNS role, considering the complex needs of patients and the future direction of nursing practice, we believe that DNP preparation for practice in the CNS role will better position the CNS to meet the demands of an evolving healthcare system. Consistent with the strategic recommendations proposed to facilitate health care transformation, NACNS believes it is imperative to increase the number of doctorally-prepared Advanced Practice Registered Nurses (APRNs), which will increase the number of doctorally prepared nurses overall. (para. 1)

The American College of Nurse Midwifery (ACNM), while seeing the value of the DNP, decided not to require it for entry to practice for CNMs or CMs (certified midwives), for the ACNM believes that midwives, "regardless of terminal degree, are safe, cost-effective providers of maternity and women's health care" (ACNM, 2012, para. 3). At last count, 4.8% of CNM's held doctoral degrees (ACNM, 2016). The AANA commissioned a task force in 2007 that extensively studied the issues and advocated for mandating the DNP but decided that the timeline should be extended to 2025 based on concerns about feasibility (AANA, 2007). The AANA has since increased its commitment to a doctorally prepared workforce, with a mandate that all CRNA programs transition to the doctoral level by January 2022 (Council on

---

BOX 4.2   **The Essentials of Doctoral Education for Advanced Practice Nursing**

1. Scientific underpinnings for practice
2. Organizational and systems leadership for quality improvement and systems thinking
3. Clinical scholarship and analytic methods for evidence-based practice
4. Information systems/technology and patient care technology for the improvement and transformation of health care policy for advocacy in health care
5. Interprofessional collaboration for improving patient and population health outcomes
6. Clinical prevention and population health for improving the nation's health
7. Advanced nursing practice

Source: American Association of Colleges of Nursing. (2006). *The essentials of doctoral education for advanced practice nursing.* Retrieved from http://www.aacnnursing.org/Portals/42/Publications/DNPEssentials.pdf

Accreditation, 2018). The ANA has taken the stance that it "supports both master's and doctoral level of preparation as entry into APRN practice through a period of transition" (American Nurses Association [ANA], 2010, p. 9).

> *Consider This* Does the mandate to make doctoral education the entry level for APRN create barriers for students from disadvantaged backgrounds to pursue their APRN degree? If so, what measures can be taken to increase diversity in APRN and support the DNP?

Although the movement to standardize the doctoral degree as the required education for APRNs has not been met, schools have adopted the recommendations with more enthusiasm than previously seen in nursing education. As of June 2017, there were 303 active DNP programs in the United States, with over 25,000 students enrolled. Additionally, 124 new DNP programs were in the planning stages (AACN, 2017). DNP programs saw a 259% enrollment increase from 2010 to 2016, and as of 2015, the goal of doubling the number of doctorally prepared nurses was realized (Campaign for Action, 2018). This is certainly cause for celebration.

Differences Between DNP/ND and PhD/DNS

There remains some confusion regarding the differences between a research doctorate (PhD or DNS/DNSc) and a practice doctorate (DNP or ND). Back in 2006, the AACN provided an excellent explanation in its introduction to the *DNP Essentials* document:

> *Doctoral programs in nursing fall into two principal types: research-focused and practice-focused. Most research-focused programs grant the Doctor of Philosophy degree (PhD), while a small percentage offers the Doctor of Nursing Science degree (DNS, DSN, or DNSc). Designed to prepare nurse scientists and scholars, these programs focus heavily on scientific content and research methodology; and all require an original research project and the completion and defense of a dissertation or linked research papers. Practice-focused doctoral programs are designed to prepare experts in specialized advanced nursing practice. They focus heavily on practice that is innovative and evidence-based, reflecting the application of credible research findings. The two types of doctoral programs differ in their goals and the competencies of their graduates. They represent complementary, alternative approaches to the highest level of educational preparation in nursing.* (p. 3)

The key focus of PhD programs is the development of research, but this may not include the implementation of the research. The primary focus of DNP graduates is to utilize the research work of the PhD or DNS nurse to effect change and improve care through clinical implementation and systems change. The two disciplines are quite complementary in their scopes and foci, with the overarching goal being safe-effective health care delivery. Key differences between DNP and PhD programs are summarized in Box 4.3.

For some time, there has been controversy in the literature regarding the value and scope of the DNP degree. In their early comments on the DNP, Meleis and Dracup (2005) stated "all doctoral education must be designed to help define, generate, develop, translate and test the substantive base of knowledge in nursing" (para. 12). This statement implies that practice doctorates will not contribute to this knowledge base. Edwardson (2010) agrees, arguing,

> *The scholarship (of the DNP) focuses on integration, application, and teaching of knowledge. The scholarship of the DNP graduate may add to the store of generalizable knowledge, but in most cases will be more local and practical in nature than that developed by the PhD-prepared nurse. They will be able to exploit the evidence base to strengthen evidence-based practice.* (p. 138)

Melnyk (2013) stated that part of the issue arises from differing PhD and DNP pedagogy. The curriculum for many DNP programs was initially developed and instructed by PhD faculty. These PhD-prepared faculty, therefore, may not understand the difference between evidence-based practice and translational research from the DNP perspective. Instead of having DNP students conduct rigorous research, which was not the original intent of the DNP, faculty need to help DNP students understand how to use the evidence "that was generated through research to improve practice" (para. 9).

Should DNP Graduates Hold Faculty Roles and Earn Tenure in Academia?

Some concern has also been raised that DNP graduates, though doctorally prepared and eligible to fill the gap of needed faculty in nursing programs, may not be able to obtain tenure and equal status with PhDs in academia. According to the AACN (2012):

> *Though primarily an institutional decision, AACN is confident that a DNP faculty member will compete favorably with other practice doctorates in tenure and promotion decisions, as is the case in law, education, audiology, physical therapy, pharmacy, criminal justice, public policy and administration, public health, and other disciplines.* (para. 11)

BOX 4.3	**Key Differences Between DNP and PhD/DNS Programs**

	DNP	PhD/DNS
Program of study	*Objectives:* Prepare nurse leaders at the highest level of nursing practice to improve patient outcomes and translate research into practice	*Objectives:* Prepare nurses at the highest level of nursing science to conduct research to advance the science of nursing
	Competencies: See AACN's *Essentials of Doctoral Education for Advanced Nursing Practice* (2006)	*Content:* See *The Research-Focused Doctoral Program in Nursing: Pathways to Excellence* (AACN, 2010)
Students	Commitment to practice career	Commitment to research career
	Oriented toward improving outcomes of patient care and population health	Oriented toward developing new nursing knowledge and scientific inquiry
Program faculty	Practice or research doctorate in nursing, with expertise in area of teaching	Research doctorate in nursing or related field
	Leadership experience in area of role and population practice	Leadership experience in area of sustained research funding
	High level of expertise in practice congruent with focus of academic program	High level of expertise in research congruent with focus of academic program
Resources	Mentors and/or preceptors in leadership positions across practice settings	Mentors and/or preceptors in research settings
	Access to diverse practice settings with appropriate resources for areas of practice	Access to research settings with appropriate resources
	Access to financial aid	Access to dissertation support dollars and financial aid
	Access to information and patient care technology resources congruent with areas of study	Access to information and research technology resources congruent with program of research
Program assessment and evaluation	*Program Outcome:* Health care improvements and contributions via practice, policy change, and practice scholarship	*Program Outcome:* Contributes to health care improvements via the development of new knowledge and scholarly products that provide the foundation for the advancement of nursing science
	Oversight by the institution's authorized bodies (i.e., graduate school) and regional accreditors	Oversight by the institution's authorized bodies (i.e., graduate school) and regional accreditors

Source: Reprinted with permission from William O'Connor, Director of Publications, American Association of Colleges of Nursing, April 14, 2015 via electronic mail.

It goes on to say that,

> *AACN data from 2011 show that doctoral students who also teach are just as likely to have a DNP as a PhD. This indicates that graduates of both types of doctoral programs are finding teaching positions.* (para. 11)

However, not all academic institutions have been as accepting of the DNP-prepared nursing faculty. In 2012, Nicholes and Dyer conducted an Internet-based survey inviting 200 randomly chosen faculty of schools of nursing around the United States. There was a 33.8% response rate of 65 participants. These participants included PhD faculty, DNP faculty, and deans. In 61.3% (n = 38) of the institutions, DNP faculty were eligible for tenure (p. 15). Three themes emerged as benefits for allowing DNPs to achieve tenure (Nicholes & Dyer, 2012). The most common benefit stated was the ability to recruit and retain greater numbers of quality, doctorally prepared nursing faculty. The other two benefits were the clinical expertise that DNPs bring to nursing programs and the educational impact of rigorous evidence-based practice scholarship seen in DNP capstone projects (Doctors of Nursing Practice [DNP], 2015).

Concerns that surfaced in the Nicholes and Dyer (2012) study were the beliefs that "DNP faculties lack the preparation for contributing to the body of scholarly research" (p. 17); that "allowing DNP faculty eligibility for tenure will diminish the progress nursing has made in academia" and "concern regarding success of DNP faculty in producing traditional research and the notion that a practice degree is not viewed as an academic equivalent to PhD" (p. 17). In the authors' final evaluation, DNP faculty were held to the same standards as the PhD faculty. "The requirements are the same as any other terminal degree in regard to teaching and service, but the research component may differ," with DNPs focusing on "clinical practice and the use of evidence-based research" (p. 17).

Similar concerns were raised in research undertaken by Udlis and Mancuso (2015), although they suggested that the role ambiguity in research, academia, and academic leadership tends to obscure the distinctness and individuality of the DNP degree, thus impacting role identity (see Research Fuels the Controversy 4.2).

Though the discussions continue, the evidence is clear that schools of nursing are adopting the DNP at record speed and nurses are flocking to these programs to obtain practice doctorates (Fang, Kennedy, & Trautman, 2017). The number of students enrolled in DNP programs increased from 10,331 in 2012 to 59,872 in 2015 (Campaign for Action, 2018). These doctorally prepared nurses are moving into leadership roles as well as serving as nursing faculty and are helping to shape health care practice. Clearly, DNPs will continue to gain respect and acceptance within academia for the unique perspective they bring to nursing education as well as for their clinical expertise in educating the next generation of nursing professionals.

Physicians and Advanced Practice Nursing

As APRNs have become more visible and utilized within health care delivery systems, there has been some pushback by physician counterparts. Key physician groups including the American Medical Association (AMA), American Academy of Family Physicians (AAFP), and others have opposed the IOM recommendations for removal of barriers to practice from APRNs, claiming patient safety concern (Health Policy Brief: Nurse Practitioners and Primary Care updated, 2013). In 2009, the American College of Physicians stated that the education of physicians and NPs is not equivalent and therefore NPs cannot function in the same capacity as physicians. The document stated,

Training of physicians involves 4 years of premedical college education, 4 years of medical school that includes 2 years of clinical rotations, 3 years or more of clinical

residency training with up to 80-hour workweeks, additional fellowship subspecialty training, and continuing medical education. (p. 9)

This statement proposes that NPs do not spend an equivalent amount of time in their education and suggests they cannot function at the expected level needed for their chosen area of practice. However, APRNs spend 4 years in the baccalaureate nursing education, plus two to three additional years obtaining a master's degree and/or 2 to 4 years to obtain their DNP. They also typically work as a registered nurse and gain needed clinical experience. The question must be asked whether APRNs need additional years of education and advanced clinical training to perform the role. Since APRNs have been providing patient care for nearly 50 years with exceptional outcomes in safety, cost-effectiveness, and patient satisfaction (Parker & Hill, 2017), it is clear that nursing is providing the level of education for these health care providers and is responsive to changing roles and requirements, as is seen in the increasing movement toward acceptance of the DNP.

Most NP programs require applicants to have at least 1 year of clinical experience as a registered nurse before applying to the NP program, and applicants must hold at least a bachelor's degree in nursing. However, many NP students have significantly more years of clinical experience prior to starting their Advanced Practice degree. It is not unusual for an NP to have seven to nine or more years of collegiate education and many more years of practice as a registered nurse before taking on the APRN role.

> *Consider This* Why might physicians have concerns regarding the independent practice of APRNs? How can APRNs best address those concerns? How does legislative lobbying come into play, both positively and negatively?

Most concerns over the quality of care provided by APRNs have been eliminated in multiple studies (Dulisse & Cromwell, 2010; Horricks, Anderson, & Salisbury, 2002; Mundinger et al., 2000; Newhouse et al., 2011; Oliver, Pennington, Revelle, & Rantz, 2014; Swan, Ferguson, Chang, Larson, & Smaldone, 2015; Weinberg et al., 2014). An extensive study by Newhouse et al. (2011) reviewed the literature from 1990 to 2008 on care provided by APRNs in comparison with physician care. The results indicated that APRNs provide cost-effective, high-quality patient care and have an important role in improving the quality of health care in the United States. More recent reviews have confirmed the quality and efficacy of APRN care

Research Fuels the Controversy 4.2

Perceptions of the Role of the Doctor of Nursing Practice–Prepared Nurse

A quantitative, descriptive, cross-sectional design study was conducted in the spring of 2013. Questionnaires were used at two large Midwestern conferences where one consisted of mostly PhD-prepared, academic and research nurses while the other was attended by mostly master's-prepared advance practice nurses. The survey consisted of 21 items, which questioned the clarity of the role of the DNP-prepared nurse, using a 4-point scale. The researchers also collected demographic information of each respondent.

There were 340 participants, mostly white women, who held at least an MSN degree. Slightly more than half of the respondents worked in an academic setting and two thirds of them identified themselves as faculty. Sixty-eight percent of the participants said they were APRNs.

Source: Udlis, K. A., & Mancuso, J. M. (2015, February). Perceptions of the role of the Doctor of Nursing Practice-prepared nurse: Clarity or confusion. *Journal of Professional Nursing, 31*(4), 274–283. doi:10.1016/j.profnurs.2015.01.004

Study Findings

Seventy-three percent of respondents felt that both the PhD and the DNP are terminal degrees with the majority (85%) agreeing that DNPs "will be able to articulate nursing's contribution to health care" (p. 6). About half had concerns about DNPs helping to "unify and strengthen the profession" (p. 6).

A large majority (81%) felt that DNPs were prepared to be successful in "complex leadership roles that influence change in health care delivery systems, policy, and interprofessional collaboration" (p. 6). At the same time, slightly less than half of the respondents felt that DNPs would be able to hold leadership positions in the academic setting.

Only slightly more than half (55%) felt that DNPs would help improve the faulty shortage and less than half (46%) felt they were prepared to teach. Interestingly, though, 63% believed that tenure requirements should be the same for both degrees. It was also believed that the DNP faculty would replace master's-prepared faculty. There was also great support (88%) that DNPs would "bridge the gap between science and practice and substantially contribute to nursing scholarship" (p. 6). More than half of the respondents (57%) felt that the "DNP degree prepares individuals to develop knowledge generating research" (p. 6).

There was much agreement that the DNP degree was similar to those of physicians, dentists, and pharmacists and that it will improve health care outcomes. There was also agreement that the DNP will help increase salaries and professional respect but some (19.5%) felt that "employers would prefer DNP graduates over MSN graduates in the clinical setting" (p. 7).

The researchers then divided the respondents by degree and analyzed the results again. In the understanding category, it was found that 80% of DNPs felt there was substantial overlap in the expectations for DNPs and PhDs as compared to only 24% of PhD-prepared nurses, 53% of MSN nurses, and 33% of PSN participants (p. 7). Further, almost all (97%) of DNPs versus only 51% of PhDs felt the DNP is a terminal degree. There was also disparity that DNPs will "strengthen and unify the profession," and 80% DNPs agree compared to 34% for PhDs and 45.5% for MSNs (p. 7).

For leadership, the greatest concern was over the ability of DNP nurses to assume academic leadership roles. Eighty-four percent of DNPs versus only 19% of PhD participants felt DNPs were prepared for these positions.

There were great disparities related to the faculty role for DNPs. The majority (84%) of DNPs believed they could help relieve the faculty shortage while only 50% of PhDs, 54% of MSNs, and 38.5% of BSN nurses agreed (p. 7). PhDs did not feel that DNP graduates are prepared for "the rigors of the faculty role" (p. 7) with only a 19% responding in the positive. At the same time, 76% of DNPs felt they could meet the requirements. There was further disagreement about whether the requirements for tenure should be the same for both degrees. Only 35% of PhDs compared to 84% of DNPs felt the requirements should be the same. The majority of all nurses in the study believed that DNPs would contribute to nursing scholarship.

When the participants were asked whether employers would prefer DNP graduates over MSNs, only 13% of MSNs agreed. Even DNPs did not fully agree. . .only 30%. Only 23% of PhDs participants agreed. Interestingly, the BSN nurses were more accepting of this premise at 46% (p. 7). Slightly less than half (49%) of MSNs agreed with the idea that DNP is an "entry-level advanced practice degree parallel to physicians, dentists and pharmacists" (p. 7). Finally, the overall majority of all nurses, irrespective of their degree, believed that DNPs would improve health outcomes.

The authors concluded that "role ambiguity was prevalent among the sample of nurses surveyed. There are multiple levels of confusion concerning research, academia, and academic leadership, and scholarship, which tend to obscure the distinctness and individuality of the DNP degree, thus impacting role identity. The roles of the DNP-prepared nurse are forming and evolving" (pp. 8–9). "To further reduce role stress, strain, and ambiguity and successfully function. . .the distinctive and necessary contributions of the DNP-prepared nurse must be embraced, valued, and operationalized" (p. 9). The authors believe the degree will continue to be challenged if these contributions are not accepted.

(Parker & Hill, 2017). In addition to achieving primary care health outcomes equal to or greater than their physician counterparts, APRNs have been shown to reduce cost with no decrease in patient satisfaction (Spetz, Skillman, & Andrilla, 2016). The abundance of data should eliminate concerns about whether care provided by APRNs can safely augment the physician supply to support reform efforts aimed at expanding access to care.

It should be clarified, however, that NPs and physicians do not strive to practice identically. Physicians practice from a medical model while APRNs practice from the nursing model which emphasizes health promotion and disease prevention. This key component of NP practice is one that many patients value. It is also supported by Healthy People 2020. It is interesting to note that in recent years, medical schools have increased education about the importance of health promotion and disease prevention, partially in response to the quality and safety movement (IOM, 2001, 2003).

As stated in the IOM report, *Health Professions Education: A Bridge to Quality (2003)*, health care professionals must "work in interdisciplinary teams – cooperate, collaborate, communicate and integrate care in teams to ensure that care is continuous and reliable" (p. 45). NPs have always advocated that all health care providers, including physicians, NPs, physical therapists, pharmacists and respiratory therapists, among others, work together to provide the highest quality of care. Shared leadership, with a patient-centered focus, gives an opportunity for all disciplines to bring their expertise with the goal of best outcomes. However, the paradigm is shifting from physician-led care to collaborative care, and doctorally prepared APRNs are poised to bring their knowledge and expertise to the table.

Increasing Diversity in Advanced Practice Nursing

Healthy People 2020 defines health equity as "attainment of the highest level of health for all people" (Office of Disease Prevention and Health Promotion [ODPHP], n.d., para. 5), yet minorities in the United States continue to experience less access to health care and lower quality than their white counterparts (Agency for Healthcare Research and Quality [AHRQ], 2012). The National Advisory Council on Nurse Education and Practice (NACNEP, 2013) compiled a report to the Secretary of the Department of Health and Human Services and Congress titled *Achieving Health Equity through Nursing Workforce Diversity*. In this report, the authors put forth the goal of creating a nursing workforce that better mirrors the diversity of the U.S. population. Studies have demonstrated better health outcomes when language

and culture of the patient match that of the provider, a term called "concordance" (NACNEP, 2013, p. 7). The report also notes that APRNs are more likely to practice in rural, underserved areas than physician counterparts.

One concern raised by several APRN organizations regarding mandating the DNP as the entry level for APRNs is that minority students may have less resources and support for doctoral studies (ACNM, 2012; NACNS, 2009). In the NACNEP Congressional report, the authors presented policy strategies to encourage diversity in the nursing workforce, faculty, and advanced practice. Specifically, they encouraged "pipe-line" K-12 programs to direct underrepresented students into science, technology, engineering, and math (STEM) programs, specifically health care and nursing. Additionally, the report called for continued HRSA Nursing Workforce Diversity Grants to be funded through the Public Health Service Act. These grants provide financial support to minority students as well as encourage schools of nursing and hospitals to promote diversity in the workplace (NACNEP, 2013, p. 6). Intentional programs of financial and mentoring support can help enhance diversity in the nursing workforce, which translates to increased access and quality of care in underserved populations (AHRQ, 2012; NACNEP, 2013).

Discussion Point

What are some innovative ways that nursing can increase its diversity?

LOOKING TOWARD THE FUTURE

The controversy over the clinical practice doctorate in nursing will likely continue for many years, but advanced practice registered nursing must continue to self-evaluate the level of education needed to provide top quality care to patients in today's health care system. Of equal importance, APRNs must develop the advocacy skills needed to survive as a vital constituent of the current evolving health care system. There is no question that APRN makes valuable contributions to the health care system. The movement to the DNP is a crucial part of that process. Continued advocacy and policy support for APRN will be critical for APRNs to most significantly impact the health of our patients. The nursing profession must continue to be vigilant about attempts to encroach on its right to practice.

The integration of APRNs into the workforce is a dynamic change in the provision of healthcare services requiring a mind shift by policy makers and healthcare professionals. . .The development of policy to support this new nursing role to its full potential was found to be essential. (Schober et al., 2015, p. 1322)

Nearly a decade ago, the IOM (2010) recommended that all levels of nursing be allowed and encouraged to perform to the full scope of their practice. Nurses must be strong advocates for the profession by joining and being actively involved in professional associations that focus on monitoring practice issues and voting for legislators who will support APRN roles. Legislators must be kept informed of nursing practice as well as provided with documentation of the outstanding patient outcomes from APRN care. The protection of nursing's freedom to practice without undue restrictions and barriers must be insured, not just for the profession, but more importantly for the health and wellness of the patients served. In collaboration, all members of the health care team must strive to enhance the health of our nation's population, especially its most vulnerable members.

For Additional Discussion

1. Compare and contrast the skill sets of PhD- and DNP-trained nurses bring to nursing education and curriculum development. How can both doctoral degrees best work together to impact the profession?

2. Give examples of barriers and facilitators for increasing diversity in advanced practice nursing. Why is diversity important?

3. Should physicians be reimbursed more than advanced practice nurses for the same services rendered? Why or why not?

4. Would you consider pursuing an advanced practice nursing degree? If not, why? If so, which of the four roles most interests you and why? Provide examples of personality traits you feel are beneficial for the different roles.

5. Do you support the NCSBN Consensus Model for APRNs? What benefits does the model provide for APRNs and consumers? Are there any benefits for physicians? What o you see as potential disadvantages of the Consensus Model?

References

Agency for Healthcare Research and Quality. (2012). *National healthcare disparities report*. U.S. Department of Health and Human Services. Washington, DC: Author. Retrieved from https://archive.ahrq.gov/research/findings/nhqrdr/nhqr12/index.html

American Association of Colleges of Nursing. (2004). *AACN position statement on the practice doctorate in nursing*. Retrieved from http://www.aacnnursing.org/Portals/42/News/Position-Statements/DNP.pdf

American Association of Colleges of Nursing. (2006). *The essentials of doctoral education for advanced nursing practice*. Retrieved from https://www.pncb.org/sites/default/files/2017-02/Essentials_of_DNP_Education.pdf

American Association of Colleges of Nursing. (2008). *The essentials of baccalaureate education for professional nursing practice*. Retrieved from http://www.aacnnursing.org/Portals/42/Publications/BaccEssentials08.pdf

American Association of Colleges of Nursing (2010). *The research-focused doctoral program in nursing: Pathways to excellence*. Retrieved from http://www.aacnnursing.org/Portals/42/Publications/PhDPosition.pdf, August 29, 2018.

American Association of Colleges of Nursing. (2015). *White Paper: Re-envisioning the clinical education of advanced practice registered nurses*. Retrieved from http://www.aacnnursing.org/Portals/42/News/White-Papers/APRN-Clinical-Education.pdf?ver=2017-08-07-093004-913

American Association of Colleges of Nursing. (2017, June). *Fact sheet: The Doctor of Nursing Practice (DNP)*. Retrieved from http://www.aacnnursing.org/News-Information/Fact-Sheets/DNP-Fact-Sheet

American Association of Nurse Anesthetists. (2007). *AANA Position on doctoral preparation of nurse anesthetists*. Retrieved from https://home.coa.us.com/accreditation/Documents/Standards%20for%20Accreditation%20of%20Nurse%20Anesthesia%20Programs%20-%20Practice%20Doctorate,%20rev%20June%202016.pdf

American Association of Nurse Anesthetists [AANA] (2015). *Who we are*. Park Ridge, IL: American Association of Nurse Anesthetists.

American Association of Nurse Anesthetists. (2018). *Certified Registered Nurse Anesthetists fact sheet.* Retrieved from https://www.aana.com/membership/become-a-crna/crna-fact-sheet

American Association of Nurse Practitioners. (2018a). *NP fact sheet.* Retrieved from http://www.aanp.org/all-about-nps/np-fact-sheet

American Association of Nurse Practitioners. (2018b). *State practice environment.* Retrieved from https://www.aanp.org/legislation-regulation/state-legislation/state-practice-environment

American College of Nurse-Midwives. (2012). *Midwifery education and the Doctor of Nursing Practice (DNP).* Retrieved from http://www.midwife.org/ACNM/files/ACNMLibrary-Data/UPLOADFILENAME/000000000079/Midwifery%20Ed%20and%20DNP%20Position%20Statement%20June%202012.pdf

American College of Nurse-Midwives. (2016). *Essential facts about midwives.* Retrieved from http://www.midwife.org/Essential-Facts-about-Midwives

American College of Nurse-Midwives. (2017). *Certified Nurse-Midwife state practice environment map 2017.* Retrieved from http://us16.campaign-archive1.com/?u=c80fd060458439222525f1852&id=2fe244a0df

American College of Physicians. (2009). *Nurse practitioners in primary care [policy monograph].* Philadelphia, PA: Author.

American Nurses Association. (2010). *Position statement on DNP as a terminal degree.* Retrieved from http://www.doctorsofnursingpractice.org/wp-content/uploads/2014/08/ANA_Position_Statement_on_DNP_as_a_Terminal_Degree_6_14_2010.pdf

APRN Consensus Work Group & National Council of State Boards of Nursing APRN Advisory Committee. (2008). *Consensus model for APRN regulation: Licensure, accreditation, certification and education.* Retrieved from https://www.ncsbn.org/Consensus_Model_for_APRN_Regulation_July_2008.pdf

Auerbach, D. I. (2012). Will the NP workforce grow in the future? New forecasts and implications for healthcare delivery. *Medical Care, 50*(7), 606–610.

Beaver, L. & Cahill, M. (2013). *The 2013 Legislative Session, a look back and a look ahead.* National Council of State Boards of Nursing. Retrieved from https://www.ncsbn.org/0413_APRN_LBeaver_MCahill.pdf

California Assembly AB 1308. (2013). Retrieved from http://leginfo.legislature.ca.gov/faces/billVotesClient.xhtml?bill_id=201320140AB1308

Campaign for Action. (2018). *Transforming nursing education.* Retrieved from https://campaignforaction.org/issue/transforming-nursing-education/

Chesney, M. L. (2015). Increasing families' health care access and choice through full practice authority. *Journal of Pediatric Health Care, 29*, 219–221.

Council on Accreditation (2018). *Nurse anesthesia programs awarding Master's and Doctoral degrees for entry into practice.* Retrieved from https://www.coacrna.org/Pages/default.aspx, August 29, 2018.

Doctors of Nursing Practice. (2015). *DNP scholarly projects.* Retrieved from http://www.doctorsofnursingpractice.org/resources/dnp-scholarly-projects/

Dulisse, B., & Cromwell, J. (2010). No harm found when nurse anesthetists work without supervision by physicians. *Health Affairs, 29*, 1469–1475.

Edwardson, S. (2010). *Doctor of philosophy and doctor of nursing practice as complementary degrees.* Retrieved from http://www.doctorsofnursingpractice.org/cmsAdmin/uploads/EDWARDSON2010.pdf doi:10.1016/j.profnurs.2009.08.004

Fang, D., Li, Y., Kennedy, K. A., & Trautman, D. E. (2017). *2016-2017 Enrollment and graduations in baccalaureate and graduate programs in nursing.* Washington, DC: American Association of Colleges of Nursing.

Hawkins, J. W., & Bellig, L. L. (2000). The evolution of advanced practice nursing in the United States: Caring for women and newborns. *Journal of Obstetric, Gynecologic, & Neonatal Nursing, 29*(1), 83–89.

Health policy brief: Nurse practitioners and primary care. Updated (2013, May 15). Retrieved from Health Affairs: http://www.healthaffairs.org/healthpolicybriefs/brief.php?brief_id=92

Horricks, S., Anderson, E., & Salisbury, C. (2002). Systematic review of whether nurse practitioners working in primary care can provide equivalent care to doctors. *British Medical Journal, 324*, 819–823.

HRSA's National Advisory Council on Nurse Education and Practice. (2013). Achieving health equity through nursing workforce diversity, Eleventh report to the secretary of the Department of Health and Human Services and the Congress. Retrieved from https://www.hrsa.gov/advisorycommittees/bhpradvisory/nacnep/Reports/eleventhreport.pdf

Institute of Medicine of the National Academies. (2001). *Crossing the quality chasm.* Washington, DC: National Academies Press.

Institute of Medicine of the National Academies. (2003). *Health professions education: A bridge to quality.* Washington, DC: National Academies Press. Retrieved from http://books.nap.edu/openbook.php?record_id=10681&page=45

Institute of Medicine of the National Academies. (2010a). *The future of nursing: Leading change, advancing health.* Washington, DC: National Academies Press.

Institute of Medicine of the National Academies. (2010b). *The future of nursing: Leading change, advancing health—Report recommendations.* Retrieved from http://nationalacademies.org/hmd/~/media/Files/Report%20Files/2010/The-Future-of-Nursing/Future%20of%20Nursing%202010%20Recommendations.pdf

Kleiner, M. M., Marier, A., Park, K. W., & Wing, C. (2014). Relaxing occupational licensing requirements: Analyzing wages and prices for a medical service. *National Bureau of Economic Research (NBER) Working Paper No. 19906.*

Kuo, Y. F., Loresto, F. L., Rounds, L. R., & Goodwin, J. S. (2013). States with the least restrictive regulations experienced the largest increase in patients seen by nurse practitioners. *Health Affairs, 32,* 1231–1243.

Kurtzman, E. T., Barnow, B. S., Johnson, J. E., Simmens, S. J., Infeld, D. L. & Mullan, F. (2017). Does the regulatory environment affect nurse practitioners' patterns of practice or quality of care in health centers? *Health Services Research, 52,* 437–458. Retrieved from http://www.hsr.org/hsr/abstract.jsp?aid=52861589753

Martsolf, G. R., Auerbach, D. I., & Arifkhanova, A. (2015). *The impact of full practice authority for Nurse Practitioners and other Advanced Practice Registered Nurses in Ohio.* Santa Monica, CA: RAND Corporation.

McLean Hospital. (2018). *History and progress.* Retrieved from http://www.mcleanhospital.org/about/history-and-progress

Meleis, A. I., & Dracup, K. (2005). The case against the DNP: History, timing, substance, and marginalization. *Online Journal of Issues in Nursing,* September 30, 2005. Retrieved from http://www.nursingworld.org/MainMenuCategories/ANAMarketplace/ANAPeriodicals/OJIN/TableofContents/Volume102005/No3Sept05/tpc28_216026.aspx

Melnyk, B. M. (2013). Distinguishing the preparation and roles of Doctor of Philosophy and Doctor of Nursing Practice graduates: National implications for academic curricula and health care systems. *Journal of Nursing Education, 52*(8), 442–448. doi:10.3928/01484834-20130719-01

Mundinger, M. O., Kane, R. L., Lenz, E. R., Totten, A. M., Tsai, W. Y., Clearly, P. D., & Shelanski, M. L. (2000). Primary care outcomes in patients treated by nurse practitioners or physicians: A randomized trial. *Journal of the American Medical Association, 283*(1), 59–68.

National Association of Clinical Nurse Specialists. (2009). *Position statement on the nursing practice doctorate.* Retrieved from http://www.nacns.org/docs/DNP-Statement1507.pdf

National Association of Clinical Nurse Specialists. (2014). *Who are clinical nurse specialists?* Retrieved from https://nacns.org/2014/08/who-are-clinical-nurse-specialists/

National Association of Clinical Nurse Specialists (2018). *Position statement on the Doctor of Nursing Practice.* Retrieved from https://nacns.org/advocacy-policy/position-statements/position-statement-on-the-doctor-of-nursing-practice/

National Certification Corporation (NCC) (2018). *Certification exams. How do I apply?* Retrieved from https://www.nccwebsite.org/Certification, August 29, 2018.

National Council of State Boards of Nursing. (2017, September 30). *National nursing data base.* Retrieved from https://www.ncsbn.org/national-nursing-database.htm

National Organization of Nurse Practitioner Faculties. (2012). *Nurse practitioner core competencies.* Retrieved from http://c.ymcdn.com/sites/www.nonpf.org/resource/resmgr/competencies/npcorecompetenciesfinal2012.pdf

Newhouse, R., Stanik-Hutt, J., White, K., Johantgen, M., Bass, E., Zangaro, G., . . . Weiner, J. (2011). Advance practice nurse outcomes 1990–2008: A systematic review. *Nursing Economics, 29*(5), 1–22. Retrieved from https://www.nursingeconomics.net/ce/2013/article3001021.pdf

Nicholes, R. H., & Dyer, J. (2012). Is eligibility for tenure possible for the doctor of nursing practice-prepared faculty? *Journal of Professional Nursing, 28*(1), 13–17.

Office of Disease Prevention and Health Promotion. (n.d.). *HealthyPeople2020—disparities.* Retrieved from https://www.healthypeople.gov/2020/about/foundation-health-measures/Disparities

Oliver, G. M., Pennington, L., Revelle, S., & Rantz, M. (2014). Impact of nurse practitioners on health outcomes of Medicare and Medicaid patients. *Nursing Outlook, 62*(6), 440–447. doi:10.1016/j.outlook.2014.07.004

Parker, J. M., & Hill, M. N. (2017). A review of advanced practice nursing in the United States, Canada, Australia and Hong Kong Special Administrative Region (SAR), China. *International Journal of Nursing Sciences, 4,* 196–204.

Perloff, J., DesRoches, C. M., & Buerhaus, P. (2016). Comparing the cost of care provided to Medicare beneficiaries assigned to primary care nurse practitioners and physicians. *Health Services Research, 51*(4), 1407–1423. doi:10.1111/1475-6773.12425

Phillips, S. J. (2018). 30th Annual APRN Legislative Update: Improving access to healthcare one state at a time. *The Nurse Practitioner, 43*(1), 27–54.

Poghosyan, L., Boyd, D., & Knutson, A. (2014). Nurse practitioner role, independent practice, and teamwork in primary care. *The Journal for Nurse Practitioners, 10,* 472–479. doi:10.1016/j.nurpra.2014.05.009

Robert Wood Johnson Foundation. (2013, June 10). *Robert Wood Johnson Foundation announces $20 million grant to support nurse PhD scientists.* Retrieved from https://www.rwjf.org/en/library/articles-and-news/2013/06/a-new-generation-of-nurse-scientists--educators--and-transformat.html

Robert Wood Johnson Foundation. (2017). *Charting nursing future: The case for removing barriers to APRN practice.* Retrieved from http://campaignforaction.org/wp-content/uploads/2017/03/CNF30-online-brief.pdf

Rounds, L. R., Zych, J. J., & Mallary, L. L. (2013). The consensus model for regulation of APRNs: Implications for nurse practitioners. *Journal of American Academy of Nurse Practitioners, 25*(4), 180–185.

Schober, M., Gerrish, K., & McDonnell, A. (2016). Development of a conceptual policy framework for advanced practice nursing: an ethnographic study. *Journal of Advanced Nursing, 72*(6), 1313–1324.

Spetz, J., Skillman, S. M., & Andrilla, C. H. A. (2016). Nurse practitioner autonomy and satisfaction in rural settings. *Medical Care Research and Review, 74*(2), 227–235. Retrieved from https://healthforce.ucsf.edu/publications/nurse-practitioner-autonomy-and-satisfaction-rural-settings

Swan, M., Ferguson, S., Chang, A., Larson, E., & Smaldone, A. (2015). Quality of primary care by advanced practice nurses: A systematic review. *International Journal for Quality in Health Care, 27*(5), 396–404. doi:10.1093/intqhc/mzv054

Udlis, K. A., & Mancuso, J. M. (2015). Perceptions of the role of the Doctor of Nursing Practice-prepared nurse: Clarity or confusion. *Journal of Professional Nursing, 31*(4), 274–283. doi:10.1016/j.profnurs.2015.01.004

US Department of Labor: US Bureau of Labor Statistics. (2018). *Occupational employment statistics.* Retrieved from https://www.bls.gov/oes/current/oes291171.htm

Weinberg, M., Kallerman, P., & Spetz, J. (2014). *Full practice authority for Nurse Practitioners increases access and controls cost.* Bay Area Council Economic Institute. Retrieved from https://canpweb.org/canp/assets/File/Bay%20Area%20Council%20Report%204-30-14/BAC%20NP%20Full%20Report%204-30-14.pdf

Evidence-Based Practice

Suzanne S. Prevost and Cassandra D. Ford

ADDITIONAL RESOURCES

Visit thePoint® for additional helpful resources
• eBook
• Journal Articles
• WebLinks

CHAPTER OUTLINE

LEARNING OBJECTIVES

The learner will be able to:

1. Differentiate between evidence-based practice and best practices.

2. Explain why the identification and implementation of evidence-based practice is important both for ensuring quality of care and in advancing the development of nursing science.

3. Identify personal, professional, and administrative strategies, as well as support systems, that promote the identification and implementation of evidence-based practice.

4. Describe the types of knowledge and education that nurses need to prepare them for conducting research and leading best practice initiatives.

5. Recognize the need to ask critical questions in the spirit of looking for opportunities to improve nursing practice and patient outcomes.

6. Delineate research and nonresearch sources of evidence for answering clinical questions.

7. Describe and compare practices that have evolved in the workplace as a result of tradition-based and research-based inquiry.

8. Compare the efficacy of randomized controlled trials, integrative reviews, and meta-analyses as reference sources to answer clinical research questions.

9. Specify institutions, units, teams, or individuals that could be considered regional or national benchmark

leaders in the provision of a specialized type of medical or nursing care.

10. Explore reasons for the disconnect that often exists between nurse researchers and educators studying evidence-based practice and nurses who seek to implement research into their practice.

INTRODUCTION

Nurses and other health care providers constantly strive to provide the best care for their patients. As new medications and health care innovations emerge, determining the best options can be challenging. This process becomes more difficult as health care administrators, insurance companies, and other payers, accrediting agencies, and consumers demand the latest and greatest health care interventions. Nurses and physicians are expected to select health care interventions that are supported by research and other credible forms of evidence. They may also be expected to provide evidence to demonstrate that the care they deliver is not only clinically effective but also cost-effective, and satisfying, to patients. In light of these challenges, the term *evidence-based practice* has emerged as a descriptor of the preferred approach to health care delivery.

This chapter begins by defining the concept of evidence-based practice. Examples of when and where nurses are using evidence-based practice are provided, as are strategies for determining and applying these practices. In addition, the *who* of evidence-based practice is addressed regarding how nurses in various roles can support this approach to care. Finally, future implications are discussed.

WHAT IS EVIDENCE-BASED PRACTICE?

The term "evidence-based practice" is part of the daily discourse among health care providers in progressive clinical environments. Evidence-based practice has a variety of definitions and interpretations. The term "evidence-based practice" evolved in the mid-1990s when discussions of evidence-based medicine were expanded to apply to an interdisciplinary audience, which included nurses. David Sackett, one of the original leaders of the movement, defined evidence-based medicine as "the conscientious and judicious use of current best evidence from clinical care research in the management of individual patients" (Sackett, Rosenberg, Gray, Haynes, & Richardson, 1996, p. 71). The Honor Society of Nursing, Sigma Theta Tau International (STTI, 2005) expanded this definition to address a broad nursing context with the following definition of evidence-based nursing practice: "An integration of the best

evidence available, nursing expertise, and the values and preferences of the individuals, families and communities who are served" (p. 1).

Historically, various industries, in health care and beyond, have used the term *best practice* to describe the strategies or methods that work most efficiently or achieve the best results. This concept is often associated with the process of *benchmarking*, which involves identifying the most successful companies or institutions in a particular sector of an industry, examining their methods of doing business, using their approach as the goal or gold standard, and then replicating and refining their methods. Today, benchmarking data is one of the less scientific forms of evidence that is used, along with the results of formal research studies, to identify evidence-based nursing practices.

> **Consider This** Today, most nurse experts agree that the best practices in nursing care are also evidence-based practices.

Although this process of identifying the best evidence-based practices has become more scientific, the ultimate goal remains to provide optimal patient care, with the goal of enhancing nursing practice and, in turn, improving patient or system outcomes.

> **Discussion Point**
> Are there any situations in which an evidence-based practice might not be considered the best practice?

WHY, WHEN, AND WHERE IS EVIDENCE-BASED PRACTICE USED?

Each week, new developments and innovations occur and are reported in health care—not only in research publications but also in the public media. Contemporary health care consumers are knowledgeable and demanding. They expect the most current, effective, and efficient interventions.

Why Is Evidence-Based Practice Important?

In their quest to provide the highest quality care for their patients, nurses are challenged to stay abreast of new developments in health care, even within the limits of their areas of specialization. Simultaneous with the growth of health care knowledge, health care costs have increased, and patient satisfaction has taken on greater importance. Administrators expect health care providers to satisfy their customers and to do it in the most clinically effective and cost-effective manner.

Control of health care costs was one of the early drivers of the evidence-based practice movement. As contracted and discounted reimbursement systems decreased revenue to hospitals and providers, it became increasingly apparent that some providers were capable of providing high-quality care in a more efficient and cost-effective manner than their peers. The practices of these industry leaders were quickly identified and emulated. Within the current litigious and cost-conscious health care environment, there remains a sense of urgency to select and implement the most effective and efficient interventions as quickly as possible.

Nurses are increasingly accepted as essential members, and often as leaders, of interdisciplinary health care teams. To effectively participate and lead a health care team, nurses must have knowledge of the most effective and reliable evidence-based approaches to care, and as nurses increase their expertise in critiquing research, they are expected to apply the evidence of their findings to select optimal interventions for their patients.

The processes and tools of evidence-based practice can help nurses respond to these challenges. This approach to care is based on the latest research and other forms of evidence, as well as clinical expertise and patient preferences. All of these factors contribute to providing quality care that is clinically effective, cost-effective, and satisfying to health care consumers.

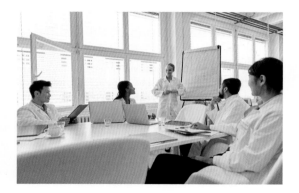

Discussion Point

What type of knowledge and education do nurses need to prepare them for leading evidence-based practice initiatives as described?

When and Where Is Evidence-Based Practice Used?

In recent years, the implementation of evidence-based practice has been identified as a priority across nearly every nursing specialty. Over the past decade, STTI, International Honor Society of Nursing (now known as Sigma), has consistently received feedback from their membership surveys asking for support systems and resources to help nurses implement evidence-based practice. This feedback has been consistent across nursing specialties and across nursing roles and positions. Initiatives to help nurses understand and implement evidence-based practice have become a priority since that time. A review of recent literature yields case studies and recommendations for evidence-based practice implementation across several nursing specialties. These are shown in Table 5.1.

In addition to the universal application across nursing specialties, the concept of evidence-based practice is also valued across nursing roles and responsibilities. Bissett, Cvach, and White (2016) discussed strategies used by nurse administrators to prepare nurse clinicians to lead evidence-based practice initiatives. Kincaid and Parks (2017) described the mentoring role of advanced practice nurses in promoting evidence-based practice. Nursing faculty are expected to use evidence-based practices to refine nursing curricula as described by Clark (2017). Last but not least, staff nurses are frequently expected to participate in evidence-based practice initiatives as described by Wright (2017).

Evidence-Based Practice Around the World

A commitment to evidence-based practice is not limited to the United States. A few countries—in particular, Australia, Canada, and the United Kingdom—adopted this approach to care several years before it became popular in the United States. The Joanna Briggs Institute, which started at the University of Adelaide, Australia, in 1996, now has over 70 centers collaborating to provide evidence-based resources to health care providers around the world. The Registered Nurses Association of Ontario has been developing and distributing evidence-based nursing practice guidelines for more than a decade. Nursing Knowledge International, a subsidiary of Sigma, also

TABLE 5.1   Evidence-Based Practice Across Nursing Specialties

Area of Specialization	Author and Year	Title or Theme	Type of Report
Administration	Fleiszer, Semenic, Ritchie, Richer, and Denis (2016)	Nursing unit leaders' influence on EBP	Qualitative research study
Critical care	Richards et al. (2017)	Reduction of catheter-associated urinary tract infections (CAUTIs) with EBP strategies	Research study implementing EBPs to decrease CAUTIs
Education and staff development	Bissett et al. (2016)	Promoting EBP	Educational intervention to enhance EBP competency among staff nurses
Gerontology	Cornelius, Herr, Gordon, and Kretzer (2017)	EBP for acute pain in older adults	Summary of evidence-based guideline for acute pain management
Medical–surgical	Case (2017)	Educational intervention to demonstrate translation to practice at primary stroke center	Quality improvement project
Mental health	Ferrara, Davis-Ajami, Warren, and Murphy (2017)	Evidence-based protocol for de-escalation training	Educational intervention
Oncology	Conley (2016)	EBP strategies for standardized care of central lines	Describes implementation of EBP project
Pediatrics	Liu, Mo, Tang, Wang, and Huang (2017)	Evaluation of evidence-based clinical nurse path for pediatric surgery patients	Randomized controlled trial
Urgent care	Kim, Brathwaite, and Kim (2017)	EBP pain management for sickle cell disease in urgent care	Quality improvement study
Women's health	Ben-David, Jonson-Reid, and Tompkins (2017)	Implementing EBP screening tool for postpartum depression	Describes EBP screening tool adoption

Note: EBP, evidence-based practice.

serves as an international clearinghouse and facilitator to promote international nursing communication, collaboration, and sharing of resources in support of evidence-based practice.

Consider This   In the past decade, the concept of evidence-based practice has evolved and been embraced by nurses in nearly every clinical specialty, across a variety of roles and positions, and in locations around the globe.

How Do Nurses Determine Evidence-Based Practices?

Evidence-based practice begins with questions that arise in practice settings. Nurses must be empowered to ask critical questions in the spirit of looking for opportunities to improve nursing practice and patient outcomes. In any specialty or role, nurses can regard their work as a continuous series of questions and decisions.

In a given day, a staff nurse may ask and answer questions such as "Should I give the analgesic only when the patient requests it, or should I encourage him to take it every

4 hours? Will aggressive ambulation expedite this patient's recovery, or will it consume too much energy? Will open family visitation help the patient feel supported, or will it interrupt his or her rest?"

A nurse manager or administrator might ask, "Who is the most qualified care provider for our sickest patient today? What is the optimal nurse-to-patient ratio for a specific unit? Do complication rates and sentinel events increase with less-educated staff? Do longer shifts result in greater staff fatigue and medication errors? Will higher-quality and more expensive mattresses decrease the incidence of pressure ulcers? What benefits promote nurse retention? How does the use of supplemental (or agency) staffing affect the morale of existing staff? Can this population be treated on an outpatient, rather than an inpatient, basis? What is the optimal length of time for a comprehensive home care assessment? How many patients can a nurse practitioner see in 8 hours?"

Likewise, a nurse educator may ask, "Is it more effective to teach a procedure in the simulation laboratory rather than on an actual patient? What are the most efficient methods of documenting continued competency? Do Web-based students perform as well on standardized tests as students in traditional classrooms?"

Each type of question can lead to important decisions that affect outcomes, such as patient recovery, organizational effectiveness, and nursing competency. The best answers and, consequently, the best decisions come from informed, evidence-based analysis of each situation. See Box 5.1 for a list of questions to assist the nurse in the process of evidence-based decision making for various nursing scenarios.

FINDING EVIDENCE TO ANSWER NURSING QUESTIONS

Nurses rely on various sources to answer clinical questions such as those cited previously. A practicing staff nurse might consult a nurse with more experience, more education, or a higher level of authority to get help in answering such questions. Institutional standards or policy and procedure manuals are also a common reference source for nurses in practice. Nursing coworkers or other health care providers, such as physicians, pharmacists, or therapists, might also be consulted. Although all of these approaches are extremely common, they are more likely to yield clinical answers that are *tradition based* rather than *evidence based*.

If evidence-based practice is truly based on best evidence, nursing expertise, and the values and preferences of patients, then local expertise and tradition is not sufficient. However, the optimal source of best evidence is often a matter of controversy.

> **Discussion Point**
>
> In your preferred area of nursing specialization, what are some key questions and decisions that nurses address on a daily basis?

> **Discussion Point**
>
> What are the best sources of evidence for answering clinical questions?

Research is generally considered a more reliable source of evidence than traditions or the clinical expertise of individuals. However, many experts argue that some types of research are better, or stronger, forms of evidence than others. In medicine and pharmacology, the *randomized controlled trial* (RCT) has been considered the gold standard of clinical evidence. RCTs yield the strongest statistical evidence regarding the effectiveness of an intervention in comparison with another intervention or placebo. For many clinical questions in medicine and pharmacy, there may be multiple RCTs in the literature addressing a single question, such as the effectiveness of a particular drug. In such situations, an even stronger form of evidence is an *integrative review or meta-analysis* wherein the results of several similar research studies are combined or synthesized to provide the most comprehensive answer to the question.

In nursing literature, RCTs, meta-analyses, and integrative reviews are significantly less common than in medical or pharmaceutical literature. For many clinical questions in nursing, RCTs may not exist, or they may not even be appropriate. For example, if a nurse is considering how best to prepare a patient for endotracheal suctioning, it would be helpful to inform the patient what suctioning feels like. This type of question does not lend itself to an RCT, but rather to descriptive or qualitative research. In general, qualitative, descriptive, or quasi-experimental studies are much more common methods of inquiry in nursing research than RCTs or meta-analyses. Furthermore, the body of nursing research overall is newer and less developed than that of some other health disciplines. Thus, for many clinical nursing questions, research studies may not exist.

Although research results are usually considered the optimal form of evidence, many other data sources have been used to support the identification of optimal interventions for nursing and other health care disciplines. Some of the additional sources are as follows:

- Benchmarking data
- Clinical expertise
- Cost-effectiveness analyses
- Infection-control data
- Medical record review data
- National standards of care
- Pathophysiologic data
- Quality improvement data
- Patient and family preferences

Another dilemma for the practicing nurse is the time, access, and expertise needed to search and analyze the research literature to answer clinical questions. Few practicing nurses have the luxury of leaving their patients to conduct a literature search. Many staff nurses practicing in clinical settings have less than a baccalaureate degree; therefore, many have not been exposed to a formal research course. Findings from research studies are typically very technical, difficult to understand, and even more difficult to translate into applications. Searching, finding, critiquing, and summarizing research findings for applications in practice are high-level skills that require substantial education and practice.

Discussion Point

If a practicing nurse has no formal education or experience related to research, what strategies should she or he use to find evidence that answers clinical questions and supports evidence-based practice?

SUPPORTING EVIDENCE-BASED PRACTICE

In light of the challenges of providing or implementing evidence-based practice, nurses must consider some alternative support mechanisms when searching for the best evidence to support their practice. Recommended mechanisms of support are summarized in Box 5.2.

Garner Administrative Support

The first strategy is to garner administrative support. The implementation of evidence-based practice should not be an individual, staff nurse–level pursuit. Administrative support is needed to access the resources, provide the support personnel, and sanction the necessary changes in policies, procedures, and practices. Recently, nursing administrators have had increased incentives to support evidence-based practice because this approach to care has become recognized as the standard expectation of organizations, such as the Joint Commission (formerly Joint Commission on Accreditation of Healthcare Organizations [JCAHO]), which accredits hospitals and other health care institutions. Evidence-based practice is also one of the expectations associated with the highly regarded Magnet Hospital Recognition program. Most nursing administrators who want their institutions to be recognized for providing high-quality care will understand the value of evidence-based practice and should therefore be willing to provide resources to support it.

BOX 5.2   Mechanisms to Promote Evidence-Based Practice

- Garner administrative support
- Collaborate with a research mentor
- Seek assistance from professional librarians
- Search for sources that have already reviewed or summarized the research
- Access resources from professional organizations
- Benchmark with high-performing teams, units, or institutions

Collaborate With a Research Mentor

One way nurse administrators can support the use of evidence-based practice is through the provision of nurse experts who can function as research mentors. Advanced practice nurses, nurse researchers, and nursing faculty are examples of nurses who may provide consultation and collaboration to support the process of searching, reviewing, and critiquing research literature and databases to answer clinical questions and identify best practices. Most staff nurses do not have the educational background, research expertise, or time to effectively review and critique extensive research literature in search of the evidence to support evidence-based practice. Research mentors can assist with these processes, whereas staff nurses can often provide the best insight on clinical needs and patient preferences. Box 5.3 includes a list of strategies for the new graduate nurse to promote evidence-based practice.

Seek Assistance From Professional Librarians

Another valuable type of support that is available in academic medical centers, and in some smaller institutions, is consultation from medical librarians. A skilled librarian can save nurses a tremendous amount of time by providing guidance in the most comprehensive and efficient approaches to search the health care literature to find research studies and other resources to support the implementation of evidence-based practice.

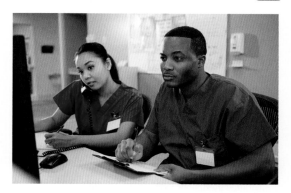

Search Already Reviewed or Summarized Research

A strategy nurses can use to expedite the search for evidence-based practice is to specifically seek references that have already been reviewed or summarized in the research literature. For example, some journals, such as *Evidence-Based Nursing* and *Worldviews on Evidence-Based Nursing*, specifically focus on providing summaries, critiques, and practice implications of existing nursing research studies. For example, recent issues of *Worldviews on Evidence-Based Nursing* included reviews and summaries on the following topics:

- Postoperative pain management in children
- Interventions to promote breast cancer screening
- Frailty as a predictor of fractures
- Psychosocial interventions for spinal cord injured patients

When conducting a literature search, use of keywords, such as "research review" or "meta-analysis," can assist the nurse in identifying published research review articles on the topic of interest.

The *Cochrane Collaboration* is a large international organization composed of several interdisciplinary teams of research scholars that are continuously conducting reviews of research on a wide variety of clinical topics. The Cochrane Collaboration promotes the use of evidence-based practice around the world. The Cochrane reviews tend to focus heavily on evaluating the effectiveness of medical interventions, for example, comparing the effects of different medications for specific conditions. Therefore, many of the Cochrane review summaries are more useful for primary care providers, such as physicians and nurse practitioners, than for staff nurse clinicians. Some of the Cochrane projects of interest to nurses in direct care positions include their reviews of products designed to prevent pressure

---

BOX 5.3 | **Strategies for the New Nurse to Promote Evidence-Based Practice**

- Keep abreast of the evidence—subscribe to professional journals and read widely
- Use and encourage use of multiple sources of evidence
- Find established sources of evidence in your specialty; do not reinvent the wheel
- Implement and evaluate nationally sanctioned clinical practice guidelines
- Question and challenge nursing traditions, and promote a spirit of risk-taking
- Dispel myths and traditions not supported by evidence
- Collaborate with other nurses locally and globally
- Interact with other disciplines to bring nursing evidence to the table

ulcers, nursing interventions for smoking cessation, interventions to help patients follow their medication regimens, and interventions to promote collaboration between nurses and physicians.

The Agency for Healthcare Research and Quality (AHRQ) is also a good resource for identifying research reviews and summaries that have been compiled by national panels of experts. The practice guidelines available through AHRQ are developed through systematic searches and reviews of research literature and scientific evidence by a professional organization, health care specialty association, or government agency. Nursing organizations that have contributed guidelines to the AHRQ include the American Association of Neuroscience Nurses; Association of Women's Health, Obstetric, and Neonatal Nursing (AWHONN); Emergency Nurses Association; the Hartford Institute for Geriatric Nursing; the Oncology Nursing Society (ONS); and the Registered Nurses Association of Ontario.

Access Resources From Professional Organizations

Professional nursing organizations can also provide a wealth of resources to support evidence-based practice. For example, the American Association of Critical Care Nurses has published several *Practice Alerts* that are relevant to nursing care in critical care units. These documents are based on extensive literature reviews conducted by national panels of nurse researchers and advanced practice nurses. They provide concise recommendations focused on areas where current common practices should change on the basis of the latest research. Some of the topics covered in the *Practice Alerts* include pain assessment in the critically ill adult, alarm management, and oral care for critically ill patients.

AWHONN (2018) also provides several resources to support evidence-based practice. For example, AWHONN produces evidence-based *Practice Briefs*, which include quick reference guides that should be incorporated into clinical practice, including the rationale for these practice changes. AWHONN also sponsors an Evidence-Based Clinical Practice Guideline Program. Each of their guidelines includes clinical practice recommendations, referenced rationale statements, quality of evidence ratings for each statement, background information describing the scope of the clinical issue, and a quick care reference guide for clinicians. Guidelines for Oxytocin Administration is an example of one of the guidelines produced through this program.

The Association of periOperative Registered Nurses (AORN), the ONS, and Sigma also provide Web-based

resources to facilitate implementation of evidence-based practice. AORN has published *Guidelines for Perioperative Practice*, the ONS provides an *Evidence-Based Practice Resource Area*, and Sigma publishes Web-based continuing education programs and several supportive publications, including *Worldviews on Evidence-Based Nursing*.

Discussion Point

What institutions, units, teams, or individuals can you identify in your region that would be considered regional or national benchmark leaders in the provision of a specialized type of medical or nursing care?

Benchmark With High-Performing Teams, Units, or Institutions

Finally, nurses can use benchmarking strategies to poll nurse experts from high-performing teams, units, or institutions to learn more about their practices for specific clinical problems or patient populations. Leaders of professional nursing organizations, such as Sigma or the National Association of Clinical Nurse Specialists, can help nurses locate and contact established nurse experts in various areas of specialization. Accrediting organizations, such as the Joint Commission, can assist in identifying institutions that are known as national leaders in providing specific types of care. The University of Iowa, Ohio State University, and McMaster University of Ontario are three North American institutions that have established reputations as leaders in evidence-based nursing practice.

Discussion Point

When the investigation reveals a need for an evidence-based change in practice, what strategies are useful for implementing change?

CHALLENGES AND OPPORTUNITIES: STRATEGIES FOR CHANGING PRACTICE

Nurses use several mechanisms for incorporating new research into current practice in the pursuit of promoting evidence-based practice. Perhaps the most common mechanism is through the development and refinement of research-based policies and procedures. Fortunately, the Joint Commission has mandated that health care institutions must implement formal processes for reviewing the latest research and ensuring that institutional policies and procedures are consistently revised in keeping with current research findings.

Protocols, algorithms, decision trees, standards of care, critical pathways, care maps, and institutional clinical practice guidelines are additional mechanisms used to incorporate new evidence into clinical practice. Each of these formats is used by health care teams to guide clinical decision making and clinical interventions. Although nurses often take the lead in developing or revising these standards and the related procedures, participation and buy-in from the interdisciplinary health care team are essential to achieve successful implementation and consistent changes in practice.

In addition to consensus from the interdisciplinary team, support from patients and their families is important. This element of the evidence-based practice process is frequently overlooked or not thoroughly considered. As previously mentioned, evidence-based nursing practice involves "an integration of the best evidence available, nursing expertise, and the values and preferences of the individuals, families and communities who are served" (STTI, 2005, p. 1).

If the review of evidence leads the health care team to recommend an intervention that is inconsistent with the patient's values and preferences (such as a specific dietary modification or transfusion of blood products), the recommendation may lead to poor adherence or total disregard by the patient. This situation can also result in loss of the patient's trust and confidence in the health care team.

> ### Discussion Point
>
> Can you think of situations in which the latest research may be inconsistent with the values of an individual or group of patients?

Challenges to Implementing Evidence-Based Practice

Although evidence-based practice is promoted by nurses around the world, several obstacles continue to inhibit the movement. Funk, Champagne, Wiese, and Tornquist (1991) originally studied this problem in 1991 and developed a survey instrument to quantify those barriers. Recently, Spiva and colleagues (2017) used this instrument in their implementation of a mentoring program to promote evidence-based practice. Practicing nurses often feel overwhelmed by the volume of research on their topics of interest; and they often lack the time and experience to be able to efficiently read and synthesize that literature. They also struggle with the political challenges of attempting to change long-standing policies and procedures in their clinical settings. Other researchers have investigated the barriers to implementing evidence-based practices and guidelines with similar findings (see Research Fuels the Controversy 5.1). Advanced practice nurses, such as clinical nurse specialists, nurse practitioners, and clinical nurse leaders, can

---

Research Fuels the Controversy 5.1

Health Professionals' Views on the Barriers and Enablers to Evidence-Based Practice for Acute Stroke Care: A Systematic Review

Evidence-based interventions used in the first 2 days after a stroke can significantly reduce the loss of brain tissue and related mortality. Several research studies support a protocol including: (1) admitting acute stroke patients to a specialized stroke unit; (2) giving thrombolytic therapy intravenously within 4.5 hours of the stroke; (3) administering aspirin within 48 hours of stroke onset; and (4) providing decompression surgery within 48 hours, if needed.

However, in many hospitals, these interventions are not routinely used. The authors conducted a systematic review of studies that address barriers and enablers related to adoption of evidence-based practice guidelines for acute stroke care. Studies conducted from 1990 to 2016 were reviewed and 10 studies were found to meet the inclusion criteria. Studies focused on the views of health care providers and allied health professionals.

Source: Baatiema, L., Otim, M. E., Mnatzaganian, G., de-Graft Aikins, A., Coombes, J., & Somerset, S. (2017). Health professionals' views on the barriers and enablers to evidence-based practice for acute stroke care: A systematic review. *Implementation Science, 12*(74). doi:10.1186/s13012-017-0599-3

Study Findings

The most commonly cited barriers to evidence based practice for acute stroke care were poor institutional support; low level of awareness, skill, or confidence with the evidence-base therapies; limited availability of specialized facilities (especially in low-income countries); and inadequate peer support.

help to educate, empower, and support staff nurses through this process.

Discussion Point

What obstacles would limit your involvement in pursuing evidence-based practice?

CONCLUSIONS

Many nurses are experiencing success in promoting evidence-based practice. Organizations such as the AHRQ and the Cochrane Collaboration provide support to help clinicians overcome some of the barriers, such as the difficulties in obtaining and understanding research reports, and the lack of time to synthesize research findings into recommended practices. The many agencies that support teams of research experts to collect, critique, and summarize the research and other forms of evidence pave the way for frontline clinicians to find and adopt evidence-based practices.

Yet challenges continue. Too few nurses understand what evidence-based practice is all about. Organizational cultures may not support the nurse who seeks out and uses research to change long-standing practices rooted in tradition rather than science. In addition, a stronger connection is needed between researchers and academics who study evidence-based nursing practice and staff nurses who must translate those findings into the art of nursing practice. Nursing cannot afford to value the art of nursing over the science. Both are critical to making sure that patients receive the highest quality of care possible.

For Additional Discussion

1. Can decision support tools such as algorithms, decision trees, clinical pathways, and standardized clinical guidelines ever replace clinical judgment?

2. What causes the disconnection between nurse researchers or faculty studying evidence-based practice and the nurses who seek to implement such research into their practice? Is the problem a lack of communication?

3. Do most nurses have access to evidence-based nursing research findings?

4. Are evidence-based practice findings consistent over time? Can you identify an evidence-based practice that was later found to be ineffective or inappropriate?

5. Should evidence-based practices be institution specific, or should they be more generalizable across different settings?

6. Is evidence-based nursing research grounded more in quantitative or qualitative research? Are both needed?

7. What can be done to increase the research knowledge base of practicing registered nurses, given that a significant proportion of those nurses have been educated at the associate-degree level?

References

Association of Women's Health, Obstetric and Neonatal Nursing. (2018). *Practice briefs*. Retrieved May 16, 2018, from https://www.awhonn.org/?page=PracticeBriefs

Ben-David, V., Jonson-Reid, M., & Tompkins, R. (2017). Addressing the missing part of evidence-based practice: The importance of respecting clinical judgment in the process of adopting a new screening tool for postpartum depression. *Issues in Mental Health Nursing, 38*(12), 989–995. doi:10.1080/01612840.2017.1347221

Bissett, K. M., Cvach, M., & White, K. M. (2016). Improving competence and confidence with evidence-based practice among nurses: Outcomes of a quality improvement project. *Journal for Nurses in Professional Development, 32*(5), 248–255. doi:10.1097/NND.0000000000000293

Case, C. A. (2017). Promoting evidence-based practice at a primary stroke center: A nurse education strategy. *Dimensions of Critical Care Nursing, 36*(4), 244–252. doi:10.1097/DCC.000000000000251

Clark, C. M. (2017). An evidence-based approach to integrate civility, professionalism, and ethical practice into nursing curricula. *Nurse Educator, 42*(3), 120–126. doi:10.1097/NNE.0000000000000331

Conley, S. B. (2016). Central line-associated bloodstream infection prevention: Standardizing practice focused on evidence-based guidelines. *Clinical Journal of Oncology Nursing, 20*(1), 23–26. doi:10.1188/16.CJON.23-26

Cornelius, R., Herr, K. A., Gordon, D. B., & Kretzer, K. (2017). Acute pain management in older adults. *Journal of Gerontological Nursing, 43*(2), 18–27. doi:10.3928/00989134-20170111-08

Ferrara, K. L., Davis-Ajami, M. L., Warren, J. I., & Murphy, L. S. (2017). De-escalation training to medical-surgical nurses in the acute care setting. *Issues in Mental Health Nursing, 38*(9), 742–749. doi:10.1080/01612840.2017.1335363

Fleiszer, A. R., Semenic, S. E., Ritchie, J. A., Richer, M.-C., & Denis, J.-L. (2016). Nursing unit leaders' influence on the long-term sustainability of evidence-based practice improvements. *Journal of Nursing Management, 24*(3), 309–318. doi:10.1111/jonm.12320

Funk, S. G., Champagne, M. T., Wiese, R. A., & Tornquist, E. M. (1991). Barriers to using research findings in practice: The clinician's perspective. *Applied Nursing Research, 4*(2), 90–95.

Kim, S., Brathwaite, R., & Kim, O. (2017). Evidence-based practice standard care for acute pain management in adults with sickle cell disease in an urgent care center. *Quality Management in Healthcare, 26*(2), 108–115. doi:10.1097/QMH.0000000000000135

Kincaid, S., & Parks, L. (2017). Evidence-based mentoring of surgical oncology nurses by advanced practice nurses. *Oncology Nursing Forum, 44*(2). 7. doi:10.1188/17.ONF.E88

Liu, Y., Mo, L., Tang, Y., Wang, Q., & Huang, X. (2017). The application of an evidence-based clinical nursing path for improving the preoperative and postoperative quality of care of pediatric retroperitoneal neuroblastoma patients: A randomized controlled trial at a tertiary medical institution. *Cancer Nursing, 40*(4), 314–322. doi:10.1097/NCC.000000000000387

Richards, B., Sebastian, B., Sullivan, H., Reyes, R., D'Agostino, J. F., & Hagerty, T. (2017). Decreasing catheter-associated urinary tract infections in the neurological intensive care unit: One unit's success. *Critical Care Nurse, 37*(3), 42–49. doi:10.4037/ccn2017742

Sackett, D. L., Rosenberg, W. M., Gray, J. A., Haynes, R. B., & Richardson, W. S. (1996). Evidence based medicine: What it is and what it isn't. *British Medical Journal, 312*(7023), 71–72.

Sigma Theta Tau International. (2005). *Evidence-based nursing position statement*. Retrieved December 10, 2017, from http://www.sigmanursing.org/why-sigma/about-sigma/position-statements-and-resource-papers/evidence-based-nursing-position-statement

Spiva, L., Hart, P. L., Patrick, S., Waggoner, J., Jackson, C., & Threatt, J. L. (2017). Effectiveness of an evidence-based practice nurse mentor training program. *Worldviews on Evidence-Based Nursing, 14*(3), 183–191. doi:10.1111/wvn.12219

Wright, S. M. (2017). Using evidence-based practice and an educational intervention to improve vascular access management: A pilot project. *Nephrology Nursing Journal, 44*(5), 427–438, 446.

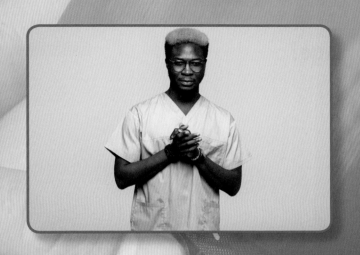

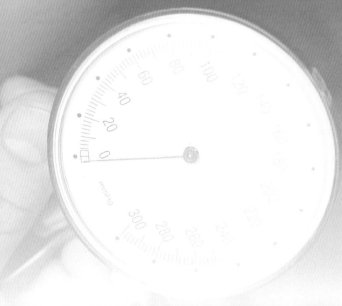

2

WORKFORCE
ISSUES

Is There a Nursing Shortage?

Carol J. Huston

CHAPTER OUTLINE

LEARNING OBJECTIVES

The learner will be able to:

1. Explore factors affecting the current supply of registered nurses (RNs) in the United States as well as the current and projected demand through 2024.

2. Compare regional differences in the supply and demand for RNs in the United States.

3. Discuss consequences of the current shortage on quality of health care, current working conditions for RNs, and RN retention rates.

4. Identify the relationship between the current nursing shortage and the state of the national economy.

5. Analyze the impact of salary as an incentive for resolving nursing shortages.

6. Address the educational challenges inherent in solving the nursing shortage given unfilled faculty positions, resignations, projected retirements, low faculty pay schedules, and the shortage of students being prepared for the faculty role.

7. Identify specific strategies being used to recruit and retain older nurses in the workforce.

8. Differentiate between and provide examples of both short- and long-term solutions to nursing shortages.

9. Outline strategies directed at both supply and demand factors that have been proposed to reduce the current nursing shortage and analyze the efficacy of each.

10. Reflect upon his or her personal commitment to a career in professional nursing.

INTRODUCTION

As government and private insurer reimbursement declined in the 1990s and managed care costs soared, many health care organizations, and hospitals in particular, began downsizing to achieve cost containment by eliminating registered nursing jobs or by replacing registered nurses (RNs) with unlicensed assistive personnel. Even hospitals that did not downsize during this period often did little to recruit qualified RNs.

This downsizing and shortsightedness regarding recruitment and retention contributed to the beginning of an acute shortage of RNs in many health care settings by the late 1990s. The health care quality and safety movement also exacerbated this shortage in the late 1990s as research emerged to demonstrate the relationship between nurse staffing and patient outcomes and the public became aware of how important an adequately sized workforce was to patient safety. Unlike earlier nursing shortages, which typically lasted only a few years, this shortage was longer and more severe than earlier nursing shortages. Indeed, as of 2010, most states in the United States reported nursing shortages, ranging from a shortage of 200 nurses in Alabama to 47,600 nurses in California (Trust for America's Health, 2018).

When the economy soured, however, early in the second decade of this century, new graduate nurses began struggling to find jobs and vacancy rates fell at most hospitals across the country. This occurred, at least in part, because many part-time nurses sought full-time employment and some nurses delayed cutting back on their work hours or seeking retirement. Thus, the economic crisis both eased the nursing shortage and obscured its depth and breadth. As the economy continues to improve, a shortage should once again occur; however, predicting how long the nation will take to recover economically and exactly when old workforce patterns may reemerge is difficult (American Association of Colleges of Nursing [AACN], 2017a). Snavely (2016) agrees, suggesting that although a moratorium in the shortage currently exists, several causal factors will lead to a critical shortage in the supply of nursing professionals available to meet the projected demands of the next decade.

> **Consider This** The recent economic crisis both eased and obscured any nursing shortage.

To more accurately assess the depth or significance of any current nursing shortage, data must be examined regarding both the demand for RNs and the supply. Assessing the demand for RNs is, in many ways, more complicated than assessing the supply. However, from an economic perspective, the most recent nursing shortage was driven more by the supply side of the supply/demand equation than the demand side. Supply shortages are more difficult to solve than demand-induced shortages because they require longer-term solutions.

This chapter will explore whether a nursing shortage exists by examining the present and projected demand for RNs, as well as the supply. In addition, the potential consequences of an unaddressed shortage will be examined, together with strategies needed to keep the shortage from recurring.

THE DEMAND FOR NURSES

Demand is defined by *Merriam-Webster* (2018a) as the quantity of a commodity or service wanted at a specified price and time. In the case of nursing, demand would be the amount of a good or service (in this case, an RN) that consumers (in this case, an employer) would be willing to acquire at a given price. A shortage occurs when employers want more employees at the current market wages than they can get. Demand then is derived from the health status of a population and the use of health services.

The demand for professional nurses in both the short- and long-term future continues to increase. In fact, employment of RNs is expected to grow much faster than the average for all occupations through 2024. Indeed, the U.S. Bureau of Labor (2018b) projects that the RN workforce will grow 15% from 2016 to 2026. The Bureau also projects the need for 649,100 replacement nurses in the workforce, bringing the total number of job openings for nurses because of growth and replacements to 1.09 million by 2024 (AACN, 2017a).

Causes of Increased Demand

There are multiple factors driving this demand, including a growing population, medical advances that increase the need for adequately educated nurses, and the increased acuity of hospitalized patients. Other factors driving demand are the technologic advances in patient care and an increasing emphasis on health care prevention.

In addition, a growing elderly population with extended longevity and more chronic health conditions requires more nursing care. As life expectancy in the United States increases, more nurses will be needed to assist the individuals who are surviving serious illnesses and living longer with chronic diseases. The AACN (2017a) concurs, suggesting that as baby boomers enter their retirement years, their demand for care is escalating, and health care reform will soon provide subsidies for more than 32 million citizens to more fully use the health care system. As a result, the demand for health care is expected to steadily increase in the next few decades and the numbers of nurses to care for these patients will lag behind.

THE SUPPLY OF NURSES

Supply refers to the quantity of goods or services that are ready for use or purchase (*Merriam-Webster*, 2018b). Currently, hospitals employ about 61% of working nurses. Eighteen percent work in ambulatory care services, 7% in nursing and residential care facilities, 5% in government, and 3% in educational services (Bureau of Health Statistics, 2018b).

To evaluate the supply of RNs in the United States, it is necessary to look at both RNs who are currently working and those who are eligible to work, but do not. In addition, the current and potential student pool must be part of the supply discussion.

The United States currently has about 2.7 million RNs filling just under 3 million jobs (Bureau of Health Statistics, 2018a). Despite declining vacancy rates, particularly at hospitals, the RN population does not appear to be large enough to meet either short- or long-term needs in hospitals or other health care settings. This is because the supply of RNs is expected to grow minimally in the coming decade, but large numbers of nurses are expected to retire. The American Nurses Association (ANA) estimates that 23% or 187,200 RNs plan to retire in the next 2 to 3 years, and an additional 81,900 will switch to part-time status. In addition, the rising demand for Advance Practice Nurses could draw another 198,000 RNs from the bedside (Nursing Solutions Inc, 2016). In total, it is estimated that 269,100 RNs will exit the workforce or reduce hours in the immediate near future (Nursing Solutions Inc, 2016).

Faller (2018) suggests that the tsunami of retirements among Baby-Boomer nurses has already begun. In addition to workforce shortages, the retirement wave of Baby-Boomer nurses will create a particular drain on clinical expertise and institutional knowledge, which are critical to quality patient care and organizational success for health care providers. Faller suggests this impending crisis must be immediately addressed by health care employers.

> *Consider This* Supply shortages are more difficult to solve than demand-induced shortages because they require longer-term solutions.

Nursing as a "Graying" Population

Nursing is a graying population—even more so than the population at large. The median age of U.S. nurses is 46 years, and older nurses make up the largest age group in the nursing profession at around 25% ("What is the Average Age," 2018). An online nursing forum noted that most nurses expect to retire in their fifties ("What is the Average Age," 2018). This means that the nursing workforce will be retiring at a rate faster than it can be replaced.

Indeed, according to a 2015 study, almost 40% of RNs are over the age of 50 and the number of nurses leaving the workforce each year has been growing steadily from around 40,000 in 2010 to nearly 80,000 by 2020 (Montana State University, 2015). In addition, the Health Resources and Services Administration projects that more than 1 million RNs will reach retirement age within the next 10 to 15 years (AACN, 2017a).

> **Discussion Point**
>
> Why is there so little discussion about the "expertise gap" that will occur as a result of impending nursing retirements?

Given the demographics of the nursing workforce, an aging pattern is expected to continue over the next decade. Indeed, the average age of the working nurse has been increasing for some time, reflecting a two- to three-decade-long trend toward older students entering nursing education programs.

> **Discussion Point**
>
> What factors have led to the "graying" of the nursing workforce? Does there appear to be any short-term resolution of these factors?

In addition, nursing faculty are even grayer than the nursing population at large. The average age of nursing faculty members continues to increase, narrowing the number of productive years nurse educators can teach. The AACN (2017b) notes in their *2015-2016 Salaries of Instructional and Administrative Nursing Faculty* that the average ages of doctorally prepared nurse faculty holding the ranks of professor, associate professor, and assistant professor were 62.2, 57.6, and 51.1 years, respectively. For master's degree–prepared nurse faculty, the average ages for professors, associate professors, and assistant professors were 57.8, 56.6, and 50.9 years, respectively. The AACN concludes that a wave of faculty retirements is expected across the United States over the next decade.

According to a *Special Survey on Vacant Faculty Positions* released by AACN in October 2016, a total of 1,567 faculty vacancies were identified in a survey of 821 nursing schools with baccalaureate and/or graduate programs across the country (85.7% response rate). Besides the vacancies, schools cited the need to create an additional 133 faculty positions to accommodate student demand. The data show a national nurse faculty vacancy rate of 7.9%. Most of the vacancies (92.8%) were faculty positions requiring or preferring a doctoral degree.

One must question where the faculty will come from to teach the new nurses needed to solve the current shortage. In addition, given the lag time required to educate masters- or doctorally prepared faculty, the faculty shortage may end up being the greatest obstacle to solving any short-term nursing shortages.

> **Consider This** Even if enough students can be recruited to become nurses, there will likely not be enough faculty to teach them.

Cusson (2014) suggests a two-pronged approach to the nurse faculty shortage. She suggests a short-term approach of creating incentives for part-time and clinical adjunct faculty to return to school for advanced degrees and providing built-in periodic raises and use of a full-time clinical coordinator to support these faculty, so they can be more closely connected to the school's curriculum and mission.

The long-term approach is to recruit graduate students to join the ranks of their professors as well as providing scholarship support for students interested in a teaching career.

Fortunately, many foundations and funders have stepped forward to do just this. In 2011, the AACN and the Jonas Center for Nursing Excellence entered into a collaboration to increase the number of doctorally prepared faculty available to teach in nursing schools nationwide. This initiative supports 198 doctoral students in 87 schools across the United States, providing financial assistance, leadership development, and mentoring support to expand the pipeline of future nurse faculty into research-focused (PhD, DNS) and practice-focused (DNP) doctoral nursing programs (AACN, 2017b).

Enrollment in Nursing Schools

The number of students enrolled or projected to enroll in nursing programs is also an important factor in determining RN supply. Unfortunately, some schools of nursing have closed nursing programs because of funding cuts or to reduce program size. Still others have been forced to turn away potential students because of a lack of faculty. Despite this, enrollment in nursing schools steadily increased every year for almost a decade and has remained fairly stable since 2014 (only a 3.6% increase in entry-level baccalaureate programs in nursing 2016; Table 6.1). Unfortunately, however, these increases will not be adequate to replace those nurses who will be lost to retirement in

TABLE 6.1	**Number of Candidates Taking the National Council Licensure Examination for Registered Nurses: First-Time, U.S.-Educated Candidates Only**					
Program	**2012**	**2013**	**2014**	**2015**	**2016**	**2017**
Diploma	3,173	2,840	2,787	2,607	2,745	2,222
Baccalaureate	62,535	65,406	68,175	70,857	72,637	75,944
Associate	84,517	86,772	86,377	84,379	81,653	79,511
Total	150,266	155,098	157,372	157,882	157,053	157,720

Source: National Council of State Boards of Nursing. (2018, January 19). *2017: Number of candidates taking NCLEX examination and percent passing, by type of candidate.* Retrieved May 12, 2018, from https://www.ncsbn.org/Table_of_Pass_Rates_2017.pdf; National Council of State Boards of Nursing. (2017, January 23). *2016: Number of candidates taking NCLEX examination and percent passing, by type of candidate.* Retrieved May 12, 2018, from https://ncsbn.org/Table_of_Pass_Rates_2016.pdf; National Council of State Boards of Nursing. (2016, January 21). *2015: Number of candidates taking NCLEX examination and percent passing, by type of candidate.* Retrieved May 12, 2018, from https://ncsbn.org/Table_of_Pass_Rates_2015_(3).pdf; National Council of State Boards of Nursing. (2015, January 21). *2014: Number of candidates taking NCLEX examination and percent passing, by type of candidate.* Retrieved May 12, 2018, from https://ncsbn.org/Table_of_Pass_Rates_2014.pdf; National Council of State Boards of Nursing. (2014, January 21). *2013: Number of candidates taking NCLEX examination and percent passing, by type of candidate.* Retrieved May 12, 2018, from https://ncsbn.org/Table_of_Pass_Rates_2013.pdf; National Council of State Boards of Nursing. (2013, February 1). *2012: Number of candidates taking NCLEX examination and percent passing, by type of candidate.* Retrieved May 12, 2018, from https://ncsbn.org/Table_of_Pass_Rates_2012.pdf

the coming decade or to meet the increasing demand for more nurse faculty, researchers, and primary care providers (AACN, 2017a).

Unfortunately, enrollment increases are not possible without a significant boost in federal and state funding to prepare new faculty, enhance teaching resources, and upgrade nursing school infrastructure. More money is needed in the form of nursing scholarships and loans to encourage young people to enter nursing. In addition, individual nurses and professional organizations must support legislation to improve financial access to nursing education. The Tri-Council for Nursing (comprising the AACN, the ANA, the American Organization of Nurse Executives, and the National League for Nursing [NLN]) has urged nurses to advocate for increased nursing education funding under Title VIII of the Public Health Service Act, as well as other publicly funded initiatives, so that there will be the necessary capacity and resources to educate future nurses.

There have, however, been increases in federal money for nursing education over the last decade. The passage of legislation such as the 2002 Nurse Reinvestment Act encouraged more students to choose nursing as a career and helped students financially to complete their education. It also encouraged graduate students to complete their studies and assume teaching positions in nursing schools. In addition, many states introduced or passed legislation designed to improve working conditions and attract more nurses.

In addition, some hospitals have joined forces with local schools of nursing to offer scholarships in exchange for a student's willingness to work in that institution after graduation. Hospitals are also lending master's and doctorally prepared nurses such as nurse practitioners, clinical nurse specialists, and clinical nurse leaders to supplement faculty positions.

Private foundations have also stepped up to offer funding for nursing education. For example, in 2008, the Robert Wood Johnson Foundation (RWJF, 2016) joined with the AACN to create the RWJF New Careers in Nursing. Through grants to schools of nursing, the program has provided scholarships of $10,000 each annually to more than 3,500 scholars. Similarly, foundations set up by nursing organizations such as the Association of Perioperative Registered Nurses, the National Student Nurses' Association, and the ANA provide scholarships and financial assistance to students and RNs pursuing degrees in nursing.

Ironically, recruitment efforts into the nursing profession in the last decade have been very successful, and the problem is no longer a lack of nursing school applicants. Indeed, enrollment in nursing programs of education has increased steadily since 2001. The problem is that there are inadequate resources to provide nursing education to those interested in pursuing nursing as a career, including an insufficient number of clinical sites, classroom space, nursing faculty, and clinical preceptors. As a result, qualified applicants are turned away, despite the current shortage of nurses.

Indeed, the AACN (2017b) reported that U.S. nursing schools turned away 64,067 qualified applicants from baccalaureate and graduate nursing programs in 2016 because of an insufficient number of faculty, clinical sites, classroom space, clinical preceptors, and budget constraints. Most nursing schools responding to the survey pointed to faculty shortages as a reason for not accepting all qualified applicants into baccalaureate programs. Robert Rosseter, spokesman for the AACN, called it a "catch 22 situation," noting a tremendous demand from hospitals and clinics to hire more nurses as well as a tremendous demand from students who want to enter nursing programs. Yet schools cannot accommodate either demand (Kavilanz, 2018).

Educational costs are also a deterrent to increasing nursing school enrollment. Nursing is often called an "expensive major" given relatively low faculty-to-student ratios in clinical courses and the need for financially strapped states to subsidize the cost of education at state universities.

Discussion Point

Should the increased cost of nursing education be passed on to students? Would students enrolled in public universities be willing to pay more for their education than students in other majors?

The greatest challenge, however, to increasing nursing school enrollment is an inadequate number of nursing faculty to teach students interested in pursuing nursing as a career. According to a 2016 *Special Survey on Vacant Faculty Positions* released by AACN (2017b), a total of 1,567 faculty vacancies were identified in a survey of 821 nursing schools with baccalaureate and/or graduate programs across the country (85.7% response rate). Besides the vacancies, schools cited the need to create an additional 133 faculty positions to accommodate student demand. The data show a national nurse faculty vacancy rate of 7.9%. Most of the vacancies (92.8%) were faculty positions requiring or preferring a doctoral degree. Most schools identify difficulty finding doctorally prepared faculty and noncompetitive salaries as roots of the problem (AACN, 2017b).

Research conducted by the NLN (n.d.) and the Carnegie Foundation Preparation for the Professions Program supports AACN's suppositions. This research found an aging, overworked faculty earning far less than nurses entering clinical practice. In fact, this study reported that nurse faculty earned less than faculty in other academic disciplines and that they earned far less than their RN counterparts in clinical practice. This lack of competitive pay for nurse educators is a significant obstacle to recruiting new nursing faculty.

At the professor rank, nurse educators suffered the largest deficit, with salaries averaging 45% lower than those of their non-nurse colleagues. Associate and assistant nursing professors were also at a disadvantage, earning 19% and 15% less than similarly ranked faculty in other fields. Those employed as nursing instructors experienced the only advantage, with salaries averaging 8% higher than those of non-nurses (NLN, n.d., para. 2).

Increasing the number of nursing students in the pipeline as a strategy for addressing the current nursing shortage depends on having enough qualified faculty to teach them. Clearly, the same energy that was directed at recruiting young people for nursing must now be directed at recruiting nursing faculty.

In response, programs have been created both to encourage nurses to consider careers in nursing education and to support them in that role. For example, the Division of Labor Workforce Investment Act has created a Faculty Loan Repayment Program for nurses willing to serve in faculty roles after graduation. Furthermore, the National Institute of Nursing Research, the Agency for Health Care Research and Quality, Department of Veterans Affairs, and other private foundations have funds available to enhance nursing education and faculty development.

In addition, AACN and the Johnson & Johnson Campaign for Nursing's Future announced the creation of a Minority Nurse Faculty Scholars program in 2008 (AACN, 2017b). This program seeks to address the nursing faculty shortage and diversity of the faculty population by providing financial support to graduate nursing students from minority backgrounds who agree to teach in a school of nursing after graduation. In late 2012, the Jonas Nurse Leaders Scholar Program expanded nationally and now provides funding and support to 198 doctoral nursing students in 87 schools across the United States, making it one of the largest programs addressing the nation's dire shortage of doctorally prepared nursing faculty (AACN, 2017b).

To support the retention of new nursing faculty, the Elsevier Foundation awarded a grant to the Sigma Theta Tau International (STTI) (now called Sigma) Foundation for Nursing in 2009 to create a Nurse Faculty Mentored Leadership Development Program. Early career nurse educators with an advanced degree were selected to receive 18 months of leadership training designed to help them overcome the challenges of transitioning from nursing practice to faculty (Elsevier Foundation, 2015). "The program

---

BOX 6.1   **Long-Term Strategies for Addressing the Nursing Faculty Shortage**

1. Recruitment
   - Provide a positive image for a career in nursing education.
   - Provide incentives for part-time and adjunct faculty to return to school to earn doctoral degrees.
   - Provide fellowships or tuition forgiveness in exchange for teaching service.
   - Develop mentoring/support programs for new academics.
2. Retention
   - Provide salaries and benefits for nursing faculty similar to that in nonacademic settings.
   - Establish positive work environments and reasonable teaching assignments.
   - Recognize and reward teaching excellence.
   - Create academic environments that foster innovation.
   - Fund faculty development and mentorship programs.
3. Collaboration
   - Partner with health care stakeholders to create support for higher education in nursing.

---

reflects the Elsevier Foundation's effort to alleviate the nurse faculty crisis by providing knowledge, skill development opportunities and support to retain new nurse educators who have transitioned into the role" (Elsevier Foundation, 2015). Other long-term strategies for addressing the nursing faculty shortage are shown in Box 6.1.

Consider This Unfilled faculty positions, resignations, and projected retirements continue to pose a threat to the nursing education workforce.

Using Foreign-Born Nurses to Relieve the Shortage

The shortage has also been alleviated at least in part by the importation of RNs from foreign markets. Widespread, transnational nursing migration is likely to continue for some time, given the success hospitals have had with foreign recruitment and the time required to strengthen the domestic nurse supply pipeline. Such practice, however, could potentially have negative implications in terms of the domestic job market and health care quality. In addition, using foreign-born labor has complex international implications, creating a drain on some countries' health care systems while shoring up the economies of countries that purposefully export their workers. Because the importation of nurses has such complex ramifications, a separate chapter is devoted to its discussion (see Chapter 7).

ROOTS OF THE SHORTAGE

Many factors contribute to the current nursing shortage in acute care settings, including an aging workforce, high turnover because of worker dissatisfaction, inadequate long-term pay incentives, and an increasing recognition by nurses that they can make more money and act more autonomously as free agents than as full-time employees of a health care organization. These factors and others (Box 6.2) will be discussed in this section.

The Free Agent Nurse

An increase in the number of free agent nurses is another aspect that must be examined in assessing supply and demand factors of the current nursing shortage. Full-time

---

employment of nurses is decreasing. Instead, nurses are increasingly assuming the role of *free agent*, a term more common to Generation X than their older counterparts, and this contributes to a shortage in acute-care agencies. A free agent nurse is often an independent contractor who sells his or her services to an employer, with the condition that he or she maintains control over the number of hours they are willing to work and working conditions.

Per-diem and *traveling nurses* are two types of free agents. The relationship between the free agent and his or her employing organization is based on a free and open exchange, more of a partnership than an unequal dependency relationship. Typically, the free agent nurse makes a higher hourly wage than other full-time or part-time employees in a health care organization in exchange for not receiving health care and retirement benefits. Such nurses also have greater control over if and when they want to work.

Historically, health care organizations have sought to employ full-time workers (employees) so that they could better control the availability of needed human resources. However, the free agent model of nursing is gaining momentum in health care organizations as they recognize that they need to supplement their full-time employee pool with these skilled workers and that significant benefit costs can be saved from using free agent or temporary workers.

Critics of the increased use of free agent nurses, particularly traveling nurses, suggest that this practice may negatively affect the quality of care related to inconsistency of caretakers and a reduced ability to determine the competencies of the specific free agent nurse. More research is needed, however, on the effect of the free agent nurse on the current nursing shortage.

Workplace Dissatisfaction

Perhaps one of the most significant yet least addressed factors leading to the current RN shortage is workplace dissatisfaction, resulting in high turnover levels and nurses leaving the profession. Long shifts, low autonomy, mandatory overtime, and being forced to work during weekends, nights, and holidays prompt many nurses to look for other jobs.

A 2014 RWJF study found that an estimated 17.5% of newly licensed RNs leave their first nursing job within the first year and one in three (33.5%) leave within 2 years (New York University, 2014).

A literature review by Goodare (2017) suggests that more than half of the nursing profession feel they are underpaid and overworked, resulting in an increased likelihood of patient's needs not being met. In addition, the research suggested that lengthy hours, quality of working environments, a lack of leadership, and the aging population and

---

BOX 6.2	**Causes of the Current Nursing Shortage**

- Increasing elderly population (more individuals who are chronically ill)
- Increased acuity in acute care settings, requiring higher-level nursing skills
- Downsizing and restructuring of the late 1990s, which eliminated many registered nurses (RN) positions
- A relatively healthy economy in the late 1990s and early 2000s, which encouraged some nurses to change from full-time employment to part-time or to quit.
- Aging RN workforce
- Workplace dissatisfaction
- Women choosing fields other than nursing for a career
- Aging faculty for RN programs
- Inadequate nursing programs to accommodate interested applicants
- Low ceiling on wages for RNs without advanced degrees
- Future educator pool for RNs more limited than demand

workforce were all seen as influential factors in nursing turnover (see Research Fuels the Controversy 6.1).

Some organizational turnover is normal and, in fact, desirable because it infuses the organization with fresh ideas. It also reduces the probability of *groupthink*, in which everyone shares similar thought processes, values, and goals (Marquis & Huston, 2017). However, excessive or unnecessary turnover reduces the ability of the organization to produce its end product. Thus, retention becomes a critical goal when workforce shortages exist, and the achievement of desired outcomes is critical to organizational success.

> **Consider This** Retention of precious nurse resources must be a very real part of the solution to the nursing shortage; health care institutions must make a commitment to improving working conditions for nurses.

Unfortunately, many highly trained, employable nurses are *voluntarily* leaving the profession. Annual turnover in acute care hospitals for bedside nurses was 16.2% in 2016, up from 13.1% in 2012 (Nursing Solutions Inc, 2017). Personal reasons (caring for a child/parent, marriage, disability, etc.), relocation, and career advancement were the top drivers for turnover in 2016 (Nursing Solutions Inc, 2017). Other often cited reasons included salary, workload/staffing ratios, retirement, scheduling, immediate manager, commute/location, and education.

High levels of turnover are disruptive to organizational functioning and threaten the quality of patient care. High turnover rates are also generally expensive. It costs roughly $60,000 to replace a nurse, including recruitment and training downtime ("What is the Average," 2018). In addition, the average time to fill an RN vacancy in 2015 was 85 days, ranging from 53 to 110 days, given specialty (Nursing Solutions Inc, 2016).

Not all health care organizations, however, have high turnover rates. Organizations perceived to be employers of choice, such as magnet hospitals, retain their employees and are more capable of replacing losses than less-sought-after employers. Therefore, having a healthy work environment provides an advantage in the competition for scarce nursing resources. Clearly, organizations that pay attention to the employee market and understand what people are looking for in the work environment have a better chance to recruit and retain top talent.

> **Consider This** Nursing shortages cannot be resolved until we address the underlying issues of worker dissatisfaction that caused them in the first place.

Is Pay an Issue?

Salaries also provide mixed incentives for young people to become nurses and for nurse retention. The economy at the end of the 20th century was fairly strong, with low unemployment and rising consumer confidence. This resulted in some RNs, who were often the second breadwinner in the

---

Research Fuels the Controversy 6.1

This literature review exploring the causes of nurses reducing their hours in the workplace or leaving the profession involved a search of three electronic databases: CINAHL (Cumulative Index for Nursing and Allied Health Literature), PubMed, and Medline via PubMed. In addition, semi-structured interviews played a sizeable part in this investigative process centered around social science.

Source: Goodare, P. (2017, June 1). Literature review: Why do we continue to lose our nurses? *Australian Journal of Advanced Nursing, 34*(4), 50–56.

Study Findings

The literature review suggested that the shortage of nursing professionals has been a known and ongoing crisis worldwide for the past decade. A multitude of reasons were identified for nurses leaving the profession, with multiple groups and subgroups of identified issues. High stress, low monetary compensation, and unrealistic workloads were major factors in nurse turnover. Indeed, the researcher noted that the image of a nurse has changed from that of a "caring and calm" health care professional to a "caring but stressed" health care professional. Conclusions highlighted the need to make nurses a central focus in the health care industry. In addition, reductions in workload were recommended as was an assurance of strength in support and guidance, within leaders in the profession. Furthermore, the researcher suggested more support for older and more experienced nurses, in order to maintain and perhaps revive the values of nursing.

family unit, reducing their work hours or leaving the workplace entirely. Many of these same RNs, however, returned to work in the past decade because of declining stock market values, a rising recession, and lower levels of consumer confidence.

Wages for RNs have, however, increased with rising demand and progression of the shortage. The median annual wage of RNs as of May 2017 was $70,000 (Bureau of Health Statistics, 2018c). Another source suggests that experience nurses (more than 20 years), on average, earn more than those at entry level ($68,000 median annual salary as compared to $55,000; PayScale, 2018a).

Current average base salaries for nurse practitioners range from $73,233 to $116,431 with bonuses and profit sharing often adding up to $20,000 additional wages annually (PayScale, 2018b). Similarly, according to the American Academy of Nurse Practitioners, the average salary of a nurse practitioner, across settings and specialties, was $94,050 (AACN, 2017a).

> ### Discussion Point
> Historically, nursing has been considered an altruistic profession. How critical do you think pay is as a motivator for people who want to become nurses today?

In contrast to the findings for staff nurses, salary is clearly a deterrent for nursing faculty, although Cusson (2014) suggests that flexible hours, the ability to work from home, generous benefit packages (particularly at state institutions), and academic calendars provide opportunities for a better lifestyle than do many clinical positions. PayScale (2018c) reported that the median salary in 2018 for a nurse educator was $72,570 (PayScale, 2018c). Similarly, AACN (2017b) reported that master's-prepared assistant professor earned an annual average salary of $77,022 in 2016.

One reason that nursing faculty salaries are poorer comparatively than nurses with graduate degrees in advanced practice roles is that nursing education has never had the same federal funding support as medical education. In addition, securing advanced academic degrees is costly. Indeed, many graduate students who may have become educators in the past are now opting instead for better-paying positions in clinical and private practice. Clearly, increasing faculty salaries and providing tuition support for graduate students considering a career as a nursing faculty will be an essential part of addressing the increasing faculty shortage.

> ### Discussion Point
> What incentives should be offered to nurses who earn a master's or doctoral degree to become nursing faculty members rather than advanced practice nurses engaged in clinical practice?

CONSEQUENCES OF NURSING SHORTAGES

What are the consequences of a nursing shortage? To answer this question, it is critical first to recognize that patient outcomes are sensitive to nursing interventions and that, as a result, nurse staffing (total hours of care as well as staffing mix) affects patient outcomes. This supposition is certainly supported by a review of the literature, which increasingly suggests that RN staffing affects patient outcomes such as inpatient mortality and other measures of quality of hospital care. Indeed, numerous studies have been conducted to describe the relationship between nurse staffing levels and clinical outcomes of patients at both the hospital and unit levels. These studies are summarized in Chapter 9.

ADDITIONAL STRATEGIES FOR SOLVING A NURSING SHORTAGE

Just as the issues that caused nursing shortages are complex, so too must be the solutions. Only some of the solutions that have been presented to address the current nursing shortage are included here, including redesigning the workplace, increasing the number of nursing students in the pipeline, importing foreign nurses, improving nursing's image, and increasing the faculty pool. In addition, Box 6.3 includes a list of 11 strategies created by Sigma (STTI, 2018) for reducing the current shortage.

Redesigning the Workplace for an Older Workforce

The age of the current nursing workforce is an important factor in the current nursing shortage because nursing can be both physically and mentally taxing, even to the young. Some experts have suggested that more attention should be given to retaining older workers or bringing retired nurses back into the workforce because these employees are generally more productive, more reliable, and highly experienced. Some adaptations of the working environment may be needed, however, to meet the needs and limitations of an aging workforce such as flexible work shift options and job sharing.

BOX 6.3   Strategies for Addressing Nursing Shortages

- Demonstrate to health care leaders that nurses are the critical difference in the U.S. health care system.
- Reposition nursing as a highly versatile profession in which young people can learn science and technology, customer service, critical thinking, and decision-making skills.
- Construct practice environments that are interdisciplinary and build on relationships among nurses, physicians, other health care professionals, patients, and communities.
- Create patient care models that encourage professional nurse autonomy and clinical decision making.
- Develop additional evaluation systems that measure the relationship of timely nursing interventions to patient outcomes.
- Establish additional standards and mechanisms for recognition of professional practice environments.
- Develop career enhancement incentives for nurses to pursue professional practice.
- Evaluate the effects of the nursing shortage on the preparation of the next generation of nurse educators, nurse administrators, and nurse researchers and take strategic action.
- Implement and sustain a marketing effort that addresses the image of nursing and the recruitment of qualified students into nursing as a career.
- Promote higher education to nurses of all educational levels.
- Develop and implement strategies to promote the retention of RNs and nurse educators in the workforce.

Source: Sigma Theta Tau International Honor Society of Nursing. (2018). *Facts on the nursing shortage.* Retrieved from https://www.sigmanursing.org/why-sigma/about-sigma/sigma-media/nursing-shortage-information, reprinted with permission.

Nursing Solutions Inc (2017) notes, however, that although 60.7% of hospitals have strategies in place to protect new hires, only 19.0% have a strategy on retaining older workers. With retirement being a major driver of turnover, hospitals will need to focus more energy on retaining this knowledge base.

In addition, RNs must be made to feel valued, and physician–nurse relationships reflecting collegiality and collaboration should be fostered. In addition, environments of shared governance should be created in which nurses actively participate in all decision making related to patient care. Staff nurses should feel empowered, and autonomy should be encouraged. Additional strategies for retaining older workers are shown in Box 6.4.

Changing Nursing's Image

Price and McGillis Hall (2014) note that stereotypical imaging and messaging of the nursing profession have been shown to shape nurses' expectations and perceptions of nursing as a career, which has implications for both recruitment and retention. Students interested in nursing may be dissuaded from choosing it as a career based on negative, stereotypical images, especially those that position the profession as inferior to medicine. Thus, strategies for future recruitment and socialization within the nursing and the health professions need to include contemporary and realistic imaging of both health professional roles and practice settings (Price & McGillis Hall, 2014). This will not be an easy task, given the historical roots of nursing stereotypes and the profession's long history of being unable to effectively change public perceptions regarding professional nursing roles and behaviors (see Chapter 23).

BOX 6.4   Strategies for Retaining Older Workers

- Flexible shift options with more options for shorter shifts
- Job-sharing
- Work redesign to limit physical energy expenditure
- Use lift teams, special beds, and equipment to reduce work-related injuries and strain
- Benefit packages that recognize the needs of mature workers
- Recognize and use experienced workers as mentors and preceptors

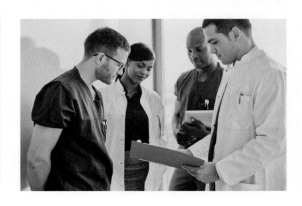

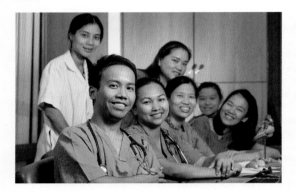

be hard-pressed to find a congressperson or senator who would not identify health care workforce shortages as one of the most serious issues affecting health care today.

Yet, efforts to proactively address the coming shortage have, to date, been few and far between. Short-term solutions to the shortage have been attempted, including importing foreign nurses and increasing federal money for nursing education. The passage of current legislation has encouraged more students to choose nursing as a career and has helped students financially to complete their education. It has also encouraged graduate students to complete their studies and assume teaching positions in nursing schools. Long-term planning and aggressive intervention, however, will be needed for some time at the national and regional levels to ensure that an adequate, highly qualified nursing workforce will be available in the future to meet health care needs in the United States.

CONCLUSIONS

Many factors led to a significant professional nursing shortage in the early 21st century and a mitigation of that shortage early in the second decade. This shortage is again recurring as the economy improves, demand increases, and an aging workforce retires. Health care providers, the public, and legislators are beginning to recognize that both the problem and the potential consequences could be severe. One would

More must be done to address the predicted future nursing shortage, and it is increasingly obvious that multiple solutions to the shortage will be needed. These solutions will require the best thinking of experts and will likely reshape fundamental core underpinnings that have been a part of the nursing work world for decades, if not centuries.

For Additional Discussion

1. In what ways do other professions do a better job of attracting younger workers—both men and women?

2. Are salaries a significant driver in the current nursing shortage? At what level would salaries not be a factor?

3. How would increasing the educational level for entry into practice affect the current nursing shortage?

4. Will the demand for RNs in the future be affected by growing technologic developments?

5. Why has the nursing workforce historically suffered some degree of a shortage every 10 to 15 years?

6. If Magnet hospital criteria (increased number of BSN-educated nurses on staff) become the baseline for organizational structure and performance, would nursing shortages exist?

7. Why are starting salaries for nurses with master's and doctoral degrees in academia so low?

8. Why do many health care organizations choose to expend more money on recruitment than on retention strategies? Which is more effective in the short term and in the long term?

9. Is implementation of mandatory minimum staffing ratios in acute care hospitals likely to reduce the nursing shortage in California?

References

American Association of Colleges of Nursing. (2017a). *Fact sheets: Nursing shortage.* Retrieved from http://www.aacnnursing.org/News-Information/Fact-Sheets/Nursing-Shortage

American Association of Colleges of Nursing. (2017b). *Fact sheet: Nursing faculty shortage.* Retrieved June 30, 2017, from http://www.aacnnursing.org/News-Information/Fact-Sheets/Nursing-Faculty-Shortage

Bureau of Health Statistics, U.S. Department of Labor. (2018a). *Registered nurses.* Retrieved May 12, 2018, from http://www.bls.gov/ooh/Healthcare/Registered-nurses.htm

Bureau of Health Statistics, U.S. Department of Labor. (2018b). *Occupational outlook handbook—Registered nurses (2016–2017 ed.).* Retrieved June 30, 2017, from https://www.bls.gov/ooh/healthcare/registered-nurses.htm#tab-6

Bureau of Health Statistics, U.S. Department of Labor. (2018c). *Registered nurses. Pay.* Retrieved May 12, 2018, from https://www.bls.gov/ooh/healthcare/registered-nurses.htm#tab-5

Cusson, R. (2014, March 20). How colleges can deal with the shortage of nursing professors. *UConn Today.* Retrieved June 29, 2017, from http://today.uconn.edu/blog/2014/03/how-colleges-can-deal-with-the-shortage-of-nursing-professors

Elsevier Foundation. (2015, February 23). *Insights into nurse faculty leadership academy.* Retrieved June 30, 2017, from http://www.elsevierfoundation.org/insights-into-our-nurse-faculty-leadership-academy-nfla-program/

Faller, M. (2018). *Retirement wave hits: Nursing shortages may worsen.* The Staffing Stream. Retrieved May 12, 2018, from http://www.thestaffingstream.com/2018/01/09/retirement-wave-hits-nursing-shortages-may-worsen/

Goodare, P. (2017, June 1). Literature review: Why do we continue to lose our nurses? *Australian Journal of Advanced Nursing, 34*(4), 50–56.

Kavilanz, P. (2018, April 30). *Nursing schools are rejecting thousands of applicants—in the middle of a nursing shortage.* CNN Money. Retrieved May 12, 2018, from http://money.cnn.com/2018/04/30/news/economy/nursing-school-rejections/index.html

Marquis, B., & Huston, C. (2017). *Leadership roles and management functions in nursing* (9th ed.). Philadelphia, PA: Wolters Kluwer.

Merriam Webster. (2018a). *Demand (definition).* Retrieved May 12, 2018, from https://www.merriam-webster.com/dictionary/demand

Merriam Webster. (2018b). *Supply (definition).* Retrieved May 12, 2018, from https://www.merriam-webster.com/dictionary/supply

Montana State University. (2015, September 21). Shortage of nurses not as dire as predicted, but challenges remain to meet America's needs. *Science Daily.* Retrieved June 30, 2017, from https://www.sciencedaily.com/releases/2015/09/150921153457.htm

National League for Nursing. (n.d.). *NLN nurse educator shortage fact sheet.* Retrieved from http://www.nln.org/docs/default-source/advocacy-public-policy/nurse-faculty-shortage-fact-sheet-pdf.pdf?sfvrsn=0

New York University. (2014, September 8). *Nearly one in five new nurses leave first job within a year, according to survey of newly-licensed registered nurses.* Retrieved June 30, 2017, from http://www.nyu.edu/about/news-publications/news/2014/09/08/nearly-one-in-five-new-nurses-leave-first-job-within-a-year-according-to-survey-of-newly-licensed-registered-nurses.html

Nursing Solutions Inc. (2016). *2016 healthcare staffing survey report.* Retrieved June 29, 2017, from http://www.nsinursingsolutions.com/Files/assets/library/workforce/Healthcare%20Staffing%20Survey%20Report%20-%202016.pdf

Nursing Solutions Inc. (2017). *2017 National health care retention & RN staffing report.* Retrieved May 12, 2018, from http://www.emergingrnleader.com/wp-content/uploads/2017/09/NationalHealthcareRNRetentionReport2017.pdf

PayScale. (2018a). *Registered nurse (RN) salary.* Retrieved May 12, 2018, from http://www.payscale.com/research/US/Job=Registered_Nurse_(RN)/Hourly_Rate

PayScale. (2018b). *Nurse practitioner (NP) salary (United States).* Retrieved May 12, 2018, from http://www.payscale.com/research/US/Job=Nurse_Practitioner_(NP)/Salary

PayScale. (2018c). *Nurse educator salary (United States).* Retrieved May 12, 2018, from http://www.payscale.com/research/US/Job=Nurse_Educator/Salary

Price, S. L., & McGillis Hall, L. (2014). The history of nurse imagery and the implications for recruitment: A discussion paper. *Journal of Advanced Nursing, 70*(7), 1502–1509. doi:10.1111/jan.12289

Robert Wood Johnson Foundation. (2016). *New careers in nursing. About.* Retrieved May 12, 2018, from http://www.newcareersinnursing.org/about-ncin.html

Sigma Theta Tau International Honor Society of Nursing. (2018). *Facts on the nursing shortage.* Retrieved May 12, 2018, from https://www.sigmanursing.org/why-sigma/about-sigma/sigma-media/nursing-shortage-information

Snavely, T. M. (2016). Data watch. A brief economic analysis of the looming nursing shortage in the United States. *Nursing Economic$, 34*(2), 98–100.

Trust for America's Health. (2018). *State data: Nursing shortage estimates (2010).* Retrieved May 12, 2018, from http://healthyamericans.org/states/states.php?measure=nursingshortage

What is the average age of retirement for nurses in the United States? (2018). Retrieved May 12, 2018, from https://www.bestmasterofscienceinnursing.com/faq/what-is-the-average-age-of-retirement-for-nurses-in-the-united-states/

Importing Foreign Nurses

Carol J. Huston

LEARNING OBJECTIVES

The learner will be able to:

1. Examine how the scope of global nurse migration has changed over the last decade.

2. Analyze "push" and "pull" factors that encourage nurses to migrate internationally.

3. Identify primary donor and recipient countries of migrating nurses.

4. Explore potential negative effects of international migration on donor countries, including "brain drain" from donor countries.

5. Apply the ethical principles of autonomy, utility, and justice in arguing for or against global nurse recruitment and migration.

6. Explore the ethical dimensions of nurse migration.

7. Outline common key components of position statements on nurse migration adopted by professional associations such as the International Council of Nurses, the International Centre on Nurse Migration, Academy Health, and the World Health Organization.

8. Explore national and international efforts to develop best practices or regulatory oversight of international nurse recruitment and migration.

9. Differentiate between the types of work visas foreign nurses use to gain entry for employment in the United States.

10. Outline the certification process required by the Commission on Graduates of Foreign Nursing Schools for migratory nurses to be able to take the NCLEX examination and obtain visas for work in the United States.

11. Discuss the need for ongoing cultural, professional, and psychological support for foreign nurses after their arrival in their importer country to assist them in successful socialization.

12. Reflect on personal beliefs and values regarding the use of widespread international recruitment and nurse migration to address nursing shortages.

INTRODUCTION

Many countries have experienced cyclical shortages of nurses, but typically they were caused by increasing demand outstripping a static or slowly growing supply of nurses. The current situation is different. Demand continues to grow, whereas supply decreases because of an aging workforce, projected increases in nursing retirements in the coming decade, and an inadequate number of new graduates from nursing education programs.

Indeed, half of the world does not have an adequate number of nurses (NurSearch, 2017). According to the World Health Organization (WHO), 48% of the member states have less than 3 nurses per 1,000 people and 27% of the world have less than 1 (NurSearch, 2017). By comparison, the United States has 10 nurses per 1,000 people. This shortage of nurses exacerbates the projected shortfall of 18 million health care workers worldwide by 2030 (Trines, 2018).

One increasingly common means of alleviating these shortages has been to recruit foreign workers. International recruitment and *nurse migration*—moving from one country to another in search of employment—has been viewed as a relatively inexpensive, "quick-fix" solution to health care worker shortages. The current situation, however, is different from the past, when nurse migration was mostly based on individual motivation and typically followed previous colonial ties. Now there is active planning of large-scale international nurse recruitment, often from developing countries that can least afford to lose their most highly educated health care workers.

This has significant local and regional implications. For example, nurse migration from developing countries has occurred at the same time that international resources were finally available to address human immunodeficiency virus and acquired immunodeficiency disease (HIV/AIDS) and improve immunization coverage around the world. This undermines efforts to address those problems in the donor countries. Another example is apparent in China, which has increasing numbers of elderly accompanied by a severe nursing shortage. The end result is that the wait time for a slot at a nursing home in Beijing amounted to 100 years in 2013 (Trines, 2018).

A recruiting onslaught affects the ability of developing countries to develop sustainable health care systems and provide appropriate care to their citizens. Indeed, few donor nations are prepared to manage the loss of their nurse workforce to such widespread migration. In addition, developing countries often recruit from each other, even within the same geographical region. Table 7.1 summarizes the

TABLE 7.1	**Effect of Push–Pull Migration on Select Countries**
Africa	Trines (2018) notes that sub-Saharan African countries bear 24% of the world's disease burden today but have only 3% of health workers and less than 1% of the world's financial resources to respond to this burden. Thus, the nursing shortage is more severe and felt more strongly in the source countries. The migration drains the source countries of desperately needed skilled personnel.
Australia	Australia has long imported foreign nurses to supplement its health care workforce and numbers are only increasing. In fact, 18.2% of nurses in Australia were foreign-trained in 2016 (up from 14% in 2009; Trines, 2018). About 3,000 registered nurses and midwives entered the Australian workforce on 457 work visas (a subclass of visa through which employers sponsor temporary skilled workers to work in Australia) in 2012–2013 (Toscano, 2015). Foreign nurses now make up 25% of all new entrants in the nation's nursing workforce each year (Toscano, 2015). In Australia, foreign-educated nurses are required to complete a 1- or 2-year pre-registration nurse course as well as language classes prior to employment. Individual nurses pay up to $20,000 per year for these courses. In addition, these nurses pay for their basic living costs. Thus, training migrant nurses is a profitable industry and contributes to the national economy.

(continued)

TABLE 7.1	**Effect of Push–Pull Migration on Select Countries (*continued*)**
Canada	Canada is both a source and a destination country for international nurse migration, with an estimated net loss of nurses. The United States is a major beneficiary of Canadian nurse emigration, resulting from the reduction of full-time jobs for nurses in Canada because of health system reforms. FWCanada Inc. (2014) notes there are two Canadian immigration programs foreign RNs can qualify for without the need of a job offer from a Canadian employer. The Quebec Skilled Worker program has long allowed foreign nurses to qualify for permanent residence. In August 2013, the Quebec government made changes to the program to allow nurses to earn even more points under this program. The other program is the Nova Scotia Provincial Nominee Program known as the Regional Labor Market Demand Stream. This program has designated 26 occupations that are in high demand in the province and has imposed relatively low barriers to apply.
China	Many Chinese nurses intend to migrate because of limited job opportunities, low salary, and low job satisfaction. Commercial recruiters have expressed a strong interest in recruiting Chinese nurses, but there are limited examples of successful ventures. It is likely that China will become an important source of nurses for developed nations in the coming years.
India	Despite an extremely low nurse-to-population ratio in India, large-scale nurse migration to other countries is increasing. Low wages, heavy workloads, poor working conditions, and a lack of respect are push factors for many Indian nurses to migrate.
Indonesia	Indonesia is recognized as an exporting country, with policies that encourage nursing professionals to emigrate abroad. Indonesia itself, however, is suffering from a crisis in nursing capacity and struggles with ensuring adequate health care access for its own populations (Efendi et al., 2017).
Ireland	As late as 25 years ago, Ireland had an abundant pool of nurses. Ireland now though actively recruits nurses from overseas. Thus, Ireland has moved from being a traditional exporter of nurses to an importer.
Lebanon	Lebanon is a source/donor country to the Persian Gulf, North America, and Europe. The primary push factors are poor working conditions and a lack of autonomy in decision making.
New Zealand	New Zealand has been both a source and destination country since the beginning of the 21st century. However, it currently has 27% of internationally qualified nurses in its workforce, one of the highest rates among countries in the Organisation of Economic Co-operation and Development (O'Connor, 2016). The movement of New Zealand RNs to Australia is expedited by the Trans-Tasman Agreement, whereas the entry of foreign RNs to New Zealand is facilitated by nursing being an identified priority occupation.
Pakistan	The burden of chronic and infectious diseases is very high in Pakistan, whereas the number of nurses is sixfold less than what is needed (Abbasi &Younas, 2016). Nurse migration from Pakistan to developed countries has contributed to adverse capacity development of nursing in Pakistan.
Philippines	The Philippines is a source country for nurse migration. National opinion has generally focused on the improved quality of life for individual migrants and their families and on the benefits of remittances to the nation; however, a shortage of highly skilled nurses and the massive retraining of physicians to become nurses elsewhere has created severe problems for the Filipino health system, including the closure of some hospitals.
Saudi Arabia	Saudi Arabia now gets most of its nurses from the Philippines—the same place where most countries, including the United States, are doing the majority of their recruiting.
South Korea	In line with the increasing significance of the role of transnational migration in health care provision especially in the West, slightly over 11,000 nurses and nurse assistants from South Korea were sent to former West Germany between the 1950s and the 1970s (Ahn, 2017).
United Kingdom	Both a donor and recipient county, nurse migration is common in the UK. A significant uptick in Bulgarian and Romanian nurse migration to the UK occurred in 2014 as a result of changes in immigration restrictions. Bulgaria and Romania were no longer subject to transitional employment restrictions as of January 1, 2014 (Office for National Statistics, 2014).
United States	Nurse immigration to the United States has tripled since 1994. "Foreign nurses" make up about 15% of registered nurses in the United States (Esposito, 2017). Foreign-educated nurses are located primarily in urban areas, most likely to be employed by hospitals, and somewhat more likely to have a baccalaureate degree than native-born nurses.

current dynamic nature of nurse migration in select countries around the world.

GLOBAL MIGRATION OF NURSES: "PUSH" AND "PULL" FACTORS

To understand what is driving the global migration of nurses, it is first necessary to examine what are known as the "push" and "pull" factors of nursing migration. *Push factors* are those factors that push or drive nurses to want to leave their countries to go to another. Low pay, inadequate opportunities for career advancement or continuing education, sociopolitical instability, and unsafe workplaces are examples of push factors. Other factors that act as push factors in some countries include the risk of HIV/AIDS to health system workers, concerns about personal security in areas of conflict, and economic instability.

> **Consider This** Nurses migrate for many reasons and the push/pull factors to migrate are in constant imbalance.

Pull factors are those factors that draw the nurse toward a different country. Pull factors typically include higher pay, more-developed career structures, opportunities for further education and professional development, and, in some cases, safety from the threat of violence (more prevalent in less-developed countries). Other pull factors, such as the opportunity to travel or to participate in foreign aid work, also influence some nurses. A summary of push and pull factors for nurse migration is given in Table 7.2.

It is important to remember that developed countries, such as Australia, the United Kingdom, the United States, Norway, Australia, Ireland, and Saudi Arabia, are the primary destinations of most migrant nurses, and developing nations are primarily the donors. Some developed countries are both a source and a recipient for the migrating nurses. Destination countries can recruit nurses as a result of a large number of pull factors. Many internationally recruited nurses suggest they would have preferred to remain in their home country with family and friends and in a familiar culture and environment, but push and pull factors overwhelmingly influenced their decision to migrate.

> **Consider This** Developed countries are often the recipients of migrant nurses and developing countries are often the donors. In essence then, developing countries are supporting the health care infrastructure of more developed countries, often at the expense of their own country.

TABLE 7.2   Push and Pull Factors for Nurse Migration

Push Factors	Pull Factors
Low pay	High pay
Inadequate opportunities for career advancement or continuing education	More developed career structures or opportunities for further education and professional development
Sociopolitical instability	Increased quality of life
Unsafe workplaces	Safety from the threat of violence
Practice restrictions	Family members in destination country
High workloads	Adventure/love of travel
Poor living conditions (housing, food, water)	Humanitarian motives
Remittance income	Recognition and status
Economic instability	Political stability

EFFECTS OF GLOBAL MIGRATION ON DEVELOPING COUNTRIES

A review of the literature suggests that different countries have experienced different effects because of the push–pull of international nurse migration. In some cases, aggressive recruitment, by which large numbers of recruits are sought, may significantly deplete a single health facility or contract an important number of newly graduated nurses from a single educational institute. This has significant local and regional implications because not only is critical intellectual capital taken away from the developing country but that country's health outcomes are likely to worsen.

The Philippines (see Fig. 7.1) has long been the number one exporter of nurses worldwide. China, with the second largest nursing workforce in the world (2.2 million nurses), is another country actively seeking to export nurses. Yet, a shortage of nurses has haunted China for years. Because of the large land mass, large population, and lack of retention in nursing, China's nursing shortage is more severe than in most developed countries and is getting worse (Wang, Whitehead, & Bayes, 2016). Only a small number of graduates are hired as permanent staff, with the majority of graduates placed on temporary contracts. This leads to instability and uncertainty among the nursing workforce, encouraging many graduates to migrate to other countries (Wang et al., 2016).

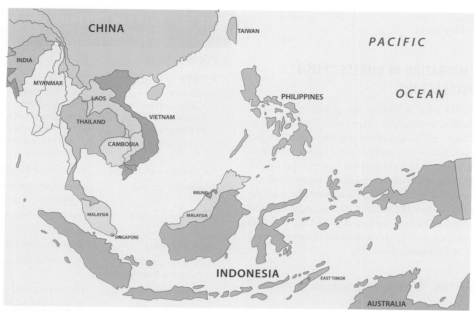

Figure 7.1 Map of Southeast Asia.

India is also gaining ground as one of the world's leading nurse exporters, despite having an extremely low nurse-to-population ratio. Surveys have shown that Indian migrant nurses, like their counterparts in other countries, are motivated to emigrate by better income prospects abroad, where they can easily earn 10 times as much than at home, as well as poor working conditions in India (Trines, 2018).

Nonetheless, recent reports from South Africa, Ghana, China, and the Caribbean highlight that such a significant outflow of nurses has had negative effects, including reductions in the level and quality of services and the loss of specialist skills. Similarly, African countries, particularly those in sub-Saharan Africa, have lost a substantial proportion of their skilled workforce through migration. Poor working conditions within the health sector, such as long work hours, high patient loads, inadequate resources, and occupational hazards, influence these nurses to consider migration.

Even the Philippines, an intentional exporter, is suffering from its migration practices. Castro-Palaganas et al. (2017) suggest that the massive expansion in education and training designed specifically for outmigration creates a domestic supply of health workers who cannot be absorbed by a system that is underfunded. This results in a paradox of underservice, especially in rural and remote areas, at the same time as underemployment and outmigration (Research Fuels the Controversy 7.1).

The economic cost of donor countries exporting their mostly highly educated workforce is staggering. Straehle (2017) notes that it costs approximately $65,997 to educate a doctor in Kenya and about $43,180 to educate a nurse. If a doctor leaves, the losses in returns for the training country's investment are estimated to be nearly eight times the cost for training the individual health care practitioner. Public finances deteriorate as a result of the loss in investment return, and the end result is that health professionals in the country may not be able to be employed because of a lack of funds.

> **Consider This** The positive global economic/social/professional development associated with international migration must be weighed against the substantial brain and skills drain experienced by donor countries.

Remittance Income

Some national governments and government agencies have, however, actually encouraged the outflow of nurses from their country, including Fiji, Jamaica, India, Mauritius, South

Research Fuels the Controversy 7.1

The Impact of Migration From the Philippines

This mixed-methods study employed a decentered, comparative approach that involved three phases: (a) a scoping review on health workers' migration of relevant policy documents and academic literature on health workers' migration from the Philippines; and primary data collection with (b) 37 key stakeholders and (c) household surveys with 7 doctors, 329 nurses, 66 midwives, and 18 physical therapists.

Source: Castro-Palaganas, E., Spitzer, D. L., Kabamalan, M. M., Sanchez, M. C., Caricativo, R., Runnels, V., . . . Bourgeault, I. L. (2017, March 31). An examination of the causes, consequences, and policy responses to the migration of highly trained health personnel from the Philippines: The high cost of living/leaving-a mixed method study. *Human Resources for Health, 15*, 1–14. doi:10.1186/s12960-017-0198-z

Study Findings

The migration of health workers has both positive and negative consequences for the Philippine health system and its health workers. Positive consequences include new opportunities for knowledge and technology transfer. Negative consequences include brain drain and the loss of investment in human capital. In addition, the gap in the supply of health workers has affected the quality of care delivered, especially in rural areas. At the household level, migration has engendered increased consumerism and materialism and fostered dependency on overseas remittances.

The researchers concluded that unless socioeconomic conditions are improved and health professionals are provided with better incentives, staying in the Philippines will not be a viable option. The massive expansion in education and training designed specifically for outmigration creates a domestic supply of health workers who cannot be absorbed by a system that is underfunded. This results in a paradox of underservice, especially in rural and remote areas, at the same time as underemployment and outmigration. Policy responses to this paradox have not yet been appropriately aligned to capture the multilayered and complex nature of these intersecting phenomena.

Africa, and the Philippines. For many years, the Philippine government actively endorsed and facilitated initiatives aimed at educating, recruiting, training, and placing nurses around the world. This was likely the result of a financial imperative, to encourage the generation of *remittance income*.

The International Centre on Nurse Migration (ICNM, 2014, para. 2) agrees, noting that "nurses' remittances represent an important course of added income and stability for individuals, families, and communities around the world. These funds lessen the burden on health systems by improving access to food, housing, and education—all three significant social determinants of health." In fact, the ICNM (2014) notes that migrants sent more than $414 billion back home in 2013.

Indeed, labor is the most profitable export of Philippines, with about 10 million citizens working around the globe and generating remittance income annually (Philippines Economy, 2018). Similarly, remittances from migrants are recognized as an important source of resilience for households in African countries.

> **Consider This** Migrating nurses often send remittances back home to support their families and bolster the economy; in addition, some workers later return home with enhanced skills and experience.

In addition, some donor countries overproduce nurses with the intent of export. For example, the mass export of nurses from the Philippines is a response to a labor market oversupply. Starting in the 1960s, the Philippine government created a systematic, state-sponsored system of labor exportation designed to foster economic development through remittances from overseas workers (Trines, 2018). Nurses played a central role in that strategy and were encouraged to emigrate. The end result was that the Philippines became the world's largest supplier of foreign-trained nurses. In addition poorly paid Filipino medical doctors, particularly from rural regions, began in the early 2000s to retrain as nurses to emigrate (Trines, 2018).

Brain Drain

It is *brain drain* that is one of the most critical negative consequences of widespread nursing migration from developing countries. Brain drain refers to the loss of skilled personnel and the loss of investment in education that is experienced when those human resources migrate elsewhere. Thus, brain drain typically occurs when the skilled professionals from less-developed countries migrate to more-developed countries, resulting in these developing countries losing their most highly skilled and educated workforce. In addition, resource-limited nations have overwhelmingly become donor countries. This is especially true for countries like South Africa, Ghana, India, and Pakistan where nurses are central to the health care systems and indeed are the most visible health care providers in those systems (Delucas, 2014). The consequences of this large-scale and nonstrategic migration are far-reaching, including a breakdown of national health care infrastructures and the inability of many donor countries to meet the health care needs of their own citizens.

For example, Jamaica's Minister of Health noted in 2017 that the brain drain of nurses has "virtually crippled the delivery of certain health care services and has had a dramatic effect on the overall quality of healthcare" (Trines, 2018, para. 39). He added that the English-speaking Caribbean at large will be facing a shortage of 10,000 nurses over the next 10 years.

Complaints of brain drain are heard from donor countries such as India, the Philippines, South Africa, and Zimbabwe. These nations argue that their human health care resources are being extracted at a time when they are needed most. This is the case even in many of the countries that have historically encouraged the exportation of their nurses. This suggests that the individual's right to choose cannot be easily negated simply because the donor country does not want to lose its highly educated human resources. Clearly, many nursing organizations and nursing leaders have begun to recognize the negative effects of international migration on "supplier" countries, but efforts to address the problem have been inadequate.

Finally, one must consider whether recruiting foreign nurses to solve acute staffing shortages is simply a poorly thought-out quick fix to a much greater problem and whether, in doing so, not only are donor nations harmed but also the issues that led to the shortage in the first place are never addressed. Certainly, one must at least question whether wholesale foreign nurse recruitment would even be necessary if importer nations made a more concerted effort to improve the working conditions, salaries, empowerment, and recognition of the home-born nurses they already employ.

Consider This Importing foreign nurses to solve the nursing shortage only puts a Band-Aid on the problem. The factors that led to the nursing shortage in the first place still need to be resolved.

Discussion Point

If the money that is being spent on recruitment and immigration of foreign nurses was instead spent on resolving the domestic nursing issues that led to a shortage in the first place, would international nurse recruitment even be necessary?

GLOBAL NURSE RECRUITMENT AND MIGRATION AS AN ETHICAL ISSUE

Controversy regarding the ethics of international recruitment of nurses is not new. Whenever resources are limited, ethical issues regarding their allocation are likely to arise. In the case of global nurse recruitment and migration, the ethical principles of autonomy, utility, and justice seem most relevant. Certainly, there must be some sort of a balance between the right of individual nurses to choose to migrate (autonomy), particularly when push factors are overwhelming, and the more utilitarian concern for the donor nations' health as a result of losing scarce nursing resources.

International law clearly guarantees an individual the right to freedom of movement and residence (as established in the Universal Declaration of Human Rights; United Nations General Assembly, 1948) and the International Covenant on Civil and Political Rights (Office of the United Nations High Commissioner for Human Rights, 1976). The individual's right to migrate is central to self-determination. Yet, how do countries experiencing institutional anemia balance the need for self-preservation with the right to freedom of movement?

Discussion Point

Should the right for the individual nurse to migrate (autonomy and self-determination) override what might be best for the donor nation (utilitarianism)?

Justice, or fairness, however, is another ethical principle that seems appropriate to this discussion because it examines how social and material goods are distributed to or withheld from members of a group or society, particularly in relation to fairness. Both recipient and donor countries have strong moral obligations to work toward fairer distributions of health care services as the fate of other communities cannot be ignored. Straehle (2017) concurs, suggesting that the right to migrate should be tied to the duties of justice that need to be satisfied before benefiting from migration. Societies would then be justified in restricting individuals in their exercise of freedom of movement if the unfettered exercise risks minimum access to health care for all.

Consider This The majority of countries importing foreign nurses are primarily White, and donor nations typically export nurses of color. The issue of race and the global economics of nursing should be examined in terms of effect on both supplier and donor countries.

Wild (2012) concurs, suggesting that there are many issues related to migration that have profound ethical relevance. For example,

Who deserves what in terms of health (care), and which role does citizenship or nationality play? How far should the responsibility of the receiving country go in terms of the health of migrants and why? Can restrictions to health care as a political instrument of deterrence be morally justified? Should there be a difference regarding health care between subgroups of migrants, for example, between forced and economic migrants, between legal and undocumented migrants, or between children and adults? (p. 12)

The ethical significance of these questions becomes especially salient in times of rising pressure on political parties to protect nation's citizens' resources.

Wild (2012) goes on to suggest that

there are bioethical justice theories for societies and, increasingly, theories on global health ethics that consider affluent countries' obligations toward developing countries. But there seems to be a blind spot when it comes to the specific question of what happens if people move into the boundaries, that is, into the sphere of responsibility of a country. There is no wider debate in bioethics on moral responsibilities that explicitly addresses the different groups of migrants, whether differential treatment for citizens can ever be morally justified, and how these moral evaluations should find their way into public and institutional policies. (p. 12)

In addition, migration numbers have increasingly become feminized. This impacts negatively on key education and health indicators including infant and child mortality and school enrollment rate by gender.

The following question then must be asked: Does global recruitment violate the principle of justice, particularly if such migration does not solve the underlying shortage and when such retention is done at the expense of the donor country? Clearly, donor countries have an ethical obligation to do what they can to provide their nurses with a safe, satisfying, and economically rewarding work environment. Importer countries have an ethical obligation to do what is necessary to be more self-reliant in meeting their professional workforce needs and to avoid recruiting nurses from those countries that can least afford to experience brain drain. Finally, professional health care associations must lead the way in addressing how best to respond to these ethical concerns.

PROFESSIONAL ORGANIZATIONS RESPOND

Given the current extent of nurse migration and the multiplicity of ethical dilemmas associated with it, many professional organizations, representing nurses from around the world, have weighed in on the issue. Some have provided formal position statements to guide both donor and importer countries. Others have attempted to provide guidance to the individual nurse considering global migration.

The International Council of Nurses

One international agency, the International Council of Nurses (ICN, 2017), has issued several position statements arguing for ethics and good employment practices in international recruitment (Box 7.1). The ICN, a federation of more than 130 national nurses' associations, represents more than 16 million nurses worldwide. The *ICN Position Statement: Nurse Retention and Migration* authored in 1999 and revised in 2007 confirms the right of nurses to migrate, as well as the potential beneficial outcomes of multicultural practice and learning opportunities supported by migration, but acknowledges potential adverse effects on the quality of health care in donor countries (ICN, 2007b).

The ICN (2007b) position statement also condemns the practice of recruiting nurses to countries where authorities have failed to implement sound human resource planning and to seriously address problems that cause nurses to leave the profession and discourage them from returning to nursing. The position statement also denounces unethical recruitment practices that exploit nurses or mislead them into accepting job responsibilities and working conditions that are incompatible with their qualifications, skills, and experience. The ICN and its member national nurses' associations call for a regulated recruitment process based on ethical principles that guide informed decision making and reinforce sound employment policies on the part of governments, employers, and nurses, thereby supporting fair and cost-effective recruitment and retention practices.

In addition, the ICN adopted a second position paper on ethical nurse recruitment in 2001 that was also revised and reaffirmed in 2007 (ICN, 2007a). This document identifies principles (Box 7.2) necessary to create a foundation for ethical recruitment, whether international or intranational contexts are being considered. The ICN suggests that all health sector stakeholders—patients, governments, employers, and nurses—will benefit if this ethical recruitment framework is systematically applied.

BOX 7.1   **ICN Position Statement on Nurse Retention, Transfer, and Migration (1999)**

ICN and its member associations firmly believe that quality health care is directly dependent on an adequate supply of qualified nursing personnel.

ICN recognizes the right of individual nurses to migrate, while acknowledging the possible adverse effect that international migration may have on health care quality.

ICN condemns the practice of recruiting nurses to countries where authorities have failed to address human resource planning and problems that cause nurses to leave the profession and discourage them from returning to nursing.

   In support of the above, ICN does the following:

- Disseminates information on nursing personnel needs and resources and on the development of fulfilling nursing career structures
- Provides training opportunities in negotiation and socioeconomic welfare–related issues
- Disseminates data on nursing employment worldwide
- Takes action to help reduce the serious effects of any shortage, maldistribution, and misutilization of nursing personnel
- Advocates adherence nationally to international labor standards
- Condemns the recruitment of nurses as a strike-breaking mechanism
- Advocates for open and transparent migration systems (recognizing that some appropriate screening is necessary to ensure public safety)
- Supports a transcultural approach to nursing practice
- Promotes the introduction of transferable benefits, for example, pension
     National nurses' associations are urged to do the following:
- Encourage relevant authorities to ensure sound human resources planning for nursing
- Participate in the development of sound national policies on immigration and emigration of nurses
- Promote the revision of nursing curriculum for basic and postbasic education in nursing and administration to emphasize effective nursing leadership
- Disseminate information on the working conditions of nurses
- Discourage nurses from working in other countries where salaries and conditions are not acceptable to nurses and professional associations in those countries
- Ensure that foreign nurses have conditions of employment equal to those of local nurses in posts requiring the same level of competency and involving the same duties and responsibilities
- Ensure that there are no distinctions made among foreign nurses from different countries
- Monitor the activities of recruiting agencies
- Provide an advisory service to help nurses interpret contracts and assist foreign nurses with personal and work-related problems, such as institutional racism, violence, and sexual harassment
- Provide orientation for foreign nurses on the local cultural, social, and political values and on the health system and national language
- Alert nurses to the fact that some diplomas, qualifications, or degrees earned in one country may not be recognized in another
- Assist nurses with their problems related to international migration and repatriation

---

Note: ICN, International Council of Nurses.
Source: International Council of Nurses. (2007b). *Position statement: Nurse retention and migration*. Retrieved July 1, 2017, from http://www.icn.ch/images/stories/documents/publications/position_statements/C06_Nurse_Retention_Migration.pdf

The International Centre on Nurse Migration

Another organization, the ICNM, established in 2005, represents a collaborative project launched by the ICN and the Commission on Graduates of Foreign Nursing Schools (CGFNS). The ICNM (2016) serves as a global resource for the development, promotion, and dissemination of research, policy, and information on global nurse migration. The ICNM Web site includes commissioned papers on nurse migration, publication links, fact sheets, and e-newsletters.

BOX 7.2   **International Council of Nurses Principles of Ethical Nurse Recruitment**

Effective planning and development strategies must be introduced, regularly reviewed, and maintained to ensure a balance between supply and demand of nurse human resources.

1. Nursing legislation must authorize regulatory bodies to determine nurses' standards of education, competencies, and standards of practice and to ensure that only individuals meeting these standards are allowed to practice as a nurse.
2. Because the provision of quality care relies on the availability of nurses to meet staffing demand, nurses in a recruiting region/country and seeking employment should be made aware of job opportunities.
3. Nurses should have the right to migrate if they comply with the recruiting country's immigration/work policies (e.g., work permit) and meet obligations in their home country (e.g., bonding responsibilities, tax payment).
4. Nurses have the right to expect fair treatment (e.g., working conditions, promotion, and continuing education).
5. Nurses and employers are to be protected from false information, withholding of relevant information, misleading claims, and exploitation (e.g., accurate job descriptions, benefits/allocations/bonuses specified in writing, authentic educational records).
6. There should be no discrimination between occupations/professions with the same level of responsibility, educational qualification, work experience, skill requirement, and hardship (e.g., pay, grading).
7. When nurses' or employers' contracted or acquired rights or benefits are threatened or violated, suitable machinery must be in place to hear grievances in a timely manner and at reasonable cost.
8. Nurses must be protected from occupational injury and health hazards, including violence (e.g., sexual harassment), and made aware of existing workplace hazards.
9. The provision of quality care in the highly complex and often stressful health care environment depends on a supportive formal and informal supervisory infrastructure.
10. Employment contracts must specify a trial period when the signing parties are free to express dissatisfaction and cancel the contract with no penalty. In the case of international migration, the responsibility for covering the cost of repatriation needs to be clearly stated.
11. Nurses have the right to affiliate to and be represented by a professional association and/or union to safeguard their rights as health professionals and workers.
12. Recruitment agencies (public and private) should be regulated, and effective monitoring mechanisms, such as cost-effectiveness, volume, success rate over time, retention rates, equalities criteria, and client satisfaction, should be introduced.

Source: Adapted from International Council of Nurses. (2007a). *Position statement: Ethical nurse recruitment*. Retrieved June 30, 2017, from http://www.icn.ch/images/stories/documents/publications/position_statements/C03_Ethical_Nurse_Recruitment.pdf

The AcademyHealth Project: Achieving Consensus on Ethical Standards of Practice for International Nurse Recruitment

AcademyHealth, a professional society of individuals and affiliated organizations throughout the United States and abroad, has also taken an active role in working to assure the ethical recruitment of international nurses (Academy-Health, n.d.). Funded through a grant from the John D. and Catherine T. MacArthur Foundation in collaboration with the O'Neill Institute for National and Global Health Law at Georgetown University, AcademyHealth convened a task force of recruiters, hospitals, and foreign-educated nurses to develop draft standards of practice about global nurse recruitment, as well as recommendations on how to institutionalize these standards. This collaboration led to the release of a *Voluntary Code of Ethical Conduct for the Recruitment of Foreign Educated Nurses to the United States*. The code was designed to increase transparency and accountability throughout the process of international recruitment and ensure adequate orientation for foreign-educated nurses. It also provided guidance on ways to ensure recruitment is not harmful to source countries. This document was endorsed by the National Council of State Boards of Nursing (NCSBN).

The World Health Organization

Another international organization involved in establishing guidelines for nurse migration is the WHO (2018) (see Fig. 7.2). In an effort to balance the right of workers to

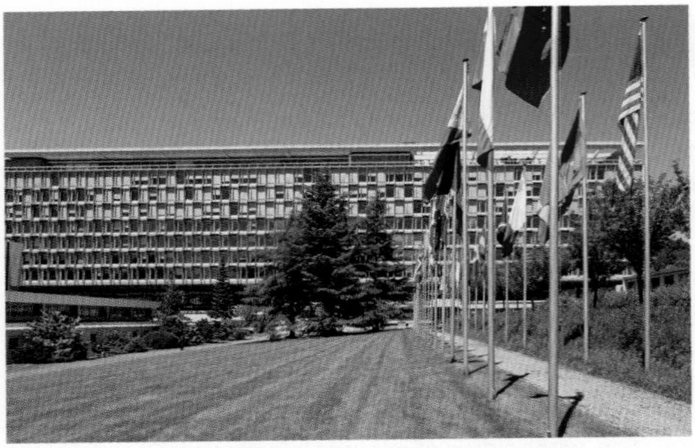

Figure 7.2 Headquarters of the World Health Organization in Geneva, Switzerland.

migrate with a need to assure that global health care needs are met, the WHO launched the *Health Worker Migration Policy Initiative* in 2007. The initiative brought together professional organizations and other groups to create a code, which emphasized the positive benefits of health worker migration and minimized its negative impacts, and that spread the benefits of health worker migration more equitably among developed and developing nations.

The code, as called for by a resolution of the World Health Assembly in 2004, promoted ethical recruitment, protects migrant health workers' rights, and encourages governments in both developed and developing nations to actively address the push and pull factors that promote nurse migration (WHO, 2018). The Code of Practice was the first of its kind on a global scale for migration. In 2011, the Sixty-Third World Health Assembly unanimously passed a resolution to adopt the *Global Code of Practice on the International Recruitment of Health Personnel*, acknowledging the global dimension and complexities of the health workforce crisis and the interconnected nature of both the problems and the solutions (WHO, 2018). In addition, the 2004 WHO Resolution 57.19 urged member states to mitigate the adverse effects of health care worker migration by forming country and regional agreements such as the South Africa/United Kingdom Memorandum of Understanding, the Pacific Code, and the Caribbean Community agreement.

Yet, research by Squires, Ojemeni, and Jones (2016) suggests that although the WHO Code has had an influence on overall foreign nurse migration dynamics to the United States by decreasing candidate numbers, in most cases, the WHO Code was not the single cause of these fluctuations. Indeed, the impact of the National Council Licensure Examination for Registered Nurses (NCLEX-RN) examination changes appears to have exerted a larger influence.

THE MISTREATMENT OF FOREIGN NURSES

Despite the costs and investment of time and energy that goes into recruiting foreign nurses, some health care organizations treat imported nurses poorly once they arrive. Some migrant nurses receive substandard jobs or wages or are subjected to illegal practices by their employers.

In addition, some recruiting firms charge foreign nurses an upfront fee, a practice that has been found illegal in connection with the recruitment of temporary farm workers in the United States and that is prohibited in the U.K. Code of Practice for the International Recruitment of Health Care Professionals. In addition, many recruiters charge migrant nurses a "buyout" or breach fee for resigning before the end of their employment contract. This is because placement agencies often charge health care organizations a significant fee, depending on the state and the nurse's experience, to bring in a foreign nurse.

> **Consider This** Recruiting internationally may be a quick-fix solution, but it is far from clear that it is always a cost-effective solution.

There are also reports that overzealous recruiters have made false promises to foreign nurses regarding job opportunities and wages and virtually forced the newly migrated RNs to work long hours in substandard working conditions. Part of the reason for this is that private for-profit agencies have increasingly become involved in the search for nursing personnel, and there is generally no designated body that regulates or monitors the content of contracts offered. Internationally recruited nurses may be particularly at risk of exploitation or abuse because of the difficulty of verifying the terms of employment as a result of distance, language barriers, cost, and naiveté. These questionable hiring or employment practices are shown in Box 7.3.

> **Consider This** Because of the lack of regulatory oversight of global nurse migration contracting, foreign nurses are at increased risk for employment under false pretenses and may be misled as to the conditions of work, remuneration, and benefits.

Discussion Point

Should there be greater regulatory oversight of foreign nurse recruitment? If so, who should be charged with this responsibility?

BOX 7.3	**Questionable Practices Reported by International Nurses**

- Changing contracts from the time a nurse departs his/her home country and on arrival in sponsor country without consent
- Paying lower wages than the prevailing rate or less than the hours worked
- Charging high breach fees
- Inadequate orientation to clinical agencies
- Imposing excessive work demands or mandatory overtime
- Retaining green cards, delays in processing social security numbers and RN permits
- Threats that nurses will be reported to immigration authorities
- Providing substandard housing

BOX 7.4	**Broad Categories of Transitional Challenges Facing International Nurse Migrants**

1. Difficulty orientating (cultural disorientation)
2. Communication barriers
3. A longing for what is missing
4. Professional development and devaluing
5. Discrimination and marginalization
6. Personal and professional differences
7. Lack of a meaningful support system

Source: Pung, L. X., & Goh, Y. S. (2017, March). Challenges faced by international nurses when migrating: An integrative literature review. *International Nursing Review, 64*(1), 146–165.

ASSIMILATING THE FOREIGN NURSE THROUGH SOCIALIZATION

The ethical obligation to the foreign nurse does not end with his or her arrival in a new country. The move from one cultural context to another can be very stressful. Many migrant nurses are afraid to express dissatisfaction or to ask for help for fear they will no longer have a job or because they fear being sent home. In addition, many of the families left behind in donor countries count on the migrant RN sending money home to improve their living standard. All of these factors place migrated nurses at increased risk for abuse and failure to assimilate. As a result, sponsoring countries must do whatever they can to see that migrant nurses are assimilated into new work environments.

Pung and Goh (2017) suggest there are seven broad categories of transitional challenges faced by international nurses who migrate: difficulty orientating (cultural disorientation); a longing for what is missing; professional development and devaluing; communication barriers; discrimination and marginalization; personal and professional differences; and a meaningful support system (Box 7.4).

Difficulty orientating and executing routine daily activities (shopping, banking, transportation, paying bills, etc.) in their host countries may be difficult for newly assimilated foreign nurses. In addition, orientation programs offered by their new workplaces may be insufficient in helping them to adjust to their new work environments.

A longing for what is missing can result from cultural uprooting. The sudden change in the social environment often brings some yearning as well as sadness for what has been left behind.

Professional development and devaluing is a reality for many migrant nurses in their host countries. Some migrant nurses suggest feeling undermined, belittled, and disrespected. In addition, they report a drop in occupational status after arriving in their host countries.

Communication barriers, however, may be the most challenging issue facing international nurses. Not only do most foreign nurse migrants have an inadequacy of language preparation they are also unfamiliar with accent, slang, and other language nuances. As a result, they find it difficult to relate to patients, families, and other health care team members, to speak up for themselves, and to advocate for their patients.

Discrimination and marginalization are also challenges for the migrant nurse. Moyce, Lash, and de leon Siantz (2016) concur, arguing that many foreign nurses experience racism and discrimination as well as skill underutilization. In addition, some migrant nurses experience unfair treatment (such as higher patient loads than others or being passed over for promotions) and racism, which results in stereotyping and rejection by patients and peers. In addition, the risk of being bullied is higher in this population.

In addition, personal and professional differences among international nurses and native nurses often result in disagreements and conflicts. Professional differences may include differences in nursing expectations, communication expectations, and values and beliefs toward patient care. In Asia, family members are expected to provide basic care to patients, and nurses usually follow doctors' orders with little questioning, whereas critical thinking and independent decision making are stressed in Western countries.

Finally, the migrant nurse often experiences the lack of a meaningful support system. With family and friends left behind, adjustment may be slow and lonely. Hongyan, Wenbo, and Junxin (2014) agree, suggesting that it is often difficult for foreign RNs to form working relationships with the host nurses in a health care organization because of feelings of isolation, loneliness, and depression. Long-term geographical separation from their family leads many of these nurses to have feelings of insecurity regarding their marriages and sadness over the lost emotional connection with their children. When immigrant nurses can establish a good relationship with their colleagues, the nurses are more motivated to stay in their work and the safety and quality of care is increased.

THE INTERNATIONAL COMMUNITY ADDRESSES THE PROBLEM

The nursing shortage and resulting global migration issues have led several national governments to intervene, and, as a result, some countries have made progress in tackling the ethical issues associated with global recruitment and migration of nurses.

Some Governments Respond

Within the last few years, many countries, including the United States, have published national nursing strategies for dealing with staff shortages. Norway has issued a policy statement on the ethics of international recruitment. The Netherlands, Ireland, and the Scandinavian countries also have good practice guidelines on international recruitment or are looking at developing guidelines. The United Kingdom, although allowing all nurses free movement rights, has implemented tight immigration and professional registration policies. Indeed, in 2005, the UK began limiting nurse recruitment to the European Union (EU) countries and only granting work permits to nurses from non-EU countries if National Health Services institutions showed that jobs could not be filled by UK or EU applications. This UK Code of Practice is one of the oldest Codes of Practice in existence.

Other countries have initiated or examined various policy responses to reduce outflow, such as requiring nurses to work in their home countries for a certain amount of time after education completion or by charging the nurse a fee to migrate to another country. Another response has been to recognize that outflow cannot be halted if principles of individual freedom are to be upheld, but that the outflow that does occur must be managed and moderated. The "managed migration" initiative being undertaken in the Caribbean, which has provided regional support for addressing the nursing shortage crisis and developed initiatives such as training for export and temporary migration,

is one example of a coordinated intervention to minimize the negative effects of outflow while realizing at least some benefit from the process.

Indonesia has adopted international principles in an effort to protect Indonesian nurses who migrate as well as the country's own participation in a bilateral trade and investment agreement, known as the Indonesia–Japan Economic Partnership Agreement (Efendi, Mackey, Huang, & Chen, 2017). Despite the potential trade and employment benefits from sending nurses abroad, Indonesia itself is suffering from a nursing shortage and cannot ensure adequate health care access for its own populations. The Indonesia–Japan Economic Partnership Agreement attempts to balance domestic health workforce needs, employment, and training opportunities for Indonesian nurses and yet acknowledge the rights of nurses to freely migrate abroad (Efendi et al., 2017).

U.S. Immigration Policy

Currently, foreign nurses who want to work in the United States must have a valid job offer from an employer, and the employer must obtain Department of Labor approval for that hire. In addition, the employer must file a special petition with the U.S. Citizenship and Immigration Services.

In addition, like most national governments, the U.S. government continues to play a pivotal role in the nurse migration issue by its ability to issue travel visas. The reality is that a finite number of visas are available and caps exist on how many green cards are issued. Clearly, commercial recruiters and employers would like to see fewer restrictions on nurse migration, but labor certification laws and rules regarding the issuance of visas are complex and ever changing.

Labor certification laws in the United States suggest that under normal circumstances, the Department of Labor is required by law to certify to the Department of State and the Immigration and Naturalization Service (INS) when a foreigner is hired that (1) an inadequate number of U.S. citizens and permanent residents are available or qualified for a given job and (2) that employment of the foreign worker will not adversely affect the wages and working conditions of similarly employed U.S. workers (U.S. Department of Labor, 2018).

The main purpose of this legal provision has been to protect the domestic labor market; however, the immigration laws have provided preferential provisions for members of certain professions in the national interest of the United States, and, as a result, the government has created a list of occupations and professions, including nursing, that do not require labor certification. Because nursing has been classified as one of the shortage areas in the U.S. economy, a so-called *blanket waiver* of the labor certification is in place.

In addition, from 1962 to 1989, foreign nurses were regarded as "professionals" under U.S. immigration laws and could therefore seek an H1 temporary work visa in the United States. In 1989, the Immigration Nursing Relief Act (INRA) created a 5-year pilot program. The INRA stipulated that only health care facilities with "attestations" approved by the Department of Health could obtain H1A occupation visas to employ nurses on a temporary basis. Consequently, other occupations that formerly fell into the H1 category became part of the new H1-B category. In addition, in 1990, Congress passed the Immigration and Nationality Act, which is the legal foundation for current immigration policies. In this act, nursing continued to be listed as a shortage area.

In 1999, the Nursing Relief for Disadvantaged Areas Act created H1-C occupational visas, which were perceived largely as an effort to renew the INRA of 1989 but with more restrictions. These temporary visas were created for foreign nurse graduates seeking employment in designated U.S. facilities (serving primarily poor patients in inner cities and some rural areas). This visa classification expired in 2009.

Currently, there are no specific nurse visas available in the United States; however, some foreign nurses apply to work under the H1-B visa for skilled workers (open to individuals from countries other than Canada or Mexico) or the TN North American Free-Trade Agreement (NAFTA) work visa (available only to Canadian and Mexican citizens). The H1-B is a nonimmigrant visa that allows recruiting of shortage professionals into jobs that require theoretical and practical application of a body of highly specialized knowledge requiring completion of a specific course of higher education (at least a bachelor's degree).

At first glance, the H1-B might look like a good match for foreign nurses because they are for temporary workers in specialty occupations, and nurses are both educated and specialized (Knapp, 2018). In addition, the United States has nursing jobs that need to be filled. The reality, however, is that many RNs do not qualify for the H1-B visa: A Fifth Circuit Court ruled in 2000 that RN hospital jobs do not currently require a bachelor's degree in nursing, regardless of recruiter requirements. Nurses can still apply for the H1-B status, however, if they have a specialized skill, particularly in intensive care, management, and specialty nursing areas or if U.S. employers can convince immigration officials that specific jobs do meet the H1-B requirement on a case-by-case basis. Other nurses more likely to earn an H1-B visa are those prepared for nurse manager or advanced practice roles, which require a Bachelor of Science in nursing or a Master of Science degree (Knapp, 2018).

In addition, the H1-B visa has an annual numerical limit "cap" of 65,000 visas each fiscal year. The first 20,000 petitions filed on behalf of beneficiaries with a U.S. master's degree or higher will be exempt from this cap in 2019 (U.S. Citizenship and Immigration Requirements, 2018).

> ### Discussion Point
> Does the increased importation of foreign nurses directly or indirectly affect the prevailing wages of domestic RNs?

Still, other foreign nurses have sought employment in the United States in accordance with NAFTA, enacted in December 1993. NAFTA established a reciprocal trading relationship between the United States, Canada, and Mexico and allowed for a nonimmigrant class of admission exclusively for business and service trade individuals entering the United States. Yet, several Canadian advanced practice registered nurses (APRNs) were prevented from reporting for work in Michigan by Customs and Border Patrol personnel in March 2017.

> *At issue was the APRNs' eligibility for TN visas, a visa category for professionals under NAFTA. A new hire was applying for a TN visa and the other nurses needed TN visa renewals. The applications were denied based on border patrol agents' interpretation—later overruled—of NAFTA rules.* (Carter, 2017, p. 12)

To complicate the matter further, on July 26, 2003, the U.S. Bureau of Citizenship and Immigration Services ruled that foreign-educated health care professionals, including nurses who are seeking temporary or permanent occupational visas, as well as those who are seeking NAFTA status, must successfully complete a screening program before receiving an occupational visa or permanent (green card) visa. This screening, completed by the CGFNS, includes an assessment of an applicant's education to ensure that it is comparable to that of a nursing graduate in the United States, verification that licenses are valid and unencumbered, successful completion of an English-language proficiency examination, and verification that the nurse has either earned certification by the CGFNS or passed the NCLEX-RN.

Another way nurses get work visas in the United States has been under the immigrant E3 to I-140 status ("green card" or Alien Registration Receipt Card). Migrant RNs enter into the United States and become permanent residents through petition to the INS. A problem with this visa status is that it does not require labor certification, so the Department of Labor does not have to certify that the wage offered to the nurse is the prevailing wage. However, the law does state that foreign nurses entering under I-140 cannot have a negative effect on domestic wages.

Further clouding the issue of immigration for foreign nurses are new or expected rulings under the Trump administration, including future restrictions on H1-B visas (Trines, 2018). In addition, the possibility of far-reaching changes to the NAFTA treaty could curtail the labor migration of RNs from Canada and Mexico, which can currently work temporarily in the United States on TN work visas and the travel ban on Muslim-majority countries will further bar health professionals from affected countries from entering the United States (Trines, 2018).

ENSURING COMPETENCY OF FOREIGN NURSES COMMISSION ON GRADUATES OF FOREIGN NURSING SCHOOLS AND THE NCLEX-RN EXAMINATION

Nursing is one of the most highly regulated health professions in the United States, and a license is required to practice in all 50 states and U.S. territories. Before 1977, endorsement and taking the State Board Test Pool Examination (SBTPE) were the two ways for foreign nurses to obtain a license. The SBTPE tested the foreign graduate's English-language proficiency and knowledge of U.S. nursing practice, but, alarmingly, only a small percentage (15%–20%) of foreign RNs typically passed the NCLEX-RN.

As a result of this high failure rate and a concern for patient safety, the ANA and the NLN, with collaboration from the Department of Labor and the INS, established CGFNS in 1977 as an independent, nonprofit organization. CGFNS is an immigration neutral nonprofit organization that helps foreign-educated health care professionals live and work in their country of choice by assessing and validating their academic and professional credentials. They also protect migrating health care professionals by advocating for ethical recruitment practices and continually monitoring the global landscape for developing trends in employment recruitment and workplace norms (Commission on Graduates of Foreign Nursing Schools [CGFNS], 2018a, para. 1–3).

The strategies CGFNS uses to accomplish this mission are to evaluate and test foreign graduates via a certification program before they leave their home countries to ensure that there is a reasonable chance for them to pass the NCLEX-RN needed for licensure in the United States. Through a contract with the NLN, which designed the NCLEX-RN, a CGFNS-qualifying examination was developed. The examination consists of two parts to test the applicant's knowledge of nursing and the English language (both written and oral).

To be eligible to take the examination, RNs must have completed sufficient classroom instruction and clinical practice and hold an initial as well as current license/registration as a first-level general nurse in their country of education (CGFNS, 2018b). In addition, a credentials review of secondary and nursing education, registration, and licensure is required to earn the CGFNS certificate. Earning CGFNS certification meets one of the immigration requirements for securing an occupational visa to work in the United States and helps to meet licensure and NCLEX eligibility requirements in many states (CGFNS, 2018b).

The CGFNS examination, however, should not be mistaken as a substitute for the state board licensing examination. Indeed, most states in the United States require foreign nurses to pass the CGFNS certification before they are allowed to take the NCLEX-RN. Of the 11,569 internationally educated nurses who took the NCLEX-RN as first-time test takers in 2016, the pass rate was only 38.85% (National Council of State Boards of Nursing, 2017). The examination specifications and passing standards are the same for foreign nurses as they are for students taking the NCLEX in the United States.

The NCSBN has also taken steps to make it easier for foreign RNs to take the NCLEX-RN. Until 2005, the NCLEX-RN was offered only in the United States and its territories. In fact, before 2005, the only option foreign nurses had was to earn the CGFNS certificate, secure a job offer from a U.S. employer, and take the NCLEX-RN only after they arrived in the United States with their green cards. Now the examination is offered in numerous countries and nonmember board territories. These locations were selected based on national security, examination security, and similarity with U.S. Intellectual Property and Copyright Laws.

CONCLUSIONS

Nurse migration and its associated ethical dilemmas are among the most serious issues facing the nursing profession, and there is little sign that the issue will abate anytime soon. Clearly, developed countries have an advantage in terms of pull factors to recruit migrant nurses from less-developed countries, and less-developed countries are the ones most likely to suffer the devastating effects of brain drain. One must ask, however, whether this quick-fix solution to the nursing shortage has become too commonplace and too easy. Does it keep recruiter countries from dealing with the issues that led to their shortage in the first place? Does it negatively affect prevailing domestic wages and artificially alter what should be normal supply/demand curves in the health care marketplace? Of even greater concern is the lack of regulatory oversight of contracting with foreign nurses, placing them at risk for unethical, if not illegal, employment practices in their host country.

Delucas (2014) agrees, suggesting that both destination and source countries are challenged by poorly controlled nurse migration. Destination countries must address the ethical implications of aggressive recruitment and their lack of developing a sustainable self-sufficient domestic workforce. Source countries struggle to fund and educate adequate numbers of nurses for domestic needs and migrant replacement.

Some countries and professional nursing organizations are beginning to address these issues. So too are national governments and regulatory agencies in an effort to protect both the migrant nurses and the public those nurses will serve. Delucas (2014) argues passionately, however, that more work must be done to engage nurses at leadership and grassroots levels to establish international treaties regarding foreign nurse migration that work collaboratively for justice and health equity. She suggests that inertia is not an option as nurses must adopt a broader sense of responsibility in addressing global disparities of health and health care and the need to develop a sustainable nursing workforce.

Yet, in the meantime, large numbers of nurses are migrating internationally, and the potentially negative effects of this increasing trend on both the migrant nurse and the donor nation are becoming ever more apparent. Jones and Sherwood (2014) note that "nurse mobility and migration will require nations and health care organizations to continue working to better understand workforce models and the employment, integration, assimilation, and regulation of an international nursing workforce" (p. 62).

For Additional Discussion

1. Are the requirements for foreign nurses to get visas in the United States adequate?

2. Does achieving CGFNS certification and passing the NCLEX-RN examination in the United States assure competency of the foreign nurse graduate?

3. As long as international nurse recruitment is a viable option, will the problems that lead to a nursing shortage in the first place be addressed?

4. Should donor countries develop nurse migration policy efforts that limit human resource exports?

5. How can government and professional nursing organizations work together to ensure that recruitment practices of foreign nurses are both ethical and appropriate?

6. How does the ethical principle of veracity (truth telling) apply to the zealous recruiting efforts of foreign nurses, particularly in developing countries?

7. Is government regulatory oversight of foreign nurse recruitment efforts in conflict with America's value of capitalistic, free enterprise?

References

Abbasi, S., & Younas, M. (2016). Brain drain of nurses from Pakistan. *Journal on Nursing, 6*(2), 7–11.

AcademyHealth. (n.d.). *About us.* Retrieved May 15, 2018, from http://www.academyhealth.org/about

Ahn, Y. (2017, March 3). *Korean nurse "guest workers" in Germany.* Retrieved July 1, 2017, from http://humanities.ku.dk/calendar/2017/march/korean-nurse/

Carter, D. (2017). Canadian nurses caught up in immigration policy confusion: In March, Canadian APRNs were prevented from working in Michigan. *American Journal of Nursing, 117*(6), 12.

Castro-Palaganas, E., Spitzer, D. L., Kabamalan, M. M., Sanchez, M. C., Caricativo, R., Runnels, V., . . . Bourgeault, I. L. (2017, March 31). An examination of the causes, consequences, and policy responses to the migration of highly trained health personnel from the Philippines: The high cost of living/leaving-a mixed method study. *Human Resources for Health, 15*, 1–14.

Commission on Graduates of Foreign Nursing Schools. (2018a). *About.* Retrieved May 15, 2018, from http://www.cgfns.org/sections/about/

Commission on Graduates of Foreign Nursing Schools. (2018b). *CGFNS certification program.* Retrieved May 15,

2018, from http://www.cgfns.org/services/certification-program/

Delucas, A. C. (2014). Foreign nurse recruitment: Global risk. *Nursing Ethics, 21*(1), 76–85. Retrieved July 1, 2017, from http://nej.sagepub.com/content/21/1/76.full.pdf+html

Efendi, F., Mackey, T. K., Huang, M., & Chen, C. (2017). IJEPA: Gray area for health policy and international nurse migration. *Nursing Ethics, 24*(3), 313–328. doi:10.1177/0969733015602052

Esposito, L. (2017, March 29). *Immigrant nurses: Filling the next U.S. shortage.* Retrieved May 15, 2018, from https://health.usnews.com/wellness/articles/2017-03-29/immigrant-nurses-filling-the-next-us-shortage

FWCanada Inc. (2014, April 3). *Canada: Canada offers registered nurses immigration programs to become permanent residents; No offers of employment necessary.* Montréal, QC: Author. Retrieved June 31, 2017, from http://www.mondaq.com/canada/x/304386/work+visas/Canada+Offers+Registered+Nurses+Immigration+Programs+To+Become+Permanent+Residents+No+Offers+Of+Employment+Necessary

Hongyan, L., Wenbo, N., & Junxin, L. (2014, September). The benefits and caveats of international nurse migration. *International Journal of Nursing Sciences, 1*(3), 314–317. Retrieved July 1, 2017, from http://www.sciencedirect.com/science/article/pii/S2352013214000787

International Centre on Nurse Migration. (2014). *Fact sheet 2014. International nurse migration and remittances.* Retrieved May 15, 2018, from http://www.intlnursemigration.org/wp-content/uploads/2014/10/NurseMigrationRemitfactsheet2014.pdf

International Centre on Nurse Migration. (2016). *About us.* Retrieved May 15, 2018, from http://www.intlnursemigration.org/about/

International Council of Nurses. (2007a). *Position statement: Ethical nurse recruitment.* Retrieved July 1, 2017, from http://www.icn.ch/images/stories/documents/publications/position_statements/C03_Ethical_Nurse_Recruitment.pdf

International Council of Nurses. (2007b). *Position statement: Nurse retention and migration.* Retrieved July 1, 2017, from http://docplayer.net/25478011-Nurse-retention-and-migration-position-statement.html

International Council of Nurses. (2017). *Who we are.* Retrieved June 30, 2017, from http://www.icn.ch/who-we-are/who-we-are/

Jones, C. B., & Sherwood, G. (2014). The globalization of the nursing workforce: Pulling the pieces together. *Nursing Outlook, 62*(1), 59–63. doi:10.1016/j.outlook.2013.12.005

Knapp, K. (2018). *When nurses can qualify for an H-1B visa to the U.S.* Nolo. Retrieved May 15, 2018, from https://www.nolo.com/legal-encyclopedia/when-nurses-can-qualify-h-1b-visa-the-us.html

Moyce, S., Lash, R., & de Leon Siantz, M. L. (2016). Migration experiences of foreign educated nurses. *Journal of Transcultural Nursing, 27*(2), 181–188. doi:10.1177/1043659615569538

National Council of State Boards of Nursing. (2017, January 23). *2016: Number of candidates taking NCLEX examination and percent passing, by type of candidate.* Retrieved July 1, 2017, from https://www.ncsbn.org/Table_of_Pass_Rates_2016.pdf

NurSearch. (2017, April 4). *Worldwide nursing shortage—10 countries with a nursing shortage crisis.* Retrieved May 15, 2018, from https://nursearch.org/worldwide-nursing-shortage-10-countries-with-a-nursing-shortage-crisis/

O'Connor, T. (2016). Nurse migration raises complex issues. *Kai Tiaki Nursing New Zealand, 22*(5), 18–19.

Office for National Statistics. (2014, January 17). *Bulgarian and Romanian migration to the UK in 2014.* Retrieved June 30, 2017, from http://www.ons.gov.uk/ons/rel/migration1/migration-statistics-quarterly-report/november-2013/sty-bulgaria-and-romania.html

Office of the United Nations High Commissioner for Human Rights. (1976). I*nternational covenant on civil and political rights.* Retrieved July 1, 2017, from http://www.ohchr.org/EN/ProfessionalInterest/Pages/CCPR.aspx

Philippines Economy 2018. (2018, February 28). *Economy overview.* Retrieved May 15, 2018, from http://www.theodora.com/wfbcurrent/philippines/philippines_economy.html

Pung, L. X., & Goh, Y. S. (2017, March). Challenges faced by international nurses when migrating: An integrative literature review. *International Nursing Review, 64*(1), 146–165.

Squires, A., Ojemeni, M. T., & Jones, S. (2016, June 30). Exploring longitudinal shifts in international nurse migration to the United States between 2003 and 2013 through a random effects panel data analysis. *Human Resources for Health, 14*, 11–21. doi:10.1186/s12960-016-0118-7

Straehle, C. (2017, April). Debating brain drain—May governments restrict emigration? *Developing World Bioethics, 17*(1), 59–60.

Toscano, N. (2015, July 7). *Nurse graduates 'locked out' of workforce as migrants get jobs.* The Sydney Morning Herald. Retrieved July 1, 2017, from http://www.smh.com.au/business/workplace-relations/nurse-graduates-locked-out-of-workforce-as-migrants-get-jobs-20150606-ghi9c8.html

Trines, S. (2018, March 6). *Mobile nurses: Trends in international labor migration in the nursing field.* World Education News + Review. Retrieved May 15, 2018, from https://wenr.wes.org/2018/03/mobile-nurses-trends-in-international-labor-migration-in-the-nursing-field

United Nations General Assembly. (1948). *The universal declaration of human rights.* Retrieved May 15, 2018, from http://www.un.org/en/documents/udhr/

U.S. Citizenship and Immigration Requirements. (2018). *H-1B fiscal year (FY) 2019 cap season.* Retrieved July 1, 2017, from https://www.uscis.gov/working-united-states/temporary-workers/h-1b-specialty-occupations-and-fashion-models/h-1b-fiscal-year-fy-2019-cap-season

U.S. Department of Labor. (2018, May 15). *Permanent labor certification.* Retrieved May 15, 2018, from https://www.foreignlaborcert.doleta.gov/perm.cfm

Wang, C. C., Whitehead, L., & Bayes, S. (2016, March). Nursing education in China: Meeting the global demand for quality healthcare. *International Journal of Nursing Sciences, 3*(1), 131–136.

Wild, V. (2012). Migration and health: Discovering new territory for bioethics. *American Journal of Bioethics, 12*(9), 11–13.

World Health Organization. (2018). *Task force on migration: Health worker migration policy initiative.* Retrieved May 15, 2018, from http://www.who.int/workforcealliance/about/taskforces/migration/en/

Unlicensed Assistive Personnel and the Registered Nurse

Carol J. Huston

LEARNING OBJECTIVES

The learner will be able to:

1. Identify driving forces leading to the increased use of unlicensed assistive personnel (UAP) beginning in the early 1990s.

2. Name common job titles for UAP.

3. Differentiate between the minimum mandated educational preparation of certified nurse aides and UAP.

4. Analyze current research that explores the effect of increased UAP use on costs and patient outcomes.

5. Discuss how the role of the registered nurse (RN) as delegator has changed with the increased use of UAP.

6. Examine how the role of delegator and supervisor of UAP increases the scope of liability for the RN.

7. Explore strategies for restructuring work environments and clarifying role expectations so that professional nurses spend less time on non-nursing tasks and UAP have role clarity.

8. Identify safeguards that health care organizations can use to increase the likelihood that UAP are used both effectively and appropriately as members of the health care team.

9. Outline current efforts seeking to regulate minimum UAP education and competencies.

10. Discuss factors contributing to both the current and projected shortages of UAP, particularly in long-term care settings.

11. Reflect on the self-confidence and skill that an RN might need to successfully delegate to a UAP.

12. Identify the sources of increased legal liability an RN and his or her employer face when health care institutions allow RNs to work beneath their scope of practice as UAP.

INTRODUCTION

In an effort to contain spiraling health care costs, many health care providers in the 1990's restructured their organizations by eliminating registered nurse (RN) positions and/or by replacing licensed professional nurses with unlicensed assistive personnel (UAP). UAP are unlicensed individuals who provide low-risk, assistive care not requiring the judgment or training of a licensed professional, while working under the direct supervision of an RN. The term includes, but is not limited to, nurse aides, nurse extenders, health care aides, technicians, patient care technicians, orderlies, assistants, and attendants. Although the term UAP will generally be used throughout this chapter, it is noteworthy that in 2007, the American Nurses Association (ANA) stopped using the term UAP and replaced it with *nursing assistive personnel* (NAP), suggesting that many NAP are now licensed or formally recognized in some manner.

Regardless of nomenclature, unlicensed workers are a significant part of the health care landscape and have been for some time. By the late 1990s, hospitals began actively recruiting the RNs who had been let go just a few years before. RNs who lost their jobs, however, were slow to return to the acute-care setting, despite a widespread, worsening nursing shortage. As a result, hospitals again increased their use of UAP early in the 21st century in an attempt to supplement their licensed nursing staff.

Both as a result of the restructuring of the 1990s and subsequent nursing shortages, the skill mix in some hospitals still includes a significant percentage of UAP. According to the U.S. Department of Labor, Bureau of Labor Statistics (2018a), 1.5 million nursing assistants (NAs) were employed in the United States in 2016. Twenty six percent of UAP worked in hospitals, 40% worked in skilled nursing facilities, 11% worked in continuing care retirement communities and assisted living facilities for the elderly, 5% in home care, and 4% for the government (U.S. Department of Labor, Bureau of Labor Statistics, 2018a).

Several reasons are commonly cited for the increased use of UAP. The primary argument for using UAP instead of licensed personnel is usually cost savings, although professional nursing shortages are a contributing factor (Marquis & Huston, 2017). Another widely recognized benefit of using UAP is that they can free professional nurses from tasks and assignments (specifically, non-nursing functions) that can be completed by less well-trained personnel at a lower cost.

So why has the increased use of UAP created so much controversy? The answer is that in many institutions, UAP are not supplements to, but replacements of, professional RN staff. This is of concern because empirical research exists regarding what percentage of the staffing mix can safely be represented by UAP without negatively affecting patient outcomes. In addition, minimum national educational and training requirements have not been established for UAP, and their scope of practice varies from institution to institution. These issues raise serious questions as to whether greater use of UAP represents an effective solution to dwindling health care resources or whether it is an economically driven, short-term response that could lead to compromised patient outcomes.

This chapter, however, does not argue for the elimination of UAP. Instead, it addresses what safeguards must be incorporated in the use of UAP so that safe, accessible, and affordable nursing care is possible.

MOTIVATION TO USE UAP

Maximizing RN Time With Patients

UAP can maximize human resources because they free professional nurses from tasks and assignments that do not require independent thinking and professional judgment. This is significant because much of a typical nurse's time is spent on non-nursing tasks and functions. Non-nursing tasks and functions are those routine or standardized activities that can be done by an individual with minimal training and do not require a great deal of individual client assessment, independent thought, or decision making. Examples of non-nursing activities include making a bed, doing vital signs, feeding clients, measuring intakes and outputs, and obtaining a weight or height.

Just how much time is spent by nurses doing non-nursing activities is unclear. Research by Jackson Healthcare, a health care staffing and management company, found that between 73% and 75% of nurses spend one-quarter of a 12-hour shift on indirect patient care services ("Nurses Spending," 2018). The top reasons for being pulled away from patient care included the following:

- Documenting information in multiple locations
- Completing logs, checklists, and other unnecessary paperwork/data collection
- Filling out regulatory documentation
- Entering/reviewing orders
- Walking to equipment/supply areas, utility rooms, etc.

Discussion Point

Why are professional RNs still completing so many non-nursing tasks? Are they reluctant to delegate them to ancillary personnel or are there inadequate support personnel to take on these tasks?

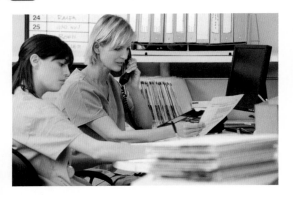

Cost Savings

Cost savings associated with UAP use—the second argument for increased UAP use—are less clear. Studies completed early in the 21st century showed conflicting findings, with some suggesting significant cost savings with UAP and others suggesting no cost savings as a result of the costs of supervision, high UAP turnover rates, and medical errors. Current research is limited. It is this lack of evidence, however, that has led some hospitals to resume reliance on UAP as the primary component of their staffing mix.

EDUCATIONAL REQUIREMENTS FOR UAP

Some monitoring of the regulation, education, and use of UAP has been ongoing since the early 1950s; however, most of this has been for *certified nurse's aides*. The Omnibus Budget Reconciliation Act of 1987 established regulations for the education and certification of nurse's aides (minimum of 75 hours of State-approved theory and practice and successful completion of a competency examination in both areas).

No federal or community standards have been established, however, for training the more broadly defined UAP. Indeed, the health care industry provides many job opportunities for individuals without specialized training. This does not mean, however, that all UAP are undereducated and unprepared for the roles they have been asked to fill. Indeed, UAP educational levels vary from less than that of a high school graduate to those holding advanced degrees. It does suggest, however, that RNs, in delegating to UAP, must make no assumptions about the educational preparation or training of that UAP. Instead, the RN must carefully assess what skills and knowledge each UAP has or risk increased personal liability for the failure to do so.

The reality is that UAP training is often completed by the employing facility and occurs without formal certification. Formal training programs that do exist are typically completed at vocational schools and community colleges and focus on long-term care, providing certifications only as necessary to meet state requirements. Often, this training is inadequate and does not prepare UAP with the competencies they need to work in a dynamic health care environment, which is very different from that existed even a decade ago. For efficiency and safety, standardized curricula that address the skill sets needed in the many settings where nurse aides are used should be implemented.

Similar to long-term care, the education and training of UAP in acute-care settings is often inadequate. In fact, there are no required educational standards or guidelines for the use of UAP in acute-care settings. Instead, UAP educational and training requirements for acute-care settings are generally facility based. This is important to remember when UAP transfer from one facility to another because no assumption should be made about UAP competency levels to perform certain tasks, despite their work experience.

> **Discussion Point**
>
> Is work experience an appropriate substitution for formal education and training for UAP? Can this be determined by an experienced RN?

UAP SCOPE OF PRACTICE

In some health care agencies, UAP assist with dressing changes, parenteral therapy, and urinary catheter insertion and perform numerous other tasks typically reserved for licensed personnel. The skill assumed by UAP, however, that has garnered the greatest concern, is administering medications. UAP who administer medications are also known as *unlicensed medication administration personnel, medication aides,* or *medication assistant technicians.*

For years, medication administration was considered a professional nursing function, requiring assessment and clinical judgment, but during the past decade, many states granted unlicensed personnel the right to pass medications, particularly in schools, assisted living facilities, and correctional institutions. In addition, *certified medicine aides* have worked in licensed nursing home settings, residential care settings, and adult day services in this country for almost four decades. Currently, at least 36 states permit the administration of medications in select settings by assistive personnel, once the requisite training is complete (American Nurses Association [ANA], 2018).

The ANA (2018) suggests, however, that despite the number of states that recognize this practice, there remains sufficient concern that the training is inadequate to ensure safe administration. Indeed, the delegation of medication administration to UAP may be perceived by the supervising RN as "handing over a crucial nursing responsibility under jeopardizing circumstances" (Gransjön Craftman, Grape, Ringnell, & Westerbotn, 2016, p. 3197; see Research Fuels the Controversy 8.1). Indeed, Carder and O'Keeffe (2016) found that most states lack clear and adequate provisions for nurse oversight of UAP who administer medications, although adult day service regulations provide a greater level of nurse oversight than residential care settings. Specifically, 32 states require residential care to hire a nurse, but only 6 include provisions regarding nurse availability (e.g., on-call, on-site, number of hours). In contrast, 10 of 20 states that require adult day service programs to hire a nurse provide availability provisions. Also disconcerting was the finding that only 18 of 24 states in which UAP can administer medications in adult day services require any training on the part of the UAP to do so, or nurse delegation (Carder & O'Keeffe, 2016).

UAP also administer drugs in school settings when a school nurse is not present. National data indicate that 11% of children age 5 to 11 years and 13% of those 12 to 17 years have a problem for which medication is taken regularly for at least 3 months ("Medication Administration in Schools," 2017).

It is the position of the National Association of School Nurses that the use of UAP to perform delegated nursing tasks in the school setting is appropriate, however, only if the school nurse can control the decision to delegate a health care task and if he/she supervises or periodically monitors and assesses the capabilities and competencies of the UAP to safely perform the delegated task (National Association of School Nurses, 2018; "Unlicensed Assistive Personnel," 2016).

As a result, many school nurses and the organizations that represent them are waging a battle to stop the expansion of UAP practice in terms of the drugs they can administer (e.g., currently only licensed school nurses can administer insulin). They argue that the administration of medications is much more than dispensing a pill, handing a student an inhaler, or giving a subcutaneous injection. It requires high-level assessment skills; an understanding of drug actions, interactions, and side effects; and the highly developed critical thinking skills needed to intervene when problems occur. In addition, the practice of nursing clearly requires a license under the Nurse Practice Act.

Research Fuels the Controversy 8.1

The Delegation of Medication Administration to UAP

The aim of this qualitative, inductive, descriptive study was to describe registered nurses' (RNs) experience in the context of delegating the administration of medication to unlicensed personnel in residential care homes. Patients in residential care homes often take large numbers of medications and this task is frequently delegated by the RN to the UAP. Data were collected using audio-recorded semistructured interviews with a purposive sample of 18 RNs and interpreted using manifest content analysis.

Source: Gransjön Craftman, Å., Grape, C., Ringnell, K., & Westerbotn, M. (2016, November). Registered nurses' experience of delegating the administration of medicine to unlicensed personnel in residential care homes. *Journal of Clinical Nursing, 25*(21/22), 3189–3198. doi:10.1111/jocn.13335

Study Findings

RNs reported feeling pressured to delegate the responsibility for medication administration to UAP because of inadequate organizational personnel and finances, even though they regarded it as part of the professional role of an RN working in a residential care home. In addition, RNs found the organization unsupportive about the delegation of nursing interventions. The RNs argued that the policymakers did not know much about the context of their task of delegating medicine administration to unlicensed personnel, and how complex the task was, but, most importantly, the challenge it presented to the quality of care and the patients' safety.

In addition, the delegation context was experienced as a gray zone and the rules and regulations were not in line with the unspoken expectation to delegate the administration of medicine to unlicensed personnel, to be able to manage their daily work. As a result, delegation to the UAP was perceived as *handing over a crucial nursing responsibility under jeopardizing circumstances*. The researchers concluded that RNs regard the responsibility of delegating the administration of medicines, follow-up, and tutoring of UAP as something important but, at the same time, a heavy responsibility to bear.

Note: UAP, unlicensed assistive personnel.

As a result, numerous lawsuits have been filed in the last 5 years questioning the use of UAP to administer drugs such as insulin to schoolchildren. In fact, in May 2013, the California Supreme Court was asked to make a ruling on whether allowing UAP to administer insulin to schoolchildren was unlawful since it sidestepped the Nurse Practice Act (California Healthline, 1998-2018). The California Nurse Practice Act specifically defines the act of medication administration as a licensed nursing function. The Court ruled that California law does permit trained UAP to administer prescription medications, including insulin, in accordance with written statements of individual students' treating physicians, with parental consent (California Healthline, 1998-2018; ANA, 2018). The Supreme Court then remanded the case back to the Court of Appeals to resolve any outstanding claims.

There are those, however, who suggest that the use of UAP to administer drugs to schoolchildren is not only appropriate but also essential in today's economic climate with limited resources and increasing health care needs. The American Academy of Pediatrics (AAP, 2009), the National Association of School Nurses, and the ANA suggest that trained and supervised UAP, who have the required knowledge, skills, and composure to deliver specific school health services under the guidance of a licensed RN, should be allowed to do so. The AAP suggests that UAP can provide standardized, routine health services under the supervision of the nurse and on the basis of physician guidance and school nursing assessment of the unique needs of the individual child and the suitability of delegation of specific nursing tasks. Any delegation of nursing duties must be consistent with the requirements of state Nurse Practice Acts, state regulations, and guidelines provided by professional nursing organizations (AAP, 2009).

> **Consider This**　Many patients given direct care by UAP assume that UAP are licensed nurses. This confusion is promulgated when health care professionals do not include their credentials on their nametags or introduce themselves to patients according to their actual job title.

A similar debate is occurring in hemodialysis clinics and nephrology centers. As of 2014, 22 states allowed dialysis technicians or UAP to administer heparin as ordered to initiate or terminate a hemodialysis treatment (O'Keefe, 2014). In most cases, the express authority for this practice lies in dialysis technician laws or Board of Nursing position statements. With several exceptions, most of these states also permit UAP to administer saline to correct hypotension during hemodialysis. Some states require such duties

be under the direct, on-site supervision of an RN or a physician, whereas other states require that administration of heparin or saline by a dialysis technician be pursuant to established facility protocol. In 10 states, the nursing delegation language may permit the RN to delegate IV medication administration through a central line access to UAP. One state, Arizona, permits UAP to administer anticoagulants. O'Keefe (2014) suggests that in the absence of nursing rules that either clearly permit or prohibit the administration of IV medications by UAP, RNs must look to their delegation authority under the state Nurse Practice Act.

Similarly, the Association of Women's Health, Obstetric and Neonatal Nurses (AWHONN) recognizes that UAP can function as supportive members of the health care team under the direction of the professional RN but notes that it is the professional RN who is ultimately responsible for the coordination and delivery of nursing care to women and newborns (Association of Women's Health, Obstetric and Neonatal Nurses, 2016).

The reality, then, is that in many settings, some UAP are performing functions that are within the legal practice of nursing. This may be a violation of the state nursing practice act and poses a possible threat to public safety. Clearly, certain professional responsibilities related to nursing care must never be delegated.

It is critical, then, that the RN never lose sight of his or her ultimate responsibility for ensuring that patients receive appropriate, high-quality care. This means that although the UAP may complete non-nursing functions such as bathing the patient, taking vital signs, and measuring and recording intake and output, it is the RN who must analyze that information using highly developed critical thinking skills and then use the nursing process to see that desired patient outcomes are achieved. Only RNs have the formal authority to practice nursing, and activities that rely on the nursing process or require specialized skill, expert knowledge, or professional judgment should never be delegated.

Regulatory Oversight of UAP

The increased use of UAP, called by some the "deskilling of the nursing workforce," has raised concern among professional organizations, consumers, and legislators alike. In the early 1990s, the ANA took the position that the control and monitoring of assistive personnel in clinical settings should be performed using existing mechanisms that regulate nursing practice. Typically, this includes the State Board of Nursing, institutional policies, and external agency standards.

Legislation has been introduced at the state level to regulate UAP use and scope of practice. Some states have attempted to regulate UAP practice through registration and certification. Others have proposed direct regulation of UAP by passing legislation that requires UAP to be certified by meeting education and competency requirements. Still others require the state boards of nursing or the Department of Health to register or certify UAP. Thus, regulation by state and jurisdiction varies widely and getting all states to agree to uniform regulations is unlikely.

Discussion Point

Why has the movement to regulate UAP education and training occurred primarily at the state level? Why has there been no national movement to do the same?

Some state boards of nursing have issued recommendations regarding scope of practice for UAP or attempted to delineate the relationship between RNs and UAP. Few states, however, used the ANA or National Council of State Boards of Nursing definitions for delegation, supervision, or assignment. Most states also report that there are no standardized curricula in place for UAP employed in acute-care hospitals. The states have not been able to reach a consensus regarding the education, training, and scope of practice needed for UAP to safely practice either. The end result, then, is that there is no universally accepted scope of practice for UAP.

In addition to existing state regulations regarding UAP education and training, as well as required competencies, many professional nursing organizations have studied the use and effect of UAP and are adopting position statements regarding their use. One national effort to define the scope of practice for UAP was undertaken by the ANA in their delineation of tasks appropriate for UAP practice in the early 1990s. Multiple revisions have followed. In 2007, the ANA suggested six actions that should be taken to create a national and/or state policy agenda about the educational preparation of UAP or NAP and the competencies they should have for safe practice. These are shown in Box 8.1.

In addition, to address the problem, some state boards of nursing have issued task lists for UAP (lists of activities considered to be within the scope of practice for UAP). However, in creating such a list, an unofficial scope of practice is created, and this suggests that such individuals will be performing activities independently. Task lists also suggest that there is no need for delegation, in that the UAP already has a list of nursing activities that he or she may perform without waiting for the delegation process (Marquis & Huston, 2017).

Yet, despite the efforts by the ANA and state boards of nursing, at the institutional level, most health care organizations interpret regulations broadly, allowing UAP a broader scope of practice than that advocated by professional nursing associations or state boards of nursing. In addition, although some institutions limit the scope of practice for UAP to non-nursing functions, many organizations allow the UAP to perform skills traditionally reserved for the licensed nurse.

BOX 8.1   **American Nurses Association's Recommendations for a National and/or State Policy Agenda for NAP**

1. Recognize that the NAP should never be considered or used as a replacement for RNs or licensed practical nurses.
2. Aggressively promote the understanding that delegation is an integral part of professional nursing practice and not a supervisory act connected to acting on behalf of the employer.
3. Establish recognized competencies for the NAP that will guide the development of a core curriculum.
4. Promote national nursing initiatives to establish criteria and guidelines for the clinical training of the NAP through the use of evidence-based research, preparing the NAP to provide routine care in predictable patient functions.
5. Establish systems for training, certification, registry, and disciplinary monitoring of the NAP.
6. Support continued efforts to implement recommendations related to patient safety and quality and the nursing work environment articulated in reports generated by the Institute of Medicine such as *To Err Is Human: Building a Safer Health System*; *Crossing the Quality Chasm: A New Health System for the 21st Century*; and *Keeping Patients Safe: Transforming the Work Environment of Nurses*.

Note: NAP, nursing assistive personnel.
Source: Excerpted from American Nurses Association. (2007). *Position statement: Registered nurses utilization of nursing assistive personnel in all settings.* Retrieved May 15, 2018, from https://www.nursingworld.org/practice-policy/medication-aids--assistants--technicians

Consider This Given the lack of national regulatory standards regarding the scope of practice for UAP, some health care institutions allow UAP to complete tasks traditionally reserved for licensed practitioners.

UAP AND PATIENT OUTCOMES

Because UAP are often involved in providing direct patient care activities, they directly influence not only the quality of care but also the care recipient's quality of life. A well-trained, caring, and competent UAP then can be a vital and contributing member of the health care team.

Certainly, at some point though, given the increasing complexity of health care and the increasing acuity of patient illnesses, there is a maximum representation of UAP in the staffing mix that should not be breached. Those levels have not yet been determined. Considerable evidence does exist, however, that demonstrates a direct link between decreased RN staffing and declines in patient outcomes. Some of these declines in patient outcomes are nurse sensitive and include an increased incidence of patient falls, nosocomial infections, increased physical restraint use, and medication errors (see Chapter 10).

REGISTERED NURSES LIABILITY FOR SUPERVISION AND DELEGATION OF UAP

Delegation has long been a function of registered nursing, although the scope of delegation and the tasks being delegated have changed dramatically over the last three decades with the increased use of UAP in acute-care settings. As a result, the professional nurse (RN) role changed in many acute-care institutions from one of direct care provider to one requiring delegation of patient care to others.

This role of delegator and supervisor increased the scope of legal liability for the RN. Although there is limited case law involving nursing delegation and supervision, it is generally accepted that the RN is responsible for adequate supervision of the person to whom an assignment has been delegated. Although nurses are not automatically held liable for all acts of negligence on the part of those they supervise, they may be held liable if they were negligent in the supervision of those employees at the time that those employees committed the negligent acts (Marquis & Huston, 2017).

Liability is based on a supervisor's failure to determine which patient needs could safely be assigned to a subordinate or for failing to closely monitor a subordinate who requires such supervision. Experienced nurses have traditionally been expected to work with minimal supervision. The RN who delegates care to another competent RN does not have the same legal obligation to closely supervise that person's work as when the care is delegated to UAP.

Consider This The UAP has no license to lose for "exceeding scope of practice," and nationally established standards to state what the limits should be for UAP in terms of scope of practice do not exist. It is the RN who bears the legal liability for allowing UAP to perform tasks that should be accomplished only by a licensed health care professional.

In assigning tasks to UAP, then, the RN must be aware of the job description, knowledge base, and demonstrated skills of each person. Thus, the need for nurses to have highly developed delegation skills has never been greater than it is today. The ability to use delegation skills appropriately will help to reduce the personal liability associated with supervising and delegating to UAP. It will also ensure that clients' needs are met and their safety is not jeopardized. General principles for RNs to use in delegating to NAP are shown in Box 8.2.

Discussion Point

What happens when the condition of a patient changes? Is the training of UAP adequate to recognize changes in clients' conditions that warrant seeking intervention from the licensed nurse?

In addition, communication between the RN and UAP dyad is a critical factor in direct patient care and thus patient safety. The bottom line is that delegating to UAP is similar to delegating to other types of health care workers. RNs are always accountable for the care given and must be responsible for instructing UAP as to who needs care and when. The UAP should be accountable for knowing how to properly perform their segment of assigned care and for knowing when other workers should be called in for tasks beyond the limits of their knowledge and training. As such, the UAP does bear some personal accountability for their actions, despite the legal doctrine of *respondent superior* (the employer can be held legally liable for the conduct of employees whose actions he or she has a right to direct or control).

BOX 8.2   **American Nurses Association's Delegation Principles for RNs Who Work with Nursing Assistive Personnel (NAP)**

1. The RN takes accountability and responsibility for all nursing care performed by the RN or an UAP.
2. The RN directs care and determines the appropriate utilization of any assistant involved in providing direct patient care.
3. The RN may delegate components of care but does not delegate the nursing process itself. The practice pervasive functions of assessment, planning, evaluation, and nursing judgment cannot be delegated.
4. The decision of whether or not to delegate or assign is based upon the RN's judgment concerning the condition of the patient, the competence of all members of the nursing team, and the degree of supervision that will be required of the RN if a task is delegated.
5. The RN delegates only those tasks for which she or he believes the other health care worker has the knowledge and skill to perform, taking into consideration training, cultural competence, experience, and facility/agency policies and procedures.
6. The RN individualizes communication regarding the delegation to the nursing assistive personnel and client situation, and the communication should be clear, concise, correct, and complete. The RN verifies comprehension with the nursing assistive personnel and that the assistant accepts the delegation and the responsibility that accompanies it.
7. Communication must be a two-way process. Nursing assistive personnel should have the opportunity to ask questions and/or for clarification of expectations.
8. The RN uses critical thinking and professional judgment when following the Five Rights of Delegation, to be sure that the delegation or assignment is
   1. The right task
   2. Under the right circumstances
   3. To the right person
   4. With the right directions and communication; and
   5. Under the right supervision and evaluation
9. Chief Nursing Officers are accountable for establishing systems to assess, monitor, verify, and communicate ongoing competence requirements in areas related to delegation.

Note: RN, registered nurse; UAP, unlicensed assistive personnel.
Source: Excerpted from American Nurses Association, National Council of State Boards of Nursing. (n.d.). *Joint statement on delegation.* Retrieved May 15, 2018, from https://www.ncsbn.org/Delegation_joint_statement_NCSBN-ANA.pdf

Stonehouse (2014) agrees, suggesting that UAP must recognize the responsibility and accountability that exist with the support worker's role. Support workers are responsible for what they choose to do, but equally for that which they choose not to do. In addition, "support workers need to embrace the fact that they, day in and day out, are personally responsible and accountable for delivering care of the highest possible standard and should be duly proud of this, knowing that the care they deliver is evidence-based and within their scope of practice" (Stonehouse, 2014, p. 513).

Discussion Point

Do most UAP believe that they can be held legally liable and accountable for their actions if they are delegated to do something by an RN that is beyond their scope of practice or training?

Marquis and Huston (2017) suggest the bottom line is that RNs are always accountable for the care given and must be responsible for instructing NAP as to who needs care, what type of care is needed, and when that care should be provided. NAP should be accountable for knowing how to properly perform their segment of assigned care and for knowing when other workers should be called in for tasks beyond the limits of their knowledge and training. Indeed, NAP must refuse to carry out a delegated task if they feel they do not have the skills, knowledge, and experience to carry it out safely; if the task is something they haven't done before or isn't a part of their normal duties; or if the supervision provided is inadequate (Royal College of Nursing, 2015). As such, the UAP does bear some personal accountability for their actions. This does not, however, negate accountability for the RN who delegated the task(s). The RN continues to be accountable for the care they deliver and for that which is delegated.

REGISTERED NURSES WORKING AS UAP: A LIABILITY ISSUE

It must also be noted that during the recent economic downturn, some employers hired new graduate RNs into UAP positions. Many of these transitional employees secured employment in these positions while students in nursing programs. Though this practice provides employment opportunities for new graduate nurses, it does raise several matters of legality. First, these RNs are not able to provide care to the level of their expertise. Instead, they must perform only direct care duties and remain in the scope of practice of an unlicensed person. This violates numerous statutes that govern scope of practice, because these statutes suggest that licensees are held to the level of practice associated with his or her licensure, regardless of employment status. Thus, licensed nurses are held liable to provide care to the level of their existing scope of practice and yet also face risk of charges of negligence or malpractice if they provide care only to the level of the UAP. Working then in a capacity beneath the level of licensure appears to greatly increase the potential for legal liability for both the nurse and his or her employer and revocation of license for the nurse.

CREATING A SAFE WORK ENVIRONMENT

There are things that health care organizations can do to increase the likelihood that UAP are used both effectively and appropriately as members of the health care team. First, the organization must have a clearly defined organization structure in which RNs are recognized as leaders of the health care team. This organization structure must facilitate RN evaluation of UAP job performance and encourage UAP accountability to the RN.

Job descriptions must also be developed by health care agencies that clearly define the roles and responsibilities of all categories of caregivers. These descriptions should be consistent with that state's nurse practice legislation, as well as with community standards of care, and should reflect differences between the roles of licensed and unlicensed personnel. Policies should facilitate adequate supervision of UAP by RNs and restrict UAP to simple tasks that can be performed safely. In addition, worker credentials should be readily apparent on the nametags worn by nursing health care personnel.

Second, uniform training and orientation programs for UAP must be established to ensure that preparation is adequate to provide at least minimum standards of safe patient care. These training and orientation programs should be based on clearly defined job descriptions for UAP. In addition, organizational education programs must be developed for all personnel to learn the roles and responsibilities

of distinct categories of caregivers. In addition, to protect their patients and their professional license, RNs must continue to seek current information regarding national efforts to standardize scope of practice for UAP and professional guidelines regarding what can be safely delegated to UAP.

In addition, there must be adequate program development in leadership and delegation skills for RNs before UAP are introduced. Delegation is a learned skill, and much can be done to better prepare RNs for this role. Educational programs that produce graduate nurses must explore the nature of the RN role, with a focus on professional nurse leadership roles, to better prepare them to meet the challenges of working in restructured health care settings. Practicing RNs should have opportunities for continuing education in the principles of delegation and supervision. This will allow them not only to recognize the limitations of UAP scope of practice but also to gain confidence in differentiating between skills requiring licensure and those that do not.

UAP SHORTAGES

Finally, if all the issues related to the education, training, scope of practice, and delegation to UAP are resolved, there may be an even greater problem. There may not be enough UAP to meet future demand. The U.S. Department of Labor, Bureau of Labor Statistics (2018b) projects that the need for UAP will grow 11% from 2016 to 2026, faster than the average for all occupations, predominantly in response to the long-term care needs of an increasing elderly population. Yet, the population of potential workers who tend to fill these jobs, overwhelmingly women ages 25 to 64 years, will increase at a much slower rate (Graham, 2017).

In addition, the U.S. Department of Labor suggests that hospitals will continue to be pressured to discharge patients as soon as possible as a result of diminishing reimbursement and this will boost admissions to nursing and residential care facilities. Modern medical technology will also drive the demand for UAP because as technology saves and extends more lives, the need for long-term care provided by UAP increases.

The unfortunate reality is that the demand for UAP as direct caregivers is already growing and the population of persons who have traditionally filled these jobs is declining. Indeed, there is a nationwide shortage of well-trained UAP in all settings, and although many states report recruitment and retention of support personnel as a major area of concern, few are actively addressing the situation.

Graham (2017) agrees, suggesting that acute shortages of home health aides and NAs are occurring across the United States. In some states, however, the problem is worse than in others. In Minnesota and Wisconsin, nursing homes denied admission to thousands of patients in 2016 because they lacked essential staff and patients. In addition, one in seven care-giving positions in Wisconsin nursing homes and group homes remained unfilled, and 70% of administrators reported a lack of qualified job applicants. Similarly, 85% of home health agencies in Wisconsin said they didn't have enough staff to cover all shifts, and 43% reported not filling shifts at least seven times a month. In Illinois, a court monitor determined that the independence of people with severe developmental disabilities was being compromised because of agencies experiencing staff shortages of up to 30% (Graham, 2017).

UAP in Long-Term Care Settings

One problem contributing to this shortage is the high turn-over rate for UAP, particularly in long-term care. The reasons for this high turnover rate are varied, but long hours, inadequate staffing, the low status of the job, exposure to infectious agents and drug-resistant infections, and the physical and emotional demands of the job contribute to it. Working conditions are also often less than ideal. Because of high UAP turnover and absenteeism, those UAP who do work must often work short-handed, which leads to greater stress.

Preshaw, Brazil, McLaughlin, and Frolic (2016) concur, suggesting that ethical and moral dilemmas, conflicts, and distress are not uncommon for the UAP in long-term care. These issues can include respecting autonomy, how to act in the resident's best interest, how to prevent the resident from coming to harm, showing respect for residents, and how to meet professional responsibility.

In addition, Sandvoll, Kristoffersen, and Hauge (2013) suggest that nursing homes are much more complex than

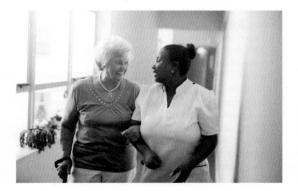

most people imagine and that a greater appreciation must be given to the need for UAP to handle a combination of working according to routines and handling unexpected events, as well as attending to the personal requirements of individual patients. The skill needed to address the complexity of these care requirements may go unnoticed or be taken for granted. Preshaw et al. (2016) agree, noting that although care within the nursing home aims to be individualized and person-centered, it may be quite difficult for the UAP to meet all patient needs on a physical, social, spiritual, and psychological level.

It is also important to note that long-term care facilities, the most common employment site for UAP, are required to meet only minimum government standards for staffing and few facilities are cited, even when understaffing occurs. For example, federal standards only require certified nursing homes that provide Medicare and Medicaid services to have a full-time director of nursing (DON), an RN on duty for 8 consecutive hours 7 days a week (this may be the DON), and one RN and licensed nurse (either an RN or licensed vocational nurse [LVN]/ licensed practical nurse [LPN]) for the two remaining shifts, regardless of its size or the acuity of its patients ("State Level Minimum," 2018). These federal regulations are out of date and do not reflect new knowledge on safe staffing levels. Many states have higher standards.

> **Consider This** The brunt of work in long-term care settings typically falls on lowly paid, unlicensed workers who have a tremendous impact on patient satisfaction and the quality of care provided.

Low pay is also an issue. The U.S. Department of Labor, Bureau of Labor Statistics (2018c) noted that the median annual wage for NAs was $27,520 (about $12/hour) in May 2017. The median wage for UAP was highest in government facilities ($32,860) followed by hospitals ($29,260). Skilled nursing facilities were lower at $26,700 (U.S. Department of Labor, Bureau of Labor Statistics, 2018c). The Governor of Nebraska announced in early 2018 that 20% pay increases would be granted to NAs at state veteran's homes, saying that their wages had fallen behind peer states (Hammel, 2018). This pay increase was the result of a staff turnover of 110% in 2017, that required mandatory overtime and the use of private staffing agencies to fill positions, which further increased costs.

In addition, few employers provide UAP employer-paid benefits such as health insurance coverage, retirement benefits, or childcare. Furthermore, there are limited career paths or advancement opportunities for UAP who do not want to achieve a licensed job category (e.g., LPN, RN), and they often have little direct input into organizational decision making.

CONCLUSIONS

The increased use of UAP presents both opportunities and challenges for the American health care system. Clearly, UAP play an increasingly integral role in safe and resource-efficient care delivery in this country (particularly in long-term care settings), and they can be successfully used to augment the health care team. With increasing patient loads and an emerging nursing shortage, however, many health care organizations and the RNs who work within them will be tempted to allow UAP to perform tasks that should be limited to professional nursing practice.

The challenge then continues to be to use UAP only to provide personal care needs or nursing tasks that do not require the skill and judgment of the RN. Nurses must remember that the responsibility for assuring that patients are protected and that UAP do not exceed their scope of practice ultimately falls on the RN. When UAP are allowed to encroach into professional nursing care, patients are placed at risk.

In addition, the blurring of the lines between the practice of RNs and UAP makes it nearly impossible for patients to make a distinction between providers. One of the most important roles then for the RN is to be a gatekeeper in assuring that care given by UAP under their supervision is always of high quality. Until answers are found, the likelihood is that UAP will continue to constitute a significant portion of the nursing workforce and the boundary between UAP and RN practice will continue to be blurred.

For Additional Discussion

1. Is cost or nursing shortages a greater driving force in increased UAP use in acute-care hospitals today?

2. Is institutional training and certification of UAP a precursor to future initiatives for institutional licensure of RNs?

3. Are the cost savings associated with increased UAP use offset by the need for greater supervision by RNs and potential declines in patient outcomes?

4. Should UAP be allowed to administer medications, perform intravenous cannulation, and change sterile dressings?

5. Do you believe that patients typically are aware whether it is the UAP or licensed nurse who is caring for them?

6. How comfortable do you believe most RNs are in the role of delegator to UAP? Do you believe most RNs are clear regarding role differentiation between the RN and the UAP?

7. Should the training and certification of UAP fall under the purview of state boards of registered nursing?

References

American Academy of Pediatrics. (2009). Policy statement—Guidance for the administration of medication in school. *Pediatrics, 124*(4), 1244–1125. Retrieved May 15, 2018, from http://pediatrics.aappublications.org/content/124/4/1244.abstract

American Nurses Association. (2018). *Medication aids, assistants, technicians.* Retrieved May 15, 2018, from https://www.nursingworld.org/practice-policy/medication-aids-assistants--technicians

Association of Women's Health, Obstetric and Neonatal Nurses. (2016, January). The role of unlicensed assistive personnel (nursing assistive personnel) in the care of women and newborns. *Journal of Obstetric, Gynecologic & Neonatal Nursing, 45*(1), 137–139.

California Healthline. (1998-2018). *Calif. Supreme Court rules school staffers can administer Rx drugs.* Retrieved July 1, 2017, from http://californiahealthline.org/morning-breakout/calif-supreme-court-rules-school-staffers-can-administer-rx-drugs

Carder, P. C., & O'Keeffe, J. (2016, November). State regulation of medication administration by unlicensed assistive personnel in residential care and adult day services settings. *Research in Gerontological Nursing, 9*(5), 209–222.

Graham, J. (2017, May 9). *Severe shortage of direct care workers triggering crisis.* Kaiser Health News. Retrieved May 15, 2018, from https://www.disabilityscoop.com/2017/05/09/severe-shortage-care-crisis/23679/

Gransjön Craftman, Å., Grape, C., Ringnell, K., & Westerbotn, M. (2016, November). Registered nurses' experience of delegating the administration of medicine to unlicensed personnel in residential care homes. *Journal of Clinical Nursing, 25*(21/22), 3189–3198. doi:10.1111/jocn.13335

Hammel, P. (2018, January 9). *Ricketts announces 20 percent pay bump for nursing assistants at state veterans homes.* Live Well Nebraska. Retrieved May 15, 2018, from http://www.omaha.com/livewellnebraska/ricketts-announces-percent-pay-bump-for-nursing-assistants-at-state/article_43d29e7a-f4c5-11e7-b19e-939c5efce6aa.html

Marquis, B., & Huston, C. (2017). *Leadership roles and management functions in nursing* (9th ed.). Philadelphia, PA: Wolters Kluwer.

Medication administration in schools introduction. (2017, February). Retrieved July 2, 2017, from http://www.maine.gov/education/sh/contents/MedicationAdministrationinSchools Introduction.15Feb2017.pdf

National Association of School Nurses. (2018). *Delegation, nursing delegation to unlicensed assistive personnel in the school setting (Revised June 2014).* Retrieved May 15, 2018, from https://www.nasn.org/search?executeSearch=true&SearchTerm=unlicensed+assistive+personnel&l=1

Nurses spending up to one quarter of time on indirect patient care. (2018). Strategies for Nurse Managers, Inc. Retrieved May 15, 2018, from http://www.strategiesfornursemanagers.com/ce_detail/248528.cfm#

O'Keefe, C. (2014). The authority for certain clinical tasks performed by unlicensed patient care technicians and LPNs/LVNs in the hemodialysis setting: A review. *Nephrology Nursing Journal, 41*(3), 247–255.

Preshaw, D. L., Brazil, K., McLaughlin, D., & Frolic, A. (2016). Ethical issues experienced by healthcare workers in nursing homes. *Nursing Ethics, 23*(5), 490–506. doi:10.1177/0969733015576357

Royal College of Nursing. (2015). *Delegation.* Retrieved May 15, 2018, from http://rcnhca.org.uk/46-2/accountability-and-delegation/delegation

Sandvoll, A. M., Kristoffersen, K., & Hauge, S. (2013). The double embarrassment: Understanding the actions of nursing staff in an unexpected situation. *International Journal of Nursing Practice, 19*(4), 368–373. doi:10.1111/ijn.12086

State level minimum nurse staffing requirements for nursing homes. (2018). Retrieved May 15, 2018, from http://www.countyhealthrankings.org/take-action-to-improve-health/what-works-for-health/policies/state-level-minimum-nurse-staffing-requirements-for-nursing-homes

Stonehouse, D. (2014). Who's responsible and who's accountable? You are! *British Journal of Healthcare Assistants, 8*(10), 511–513.

U.S. Department of Labor, Bureau of Labor Statistics. (2018a). *Nursing assistants and orderlies.* Retrieved May 15, 2018, from https://www.bls.gov/ooh/healthcare/nursing-assistants.htm#tab-3

U.S. Department of Labor, Bureau of Labor Statistics. (2018b). *Nursing assistants and orderlies. Job outlook.* Retrieved May 15, 2018, from https://www.bls.gov/ooh/healthcare/nursing-assistants.htm#tab-6

U.S. Department of Labor, Bureau of Labor Statistics. (2018c). *Nursing assistants and orderlies. Pay.* Retrieved May 15, 2018, from https://www.bls.gov/ooh/healthcare/nursing-assistants.htm#tab-5

Unlicensed Assistive Personnel. (2016, September). *NASN School Nurse, 31*(5), 299–301. doi:10.1177/1942602X166611928

Diversity in the Nursing Workforce

Carol J. Huston

LEARNING OBJECTIVES

The learner will be able to:

1. Examine the relationship between health disparities and a lack of diversity in the health care workforce.

2. Explore factors leading to the lack of ethnic and gender diversity in nursing.

3. Suggest individual, organizational, and professional strategies to increase ethnic and gender diversity in nursing.

4. Identify common barriers faced in both recruiting and retaining minority students and faculty in higher education.

5. Compare opportunities for career advancement at senior levels of health care management between racial/ethnic minorities and Whites.

6. Identify at least three professional nursing associations that are directed at serving the needs of a specific racial or ethnic population.

7. Investigate stereotypes of male nurses that both hinder the recruitment and retention of men into nursing and pose socialization and acceptance challenges for them.

8. Compare economic and advancement opportunities for men and women in nursing.

9. Argue for or against the need for affirmative action to bring more men into the nursing profession.

10. Analyze research exploring generational differences in work values and preferences among registered nurses and explore the challenges inherent in having up to four generations cohabitate in the same profession at the same time.

INTRODUCTION

Diversity has been defined as the differences among groups or between individuals, and it comes in many forms, including age, gender, religion, customs, sexual orientation, physical size, physical and mental capabilities, beliefs, culture, ethnicity, and skin color. Yet, despite increasing diversity (particularly ethnic and cultural) in the United States, the nursing workforce continues to be fairly homogeneous, at least in terms of ethnicity and gender, being White, female, and middle aged.

This lack of ethnic, gender, and generational diversity is a concern not only for the nursing profession but also for its clients because a lack of diversity in the workforce has been linked to health disparities. A diverse nursing workforce that understands cultural influences related to illness and wellness and is able to adapt nursing interventions accordingly increases the likelihood that clients will receive culturally competent care (Williams, Bourgalt, Valenti, Howie, & Mathur, 2018). In addition, Butcher (2017) suggests that having diversity in leadership and governance has the potential to most effectively address the call to end care disparities.

The nursing workforce then must strive to be at least as diverse as the population it serves. Rozelle (2018) agrees, suggesting that diverse health care teams are now considered critical for cultural competence and that organizations that promote diversity and inclusion are more successful than those which do not. That's because inclusion cultures accept people for who they are and send a message that no one should feel like they have to change who they are to fit into the group.

> **Consider This** For far too long, health care environments were thought of as neutral territories where patients were expected to be "good houseguests" who fit in, rather than recognizing and welcoming their diversity ("Response to Diversity," 2018, para. 1).

Indeed, a clamor for greater diversity in the profession continues to occur, and this is apparent in a review of the literature. Historically though, despite this stated need for and appreciation of the benefits of a diverse health care workforce, efforts to increase the number of minority professionals have not been as successful as hoped.

> **Consider This** Barriers to increasing the number of minority health care professionals include, but are not limited to, racism, discrimination, and a lack of commitment to changing the situation.

> **Discussion Point**
>
> For nursing care to be culturally and ethnically sensitive, must it be provided by a culturally and ethnically diverse nursing population?

This chapter focuses primarily on three aspects of diversity in the nursing workforce: ethnicity, gender, and age (generational factors). Factors leading to the lack of ethnic and gender diversity in nursing are explored, as are individual and organizational strategies to address the problem. (The importation of foreign nurses as a factor in workforce diversity is discussed in Chapter 7.) In addition, the efforts of health care stakeholders, the government, states, and current professional nursing organizations to increase diversity in the profession are examined. Finally, the effect of generational diversity on workers and workplace functioning is presented.

ETHNIC DIVERSITY IN THE UNITED STATES

Demographic data from the U.S. Census Bureau continue to show increased diversification of the U.S. population, a trend that began almost 35 years ago. As of July 2017, 61.3% of the population was White, not Hispanic or Latino origin (U.S. Census Bureau, 2018). Hispanics continue to be the largest minority group at 17.8% and are the fastest growing population group. Blacks are the second largest minority group (13.3%), followed by Asians (5.7%), American Indians and Alaska natives (1.3%), and native Hawaiians and other Pacific Islanders (0.2%; U.S. Census Bureau, 2018). Projections suggest that current minority populations will become the majority by the year 2043 (American Association of Colleges of Nursing [AACN], 2018a).

ETHNIC DIVERSITY IN NURSING

There are significant differences between the ethnic and gender demographics of the U.S. population and those of the nursing workforce in the United States (Table 9.1). Although the number of nurses from minority backgrounds continues to rise in the United States, it is considerably lower than the minority representation in the general population.

According to 2013 data from the National Council of State Boards of Nursing and the Forum of State Nursing Workforce Centers, nurses from minority backgrounds represent just 19% of the registered nurse (RN) workforce, with the RN population comprising 83% White, 6% African-American, 6% Asian, 3% Hispanic, 1% American

TABLE 9.1	Comparison of U.S. Population and Registered Nurse Workforce in Terms of Ethnicity and Gender	
Characteristic	Year 2017 U.S. Census Data (% Representation)	Year 2013 Registered Nurse Workforce (% Representation)
Gender: Male	49.2	9.6
Gender: Female	50.8	90.4
White (non-Hispanic and non-Latino)	61.3	83.0
Black/African-American	13.3	6.0
Asian/Native Hawaiian/Pacific Islander	5.7	6.0
American Indian/Alaskan native	0.2	1.0
Hispanic/Latino	17.8	3.0
Persons responding to two or more races	2.6	1.0 (other)

Source: American Association of Colleges of Nursing. (2018a). *Enhancing diversity in the workforce.* Retrieved May 16, 2018, from http://www.aacnnursing.org/News-Information/Fact-Sheets/Enhancing-Diversity; U.S. Census Bureau. (2018). *Quick facts. United States.* Retrieved May 16, 2018, from https://www.census.gov/quickfacts.

Indian/Alaskan Native, 1% Native Hawaiian/Pacific Islander, and 1% other (with these figures showing only small increases over the past decade; AACN, 2018).

Similarly, Kovner et al. (2018) found only small increases in the number of White Hispanic nurses as well as males in the profession, when comparing 2006 and 2016 data. These small gains did not meet the Institute of Medicine's (IOM, 2010) *Future of Nursing* recommendations related to increased age, gender, ethnic, and racial diversity in the profession.

Recruiting and Retaining Minority Students in Nursing

Clearly, increasing diversity in the nursing profession must begin with the aggressive recruitment of minority students. In addition, the literature reports that underrepresented minorities (URM) in nursing programs encounter multiple barriers to academic success (Williams et al., 2018). Given that students who do not perceive any barriers to completing their nursing program are three times more likely to pass the NCLEX on the first attempt, significant attention must be given to retention efforts of URM (Williams et al., 2018).

The reality is that White students continue to dominate ethnicity on most college campuses in the United States. Only 30.1% of nursing students in entry-level baccalaureate programs 2007 to 2016 were from minority backgrounds (AACN, 2018a). In addition, about 31.9% of master's students and 29.7% of students in research-focused doctoral programs were from minority backgrounds (AACN,

2018a). These numbers reflect small percentage increases from 2010 to the present (1%–3%), suggesting that although some strides have been made in recruiting and graduating minority nurses, more must be done before equal representation is realized.

Discussion Point

Should more resources (time, energy, money) be devoted to the recruitment of or retention of minority students? Is a two-pronged approach (emphasizing both recruitment and retention) necessary? Why or why not?

The key to recruiting more minority students into nursing is likely creating learning environments that integrate diversity and cultural competence across academic programs and demonstrate an appreciation and respect of minority students themselves. Research by Sedgwick, Oosterbroek, and Ponomar (2014), however, suggests that although undergraduate nursing students quickly learn that RNs, clinical nursing instructors, and peers support the abstract notion of cultural diversity and its inclusion in nursing education in principle, their practices and behaviors often differ. Indeed, minority students often report experiencing bias and discrimination in their interactions with all groups of people involved in their learning. Thus, bias and discrimination are often a systems issue at the institutional level as well as a systemic issue, that is, biased and discriminatory behavior is not limited to one particular group.

Consider This Although most nurse educators and nursing students support the abstract notion of cultural diversity and its inclusion in nursing education in principle, their practices and behaviors often differ.

In addition, many experts suggest that recruitment and retention rates are low with underrepresented groups because such groups are at greater risk of being economically disadvantaged, and this, in turn, places them at greater risk of having received an inferior preparatory education. Students who complete their secondary education in economically disadvantaged communities or institutions may have inadequately developed reading, writing, and critical thinking skills and often lack access to advanced preparation in the natural and physical sciences. This makes them less viable as candidates for admission to a nursing program.

Consider This Recruitment and retention of minority nursing students could improve if these students were given solid secondary academic preparation and if the environments in which they are educated were more accepting of and hospitable to students from diverse backgrounds.

For some minority students, it is an inferior secondary education preparation that predisposes them to course and even program failure. In addition, because many minority students are the first in their families to attend college, it might be difficult for family members to understand and be supportive of the challenges of higher education and the rigor of academic coursework. Minority students also tend to experience more difficulty with social adjustment in the college environment, particularly when they are attending a predominantly White institution and a lack of diversity in faculty role models and mentors contributes to their social isolation.

Finances are also often a barrier to minority students, many of whom must work at least part-time to subsidize the cost of their college education. To address the need for financial support for individuals from disadvantaged backgrounds, the U.S. Health Resources and Services Administration (HRSA, 2017) began offering the *Nursing Workforce Diversity* (NWD) program in 1998. This program provides grants or contracts to projects that provide student stipends or scholarships, stipends for diploma or associate degree nurses to enter a bridge or degree completion program, student scholarships or stipends for accelerated nursing degree programs, preentry preparation, advanced education

preparation, and retention activities. In addition, the NWD program strengthens and expands the comprehensive use of evidence-based strategies shown to increase the recruitment, enrollment, retention, and graduation of students from disadvantaged backgrounds in schools of nursing (HRSA, 2017). A summary of the barriers minority students face in completing their nursing education is shown in Box 9.1.

Consider This It is the retention and graduation of minority students that will begin to change the cultural face of nursing.

To address these concerns, many universities have launched initiatives directed at both the recruitment and retention of these minority students. In addressing recruitment, Scott and Zerwic (2015) note that the University of Illinois at Chicago College of Nursing used the American Association of Medical Colleges Holistic Review Project as a platform to implement a process and paradigm shift for admissions to its nursing programs. In doing so, they argued that the use of holistic admissions can increase the diversity among nursing students and provide the first step toward a diversified nursing profession.

In addressing retention, Tab (2016) detailed the implementation of The RUN 2 Nursing program, an NWD program funded by the U.S. Department of Health and Human Services, at a regional university school of nursing in rural southeast Georgia. The RUN 2 program emphasized the use of faculty mentoring and peer tutoring to make a difference in the academic success of minority nursing students from rural and disadvantaged backgrounds. Other retention and graduation activities included NCLEX preparation for licensure, leadership and professional training, diversity training, workshops on study and time management skills, and scholarships to assist students with

BOX 9.1   **Common Barriers for Minority Students in Academic Nursing Programs**

1. Inferior academic preparation
2. Financial problems
3. Inadequate social support
4. A lack of mentoring opportunities
5. Inconsistent faculty and institutional support
6. Inadequate numbers of minority faculty role models

financial needs including cost of tuition, books, transportation to clinical sites, and other expenses.

Similarly, research by Diefenback, Michalec, and Alexander (2016) noted the importance of increasing the diversity of nursing and university faculty, staff, and administration; implementing diversity training for faculty and students; ensuring cultural competency of the curriculum; fostering formal support structures such as minority student organizations; providing academic supports; facilitating affordability of college; and engaging family support as retention measures for racially and ethnically URM students.

Minority Nurse Educators

The underrepresentation of minority nurse faculty is also well documented. Data from 2016 suggest that only 15.9% of all full-time instructional faculty come from diverse backgrounds, and only 7% are male (AACN, 2017b). Although the number of diverse nursing faculty has made small but continuous gains over the past decade, the percentage of diverse faculty is only half that of diverse nursing students (29.5%). The fact is that far too few nurses from racial/ethnic minority groups with advanced nursing degrees pursue faculty careers.

In an effort to increase the number of minority nurse scholars, the American Association of Colleges of Nursing (AACN) and the Johnson & Johnson Campaign for Nursing's Future launched a national scholarship program in 2007 to increase the number of nursing faculty from ethnic minority backgrounds (AACN, 2018b). This scholarship program supports full-time nursing students in doctoral or master's degree programs, with a preference given to those completing a doctorate. Scholarship recipients must agree to teach in a U.S. school of nursing after completing their advanced degree. Five scholarship recipients are selected annually, with each receiving a $18,000 scholarship.

Another opportunity to support minority faculty is the HRSA *Minority Faculty Fellowship Program* grants. These program grants provide stipends to educational programs to increase the number of faculty representing racial and ethnic minorities. This stipend provides up to 50% of the faculty salary, which is matched or exceeded by the employing institution.

ETHNIC DIVERSITY IN HEALTH CARE ADMINISTRATION

Rosin (2016) notes that a diverse leadership team is important to the realization of strategic goals and objectives for businesses in any industry, yet across all industries, minorities continue to be underrepresented in top leadership positions ("Diversity in C-Suite," 2018). Data from the Equal Employment Opportunity Commission showed that 119,009 minorities held executive- and senior-level positions across private industry in 2015. That's 14% out of a total of 849,503 leadership jobs reported by the agency ("Diversity in C-Suite," 2018).

Health care is struggling to increase diversity in leadership jobs as well. Although improving diversity is a priority to many health care organizations, progress is slow. Although 32% of patients are minorities, only 11% of executive leadership positions, 19% of first- and middle-level management positions, and 14% of board members are currently filled by minorities (Butcher, 2017).

The problem is typically not a lack of highly qualified minority candidates to fill these top jobs. More often, it is that organizations fail to view talented people as potential leaders. Linda Hill, a professor of business administration at Harvard Business School, suggests this may occur because there are "demographic invisibles"—people who, because of their gender, ethnicity, nationality, or even age, don't have access to the tools—the social networks, the fast-track training courses, the stretch assignments—that can prepare them for positions of authority and influence" (Hemp, 2008, p. 125). Hill also suggested that other potential leaders are missed because they are viewed as "'stylistic invisibles'—individuals who don't fit the conventional image of a leader, because they don't exhibit take charge, direction setting behavior" (Hemp, 2008, p. 125). This also may represent cultural differences more than leadership ability.

There are also differences in perceptions between Whites and minorities and between men and women as to how quickly the diversity leadership gap is narrowing. In a 2015 survey, nearly twice as many respondents felt that health care organizations had made headway compared to survey results in 2011 (Rosin, 2016). However, White respondents were more likely to say diversity has improved than racially/ethnically diverse respondents (57% and 26%, respectively) and male respondents were more likely to think diversity has improved (48%) than female respondents (32%). Results also suggested an ongoing need to further improve diversity in the C-suite since multiple barriers still exist, which are slowing efforts to diversify health care management teams (Research Fuels the Controversy 9.1).

There is hope, however. The drive to bring more diversity to the leadership ranks and reduce health care disparities spurred the American College of Healthcare Executives, American Hospital Association, Association of American Medical Colleges, Catholic Health Association,

Research Fuels the Controversy 9.1

Diversity in the Healthcare C-Suite

Witt/Kieffer distributed an online survey to a broad range of its executive clients in the summer of 2015. (The same survey had been distributed in 2011.) The company also conducted phone interviews with executives who participated in the survey. Of the 311 participants, 75% identified themselves as CEOs or other C-suite executives and vice presidents; 55% identified as Caucasian, whereas 45% identified as racially or ethnically diverse individuals; and 31% identified as female and 69% identified as male.

Source: Rosin, T. (2016, May 3). *5 findings on diversity—or lack thereof—in the healthcare C-suite.* Becker's Healthcare. Retrieved July 14, 2017, from http://www.beckershospitalreview.com/hospital-management-administration/5-findings-on-diversity-or-lack-thereof-in-the-healthcare-c-suite.html

Study Findings

- Two-thirds of respondents (66%) agreed that diversity recruiting enables an organization to reach its strategic goals, whereas 71% of respondents said cultural differences among executives support successful decision making. Another 72% of respondents agreed that a diverse workforce enhances the equity of care.
- Compared with 2011, both White respondents and racially/ethnically diverse respondents agreed health care organizations' executive teams today are more racially diverse. However, just 26% of White respondents and 10% of racially/ethnically diverse respondents agreed minority executives are well-represented today in health care management teams.
- Although slightly more respondents felt the diversity of management teams today reflect their patient demographics compared with respondents in 2011, the vast majority of respondents still disagreed. Asian respondents were most likely to disagree (90%), followed by Hispanic respondents (88%), Black respondents (77%) and White respondents (69%).

- White respondents were most likely to name lack of access to diverse candidates (indicated by 83% of White respondents), lack of diverse candidates to promote from within (81%), and lack of diverse candidates participating in the executive search process (77%) as the biggest barriers. Racially/ethnically diverse respondents were most likely to cite a lack of commitment by top management (indicated by 85% of respondents), lack of commitment by the board (72%), and individual resistance to placing diverse candidates (64%) as the primary barriers.
- White and racially diverse survey respondents agreed promoting minorities from within (indicated by 83% of all respondents), hiring minority executives for senior management jobs (73%), communicating the value of cultural differences (70%), seeking out minority candidates from professional organizations (67%), and seeking regular input about the organization's diversity initiatives (52%) could support efforts to diversify the senior management team.

and America's Essential Hospitals to form the *Equity of Care Committee* in 2011. This committee put together a set of best practices for building a leadership diversity program that includes the creation of diversity dashboards to determine how an organization is performing. Each year, the Christus board identifies a set of goals for diversity and inclusion and senior leaders are held accountable for meeting those metrics (Weinstock, 2015).

But even more effort is needed; companies need to offer minorities opportunities to shadow senior executives and should recruit at schools with diverse ethnic enrollments. Marquis and Huston (2017) agree, suggesting that health care organizations must be more open-minded about who health care's future leaders might be and begin to prepare more diverse candidates to be effective leaders. This will require the formal education and training that are a part of most management-development programs, as well as a development of appropriate attitudes through social learning.

Consider This Increasing the number of ethnic minorities in executive health care positions will require an intentional commitment to do so and a well-planned development program that includes the same type of mentoring activities that their White counterparts have long enjoyed and benefited from.

ETHNIC PROFESSIONAL ASSOCIATIONS IN NURSING

There is a professional association for almost every ethnic group in nursing. Several of the many organizations include the National Black Nurses Association, the National Association of Hispanic Nurses, the Philippine Nurses Association, the National Alaska Native American Indian Nurses Association, and the Asian American/Pacific Islander Nurses Association Incorporated. See Box 9.2 for more information on these groups.

BOX 9.2   Ethnic Professional Associations in Nursing

Support groups and professional associations abound among nurses in the United States. Some of the groups formed to address specific issues related to ethnic diversity in nursing include the following:

National Black Nurses Association
The National Black Nurses Association (NBNA, 2018), founded in 1971, represents approximately 150,000 Black nurses from the United States (with 91 chartered chapters nationwide), the Eastern Caribbean nations, and Africa. The mission of the NBNA is to "provide a forum for collective action by African American nurses to represent and provide a forum for black nurses to advocate for and implement strategies to ensure access to the highest quality of health care for persons of color" (NBNA, 2018, para. 4).

National Association of Hispanic Nurses
The National Association of Hispanic Nurses (NAHN, 2018) was founded in 1975 by Ildaura Murillo-Rohde and evolved out of the Ad Hoc Committee of the Spanish-Speaking/Spanish Surname Nurses' Caucus, which was formed during the American Nurses Association convention in San Francisco in 1974. The NAHN is committed to advancing the health in Hispanic communities and to lead, promote, and advocate the educational, professional, and leadership opportunities for Hispanic nurses. There are 2,000 members.

Philippine Nurses Association, Inc.
Founded on September 2, 1922 as the Filipino Nurses Association (FNA), the FNA was incorporated in 1924 (Philippine Nurses Association [PNA], 2018). The International Council of Nurses accepted the FNA as one of the member organizations on July 8–13, 1929. The FNA became the Philippine Nurses Association (PNA) in 1966. The mission of the PNA is to promote professional growth toward the attainment of the highest standards of nursing. Its vision is that by 2030, PNA will be the primary professional association advancing the welfare and development of globally competent Filipino nurses (PNA, 2018).

National Alaska Native American Indian Nurses Association
The National Alaska Native American Indian Nurses Association (NANAINA, 2018) was founded on its predecessor organization, the American Indian Nurses Association, and, later, the American Indian Alaska Native Nurses Association. The NANAINA is dedicated to supporting Alaska Native and American Indian students, nurses, and allied health professionals through the development of leadership skills and continuing education. It also advocates for the improvement of health care provided to American Indian and Alaska Native consumers and culturally competent health care.

Asian American/Pacific Islander Nurses Association Inc.
The Asian American/Pacific Islander Nurses Association Inc. (AAPINA, 2008–2017) serves as the unified voice for Asian American Pacific Islander (AAPI) nurses around the world. AAPINA strives to positively affect the health and well-being of AAPIs and their communities by supporting AAPI nurses and nursing students around the world through research, practice, and education; facilitating and promoting networking and collaborative partnerships; and influencing health policy through individual and community actions.

Discussion Point

If our goal is to better appreciate and merge cultural and ethnic diversity in nursing, why do culturally and ethnically diverse nurses separate themselves with their own professional nursing organizations?

GENDER DIVERSITY IN NURSING

Diversity goals in nursing are not just directed at ethnicity—they also frequently include increasing the number of men in nursing. Decades of legal barriers kept men out of the profession and some nursing schools refused to admit men until a 1981 U.S. Supreme Court ruling (Heitz, 2015). As a result, just 9.6% of U.S. nurses were men in 2013, a percentage that has climbed slowly but steadily since 1980 (AACN, 2018a). The American Assembly for Men in Nursing hopes to bump that statistic up to 20% by 2020 (Heitz, 2015).

In addition, although female nurses outnumber male nurses in every U.S. state, some state-wide variations were reported in 2015 (Rappleye, 2015). For example, in Hawaii there are five female nurses for every male nurse, whereas in Kentucky female nurses outnumber male nurses 12 to 1. The ratio of female to male nurses is greatest in Iowa, North Dakota, and South Carolina, where there are more than 15 female nurses for each male nurse. No states have an equal distribution of gender in nursing (Rappleye, 2015).

There are efforts underway to increase the number of men in nursing. Some suggest that recruitment campaigns are not enough and that affirmative action, similar to the efforts used to increase the number of women in medicine and engineering, will be required before there will be any significant increase in the number of male nurses.

Discussion Point

Affirmative action has been used successfully to increase the presence of some URMs in health care. Should the same be done to increase the number of men in nursing?

Yet, despite a call to increase the number of men in nursing, progress in this regard has been slow. Clow, Ricciardelli, and Bartfay (2014) suggest that social isolation (a lack of role models and mentors, lack of peer support); failure to acknowledge and discuss gender differences in expressions of care (e.g., physical touch used by men vs. women); sexism (professors and textbooks that refer nurses solely with feminine pronouns; antimale comments in the classroom); suppression of the contributions men have made to the field of nursing (e.g., textbooks and nursing programs that ignore the historical role of men in nursing, lectures and textbooks that only portray women as nurses); and media portrayals of male nurses as socially or sexually deviant are part of the problem. In addition, male non-nursing students hold significantly more negative attitudes toward male nurses than female non-nursing students (Clow et al., 2014).

Consider This Caregiving is not just a feminine trait.

Similarly, male scholars in the Robert Wood Johnson Foundation (RWJF) Nurse Faculty Scholars program

reported facing negative stereotypes, perceptions, and generalizations about men who pursue a nursing career (Brody et al., 2017). Some of these negative stereotypes and generalizations related to intelligence; they were not smart enough to be a physician. They also reported curiosity about their sexual orientation that some scholars perceived as a form of microaggression.

The reality is that most of the public would describe nursing as a female occupation, and young men often report they never even consider a career as a nurse. The media also perpetuates the image of the nurse as female. Many media sources, and even nursing textbooks at times, refer to the comforting caregiver nurse as "she," suggesting that male nurses are unable to demonstrate caring behavior and touch similar to their female counterparts. In addition, male nurses may be stereotyped as effeminate, homosexual, or predatory. These stigmatizing discourses may deter men's entry into nursing.

Stuesse and Stuesse (2017) suggest that notions about gender roles in the workplace need to be addressed through education at a young age. Stereotypical gender role choices need to be eliminated, and young minds need to be opened through education to career possibilities once dismissed as not for men or not for women. The difficulty of male nurses socializing into what has long been perceived as a woman's occupation is depicted in Figure 9.1.

Consider This RN Frank Poliafico says one of the first things to know about men in nursing is what to call them......"I'm not a male nurse. I'm a nurse" (English, 2017).

Clearly, stereotypes that suggest male nurses are less capable of therapeutic caring, compassion, and nurturing than female nurses hurt the profession, as well as society in general. At least partly because of these stereotypes, some patients have gender preferences (more commonly female) for their caregivers. This seems to be particularly true for nurses employed in labor and delivery settings.

Although a position statement by the Association of Women's Health, Obstetric and Neonatal Nurses (AWHONN; "Gender Bias," 2016) maintains that nurses, regardless of gender, should be employed in nursing based on their ability to provide such care, Brusie (2013) reported that in a 2005 survey of male nurses, less than 1% of male nurses work in obstetrics—the lowest percentage of any field. And as recently as 10 years ago, some states, like California, actually legally banned males from working

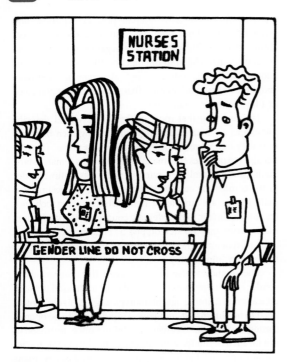

Figure 9.1 Challenges faced by men in nursing. (*Source:* © 2002, Medzilla, Inc. http://www.medzilla.com, reprinted with permission.)

as nurses on obstetrical floors. (Today, states and hospitals cannot deny a male entry into a nursing profession simply based on his gender.) Court cases have confused the issue further. In some cases, the courts have ruled that female gender is a legitimate qualification for labor and delivery nurses, yet other courts have found these qualifications to be discriminatory.

Is There a Male Advantage in Nursing?

Despite the barriers that male nurses face, their minority status may give male nurses advantages in hiring and promotion, unlike women in male-dominated professions. Despite their minority status, men in nursing often rise more rapidly into management positions and earn more money than their female counterparts. Indeed, research by Muench, Busch, Sindelar, and Buerhaus (2016) found that the mean annual salary of male nurses is $10,000 more than their female counterparts. This gap narrowed to $5,148, however, after considering demographic and employment characteristics.

Some experts have suggested that the more rapid career trajectory and relative higher pay for male nurses likely reflects the historical trend that more men are employed full-time in their career paths, whereas women tend to have career gaps related to childbearing or rearing families and often work fewer hours. There is little research, however, to support this.

Indeed, recent research by Greene, El-Banna, Briggs, and Park (2017) found that male nurse practitioners (NPs) earned $12,859 more than female NPs, after adjusting for individual differences in demographics and work characteristics. The gender gap was $7,405 for recent NP graduates and grew over time. Male NPs earned significantly more than female NPs across all clinical specialty areas.

Some differences in work motivation were noted, however, in research by Muench et al. (2016) which found that female RNs moved less often across states and changed employers less frequently than male RNs. In addition, male RNs were more likely to change jobs for pay, though no gender differences were associated with changing jobs for promotion. Gender pay differences, however, existed early in new graduate nurses' careers, negating the argument that pay differences were a result of men working more hours. This observation is disconcerting because gender differences in salary early in a career typically increase over time. In addition, the gap existed for female nurses who did not have children. Thus, a "motherhood penalty" is not a primary driver of the earnings gap in nursing (Muench et al., 2016).

> **Consider This** Many experts suggest that the power of the profession would be elevated if more men were to become nurses. Yet men in nursing hold a disproportionately large share of the high-income jobs and have higher salaries than their female counterparts.

Why Are Men Leaving Nursing?

Although increased numbers of men are joining the nursing profession, disproportionate numbers of male nurses are also leaving, as compared with female nurses. In fact, new male nurses leave the profession at a much higher rate than female nurse graduates. Wallen, Mor, and Devine (2014) suggest this may be a result of the potentially conflicting social expectations men face when they work in female-dominated professions. A scarcity of male role models and conflicting expectations regarding social approval for men in nursing and the assumption of traditional feminine values related to nurturing and caring accentuate the problem.

Research by Wallen et al. (2014) suggests that the respect nurses receive in general as a profession does mediate these conflicting social expectations for male nurses, and in fact, this respect is a significant factor in determining the job satisfaction and affective commitment of male nurses. Thus, efforts to increase occupational status among all nurses decrease the attrition of all nurses, but male nurses in particular. In addition, interventions aimed at male nurses' gender and professional identities might have positive effects on their professional outcomes. This could be as simple as paying attention to the gender neutrality of language used in job advertisements and internal communication.

In addition, although the literature has been mixed, the majority of nursing studies that examined gender and job dissatisfaction suggested that male nurses are more dissatisfied than their female counterparts. Some experts argue that more men than women leave nursing because nursing still lacks status and therefore nurses are often demeaned by other health professionals. Male nurses may be less willing to tolerate this kind of treatment.

> **Consider This** Recent graduates of the nation's nursing schools are leaving the profession more quickly than their predecessors, with male nurses leaving at a higher rate than their female counterparts.

GENERATIONAL DIVERSITY IN NURSING

Age has also become a diversity issue during the last decade. The problem is not that the nursing workforce lacks generational diversity but that typically four generations

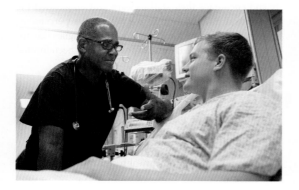

have not cohabitated at the same time in a profession. This climate offers challenges and opportunities for leaders. Opportunities include having a workforce that more closely resembles the diversity of clients served and the chance for best thinking from different perspectives. The challenges include the complexities that result when productivity and efficiency are dependent upon each team member working together effectively.

According to a 2013 survey conducted by the National Council of State Boards of Nursing and The Forum of State Nursing Workforce Centers, 55% of the RN workforce is age 50 or older (AACN, 2017a). Indeed, nurses over the age of 50 have become the largest segment of the nursing workforce. Given the need to both retain older nurses and to recruit new, young nurses into the field, generational issues must be examined further.

Defining the Generations

The research increasingly suggests that the different generations represented in nursing today may have different attitudes and value systems, which greatly impact the settings in which they work. They may also have significantly different career socialization experiences and expectations regarding their chosen profession and employer. In addition, workplace relationships are often influenced by these generational differences.

Most experts identify four generational groups in today's workforce: the veteran generation (also called the *silent generation*), the baby boomers, Generation X, and Generation Y (also called the *millennials*). The *veteran generation* is typically recognized as those nurses born between 1925 and 1942. Having lived through several international military conflicts (World War II, the Korean War, and the Vietnam War) and the Great Depression, they are often risk averse (particularly in regard to personal finances), respectful of authority, and supportive of hierarchy. They are also called the *silent generation* because they tend to support the status quo rather than protest or push for rapid change. As a result, these nurses are less likely to question organizational practices and more likely to seek employment in structured settings (Marquis & Huston, 2017). Their work values are traditional, and they are often recognized for their loyalty to their employers.

The *boom generation* (born 1943–1960) also displays traditional work values; however, they tend to be more materialistic and present oriented and are thus willing to work long hours at their jobs in an effort to get ahead. Clipper (2013) notes that overall, boomers enjoy work, often make the choice to "live to work," and put in many hours. They are personally gratified when they perform well at work. This is also a very competitive cohort by nature that insists that their work is done to the best of their ability and will often beat deadlines. Nurses born in this generation may be best suited for work that requires flexibility, independent thinking, and creativity.

In contrast, *Generation Xers* (born between 1961 and 1981), a much smaller cohort than the baby boomers who preceded them or the Generation Yers who follow them, may lack the interest in lifetime employment at one place that prior generations have valued, instead valuing greater work-hour flexibility and opportunities for time off. Indeed, Clipper (2013) suggests this generation generally works because it is a necessity. This likely reflects the fact that many individuals born in this generation had both parents working outside their home as they were growing up and they want to put more emphasis on family and leisure time in their own family units. Thus, this generation may be less economically driven than prior generations and may define success differently than the veteran generation or the baby boomers. Generation Xers don't mind working hard, but they typically expect something in return, such as job security, good pay, promotions, and flexible schedules. This group is willing to be a team player if they like the team and enjoy what they are doing (Clipper, 2013).

Generation Y (born 1982–1999) represents the first cohort of truly global citizens. They are known for their optimism, self-confidence, relationship orientation, volunteer-mindedness, and social consciousness. This generation may, however, have difficulty being accountable for their actions and work, arguing that a poor performance may not be "their fault." In addition, Clipper (2013) notes that as a whole, millennials don't need their work to define them. They do get bored easily but are willing to work hard as long as they perceive an equivalent benefit to them personally, such as career advancement or financial rewards. A good performance by this group means that all of the variables are in their favor, the right resources, the right team (no conflict among the team as this group prefers group processes/decisions), and the right reasons to do it. They are also technologically savvy, which is why some people call them "digital natives."

Joan M. Kavanagh, Associate Chief Nursing Officer for nursing education and professional development at Cleveland Clinic, notes, however, that millennials often "get a bad rap" (Krischke, 2014, para. 3). "They may tend to change jobs more frequently, but much of that has to do with growth and expansion since their work ethic is intense and committed. They also tend to be innovators, entrepreneurs and bold

risk takers. While those aren't competencies we may have been looking for in the past, they are certainly competencies that will serve us well in this time of unprecedented change" (Krischke, 2014, para. 3).

Given these attitudinal and value differences, it is not surprising that some workplace conflict results between different generations of workers. The reason for this is that each generation may use its own value system as the measurement tool when comparing themselves to their colleagues (Clipper, 2013). Baby boomers may perceive Generation Y nurses as brash or disrespectful or feel that they come to work with a sense of entitlement. There are differing levels of formality, with the older generations preferring the use of titles such as Mr. and Mrs., whereas the younger generations default to using first names, not only with peers, but with patients and supervisors (Krischke, 2014). Generation X workers also report higher levels of burnout as compared with baby boomers, related to incivility from colleagues and cynicism. In addition, there may also be conflicts related to competencies and strategies for knowledge acquisition.

Although this type of generational diversity poses management challenges, it also provides a variety of perspectives and outlooks that can enhance productivity and result in the generation of new ideas. Although the literature often focuses on differences and negative attributes between the generations, particularly for Generations X and Y, a more balanced view is needed. Generational diversity allows patients to receive care from both the most experienced nurses and those with the most recent education and likely greater technology expertise.

The key is that nurse leaders must be clear on workplace expectations so that everyone understands the goals, and so that nurses can accept their colleagues' differences in work performance (Clipper, 2013). Thus, an appreciation of differences is fostered while focusing on what the team has in common—such as common goals (Krischke, 2014). In doing so, nurse leaders must foster a culture of inclusivity and encourage their staff to learn and understand the generational differences that are behind the perceptions of work ethic and performance, so that colleagues can appreciate how the attitude and expectation has been formed (Clipper, 2013).

THE CLAMOR FOR DIVERSITY

Although the need for diversity in nursing is not new, the need to successfully address this issue has never been greater. In response, the government, professional organizations, coalitions, and other health care stakeholders have

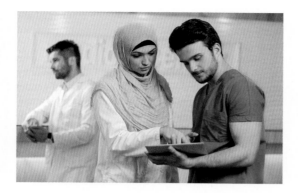

introduced initiatives/funding to address the issue and bring attention to the problem.

For example, the Joint Commission released a report in 2008 titled *One Size Does Not Fit All: Meeting the Health Care Needs of Diverse Populations* (Wilson-Stronks, Lee, Cordero, Kopp, & Galvez, 2008). This report called on health care organizations to meet the unique cultural and language needs of a diverse population and provided a tool for organizations to use that promotes patient safety and health care quality for all patients. In addition, the Institute of Medicine (IOM, 2010) report *The Future of Nursing* noted that to improve the quality of patient care, more emphasis was needed to make the nursing workforce diverse, particularly in the areas of gender and race.

In 2010, the AACN (2018a) published a new set of competencies and an online faculty toolkit at the culmination of a national initiative funded by The California Endowment titled *Preparing a Culturally Competent Master's and Doctorally-Prepared Nursing Workforce*. Working with an expert advisory group, the AACN identified a set of expectations for nurses completing graduate programs and created faculty resources needed to develop nursing expertise in cultural competency. This work complemented a similar project for undergraduate programs that resulted in the publication of the document *Cultural Competency in Baccalaureate Nursing Education* and the posting of an online toolkit for faculty.

In addition, in 2013, the AACN and the RWJF initiated the *Doctoral Advancement in Nursing (DAN) Project* to enhance the number of minority nurses completing PhD and DNP degrees (AACN, 2018a). DAN's expert committee developed a white paper featuring successful student recruitment and retention strategies to be used by schools of nursing; comprehensive approaches to leadership and scholarship development for students; and suggestions for model doctoral curriculum. The DAN project has also created faculty and student toolkits to guide the process of gaining entry into doctoral programs.

In addition, many professional nursing organizations have issued position statements or recommendations on diversity. In 2017, AACN, the national voice for baccalaureate and higher-degree education programs, drafted a position statement that recognizes diversity, inclusion, and equity as critical to nursing education and fundamental to developing a nursing workforce able to provide high-quality, culturally appropriate, and congruent health care in partnership with individuals, families, communities, and populations ("AACN Position Statement," 2017). The position statement suggests that to improve the quality of nursing education, ameliorate health inequities, and advance leadership in the profession and society at large, the values and principles of diversity, inclusion, and equity must remain mission central.

Similarly, the National League for Nursing (NLN) issued a vision statement in 2016 that suggested that diversity and quality health care are inseparable, and that together, they can create a path to increased access and improved health and the elimination of health disparities (NLN Releases a Vision, 2016). The NLN affirmed its commitment to the education of exemplary nurses who value and embody the richness of difference and inclusion to advance the health of the nation and the global community.

The ANA also issued a position statement on discrimination and racism in health care in 1998 and stated its commitment to working toward the eradication of discrimination and racism in the profession of nursing, in the education of nurses, in the practice of nursing, and in the organizations in which nurses work. The *ANA Code of Ethics for Nurses* advocates diversity in its assertion that the nurse, in all professional relationships, practices with compassion and respect for the inherent dignity, worth, and uniqueness of every individual, unrestricted by considerations of social or economic status, personal attributes, or the nature of health problems.

The American Organization of Nurse Executives also developed a diversity statement in 2005. This statement suggests that the success of nursing leadership as a profession depends on reflecting the diversity of the communities it serves and that diversity is one of the essential building blocks of a healthful practice/work environment. In contrast, the International Council of Nurses does not have a diversity statement, but rather has embedded *diversity* in its policy and practice. For example, the organization promotes the principles of equal opportunity employment, pay equity, and occupational desegregation.

CONCLUSIONS

Projections suggest that current ethnic minorities are likely to soon become the majority of the U.S. population. This diversity, however, is not reflected in the nursing workforce or in schools of nursing. Similarly, men are underrepresented in nursing, and efforts to increase the number of men in the nursing profession are even fewer than those directed at increasing ethnic diversity. Finally, generational diversity is occurring in all health care organizations;

however, few organizations have directly confronted the implications of how to deal with this diversity or examined the impact it has on the quality of care provided.

Diversity, equity, and parity are business imperatives but should also be moral imperatives. Using "change by drift" strategies to address the lack of ethnic and gender diversity in nursing has been ineffective. Clearly, proactive, well-thought-out strategies are needed at multiple levels and by multiple parties before diversity in the nursing profession mirrors that of the public it serves.

For Additional Discussion

1. What are the strongest driving and restraining forces for increasing ethnic diversity in nursing, increasing gender diversity in nursing, and having a multigenerational nursing workforce?

2. What are the advantages and disadvantages of intergenerational nurses working together?

3. Should funding for diversity initiatives come from federal or state governments, or from corporate partnerships?

4. Should the institutions that reap the benefits of a diverse workforce share the costs to make that happen?

5. Should there be different nursing school entry requirements for minority students than for their White counterparts?

6. Is an affirmative action approach needed to increase the number of both men and minorities in the nursing profession?

7. Will having more men in nursing raise the status of the profession?

8. What are the potential barriers to having more men in the nursing profession?

9. Why have women been better able to further their numbers in medicine than men have in nursing?

10. How does the use of mentors assist in both the recruitment and the retention of minority (ethnic and gender) nurses?

11. Does a multigenerational nursing workforce improve patient care? If so, how?

12. Which health disparities do you think would be more positively impacted if the nursing workforce was more diverse?

References

AACN position statement on diversity, inclusion, & equity in academic nursing. (2017). *Journal of Professional Nursing, 33*(3), 173–174. doi:10.1016/j.profnurs.2017.04.003

American Association of Colleges of Nursing. (2017a). *Nursing shortage fact sheet*. Retrieved May 16, 2018, from http://www.aacnnursing.org/News-Information/Fact-Sheets/Nursing-Shortage

American Association of Colleges of Nursing. (2017b). *Enhancing diversity in the workforce*. Retrieved May 16, 2018, from http://www.aacnnursing.org/News-Information/Fact-Sheets/Enhancing-Diversity

American Association of Colleges of Nursing. (2018a). *Enhancing diversity in the workforce*. Retrieved May 16, 2018, from http://www.aacnnursing.org/News-Information/Fact-Sheets/Enhancing-Diversity

American Association of Colleges of Nursing. (2018b). *Johnson & Johnson/AACN minority nurse faculty scholars*. Retrieved May 16, 2018, from http://www.aacnnursing.org/Students/Financial-Aid-Scholarships/Minority-Nurse-Faculty-Scholarship

Asian American/Pacific Islander Nurses Association, Inc. (2008–2017). *About us*. Retrieved July 14, 2017, from http://www.aapina.org/about-us/

Brody, A. A., Farley, J. E., Gillespie, G. L., Hickman, R., Hodges, E. A., Lyder, C., . . . Pesut, D. J. (2017, May). Diversity dynamics: The experience of male Robert Wood Johnson Foundation nurse faculty scholars. *Nursing Outlook, 65*(3), 278–288. doi:10.1016/j.outlook.2017.02.004

Brusie, C. (2013, September 10). *Would you trust a male nurse during your labor and delivery?* Retrieved May 16, 2018, from http://www.pregnancyandbaby.com/pregnancy-birth/

articles/966941/would-you-trust-a-male-nurse-during-your-labor-and-delivery

Butcher, L. (2017, September). Enhancing diversity. *H&HN: Hospitals & Health Networks, 91*(9), 18–23.

Clipper, B. (2013). *Generational diversity: Implications for nurse staffing.* Retrieved July 14, 2017, from Advance Healthcare Network—For Nurses website: http://utahcnatraining.blogspot.com/2013/04/generational-diversity-implications-for.html

Clow, K. A., Ricciardelli, R., & Bartfay, W. J. (2014). Attitudes and stereotypes of male and female nurses: The influence of social roles and ambivalent sexism. *Canadian Journal of Behavioural Science, 46*(3), 446–455.

Diefenbeck, C., Michalec, B., & Alexander, R. (2016, January). Lived experiences of racially and ethnically underrepresented minority BSN students: A case study specifically exploring issues related to recruitment and retention. *Nursing Education Perspectives (National League for Nursing), 37*(1), 41–44. doi:10.5480/13-1183

Diversity in C-suite lacking across all industries. (2018, February 26). *Modern Healthcare, 48*(9), 32.

English, T. (2017, February 1). I am not a male nurse. I am a nurse. *The Journal of Nursing.* Retrieved May 18, 2018, from https://www.asrn.org/journal-nursing/february1-2017.html

Gender bias in women's health, obstetric, and neonatal nursing. (2016, June). *Nursing for Women's Health, 20*(3), 327. doi:10.1016/S1751-4851(16)30146-5

Greene, J., El-Banna, M. M., Briggs, L. A., & Park, J. (2017, November). Gender differences in nurse practitioner salaries. *Journal of the American Association of Nurse Practitioners, 29*(11), 667–672. doi:10.1002/2327-6924.12512

Health Resources and Services Administration. (2017). *Nursing workforce diversity (NWD).* Retrieved July 13, 2017, from https://bhw.hrsa.gov/fundingopportunities/default.aspx?id=71a65b17-a6c8-45cf-a944-99b0d256fcef

Heitz, D. (2015, April 22). *Male nurses are on the rise—filling a need and making a living.* Healthline. Retrieved July 16, 2017, from http://www.healthline.com/health-news/male-nurses-are-on-the-rise-filling-a-need-and-making-a-living-042215#1

Hemp, P. (2008). *Where will we find tomorrow's leaders? A conversation with Linda A. Hill by Paul Hemp.* Harvard Business Review. Retrieved July 15, 2017, from https://hbr.org/2008/01/where-will-we-find-tomorrows-leaders

Institute of Medicine. (2010, October). *The future of nursing: Leading change, advancing health.* Retrieved July 16, 2017, from http://thefutureofnursing.org/IOM-Report

Kovner, C. T., Djukic, M., Jun, J., Fletcher, J., Fatehi, F. K., & Brewer, C. S. (2018, March). Diversity and education of the nursing workforce 2006–2016. *Nursing Outlook, 66*(2), 160–167. doi:10.1016/j.outlook.2017.09.002

Krischke, M. M. (2014, May 6). *Generational differences in nursing: Has the work ethic changed?* Retrieved July 15, 2017, from NurseZone.com website: http://essynursingservices.com/generational-differences-in-nursing-has-the-work-ethic-changed

Marquis, B., & Huston, C. (2017). *Leadership roles and management functions in nursing* (9th ed.). Philadelphia, PA: Wolters Kluwer.

Muench, U., Busch, S. H., Sindelar, J., & Buerhaus, P. I. (2016, September/October). Exploring explanations for the female-male earnings difference among registered nurses in the United States. *Nursing Economic$, 34*(5), 214–223.

National Alaska Native American Indian Nurses Association. (2018). *The National Alaska Native American Indian Nurses Association (NANAINA).* Retrieved May 16, 2018, from https://ncemna.org/ourcauses/the-national-alaska-native-american-indian-nurses-association-nanaina

National Association of Hispanic Nurses. (2018). *History.* Retrieved July 15, 2017, from http://www.nahnnet.org/NAHN/About/History/NAHN/Content/History.aspx?hkey=45d72c12-d9fb-4a57-860a-5053827c9649

National Black Nurses Association. (2018). *About NBNA.* Retrieved May 16, 2018, from http://www.nbna.org/about

NLN releases a vision for achieving diversity and meaningful inclusion in nursing education. (2016, May/June). *Nursing Education Perspectives (National League for Nursing), 37*(3), 186. doi:10.1097/01.NEP.0000000000000018

Philippine Nurses Association Inc. (2018). *About PNA. History.* Retrieved May 16, 2018, from http://www.pna-ph.org/the-company/about-pna/history

Rappyleye, E. (2015, May 29). *Gender ratio of nurses across 50 states.* Retrieved July 15, 2017, from http://www.beckershospitalreview.com/human-capital-and-risk/gender-ratio-of-nurses-across-50-states.html

Response to diversity. (2018, April). *Critical Care Nurse, 38*(2), 76–80.

Rosin, T. (2016, May 3). *5 findings on diversity—or lack thereof—in the healthcare C-suite.* Becker's Healthcare. Retrieved July 14, 2017, from http://www.beckershospitalreview.com/hospital-management-administration/5-findings-on-diversity-or-lack-thereof-in-the-healthcare-c-suite.html

Rozelle, C. (2018, Winter). Exposing students to diverse health care teams. *ABNF Journal, 29*(1), 5–7.

Scott, L. D., & Zerwic, J. (2015). Holistic review in admissions: A strategy to diversify the nursing workforce. *Nursing Outlook, 63*(4), 488–495. doi:10.1016/j.outlook.2015.01.001

Sedgwick, M., Oosterbroek, T., & Ponomar, V. (2014). "It all depends": How minority nursing students experience belonging during clinical experiences. *Nursing Education Perspectives, 35*(2), 89–93. doi:10.5480/11-707.1

Stuesse, E. R., & Stuesse, M. J. (2017). A woman's job? A man's job? *Reflections on Nursing Leadership, 43*(2), 20–23.

Tab, M. (2016). Helping minority students from rural and disadvantaged backgrounds succeed in nursing: A nursing workforce diversity project. *Online Journal of Rural Nursing & Health Care, 16*(1), 59–75. doi:10.14574/ojrnhc.v16i1.362

U.S. Census Bureau. (2018). *Quick facts. United States.* Retrieved May 16, 2018, from https://www.census.gov/quickfacts/

Wallen, A. S., Mor, S., & Devine, B. A. (2014). It's about respect: Gender-professional identify integration affects male nurses' job attitudes. *Psychology of Men & Masculinity, 15*(3), 305–312.

Weinstock, M. (2015, April 2). *NAACP grades hospital leadership diversity.* H&HN. Retrieved July 14, 2017, from http://www .hhnmag.com/articles/3594-naacp-grades-hospital-leader-ship-diversity

Williams, L., Bourgault, A., Valenti, M., Howie, M., & Mathur, S. (2018, March). Predictors of underrepresented nursing students' school satisfaction, success, and future education intent. *Journal of Nursing Education, 57*(3), 142–149.

Wilson-Stronks, A., Lee, K. K., Cordero, C., Kopp, A. L, & Galvez, E. (2008). *One size does not fit all: Meeting the healthcare needs of diverse populations.* Retrieved July 16, 2017, from http://www.jointcommission.org/assets/1/6/ HLCOneSizeFinal.pdf

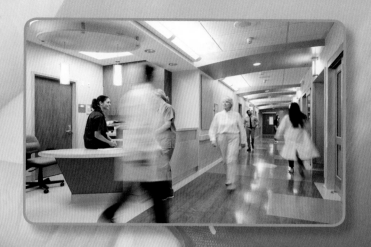

3

WORKPLACE ISSUES

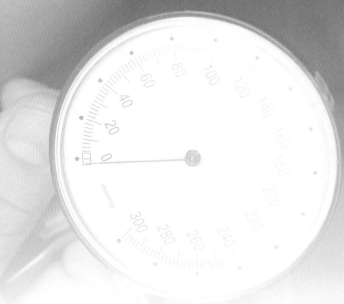

Mandatory Minimum Staffing Ratios

Carol J. Huston

LEARNING OBJECTIVES

The learner will be able to:

1. Explore factors driving legislative mandates for minimum registered nurse (RN) representation in the staffing mix.

2. Summarize current research findings regarding the effect of staffing ratios and staffing mix on patient outcomes.

3. Debate driving and restraining forces for legislating minimum licensed staffing ratios.

4. Assess the efficiency and effectiveness of the processes used by the state of California Department of Health Services to determine initial minimum RN–patient staffing ratios for different types of hospital units.

5. Describe challenges to staffing ratio implementation in California, including the need to define "licensed nurses," legal challenges to the "at all times clause," and strategies directed at delaying or rescinding the mandate altogether.

6. Investigate the movement and/or progress of states other than California to adopt minimum RN staffing ratios.

7. Discuss the effect of the current nursing shortage on the likelihood of successful passage of proposed staffing ratio legislation in states other than California.

8. Argue for or against the appropriateness of the "at all times clause" as part of California's staffing ratio mandate.

9. Assess whether California's 2004 implementation of mandatory minimum RN staffing ratios has met its goals.

10. Identify alternatives to staffing ratio mandates that seek to ensure that staffing resources are adequate to provide safe patient care.

11. Reflect on the staffing ratios used in his or her work setting and assess, using clearly defined criteria, whether they are adequate to provide quality patient care.

INTRODUCTION

For some time now, economics has been the primary driver in dictating changes in the registered nurse (RN) skill mix in hospitals. As a result, the trend early in the first decade of the 21st century was to reduce RNs in the staffing mix and to replace them with less expensive personnel. Empirical research increasingly concludes, however, that the number of RNs in the staffing mix has a direct effect on quality care and, in particular, patient outcomes (Fowler and Comeaux, 2017). In response, legislators, health care providers, and the public are increasingly demanding adequate staffing ratios of RNs in health care settings. Indeed, recent research showed that the overall use of UAP/NAP and licensed practical nurse/ licensed vocational nurse (LPN/LVN) hours per patient day declined from 2010 to 2014, whereas RN hours per patient day remained stable (Li, Pittman, Han, and Lowe, 2017).

It is noteworthy that the U.S. federal government has established minimum standards for licensed nursing in certified nursing homes but not in acute care hospitals. Several attempts have been made in Congress in the past decade to enact hospital nurse staffing laws; however, none have come close to fruition. Section 42 of the Code of Federal Regulations (42CFR 482.23[b]) does require Medicare-certified hospitals to "have adequate numbers of licensed RNs, licensed practical (vocational) nurses, and other personnel to provide nursing care to all patients as needed"; however, this "nebulous language and failure of Congress to enact a quality nursing care staffing act to date, has left it to the states to ensure that staffing is appropriate to patients' needs" (American Nurses Association [ANA], 2018, para. 4).

As a result, a national (indeed international) movement to examine the need for minimum staffing ratios has begun. Many states in the United States, with the backing of some nursing organizations, have moved toward imposing mandatory licensed staffing requirements. In fact, as of 2015, 14 states addressed nurse staffing in hospitals in law/regulations (California, Connecticut, Illinois, Massachusetts, Minnesota, Nevada, New Jersey, New York, Ohio, Oregon, Rhode Island, Texas, Vermont, and Washington) (ANA, 2018). Many of the states that have adopted legislation about staffing originally sought staffing ratio legislation.

In addition, Massachusetts has already passed a law specific to intensive care units requiring a 1:1 or 1:2 nurse-to-patient ratio, depending on stability of the patient, and Minnesota now requires a Chief Nursing Officer or designee to develop a core staffing plan with inputs from others (ANA, 2018). Seven states (Connecticut, Illinois, Nevada, Ohio, Oregon, Texas, and Washington) now require hospitals to have staffing committees responsible for plans and staffing policy (ANA, 2018).

California, however, is the only state that stipulates in law, regulations for required minimum nurse-to-patient ratios in hospitals and long-term care facilities, that must be maintained at all times, by unit. Another state, however, is close. A proposed November 2018 ballot question (yet to be voted on at the time of this writing) would mandate nurse staffing ratios in Massachusetts as well (Schoenberg, 2018). The Massachusetts Health and Hospital Association suggests that mandating nurse staffing ratios would cost the Massachusetts health care system $1.3 billion in the first year and $900 million each year after that (Schoenberg, 2018). Supporters of the ballot question say safe staffing ratios are necessary to ensure that nurses can adequately care for patients. Opponents of the ballot question argue there is already a nursing shortage, so requiring hospitals to hire more nurses will mean the nurses that are available to hire are less experienced. That could make patients less safe.

This chapter explores both the driving and the restraining forces for legislatively mandated minimum RN representation in the staffing mix. California's experience, as the first and only state to implement minimum staffing ratios, is detailed, as well as its struggle to define appropriate ratios and implement staffing ratios in an era of limited fiscal and human resources. The chapter concludes by looking at the movement of other states toward the adoption of minimum staffing ratios and strategies that have been suggested as alternatives to mandatory staffing ratios.

> **Consider This** Identifying and maintaining the appropriate number and mix of nursing staff is critical to the delivery of quality patient care.

STAFFING RATIOS AND PATIENT OUTCOMES

Linda Aiken, "undoubtedly the most influential researcher in nurse staffing, not only in the United States, but globally," suggests that although most research "has little impact on actual practice, that 20 years of research on the impact of nurse staffing on patient outcomes has made a big difference in the outcomes of patients and nurses, and managerial and clinical practice" (Kerfoot & Douglas, 2013, p. 216). Indeed, hundreds, if not thousands, of studies in the last decade have examined the link between staffing mix and patient outcomes. Many of the studies note a link between the increased representation of RNs in the staffing mix and improved patient outcomes.

Consider This There is wide variation in the skill mix (percentage of licensed to unlicensed workers) and RN-to-patient ratios across the United States.

Few studies, however, have had as much effect on determining safe staffing ratios as two benchmark research studies published in 2002. The first study was the work of Needleman, Buerhaus, Mattke, Stewart, and Zelevinsky (2002). This study of 799 hospitals in 11 states found a higher prevalence of infections, such as pneumonia and urinary tract infections, failure to rescue, and shock or cardiac arrest when the nurses' workload was high.

The second study, which is often cited as the seminal work in support of establishing minimum staffing ratio legislation at the federal or state level, was completed by Aiken, Clarke, Sloane, Sochalski, and Silber (2002). This study of more than 10,000 nurses and 230,000 patients in 168 hospitals concluded that in hospitals with higher patient-to-nurse ratios, surgical patients had a greater likelihood of dying within 30 days of admission. In addition, they experienced increased odds of failure to rescue (mortality following complications). This occurred because the time nurses have for surveillance, early detection, and timely intervention—particularly with patients who are not at high risk but who are vulnerable to other unfavorable outcomes—has a direct effect on patient outcomes.

In addition, the study found that staffing at six patients per nurse rather than four would result in an additional 2.3 deaths per 1,000 patients and an additional 8.7 deaths per 1,000 patients with complications. Staffing at eight patients per nurse rather than six would incur an additional 2.6 deaths per 1,000 patients and 9.5 deaths per 1,000 patients with complications. Uniformly staffing at eight patients per nurse rather than four was expected to entail five excess deaths per 1,000 patients and 18.2 complications per 1,000

patients. In addition, patients had a 31% higher chance of dying within 30 days of admission (Aiken et al., 2002).

Consider This There is compelling evidence to suggest that increasing the number of RNs in the staffing mix leads to safer workplaces for nurses and a higher quality of care for patients.

Within days of the study's release, Aiken's study results were summarized, repeated, and analyzed in detail in almost all relevant public forums and by most professional health care organizations. The message was clear: There was a direct link between nurse-to-patient ratios and mortality rates from preventable complications, and having an inadequate number of RNs places the public at risk.

Discussion Point

Why did the study by Aiken et al. (2002) garner so much national attention in so many public forums? Were the findings significantly different than those of earlier studies? Was it timing?

Was it how "the message" was managed?

Over the past two decades, research sophistication regarding how best to study the relationship between staffing and patient outcomes has increased dramatically. Still, there are issues related to how outcomes are defined, what operational definitions should be used, and who should be counted in nurse staffing. Perhaps that is why more recent research has raised questions about whether RN staffing levels truly do have an impact on patient outcomes. Summaries of select recent research studies are shown in Table 10.1. This has made the determination of the optimal nurse-to-patient ratio an ongoing challenge.

ARE MANDATORY MINIMUM STAFFING RATIOS NEEDED?

One proposed solution to Aiken's research findings was the implementation of minimum mandatory RN–patient staffing ratios in acute care hospitals. Numerous articles have appeared in the media attesting to grossly inadequate staffing in hospitals and nursing homes, and professional nursing organizations, such as the ANA, continue to express concern about the effect poor staffing has both on nurses' health and safety and on patient outcomes.

TABLE 10.1   Select Research on Nurse Staffing Levels and Patient Clinical Outcomes (2016–2018)

Citation	Description
Driscoll et al. (2018)	This review of 35 cross-sectional research studies, the majority utilizing large administrative databases, found that higher staffing levels were associated with reduced mortality, medication errors, ulcers, restraint use, infections, pneumonia, higher aspirin use, and a greater number of patients receiving percutaneous coronary intervention within 90 minutes. The researchers concluded that nurse-to-patient ratios influence many patient outcomes, most markedly in-hospital mortality.
Cho, Park, Choi, Lee, and Kim (2018)	This cross-sectional study of 58 hospitals with 100 or more beds in South Korea found that nurse staffing and nurse were significantly associated with the length of stay of surgical patients. A 10% increase in the average number of patients per nurse increased the length of stay by 0.284 days ($p = 0.037$).
Morita, Matsui, Fushimi, and Yasunaga (2017)	This retrospective cohort study examined the association of inpatient nurse-to-occupied bed ratio (NBR) with in-hospital fractures. Logistic regression analysis showed that the proportion of in-hospital fractures in the group with the highest NBR was significantly lower than that in the group with the lowest NBR. The researchers concluded that sufficient nurse staffing may be important to reduce postsurgical in-hospital fractures in acute care hospitals.
Hill (2017)	This systematic literature review explored the relationship between registered nurse staffing levels and patient mortality in acute secondary care settings in England. Two research articles supported the hypothesis that reduced nursing time directly affected patient mortality; two did not, although they reported that patient outcomes were affected negatively, contributing to poor patient experience, and one suggested that patient survival rates after cardiac arrest in acute care settings were directly related to nurse ratios. All studies suggested patient outcomes were likely to be underreported, and the degree of underreporting may be higher where staffing levels are low. This limits the ability to observe associations between outcomes and staffing levels.
Wolf, Perhats, Delao, Clark, and Moon (2017)	The purpose of this qualitative, exploratory study was to examine emergency nurses' perceptions of factors involved in safe staffing levels and to identify factors that negatively and positively influence staffing levels. Participants reported that staffing levels were determined by the number of beds in the department (as in inpatient units) but not by patient acuity or the number of patients waiting for treatment. Participants identified both absolute numbers of staff and experience mix as components of safe staffing. Inability to predict the acuity of patients waiting to be seen was a major component of nurses' perceptions of unsafe staffing. Researchers concluded that absolute numbers of staff, as well as skill and experience mix, should be considered to provide staffing levels that promote optimal patient and nurse outcomes.
Leary, Tomai, Swift, Woodward, and Hurst (2017)	The purpose of this research was to uncover possible associations and explore if a deeper understanding of relationships between staffing and other factors such as safety could be revealed within routinely collected national data sets in the UK. A number of associations were revealed within both the UK staffing data set and the National Health Service (NHS) benchmarking data set. However, the challenges of using these data included inconsistent data collection and quality. The researchers concluded that relationships are likely to be complex and nonlinear and that the validity, usefulness, and method of routine national data collection appear to require reexamination.
Staggs et al. (2017)	This longitudinal study of 3,101 medical, surgical, and medical–surgical units in U.S. hospitals participating in the National Database of Nursing Quality Indicators from 2006 to 2010 examined whether nurse staffing relative to a unit's long-term average was associated with restraint use. The researchers found that nursing skill mix was inversely correlated with restraint use for fall prevention and for any reason and concluded that ensuring adequate skill mix should reduce use of restraint.

(continued)

TABLE 10.1	**Select Research on Nurse Staffing Levels and Patient Clinical Outcomes (2016–2018)** (*continued*)
Citation	**Description**
Sermeus (2016)	Using data from more than 33,000 nurses and 11,000 patients in 500 hospitals from 12 European countries, from 2009 until 2011, this study found that an increase in a nurse's workload by one patient increased the likelihood of an inpatient dying within 30 days of admission by 7% and that every 10% increase in bachelor's degree nurses was associated with a decrease in this likelihood by 7%.
Schneider and Geraedts (2016)	This study investigated the association between nurse and physician staffing and the incidence of hospital-acquired pressure ulcers in acute care hospitals in Germany. The total number of nurses and physicians per 100 beds did not show significant associations with outcome variables; however, the proportion of nurses with at least 3 years of training to total nursing staff was inversely associated with the incidence of pressure ulcers at hospital level, indicating a higher efficacy of pressure ulcer prevention measures.
Giuliano, Danesh, and Funk (2016)	This study examined the relationship between nurse staffing and 30-day excess readmission ratios for patients with heart failure in the top U.S. adult cardiology and heart surgery hospitals. A significant difference ($p = 0.021$) was found between the low nurse staffing group ($n = 358$) and the high nurse staffing group ($n = 303$). Thus, hospitals with a lower nurse staffing index had a significantly higher excess readmission rate.
Neuraz et al. (2015)	This multicenter longitudinal study involving 5,718 patients who were admitted to eight adult intensive care units (ICUs) in four university hospitals in France over a 1-year period, found that ICU patient mortality increased when the number of patients was above 2.5 per nurse and above 14 per physician. Shifts with inadequate staffing occurred mostly during weekends for nurses and nights for physicians. Higher risk of death was also correlated with heavy workload.

Proponents of mandated minimum staffing ratios argue that minimum staffing ratios are absolutely essential to ensuring that staffing is adequate to promote patient safety and to achieving desired patient outcomes. They also suggest that the use of standardized ratios provides a more consistent approach than acuity-based staffing.

> **Consider This** The bottom line is that minimum staffing ratios would not have been proposed if staffing abuses and the resultant decline in the quality of patient care had not occurred in the past.

Critics, however, suggest that the overall cost of care would increase exponentially if mandatory ratios were imposed nationally and that no guarantee of quality improvement or positive outcomes exists with such ratios. In addition, there is a risk that staffing may actually decline with ratios because they might be used as the ceiling or as ironclad criteria if institutions are unwilling to make adjustments for patient acuity or RN skill level.

The American Organization of Nurse Executives (AONE) agrees, noting that it does not support mandated nurse staffing ratios because staffing is a complex issue composed of multiple variables, and ratios cannot guarantee that the health care environment is safe (Rice, 2015). Dr. Christine Cassel, CEO of the National Quality Forum, also agrees, arguing there is not enough research evidence to indicate how effective fixed staffing ratios are at improving patient outcomes (Rice, 2015). In fact, evidence regarding the benefits of staffing ratios is mixed and sometimes contradictory.

Mandatory ratios also ignore the education, experience, and skill level of the individual nurse. The Ohio Hospital Association concurs, arguing that:

> *Staffing a hospital is a complex process that continually changes according to the number of patients and severity of conditions being treated in the hospital. Mandated staffing ratios restrict hospitals' ability to adjust to the needs of their patients. Furthermore, fixed ratios improperly assume that all nurses share the same skill sets and are simply "interchangeable parts" in the treatment of patients. Hospitals must have the flexibility to respond to the dynamic state of patient needs and must focus on a variety of factors other than staffing ratios when determining staffing levels, while always keeping patient*

safety at the core of those decisions. Those factors include patient needs, volume, and acuity, patient satisfaction, resources available, nursing staff competency and skill mix, availability of medical and support staff, and a variety of staffing standards set by accrediting bodies, professional societies, and federal and state regulators (Ohio Nurses Association, 2017, last para).

Aiken also agrees, suggesting that "It's the legislative mandate aspect that is controversial—not so much the actual focus on safe staffing, or the required staffing levels. Americans tend not to like legislative mandates" (Kerfoot & Douglas, 2013, p. 217). Similarly, Corbridge (2017) argues that mandating inflexible nurse staffing ratios or stringent meal and rest break requirements do not improve patient care or outcomes.

It is cost, though, that is likely most often cited as a deterrent for implementing minimum staffing ratios. An increase in RN staffing is clearly more expensive than using unlicensed staff but if patient outcomes are better, these increased costs may be offset.

Recent evidence, however, is limited, making it difficult to assess cost-effectiveness. One study conducted by Clark, Saade, Meyers, Frye, and Perlin (2014),

examined the relationship between nurse-to-patient staffing ratios and perinatal outcomes in women receiving oxytocin during labor. The study found that adoption of universal 1:1 staffing for this patient population in the United States would result in the need for an additional 27,000 labor nurses at a cost of $1.6 billion. The researchers suggested this cost could not be justified given the lack of evidence regarding the relationship between nurse-to-patient staffing ratio and improved perinatal outcomes.

A study by Silber et al. (2016), however, of 172,225 patients in 606 hospitals across three states (Illinois, New York, and Texas) found that the total average cost of surgery remained at about $27,000 in both facilities with good staffing and those with poorer staffing (a mean ratio of about 1.5 nurses per bed vs. those with a mean of less than 1 nurse per bed), suggesting that better-staffed facilities had a formula for excellent value as well as better patient outcomes (Research Fuels the Controversy 10.1).

Still others argue that it is health care professionals—not legislators or regulators—who understand health care and are best qualified to determine staffing needs, particularly when best practices in staffing are used (Box 10.1).

Research Fuels the Controversy 10.1

Testing Outcomes and Cost of Care Based on Nurse Staffing

This study examined the outcomes and cost of care of a total of 172,225 patients in 606 hospitals across three states (Illinois, New York, and Texas). The research explored whether hospitals recognized nationally as having better nursing work environments displayed better value (lower mortality with similar costs) than those with worse nursing environments. The 35 hospitals with better nursing work environments had a mean nurse-to-bed ratio of 1.51 and the 293 hospitals with worse nursing environments had a mean nurse-to-bed ratio of 0.69.

Thirty-day mortality in better nursing work environment hospitals was 4.8% vs. 5.8% in worse environment hospitals ($p < 0.001$), whereas the cost per patient was similar.

Source: Silber, J. H., Rosenbaum, P. R., McHugh, M. D., Ludwig, J. M., Smith, H. L., Niknam, B. A., . . . Aiken, L. H. (2016, June). Comparison of the value of nursing work environments in hospitals across different levels of patient risk. *JAMA Surgery, 151*(6), 527–536. Retrieved July 29, 2017, from http://jamanetwork.com/journals/jamasurgery/fullarticle/2482670

Study Findings

Thirty-day mortality in focal hospitals was 4.8% compared to 5.8% in control hospitals, whereas the cost per patient was similar, suggesting better value in the focal group. For the focal vs. control hospitals, the greatest mortality benefit occurred in patients in the highest risk quintile, with a nonsignificant cost difference of $941 per patient. The greatest difference in value between focal and control hospitals appeared in patients in the second-highest risk quintile, with a nonsignificant cost difference of −$862.

The researchers concluded that hospitals with better nursing environments and above-average staffing levels were associated with better value (lower mortality with similar costs) compared with hospitals without nursing environment recognition and with below-average staffing, especially for higher-risk patients. These results did not suggest that improving any specific hospital's nursing environment would necessarily improve its value, but they did show that patients undergoing general surgery at hospitals with better nursing environments generally receive care of higher value.

Best Practices for Determining Nurse Staffing Ratios

1. Develop strategies to use when staffing levels are not adequate
2. Create an internal resource pool for flexibility and census adjustments
3. Communicate all action plans to staff nurses and administrative stakeholders
4. Empower staff nurses to identify solutions for staffing decisions and budget
5. Benchmark staffing ratios annually with other facilities
6. Correlate staffing with patient outcomes, adverse events, and root causes
7. Evaluate patient satisfaction feedback

Source: Nurse staffing ratios. (2013). *AORN Journal, 97*(5), 604–538. doi:10.1016/j.aorn.2013.02.011

This might be the case, but given that hospitals are no longer exempt from "big business," profit-driven motives, one must question whether what is best for patients can be separated from what is best financially for the institution. Wallace (2013) argues, then, that staffing must always take into account educational preparation, experience, and professional needs, and nurse managers must always evaluate competency levels and critical thinking skills as a basis for staffing to create a safe patient care environment.

CALIFORNIA AS THE PROTOTYPE FOR MANDATORY MINIMUM STAFFING RATIOS

Passing the Legislation

California has had a minimum ratio of licensed nurse-to-patient requirement (Title 22 of the California Code of Regulations) for intensive care and coronary care units for more than three decades; however, no minimums were initially established for other types of acute care units. Given increasing pressure from nursing unions in the state, increasing bad press about poor quality care, the increased use of unlicensed assistive personnel as direct care providers, and skyrocketing patient loads for licensed nurses in acute care, California stepped forward as the first state in the nation to implement mandatory minimum staffing ratios.

Under Assembly Bill (A.B.) 394 ("Safe Staffing Law"), passed in 1999 and crafted by the California Nurses Association (CNA), all hospitals in California were to comply with the minimum staffing ratios shown in Table 10.2 by January 1, 2004. These ratios, developed by the California Department of Health Services (CDHS) with assistance from the University of California, Davis, represented the maximum number of patients an RN could be assigned to care for, under any circumstance. In addition, this legislation prohibited unlicensed personnel from performing certain procedures such as administering medication, performing venipuncture, providing parenteral or tube feedings, inserting nasogastric tubes, inserting catheters, performing tracheal suctioning, assessing patient conditions, providing patient education, and performing moderately complex laboratory tests.

Determining Appropriate Ratios

Developing draft regulations for minimum staffing ratios was challenging for the CDHS because data were not readily accessible regarding the distribution of nurse staffing in California hospitals, the number of hospitals likely to be affected by the minimum staffing requirements, or the expected costs of this legislation. In addition, the ratios were meant to supplement valid and reliable patient classification systems (PCS), which had been required in California hospitals since 1996. The problem was that although California hospitals had been required to submit their PCS data to the state, there was no standardization and little guidance about what characterized a valid PCS or what criteria should be used in determining the PCS. Therefore, PCS data yielded little, if any, helpful information to the CDHS for determining appropriate ratios.

Discussion Point

The California Healthcare Association advocated the use of PCS as the gold standard for staffing decisions rather than staffing ratios. The CNA argued for the reverse. What motives may have driven these positions?

Cost was also not known. Initial projections by the Public Policy Institute of California suggested that many hospitals in California would experience sharp increases in cost associated with the increase in numbers of licensed staff. At least in part as a result of limited empirical data, proposals received by CDHS suggested a wide range of minimum staffing ratios and even more widely differing estimates of cost. The California Hospital Association (CHA), a hospital

TABLE 10.2   Minimum Registered Nurse (RN) Staffing Ratios for Hospitals in California in 2004 and New National Nurses United (NNU) Recommendations for 2018

Unit	Minimum RN–Patient Ratio Required in California in 2004 as a Result of AB 394	Minimum RN–Patient Ratio Recommended by NNU in 2018
Critical care/intensive care unit (ICU)	1:2	1:2
Neonatal ICU	1:2	1:2
Operating room	1:1	1:1 (plus at least one additional scrub assistant)
Postanesthesia		1:2
Labor and delivery	1:2	1:2
Antepartum	1:4	1:3
Postpartum couplets	1:4	1:3
Combined labor and delivery and postpartum		1:3
Postpartum women only	1:6	1:3
Intermediate-care nursery		1:4
Pediatrics	1:4	1:3
Emergency room (ER)	1:4	1:3
Trauma patient in ER		1:1
ICU patient in ER		1:2
Step-down	1:4 initially; 1:3 as of 2008	1:3
Telemetry		1:3
Medical–surgical	1:6 initially; 1:5 as of 2005	1:4
Oncology	1:5 initially; 1:4 as of 2008	
Coronary care		1:2
Acute respiratory care		1:2
Burn unit		1:2
Other specialty care units		1:4
Psychiatry	1:6	1:4
Rehabilitation		1:5
Skilled nursing facility		1:5

Source: National Nurses United. (2010–2018). *National campaign for safe RN-to-patient staffing ratios.* Retrieved May 16, 2018, from http://www.nationalnursesunited.org/issues/entry/ratios

trade group representing the interests of nearly 500 hospital and health system members in California at that time, called for a minimum staffing ratio of 1 nurse to 10 patients on medical–surgical units, whereas the unions representing the largest numbers of nurses in the state argued for minimum ratios in medical–surgical units of 1:4. The CNA recommended a 1:3 ratio in medical–surgical units.

Following months of waiting and almost 2 years of wrangling, the final minimum staffing ratios were announced in January 2002 (see Table 10.2). Governor Gray Davis, in a press conference at St. Vincent's Medical Center in Los Angeles, announced that his administration supported a ratio of one nurse to every six patients in medical–surgical units— twice the number of patients supported by the CNA and four fewer than that favored by the CHA. Regulations were released later that spring with 45 days allocated for public comment. Hospitals in California were also required to continue to keep a PCS in place and to staff according to the PCS if it called for a larger number of nurses than the minimum ratios set by the CDHS.

Delays in Implementation

Implementing the ratio legislation proved to be just as difficult as determining what the ratios should be. The first challenge that arose was interpreting the meaning and intent of the legislation's language in regard to what constituted "licensed nurses." Almost immediately, questions were raised about whether the minimum mandatory ratios had to reflect RN representation in the staffing mix or whether LVNs/LPNs would meet the requirement.

The CNA argued that the intent of the law was to regulate minimum RN staffing, which inflamed the labor unions representing LVNs/LPNs. Amid much controversy, the issues were aired at a public hearing before the Department of Health Services in San Francisco, and a determination was provided that the ratios referred to RNs only and that LVNs/LPNs would be authorized to practice only under the direction of licensed RN or physician.

Questions were then raised as to whether hospitals could eliminate or reduce their nonlicensed staff in an effort to save costs, given that the number of RNs would be increased. The CNA argued that the ratios were based on CDHS surveys of existing hospital staffing patterns and that nonlicensed staff should not be cut if safe patient care was to be assured. The state, however, chose not to weigh in, arguing that its position was to regulate minimum RN–patient ratios; as a result, many hospitals immediately began reducing the number of support personnel to offset the increased cost of RN staff, and many RNs were forced to assume non-nursing care tasks.

Finally, the CHA, with the help of State Senator Sam Aanestad, introduced new legislation (A.B. 847) to the California State Senate Health and Human Services committee in April 2003 in an attempt to delay implementation of the 1:5 minimum nurse–patient staffing ratio on medical–surgical units until it could be ascertained that adequate RNs were available to meet the ratios. Opponents of the delay argued that this was simply an effort to preclude implementation of the mandate altogether. The bill failed.

Then the hospitals persuaded Governor Arnold Schwarzenegger to issue an emergency regulation in November 2004 to overturn emergency room ratios and the improved medical–surgical ratios, citing financial crises (Cortez, 2008). In response, the CNA and the National Nurses Organizing Committee (NNOC) launched more than 100 protests against Schwarzenegger, which resulted in a massive grassroots movement and the stinging defeat of four Schwarzenegger ballot initiatives in a 2005 special election (Cortez, 2008). The emergency regulation was ruled illegal in March 2005 by a state superior court judge and overturned. The judge argued that the financial state of hospitals did not give the state the right to delay implementing the law because the law's intent was to improve patient safety. Hospitals were told to comply immediately.

Still, resistance to staffing ratio implementation continued. Hospitals were accused of encouraging management staff to undermine and avoid compliance with the new RN staffing ratios. Nursing unions responded with threats to close down units with inadequate staffing, to delay elective surgeries, and to wage a public relations campaign to garner public support for the nurses.

The Struggle to Implement the Ratios

Despite these efforts and a pervasive, ongoing resistance to staffing ratio implementation, the staffing ratio mandate did become effective on January 1, 2004. But were hospitals ready and willing to implement these changes? By and large, bigger hospitals in the state were ready to meet the mandate by the time of its implementation. Many smaller hospitals, however, had existing budget deficits and had to seek waivers from the CDHS because of their difficulty in meeting ratios. Waivers were allowed; however, hospitals had to be rural and meet very strict conditions.

> ### Discussion Point
>
> Should small rural hospitals be given waivers for the mandatory staffing ratios? Is this justified by the patient population characteristics, or is it simply an economic incentive to keep these hospitals viable?

The dire predictions about reductions in hospital services increased emergency room diversions, and hospitals in California having to close doors if mandatory staffing ratio legislation passed, never materialized. In fact, most hospitals in California did not have to hire more contracted RNs to comply with the ratios. Nor was there a decrease in skill mix as a result. In fact, nurses from all over the country moved to California for jobs when the staffing ratios legislation passed.

Aiken agrees, noting that the adverse, unintended consequences of mandatory nurse staffing levels, feared before the implementation of mandated staffing ratios, never materialized (Kerfoot & Douglas, 2013). Instead, a large proportion of hospitals continued to have more nurses than required, most nurses reported that their workloads decreased, and when more agency nurses were used, there did not appear to be any negative impacts on quality of care (Kerfoot & Douglas, 2013).

The "At All Times" Clause

Almost immediately after implementation of A.B. 394, legal clarification did become necessary, however, regarding interpretation of the law with regard to ratio coverage "at all times." A ruling by the CDHS blindsided many hospitals in its strict interpretation that ratios had to be maintained at all times, including breaks and lunches. For many hospitals, this meant hiring additional rotating staff to fill in for nurses when they leave the bedside for short periods (breaks, lunch, transporting patients, etc.) or face being noncompliant.

As a result, the CHA filed a lawsuit on December 30, 2003, challenging the ruling and arguing that the "at all times" ruling was impossible to implement. The motion was heard in a Sacramento court on May 14, 2004. In a 10-page ruling issued on May 26, 2004, the judge dismissed the hospital association lawsuit, saying that not adhering to the "at all times" clause would make the nurse-to-patient ratios meaningless. Again, the ruling was an effort to maintain the intent of the law—to protect patients.

Discussion Point

Is an "at all times" ruling necessary to ensure quality health care?

Have RN Staffing and Patient Outcomes Improved in California Because of Mandatory Minimum Staffing Ratios?

As of January 1, 2008, California's historic staffing law for RN staffing ratios completed its phase-in period, and almost a decade of data now exist regarding compliance with the staffing ratios, as well as changes in patient outcomes. A synthesis by Donaldson and Shapiro (2010) of 12 studies examining the impact of California's ratios on patient care cost, quality, and outcomes in acute care hospitals revealed that the implementation of minimum nurse-to-patient ratios did reduce the number of patients per licensed nurse and increase the number of worked nursing hours per patient day in hospitals. There were, however, no significant impacts of these improved staffing measures on measures of nursing quality and patient safety indicators across hospitals. Donaldson and Shapiro emphasized, however, that adverse outcomes did not increase despite the increasing patient severity reflected in case mix index and cautiously posited that this finding might actually suggest an impact of ratios in preventing adverse events in the presence of increased patient risk.

In addition, Aiken (2010) and the Center for Health Outcomes and Policy Research at the University of Pennsylvania conducted an independent evaluation of California's mandated nurse staffing requirements. This survey of more than 22,000 RNs, working in 604 hospitals in California and two comparison states without legislation—Pennsylvania and New Jersey—found that overall, nurses in California cared for an average of one patient fewer than nurses in the two comparison states. On medical and surgical units, California hospital nurses each took care of two fewer patients. In terms of patient outcomes, Aiken studied more than 1 million patients who had common surgical procedures in these hospitals in 2006, more than 2 years after mandatory nurse staffing was implemented. She found that California hospitals had significantly lower risk-adjusted mortality and were better at rescuing patients who experienced complications than the comparison states, even after taking into account factors other than differences in nurse staffing.

Similarly, a literature review conducted by Serratt (2013b) suggested mixed results, with three studies finding both positive and negative outcomes and five studies reporting no significant changes in patient outcomes. Serratt concluded that some improvements resulted from the implementation of staffing ratios, but the positives were not as significant and widespread as predicted. Another study reported by Serratt (2013a) found an increase in labor costs and some reduction in services with ratio implementation, suggesting a negative financial impact on selected outcomes of California hospitals.

In addition, Munnich (2014) reported that little evidence exists to support the idea that this law was effective in attracting more nurses to the hospital workforce or improving patient outcomes, although nurse-to-patient ratios in medical–surgical units increased substantially following the staffing mandate. Survey data from two nationally representative datasets indicate that the law had no effect on the aggregate number of RNs or the hours they worked in California hospitals, and at most a modest effect on wages. Munnich cautioned that California's experience with minimum nurse staffing legislation may not be generalizable to states considering similar policies in very different hospital markets.

Another literature review by Mark, Harless, Spetz, Reiter, and Pink (2013) also noted mixed results in terms of whether mandatory ratios in California improved patient care quality. Although the Agency for Healthcare Research and Quality (AHRQ) reported that its patient safety indicators showed a significant reduction in patient falls, pressure ulcers, and restraint use, conflicting data by California hospitals, Mark et al. found no significant differences to support AHRQ's findings.

Yet, Tellez and Seago (2013) note that nurse satisfaction and nurse retention rates did rise after passage of the California staffing law. The significance is that as the nursing workforce ages and retires, there will be a shortage of experienced nurses to care for the increasing demand for health care put forward by the Affordable Care Act. These facts place pressure on the health care system to care for more patients with fewer nurses. California's staffing legislation is serving to counter mounting pressure.

The answer as to whether mandated ratios have improved care or created new cost burdens for California is still unclear. The CNA says the ratios have improved nurse retention, raised the numbers of qualified nurses willing to work, reduced burnout, and improved morale. Aiken agrees, suggesting that there is very good scientific evidence that staffing improved even in safety-net hospitals that had long had poor staffing (Kerfoot & Douglas, 2013). Aiken also notes that prior to the California staffing legislation, all of the blue ribbon committees that looked at safe nurse staffing shied away from establishing specific patient-to-nurse ratios. Thus, communicating with stakeholders and the media was difficult without "a recommended number." "The evidence-based benchmark implemented in California of no more than five patients per nurse on medical and surgical units has become the number' against which to evaluate hospital staffing" (Kerfoot & Douglas, 2013, p. 217).

> **Consider This** The answer as to whether mandated ratios have improved care or created new cost burdens for California is still unclear.

OTHER ALTERNATIVES

Efforts are also under way, in both California and the rest of the nation, to explore alternatives to improving nurse staffing that do not require legislated minimum staffing ratios. The reality is that many leading health care and professional nursing organizations do not support the need for legislated minimum staffing ratios. For example, the Joint Commission, one of the most powerful accrediting bodies for hospitals in the United States, has been reluctant to endorse nationally mandated minimum staffing ratios, suggesting that this would not be flexible enough to encompass the diversity represented in hospitals across the United States.

In addition, the ANA does not support fixed nurse–patient ratios, arguing that evidence does not exist to support legislated ratios (ANA, 2018b). Instead, it advocates an evidence-based workload system that takes into account the many variables that exist to ensure safe staffing. In fact, the ANA (2018a) has recommended three general approaches to assure sufficient nurse staffing at the state level (Box 10.2). The ANA argues that this type of approach better accommodates changes in patients' needs, available technology, and the preparation and experience of staff. In addition, the ANA argues that what may be established through legislation today as an appropriate minimum nurse-to-patient ratio may be obsolete by the next shift or 2 years from now and that disclosure of staffing plans without evaluation and recourse for inadequate levels is futile.

Aiken also suggests that she is not necessarily an advocate of legislative mandates (Kerfoot & Douglas, 2013). Instead, she argues that there are multiple ways to achieve the objectives that have been achieved in California. She continues to support publicly reported nurse staffing and urges nurses to do the same so that greater transparency regarding hospital staffing can occur. She concludes that "even folks who are not in favor of legislative mandates should open their minds to the evidence that the California legislation did work as intended" and that "it is a mistake for nurses to reject evidence if not to their liking for some reason" (Kerfoot & Douglas, 2013, p. 217).

In addition, the Veterans Health Administration (VHA) enacted a staffing methodology model in 2011 that uses expert panels at the unit level to determine inpatient staffing levels based on acuity. These levels are then reported to the facility level. Implementation of the staffing methodology was, however, delayed in part to leadership turnover. Preliminary evaluation of the model suggests some empowerment of nurses at the unit level; however, the impact on patient outcomes is not yet available (Fowler & Comeaux, 2017; Taylor et al., 2015).

Buchan (2014) suggests that research regarding mandated staffing ratios is a "scientific exercise hampered by inadequate research, limited data, disagreement on

---

> **BOX 10.2** **Three General Approaches Recommended by the ANA (2018) to Maintain Sufficient Staffing**
>
> 1. The formation of nurse-driven staffing committees to create staffing plans that reflect the needs of the patient population and match the skills and experience of the staff.
> 2. Legislators mandate specific nurse-to-patient ratios in legislation or regulation.
> 3. Facilities are required to disclose staffing levels to the public and/or a regulatory body.

definitions in differences between organization and health system norms" (para. 1). Indeed, he argues that although proponents may have the best intentions, insufficient quality outcome evidence exists to support the imposition of mandated nurse staffing ratios. Still, he notes that in areas where there are so few nurses that patient care is unsafe, ratios do provide some type of bulwark against further erosion of staffing levels. Ratios then appear to make sense only where management and resources are most inadequate.

CONCLUSIONS

The literature suggests that increasing RN representation in the staffing mix improves at least some patient outcomes. What is less clear is what the optimal staffing levels are for various patient populations and when costs associated with staffing mix become unreasonable in terms of attempting to improve patient outcomes. In addition, given the lessons that have already been learned with the "RN/LVN debate" and the "at all times" requirement, more thought must be given to how strictly staffing ratio regulations are to be interpreted and how enforcement can be effective if there are no monetary consequences for breaking rules. In addition, the intermingling roles of state government as a legislator of minimum staffing ratios, compliance officer, disciplinary enforcer, and potential funding source to assist with mandated ratio implementation need further examination and clarification.

Finally, it must be recognized that patient acuity is continuing to rise, and the mandatory minimum staffing ratios adopted in California in 2003 were arguably inadequate just 5 years later, especially when hospitals refused to staff above the ratios when census and acuity call for it (Cortez, 2008). In fact, the New National Nurses United (NNU, 2010–2018) is advocating for even lower ratios (see Table 10.2). These ratios would pose even greater fiscal and human resource challenges to California hospitals in terms of their implementation.

The implementation and subsequent evaluation of mandatory staffing ratios in California should, however, provide some insight into these ongoing issues that will be helpful to other states that choose to follow in California's footsteps. Clearly, the enactment of California's nurse-to-patient ratio law was far from smooth, and concerns continue about the costs of hiring additional licensed staff, and the need to meet the "at all times" clause.

It is not clear yet whether California has the resources (both human and fiscal) it would need to lower the staffing ratios further. Some of the initial implementation struggles may have been related to the normal issues that arise whenever a new law takes effect; however, the reality is that California has struggled to maintain the mandate. The fact that it took 5 years from passage of the legislation to mandated implementation is telling. What is even more telling are the number of hospitals in California that continue to report difficulty in meeting staffing ratio requirements and the resistance that continues to be a part of its implementation.

Perhaps Linda Aiken said it best: "We need to address the fundamental issues, like workloads that are too great and chaotic environments. It's not to say that nothing else matters in patient safety. But it does say nurse staffing matters a lot" (Rice, 2015, para. 34).

For Additional Discussion

1. Given rising patient acuity levels and increased scope of responsibility for RNs, at what point should California reexamine the adequacy of current staffing ratios?

2. In an effort to cut the costs associated with implementing minimum RN staffing ratios, some hospitals eliminated their support staff. Have RNs gained anything when this is the case?

3. Should LVNs/LPNs be counted to meet minimum mandatory staffing ratio requirements?

4. Is allowing hospitals to determine their staffing needs a little like having the "fox guard the chicken coop?"

5. Does the implementation of mandatory staffing ratios in the midst of a severe national nursing shortage make sense? Why or why not?

6. At what point does cost related to staffing mix become so prohibitive that society will be willing to accept some increase in patient morbidity and mortality?

7. What critical lessons should other states learn from California's experience thus far in implementing mandatory staffing ratios?

References

Aiken, L. (2010). Safety in numbers. *Nursing Standard, 24*(44), 62–63.

Aiken, L. H., Clarke, S. P., Sloane, D., Sochalski, J., & Silber, J. (2002). Effects of nurse-staffing on nurse burnout and job-dissatisfaction and patient deaths. *The Journal of the American Medical Association, 288*, 1987–1993.

American Nurses Association. (2018a). *Nurse staffing*. Retrieved May 15, 2018, from http://www.nursingworld.org/MainMenuCategories/Policy-Advocacy/State/Legislative-Agenda-Reports/State-StaffingPlansRatios

American Nurses Association (Michigan) (2018b). *ANA's case for evidence-based nursing staffing*. Retrieved August 26,. 2018 from http://www.ana-michigan.org/anas-case-evidence-based-nursing-staffing/

Buchan, J. (2014). Getting staffing levels right. *Nursing Standard, 28*(49), 30.

Cho, E., Park, J., Choi, M., Lee, H. S., & Kim, E. (2018, March). Associations of nurse staffing and education with the length of stay of surgical patients. *Journal of Nursing Scholarship, 50*(2), 210–218.

Clark, S. L., Saade, G. A., Meyers, J. A., Frye, D. R., & Perlin, J. B. (2014). The clinical and economic impact of nurse to patient staffing ratios in women receiving intrapartum Oxytocin. *American Journal of Perinatology, 31*(2), 119–123.

Corbridge, I. (2017, January 31). *Requirements to nurse staffing ratios*. Retrieved July 29, 2017, from http://www.wsha.org/articles/requirements-nurse-staffing-ratios

Cortez, Z. (2008, January 4). *California's nurse-patient ratio law: Saving lives, reducing the nursing shortage*. Retrieved July 20, 2017, from http://www.californiaprogressreport.com/site/california%E2%80%99s-nurse-patient-ratio-law-saving-lives-reducing-nursing-shortage

Donaldson, N., & Shapiro, S. (2010). Impact of California mandated acute care hospital nurse staffing ratios: A literature synthesis. *Policy, Politics & Nursing Practice, 11*(3), 184–201.

Driscoll, A., Grant, M. J., Carroll, D., Dalton, S., Deaton, C., Jones, I., . . . Astin, F. (2018, January). The effect of nurse-to-patient ratios on nurse-sensitive patient outcomes in acute specialist units: A systematic review and meta-analysis. *European Journal of Cardiovascular Nursing, 17*(1), 6–22.

Fowler, D., & Comeaux, Y. (2017). The legislative role in nurse staffing ratios. *Med-Surg Matters, 26*(2), 12–13.

Giuliano, K. K., Danesh, V., & Funk, M. (2016). The relationship between nurse staffing and 30-day readmission for adults with heart failure. *Journal of Nursing Administration, 46*(1), 25–29.

Hill, B. (2017, June 22). Do nurse staffing levels affect patient mortality in acute secondary care? *British Journal of Nursing, 26*(12), 698–704.

Kerfoot, K. M., & Douglas, K. S. (2013). The impact of research on staffing: An interview with Linda Aiken, Part 1. *Nursing Economic$, 31*(5), 216–253.

Leary, A., Tomai, B., Swift, A., Woodward, A., & Hurst, K. (2017). Nurse staffing levels and outcomes—Mining the UK national data sets for insight. *International Journal of Health Care Quality Assurance, 30*(3), 235–247. doi:10.1108/IJHCQA-08-2016-0118

Li, S., Pittman, P., Han, X., & Lowe, T. J. (2017). Nurse-related clinical nonlicensed personnel in U.S. Hospitals and their relationship with nurse staffing levels. *Health Services Research, 52*, 422–436.

Mark, B., Harless, D., Spetz, J., Reiter, K., & Pink, G. (2013). California's minimum nurse staffing legislation: Results from a natural experiment. *Health Services Research, 48*(2), 435–454.

Morita, K., Matsui, H., Fushimi, K., & Yasunaga, H. (2017, June). Association between nurse staffing and in-hospital bone fractures: A retrospective cohort study. *Health Services Research, 52*(3), 1005–1023. doi:10.1111/1475-6773.12529

Munnich, E. L. (2014). The labor market effects of California's minimum nurse staffing law. *Health Economics, 23*(8), 935–950.

National Nurses United. (2010–2018). *National campaign for safe RN-to-patient staffing ratios*. Retrieved May 16, 2018, from http://www.nationalnursesunited.org/issues/entry/ratios

Needleman, J., Buerhaus, P., Mattke, S., Stewart, M., & Zelevinsky, K. (2002). Nurse-staffing levels and the quality of care in hospitals. *The New England Journal of Medicine, 346*, 1715–1722.

Neuraz, A., Guérin, C., Payet, C., Polazzi, S., Aubrun, F., Dailler, F., . . . Duclos, A. (2015, August). Patient mortality is associated with staff resources and workload in the ICU: A multicenter observational study. *Critical Care Medicine, 43*(8), 1587–1594.

Ohio Nurses Association. (2017, May 4). *Nurses say mandatory overtime puts patients at risk*. Retrieved July 30, 2017, from http://www.ohnurses.org/nurses-say-mandatory-overtime-puts-patients-risk

Rice, S. (2015, October 24). *Got enough nurses? Nurse groups cite Kentucky case to support push for staffing ratio laws*. Modern Healthcare. Retrieved July 29, 2017, from http://www.modernhealthcare.com/article/20151024/MAGAZINE/310249979

Schneider, P. P., & Geraedts, M. (2016). Staffing and the incidence of pressure ulcers in German hospitals: A multicenter cross-sectional study. *Nursing & Health Sciences, 18*(4), 457–464. doi:10.1111/nhs.12292

Schoenberg, S. (2018, May 1). *Nurse staffing ratios: What is the 2018 Massachusetts ballot question all about?* Retrieved May 16, 2018, from http://www.masslive.com/politics/index.ssf/2018/05/nurse_staffing_ratios_what_is.html

Sermeus, W. (2016). Understanding the role of nurses in patient safety: From evidence to policy with RN4CAST. *BMC Nursing, 15*, 1.

Serratt, T. (2013a). California's nurse-to-patient ratios, Part 2: 8 Years later, what do we know about hospital level outcomes? *Journal of Nursing Administration, 43*(10), 549–553.

Serratt, T. (2013b). California's nurse-to-patient ratios, Part 3. *Journal of Nursing Administration, 43*(11), 581–585.

Silber, J. H., Rosenbaum, P. R., McHugh, M. D., Ludwig, J. M., Smith, H. L., Niknam, B. A., . . . Aiken, L. H. (2016, June). Comparison of the value of nursing work environments in hospitals across different levels of patient risk. *JAMA Surgery, 151*(6), 527–536. Retrieved July 29, 2017, from http://jamanetwork.com/journals/jamasurgery/fullarticle/2482670

Staggs, V., Olds, D., Cramer, E., Shorr, R., Staggs, V. S., Olds, D. M., & Shorr, R. I. (2017). Nursing skill mix, nurse staffing level, and physical restraint use in US hospitals:

A longitudinal study. *Journal of General Internal Medicine, 32*(1), 35–41. doi:10.1007/s11606-016-3830-z

Taylor, B., Yankey, N., Robinson, C., Annis, A., Haddock, K. S., Alt-White, A., & Sales, A. (2015). Evaluating the Veterans Health Administration's staffing methodology model: A reliable approach. *Nursing Economic$, 33*(1), 36–66.

Wallace, B. C. (2013). Nurse staffing and patient safety: What's your perspective? *Nursing Management, 44*(6), 49-51.

Tellez, M., & Seago, J. (2013). California nurse staffing law and RN workforce changes. *Nursing Economic$, 31*(1), 18–28.

Wolf, L. A., Perhats, C., Delao, A. M., Clark, P. R., & Moon, M. D. (2017). On the threshold of safety: A qualitative exploration of nurses' perceptions of factors involved in safe staffing levels in emergency departments. *Journal of Emergency Nursing, 43*(2), 150–157. doi:10.1016/ j.jen.2016.09.003

Mandatory Overtime in Nursing
How Much? How Often?

Carol J. Huston

LEARNING OBJECTIVES

The learner will be able to:

1. Identify the strengths and the limitations of the Fair Labor Standards Act of 1938 in terms of protecting workers against mandatory overtime.

2. Identify how changes to federal overtime rules in the last decade and more recent court rulings have effected traditional "white-collar" employees, including salaried nurses in the United States.

3. Investigate current federal and state legislative efforts to regulate overtime limits for nurses.

4. Explore the current extent of mandatory overtime in nursing as identified in the literature.

5. Identify consequences of mandatory overtime in nursing, including fatigue, increased error rates,

increased legal liability, threats to the nurse's personal safety, and increased staff turnover rates.

6. Know and understand the provisions of the Nurse Practice Act in their state, as well as the position statements or advisory opinions that have been issued by his or her state board of nursing regarding mandatory overtime and patient abandonment.

7. Discuss the limits of the nurse's professional duty, and assess how much risk a professional nurse should assume in fulfilling a professional duty.

8. Reflect on the number of hours he or she can safely work before quality of care is potentially compromised.

INTRODUCTION

A short-term means of dealing with nursing shortages has been to require nurses to work extra shifts, often under threat of "patient abandonment" or punitive measures. *Mandatory overtime*, also called *compulsory* or *forced overtime*, occurs when employees are required to work more hours than are standard (generally 40 hours per week) or risk employer reprisals if they refuse to do so. Mandatory overtime may result from many unexpected events such as natural or human-caused disasters, sudden job vacancies, staff absences on account of illness, or rapid changes in patient care requirements; or it may be a standard staffing practice.

A review of the literature suggests that the use of mandatory overtime in nursing varies greatly from institution to institution and from state to state. Some health care employers have suggested that nursing shortages are the cause of mandatory overtime in their facilities. The consensus, however, is that working overtime among nurses is a prevalent practice used to control chronic understaffing and normal variations in the patient census. Increasingly, nurses are reporting that mandatory overtime has become standard operating procedure instead of a last resort to deal with short staffing. In fact, in some hospitals, mandatory overtime is routinely used to keep fewer people on the payroll, as well as to alleviate immediate shortages.

> ***Consider This*** Nursing overtime, both mandatory and voluntary, is prevalent in the health care industry as a solution for managing staff shortages and high census episodes (Wheatley, 2017, p. 213).

Indeed, Bae and Fabry (2014) note that 54% of the respondents to the 2008 National Sample Survey of Registered Nurses worked more than 39 hours per week, approximately 200 hours per year more than the average American worker. Furthermore, American nurses are more likely to work 12-hour shifts, and concerns are being raised about whether there is adequate time for rest and recovery between shifts.

Some nursing specialty units are known, however, to have more mandatory overtime than others, such as the operating room and postanesthesia care units. This occurs because of emergent and dynamic patient needs, unpredictable delays in surgical procedures, and significant differences in the efficiency of members of the operating room staff. To create guidelines for safe practice in the perioperative setting, the Association of Perioperative Registered Nurses (AORN, 2014) created a Position Statement on Safe Work/On-Call Practices in 2014. Excerpts from this document are shown in Box 11.1.

BOX 11.1 **Excerpts From the Association of Perioperative Registered Nurses (AORN) Position Statement on Perioperative Safe Staffing and On-Call Practices**

The AORN, recognizing the potential negative consequences of sleep deprivation and sustained work hours and further recognizing that adequate rest and recuperation periods are essential to patient and perioperative personnel safety, suggests the following strategies:

1. Perioperative registered nurses should not be required to work in direct patient care more than 12 consecutive hours in a 24-hour period and not more than 60 hours in a 7-day period. All work hours (i.e., regular hours and call hours worked) should be included in calculating total work hours.
2. The staffing plan should promote quality patient outcomes by using patient acuity and nursing workload guidelines to deliver safe patient care and support a safe work environment. The plan should identify strategies for cost-effective and efficient staffing priorities without compromising perioperative patient safety and outcomes.
3. The perioperative staffing plan should include provisions for unplanned, urgent, or emergent procedures and how to provide care for patients when procedures run over the scheduled time.
4. Arrangements should be made, in relation to the hours worked, to relieve a perioperative registered nurse who has worked on call during his or her off shift and who is scheduled to work the following shift to accommodate an adequate off-duty recuperation period.
5. On-call staffing plans should be based on strategies that minimize extended work hours, allow for adequate recuperation, and retain the perioperative RN as circulator.
6. Perioperative nurse managers should determine both direct and indirect care patient caregivers for the unit. Additionally, productive and nonproductive time should be considered.

Source: Association of Perioperative Registered Nurses. (2014). *AORN Position statement on perioperative safe staffing and on-call practices*. Retrieved July 29, 2017, from https://www.scribd.com/document/317254444/AORN-Position-Statement-on-Perioperative-Safe-Staffing-and-on-Call-Practices

MANDATORY OVERTIME AS A WAY OF LIFE IN THE UNITED STATES

Although nurses bemoan mandatory overtime in the profession, the reality is that mandatory overtime is not new, nor is it restricted to nursing. Americans typically work more hours and take fewer vacations than workers in other advanced economies. In fact, Miller (2018) calls the United States the most overworked developed nation in the world. That's because 85.8% of males and 66.5% of females in the United States work more than 40 hours per week. In comparison, Americans work 137 more hours per year than Japanese workers, 260 more hours per year than British workers, and 499 more hours per year than French workers (Miller, 2018). In addition, the United States is the only industrialized country in the world that has no legally mandated annual leave, and in every country except Canada and Japan (and the United States, which averages 13 days per year), workers get at least 20 paid vacation days. In France and Finland, they get 30—an entire month off, paid, every year (Miller, 2018).

Covert (2014) agrees, reporting that the reality of full-time American workers is not a 40-hour workweek; instead, the average full-time worker is putting in 47 hours each week, nearly an extra day's worth of time. While the workweek has been shrinking among all countries, the United States continues to be well above average in the number of hours its

people work each year, and with more worked hours than other developed countries like Australia, Canada, Germany, and the United Kingdom.

For some Americans, hard work may be a badge of honor, or it may be the means of accommodating lifestyles that increasingly require two wage earners in a household. It may also be that Americans are working this hard because they are afraid not to. In the United States, unlike most other countries, employment is *at will*, meaning that employers can dismiss employees for any reason (aside from those of gender, race, age, or disability) or for no reason at all. Thus, employees who refuse to work overtime can lose their jobs or face other reprisals.

Nurses argue, however, that mandatory overtime in nursing is not comparable with that in other fields because the consequences of being overly fatigued for the nurse may literally have life-and-death consequences. Proponents of mandatory overtime argue that it is an economic reality, given how limited labor health care resources are, particularly considering the international nursing shortage. The problem is that both positions are at times correct.

> **Consider This** Many nurses report a dramatic increase in the use of mandatory overtime to solve staffing problems and fear potential consequences for safety and quality of care for their patients.

This chapter defines mandatory overtime, examines the extent of its use in nursing, and discusses the consequences of mandatory overtime in nursing as identified in the literature.

LEGISLATING MANDATORY OVERTIME
The Fair Labor Standards Act

The definition of what constitutes overtime in the United States or how it should be calculated has historically varied from state to state and from industry to industry. There are, however, national standards in terms of the *Fair Labor Standards Act* (FLSA) of 1938. This act, which regulates overtime, does not impose limits on overtime hours or prohibit dismissal or any other sanction for declining overtime work. It does, however, require that payroll employees (those who are not "exempt" from the overtime requirements of the FLSA) be paid an overtime premium of at least one-and-a-half times the regular rate of pay for each hour worked more than 40 in a week (U.S. Department of Labor, n.d.).

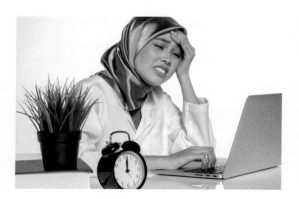

Consider This Labor laws such as the FLSA need to be amended to protect workers against excessive work hours and mandatory overtime and to protect the public from the dangers of an overburdened, stressed workforce.

The FLSA does, however, contain language that permits the health care industry to use a different overtime standard than the 40-hour workweek since scheduling occurs 24 hours a day, 365 days a year. Historically, this overtime standard required that hospitals and residential care facilities pay overtime after either 8 hours in a day or 80 hours in a 14-day pay period. It also permits employees to work more than 40 hours in a week and not be paid overtime provided they do not work more than 8 hours in a shift or if they work fewer than 40 hours in the next week. Employers are permitted to use both the 40-hour and the 80-hour standards in the same facility, depending on the scheduling patterns for employees, but they must use one standard for individual employees, and it must be applied consistently.

Recent Changes to Federal Overtime Rules

There have been changes, however, to the federal overtime rules in the last decade or so. Some changes, which became effective in 2004, defined exemptions from the FLSA for what were traditionally called "white-collar" employees. The new rules increased the amount of money employees could earn before they were no longer eligible to receive overtime pay; however, employees who directed and supervised two or more other full-time employees fell under the executive exemption. Similarly, the new rules excluded from the FLSA, employees who had the authority to hire, fire, and promote employees or whose primary duties involved the performance of office or nonmanual work and the exercise of discretion and independent judgment.

Almost immediately, nursing leaders expressed concern that the language in the new rules opened the door for employer attempts to reclassify nurses as exempt from overtime protections historically given to workers under the FLSA. This occurred because under the new regulations, "learned professionals" earning fairly low salaries (anything above US$455 per week) could not earn overtime pay (National Athletic Trainers Association, 2018).

Nurses meet the criteria of *learned professional*, which is defined in part as employees who perform work that requires advanced knowledge (work that is predominantly intellectual in character and that includes work requiring the consistent exercise of discretion and judgment;

National Athletic Trainers Association, 2018). In addition, the learned professional must have advanced knowledge in a field of science or learning, and the advanced knowledge must be customarily acquired by a prolonged course of specialized intellectual instruction.

Concerns about the exemption of health care workers from protection under the FLSA were borne out in a June 2007 Supreme Court ruling that the U.S. Department of Labor had acted appropriately in denying FLSA protection to 10 home care workers even when employed by large, third-party home care agencies (Dawson, 2007). In the case of *Long Island Care at Home, LTD. versus Coke,* "the Court ruled that Ms. Evelyn Coke, a home care aide from Queens, New York, deserved neither overtime pay nor minimum wage, although she was frequently asked to work up to 70 hours per week" (Dawson, 2007, para. 1). This ruling occurred because of an exemption to the FLSA that applies to companions and housekeepers who work in the homes of their clients. On October 7, 2014, however, the United States Department of Labor announced that it would delay enforcement of its new rules designed to narrow the companionship exemption for home care workers under the FLSA, from January 1, 2015 to January 2016 (Sabatino and Newman, 2015). The new rules extend minimum wage and overtime protections to direct care workers, which are the same protections provided to most U.S. workers, including those who perform the same work in nursing homes.

In addition, it is important to note that nurses are eligible for overtime pay and protection under the FLSA if they are classified by employers as hourly—not salaried—employees, because salaried employees are not eligible for overtime. Thus, salaried employees and nurses who are considered to be exempt under the FLSA have virtually no rights under these new overtime rules. They are entitled only to their base salary, less deductions, by law and may be held to whatever schedule an employer demands because there are no restrictions on mandatory overtime in the FLSA.

In early 2014, President Obama issued an Executive Order to the Secretary of Labor to update the regulations regarding overtime exemptions and increase the overtime exemption salary (McBrayer, McGinnis, Leslie, & Kirkland, PLLC, 2015). The White House cited the erosion of the 40-hour workweek coupled with the failure to update the salary threshold to keep current with inflation as grounds for the order. The proposed rulemaking was to take place in late 2014, but the effective date of the final rule was not until December 1, 2016. At that time, the salary exemption was raised from $23,000 annually (or $455 a week) to $47,476 annually (or $913 per week; U.S. Department of Labor, 2018). This salary represents the 40th percentile of earnings of full-time salaried workers in the lowest-wage Census Region, currently the South (U.S. Department of Labor, 2018).

As of January 2018, The Department of Labor was still undertaking rulemaking to revise the regulations that govern the exemption of executive, administrative, and professional employees from the FLSA's minimum wage and overtime pay requirements. Until the Department issues its final rule, it will enforce the part 541 regulations in effect on November 30, 2016, including the $455 per week standard salary level (U.S. Department of Labor, 2018).

McBrayer, McGinnis, Leslie, and Kirkland, PLLC (2015) note that employers should also plan for the exemption for executive, administrative, or professional roles to become somewhat more constricted, because many commentators feel that regulations regarding these roles might start to track similar regulations in other states. Those states have a minimum threshold for the amount of an employee's time that must be performed in a "white-collar" role to continue to be exempt.

In addition, a new bill (The Working Families Flexibility Act of 2017) was introduced into Congress in February 2017 to allow employees to receive compensatory time (extra paid time off) instead of overtime payments (Green, 2017). The bill was passed by the House in May, but the Senate version stalled.

If the bill passed, employees would have had to agree in writing to voluntarily receive comp time instead of overtime pay before any overtime work was performed. Comp time then would have been provided at the same rate that overtime was paid—meaning that workers receiving comp time would have received one-and-a-half hours of comp time for every hour of overtime they worked. The bill would have prohibited an employee from accruing more than 160 hours of compensatory time, and monetary compensation had to be provided for any unused compensatory time off accrued during the preceding year (Green, 2017). Opponents of the bill argued that the bill undermined protections for low wage workers because employers could coerce employees into taking comp time instead of traditional overtime compensation; however, the bill explicitly prohibited employers from intimidating, threatening, or coercing any employee regarding their rights to choose or not to choose to take the comp time option, or their right to use banked comp time (U.S. Chamber of Commerce, 2017).

Legislating Limits on Nursing Overtime

Wheatley (2017) suggests that sufficient evidence exists to show the negative impacts of mandatory overtime on nurse personal wellness and risk for workplace injury, patient outcomes, and nursing turnover to warrant the continued attention of policy makers. Despite multiple efforts, however, over the last decade to introduce national legislation directed at prohibiting employers from requiring licensed health care employees to work more than 8 hours in a single workday or 80 hours in any 14-day work period—except in the case of a natural disaster or declaration of emergency by federal, state, or local government officials—no such legislation has been passed.

States are, however, increasingly taking a role in both defining mandatory overtime and putting limits to its use. Every nurse should know and understand the provisions of the Nurse Practice Act in his or her state, as well as the position statements or advisory opinions that have been issued by the state board of nursing on mandatory overtime and patient abandonment.

Discussion Point

What position statement or advisory opinion has your state board of nursing issued regarding mandatory overtime and patient abandonment? Do you feel that it is adequate to protect both nurses and patients from unsafe working conditions?

In addition, the American Nurses Association (ANA) has added mandatory overtime to its Nationwide State Legislative Agenda, supporting the enactment of mandatory overtime legislation by state legislatures and the attention to such issues by regulatory agencies. As of 2017, 18 states had restrictions in law or regulations on the use of mandatory overtime for nurses (Alaska, California Connecticut, Illinois, Maine, Maryland, Massachusetts, Minnesota, Missouri, New Hampshire, New Jersey, New York, Oregon, Pennsylvania, Rhode Island, Texas, West Virginia, and Washington (Johnson//Becker PLLC, Monheit, and Banville Law, 2017).

Alaska passed mandatory overtime restrictions for nurses in health care settings in 2010 (became effective in 2011) preceded by Texas in 2009. In Alaska, the law states that a registered nurse or licensed practical nurse in a health care facility who is not employed in a federal or tribal facility may not be required or coerced, directly or indirectly, to work beyond his or her agreed-upon regular shift or accept overtime if in the judgment of the nurse, the overtime would jeopardize patient or employee safety ("Mandatory Overtime Limitations," 2014). In addition, the nurse cannot work more than 14 consecutive hours except under very specific conditions such as a nurse voluntarily working overtime on an aircraft in use for medical transport or a nurse participating in the performance of a medical procedure that has begun but not been completed. On-call time is not counted in the 14 hours unless the nurse is actually called back into work ("Mandatory Overtime Limitations," 2014).

Pennsylvania enacted the Prohibition of Excessive Overtime in Health Care Act (HB 834) in October 2008. This law stated that a health care facility could not require an employee to work in excess of an agreed to, predetermined, and regularly scheduled daily work shift unless there was an unforeseeable declared national, state, or municipal emergency or a catastrophic event that was unpredictable or unavoidable and that substantially affected or increased the need for health care services (American Nurses Association [ANA], 2017). This law did not preclude employees from voluntarily accepting overtime, and it did not apply to those workers compensated for "on-call" time.

New York also enacted legislation in 2008 prohibiting health care employers (excluding home care facilities) from forcing nurses to work overtime, except during health care disasters that increased the need for health care personnel unexpectedly or when a health care employer determined that there was an emergency and had made a good faith effort to have overtime covered on a voluntary basis (ANA, 2017). Another exception included an ongoing medical or surgical procedure in which the nurse is actively engaged, such as in surgery, and whose continued presence through completion is essential to the health and safety of the patient (ANA, 2017).

Although the New York legislation provides a good example of how states can reduce the risk of mandatory overtime for nurses, it should be noted that the New York Nurses Association first proposed legislation to ban mandatory overtime in 2000. Eight years were required to gain enough support from patient advocacy groups and other unions that represent nurses.

Minnesota also successfully passed legislation in 2007 that prohibited nurses from being required to work more than a "normal work period," meaning 12 or fewer consecutive hours, consistent with their predetermined work shift, but again excludes an emergency (ANA, 2017):

The definition of emergency refers to a period when replacement staff are not able to report for duty for the next shift or increase patient need, because of unusual, unpredictable, or unforeseen circumstances such as, but not limited to, an act of terrorism, a disease outbreak, adverse weather conditions, or natural disasters which impact the continuity of patient care. (para. 5)

Similar legislation became effective in New Hampshire in 2008. This legislation prohibited an employer from disciplining or removing any right, benefit, or privilege of a registered nurse, licensed practical nurse, or licensed nursing assistant for refusing to work more than 12 consecutive hours, except under specific circumstances, such as those identified in the New York and Minnesota legislation (ANA, 2017). A nurse might be disciplined for refusing to work mandatory overtime in these situations.

Finally, the Academy of Medical-Surgical Nurses (AMSN, 2018) issued a position statement in 2012 suggesting that overtime should be offered only on a voluntary basis and only after all other attempts to provide adequate staffing have failed. In addition, the AMSN notes that nurses should never be required to work beyond their individual physical and mental capacity and that mandatory overtime should not be used as a solution to chronic understaffing.

THE CONSEQUENCES OF MANDATORY OVERTIME

Research on the effects of overtime has focused largely on studies of individuals working scheduled 12-hour shifts. However, when staff *plan* to work 12-hour shifts or additional shifts on a voluntary basis, they are more likely to get plenty of rest immediately before working the extended shift. Overtime mandated by an employer, however, occurs with little or no prior notice, so higher levels of fatigue may occur. In addition, many nurses report working far more than 12 hours when mandatory overtime is involved.

How long can nurses work safely? Given the variability in each situation, there is no one answer to this question. There is little doubt, however, that after a certain point of protracted work time, fatigue becomes a factor and the likelihood of errors, near errors, mistakes, and lapses in judgment increases.

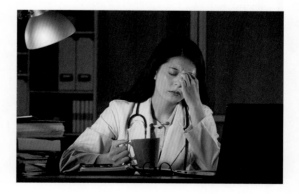

Richards, Harrison Weathers, Hassan Barwari, and Reith (2016) note that the Department of Transportation (DOT) and the Federal Aviation Administration (FAA) each regulate how long pilots, air traffic controllers, engineers, flight attendants, airline mechanics, and other employees can work in order to maintain airline safety standards and protect crew and passengers. Similarly, the DOT and the Federal Motor Carrier Safety Administration regulate the number of consecutive hours truck drivers may work. In contrast, there is no state or federal regulation of the hours a nurse may work.

> **Consider This** Federal regulations have used transportation laws to place limits on the amount of time that can safely be worked in aviation and trucking. It seems appropriate that Congress needs to go beyond the FLSA and at least examine the need to create safety parameters around mandatory overtime in nursing.

The ANA authored a position statement in 2006 arguing that nursing employers should do the same by ensuring that sufficient system resources exist to (1) provide the individual registered nurse in all roles and settings with a work schedule that provides for adequate rest and recuperation between scheduled work and (2) provide sufficient compensation and appropriate staffing systems that foster a safe and healthful environment in which the registered nurse does not feel compelled to seek supplemental income through overtime, extra shifts, and other practices that contribute to worker fatigue (ANA, 2006).

The reality, however, is that mandatory overtime is very much a part of contemporary nursing practice, and the literature increasingly suggests that fatigue can result in a host of negative consequences, including occupational injury, illness, burnout, reduced quality of care, and errors. The longer the nurse works after he or she becomes fatigued, the greater the risk of these consequences.

For example, Aveyard (2016) notes that 12-hour (or longer) shifts can be detrimental to an individual's health, causing disruptions to their circadian rhythms, altered activity-rest patterns, increased stress levels, and issues with social and domestic life. Thompson, Stock, and Banuelas (2017) agree, suggesting that nurses have one of the highest nonfatal injury rates of all occupations, which may be a consequence of long, cumulative work schedules. Fatigue may accumulate across multiple shifts and lead to performance impairments, which in turn may be linked to injury risks. These findings echo those of Chen, Davis, Daraiseh, Pan, and Davis (2014), who concluded that nurses working 12-hour shifts experienced a moderate to high level of acute fatigue and moderate levels of chronic fatigue and intershift recovery.

In addition, research by Stimpfel, Brewer, and Kovner (2015) found that more than half (61%) of new nurses worked overtime (mandatory or voluntary) weekly. This overtime work was associated with a 32% increase in the risk of a needle stick, and nurses working night shift experienced a 16% increase in the risk of a sprain or strain injury (Research Fuels the Controversy 11.1).

Research Fuels the Controversy 11.1

The Impact of Work Schedule on Occupational Injury and Illness

This study sought to describe newly licensed nurses' shift work characteristics and to determine the association between shift type and scheduling characteristics and nurse injury. The study was a secondary analysis of a nationally representative survey of newly licensed registered nurses using a cross-sectional design. The analytic sample included 1,744 newly licensed registered nurses from 34 states and the District of Columbia who reported working in a hospital and were within 6–18 months of passing their state licensure exam at the time of survey administration.

Source: Stimpfel, A. W., Brewer, C. S., & Kovner, C. T. (2015). Scheduling and shift work characteristics associated with risk for occupational injury in newly licensed registered nurses: An observational study. *International Journal of Nursing Studies, 52*(11), 1686–1693.

Study Findings

The majority (79%) of newly licensed nurses worked 12-hour shifts, a near majority worked night shift (44%), and over half (61%) worked overtime (mandatory or voluntary) weekly. Nurses working weekly overtime were associated with a 32% increase in the risk of a needle stick, and nurses working night shift were associated with a 16% increase in the risk of a sprain or strain injury. The researchers concluded that overtime and night shift work were significantly associated with increased injury risk in newly licensed nurses independent of other work factors and demographic characteristics. The findings warrant further study given the long-term consequences of these injuries, costs associated with treatment, and loss of worker productivity.

Griffiths et al. (2014) suggest as well that prolonged shifts have negative impacts on patient outcomes, noting that nurses working for ≥12 hours were more likely to report poor or failing patient safety, poor or fair quality of care, and more care activities left undone. Similarly, a literature review by Bae and Fabry (2014) found that 21 nurse outcome measures and 19 patient outcome measures correlated with work hours and overtime. These findings suggest that the positive relationships between working long hours and adverse outcomes to the nurses are strong, although more evidence is needed. Another recent study found that the odds of having a health care–associated infection were higher on days that were preceded by a high nursing overtime ratio (Beltempo, Blais, Lacroix, Cabot, & Piedboeuf, 2017).

All these findings reinforce those of a report of the Board on Health Care Services and the Institute of Medicine (2004), *Keeping Patients Safe: Transforming the Work Environment of Nurses*, which said that nurses' long working hours pose a serious threat to patient safety. In fact, the report argued that limiting the number of hours worked per day and consecutive days of work by nursing staff, as is done in other safety-sensitive industries, is a fundamental safety precaution. Similarly, Marquis and Huston (2017) argued that certain minimum criteria should always be met for safe staffing. These criteria are shown in Box 11.2.

Discussion Point

How many hours can the typical nurse work before she or he might be considered unsafe? How much individual leeway is feasible in making this determination?

BOX 11.2   Minimum Criteria for Staffing Decisions

1. Decisions made must meet state and federal labor laws and organizational policies.
2. Staff must not be demoralized or excessively fatigued by frequent or extended overtime requests.
3. Long-term as well as short-term solutions to staffing shortages must be sought.
4. Patient care must not be jeopardized.

Source: Marquis, B., & Huston, C. (2017). *Leadership roles and management functions in nursing* (9th ed.). Philadelphia, PA: Wolters Kluwer.

Discussion Point

Is increasing the use of mandatory overtime perpetuating nursing shortages? Do you think nurses who no longer work in nursing roles would be more apt to return to work if they felt they had more control over the hours they worked (i.e., if mandatory overtime were banned)?

PROFESSIONAL DUTY AND CONSCIENCE

Mandatory overtime and patient abandonment must also be examined in terms of professional duty. A *professional duty* is the direct result of others having welfare rights, such as the right to safe care. Because people have a right to such care, nurses have an associated duty to ensure that they accept patient care assignments only if they are mentally and physically able to provide, at minimum, safe care.

The problem is that there is great variability in terms of how many hours a nurse can work and still provide competent safe care. For example, the practice of mandatory overtime is grounded in the commitment to prevent harm to patients by guaranteeing adequate nurse–patient ratios, yet the overfatigued nurse may pose even greater risk of harm to patients by agreeing to work. The ANA (2018a) agrees, suggesting that regardless of the number of hours worked, each registered nurse has an ethical responsibility to carefully consider his or her level of fatigue when deciding to accept any assignment extending beyond the regularly scheduled workday or workweek. The ANA concludes that registered nurses are responsible for negotiating or even rejecting a work assignment that compromises the availability of sufficient time for sleep and recovery from work. The amount of recovery time necessary depends on the amount of work, including regularly scheduled shifts and mandatory or voluntary overtime.

Discussion Point

Who bears the risk or the consequences of risk when an overworked nurse makes errors that contribute to patient harm?

What happens when the nurse determines that he or she must refuse to work additional hours because of safety concerns related to level of fatigue? Saying no to a desperate employer, especially when the fear that short staffing may compromise patient safety, is likely much harder than it sounds. Indeed, moral dilemmas abound when health care providers feel they must refuse a patient care assignment.

When this occurs, some nurses feel compelled to file their refusal to work as a *conscientious objection*. The purpose of conscientious objection is to protect the rights of employees who refuse to participate in procedures based on conscience. The issue of whether a nurse can refuse mandatory overtime based on conscience, however, has limited case law precedent.

The ANA's (2015) *Code of Ethics* might be helpful to some nurses in resolving potential ethical conflicts between their professional duty to provide care and their conscience, or the realization that providing such care may actually place patients at risk for harm. The *Code of Ethics*, however, could potentiate the dilemma because it states that nurses should care for all people in need without discrimination. The problem is that it also says that the nurse is to maintain conditions of employment that are conducive to high-quality nursing care.

The ANA also recommends the *Nurses' Bill of Rights* as a tool for dialogue to resolve concerns that nurses may have about work environments that might not support professional practice. The Nurses' Bill of Rights was conceived to support nurses in an array of workplace situations, including mandatory overtime, and suggests that nurses must bring these workplace issues to the attention of employers to meet their responsibilities to their patients and to themselves (ANA, 2018b).

Patient Abandonment

One of the most common reasons nurses cite for working mandatory overtime is the threat that refusal to do so could be construed as *patient abandonment*, a charge that can result in loss of licensure. Therefore, many nurses believe that they have no choice when confronted by a request for overtime, even though they might be working a shift in excess of 12 hours.

> **Consider This** In some facilities, nurses are being threatened with dismissal or with the charge of patient abandonment if they refuse to accept overtime.

Despite this perception, the ANA does not support the forced overtime of nurses, and their position is that a nurse should not be held accountable for patient abandonment if the nurse turned down an assignment that could be unsafe to patients or self. In fact, most state boards of nursing maintain that refusal to work mandatory overtime is not patient abandonment; in a situation in which a nurse has accepted a patient or assignment, the nurse must simply notify the supervisor that he or she is leaving and report off to another nurse.

Usually, however, nurses would have less likelihood of losing their license or being reprimanded if an assignment (mandatory overtime) was never accepted in the first place than if the assignment was accepted and then the nurse changed his or her mind. This is because accepting the assignment suggests that a nurse–patient relationship has been established. Thus, patient abandonment is more likely when the nurse accepts a patient assignment and then ceases to provide nursing care without appropriately transferring the responsibility for the patient to another professional nurse. This then becomes a form of negligence in nursing since the termination of the provider–patient relationship was unilateral, despite the patient's continued need for care. Once a nurse begins treating a patient, she or he is legally bound to care for that patient until another nurse is available to assume responsibility for the patient (Trossman, 2016).

In addition, boards of nursing in several states have developed clear statements differentiating patient abandonment from *employment abandonment*. Typically, these statements define employment abandonment as nurses leaving their places of work to avoid injury to patients or to themselves. This definition is similar to language used by the Maryland Board of Registered Nursing (BRN) in defining patient abandonment; however, the Maryland BRN (n.d.) suggested that there are many variables to be examined in determining whether patient abandonment has occurred. The definition of patient abandonment and these variables are shown in Box 11.3.

> **Consider This** Although boards of nursing often rule that refusing mandatory overtime is not patient abandonment and thus is not cause for loss of licensure, they have no jurisdiction over employment and contract issues. Refusing to work mandatory overtime may still result in termination of a nurse's employment.

Similarly, the Vermont Board of Nursing (2018) defined abandonment as disengagement from the nurse–patient or caregiver–patient relationship without properly notifying appropriate personnel (e.g., supervisor or employer) and/or making reasonable arrangements for continuation of care, or failing to provide adequate patient care until the responsibility for care of the patient is assumed by another nurse, nursing assistant, or other approved provider. Examples of situations that may constitute abandonment are provided in Box 11.4.

UNIONS AND MANDATORY OVERTIME

Because collective bargaining agreements can require greater protections beyond those outlined in the FLSA, the position of most collective bargaining agents is that

BOX 11.3 **The Link Between Nurse–Patient Relationships and Patient Abandonment as Outlined by the Maryland Board of Registered Nursing**

Abandonment occurs when a licensed nurse terminates the nurse–patient relationship without reasonable notification to the nursing supervisor for the continuation of the patient's care.

The nurse–patient relationship begins when responsibility for nursing care of a patient is accepted by the nurse. Nursing management is accountable for assessing the capabilities of personnel and delegating responsibility or assigning nursing care functions to personnel qualified to assume such responsibility or to perform such functions.

The Variables That Need to Be Examined in Each Alleged Incident of Abandonment Include but Are Not Limited To:

1. What were the licensee's assigned responsibilities for what time frame? What was the clinical setting and what were the resources available to the licensee?
2. Was there an exchange of responsibility from one licensee to another? When did the exchange occur, that is, shift report and so on?
3. What was the time frame of the incident, that is, time licensee arrived, time of exchange of responsibility, and the like?
4. What was the communication process, that is, whom did the licensee inform of his or her intent to leave, and was it lateral, upward, downward, and so forth?
5. What are the facility's policies, terms of employment, and/or job description regarding the licensee and call-in, refusal to accept an assignment, reassignment to another unit, mandatory overtime, and the like?
6. What is the pattern of practice/events for the licensee and the pattern of management for the unit/facility, that is, is the event of a single isolated occurrence, or is it one event in a series of events?
7. What were the issues/reasons why the licensee could not accept an assignment, continue an assignment, or extend an original assignment, and so forth?

Source: Maryland Board of Registered Nursing. (n.d.) *Abandonment.* Retrieved April 12, 2018, from http://mbon.maryland.gov/Pages/practice-abandonment.aspx

the practice of mandatory overtime should be eliminated entirely. However, there are differences among union contracts, and the strategies used by unions to reduce mandatory overtime vary greatly.

The American Federation of Teachers (AFT, n.d.) has been on record since 1990, calling for a ban on mandatory overtime through a twofold approach—legislation and contract language: At the federal level, AFT is working with

legislators to require facilities receiving Medicare funding to stop mandating overtime and notes that on-call time should be treated as work time. In addition, many local unions have negotiated contract language limiting the practice of mandatory overtime.

The Service Employees International Union (SEIU) has also consistently spoken out against mandatory overtime, and in partnership with the Nurse Alliance, created an Overtime

BOX 11.4 **Sample Situations That Might Constitute Patient Abandonment**

- Leaving the patient care area without transferring responsibility for patient care to an authorized person
- Remaining unavailable for patient care for a period of time such that patient care may be compromised because of lack of available qualified staff
- Inattention or insufficient observation or contact with a patient
- Sleeping while on duty without the approval of a supervisor in accordance with written facility policy
- Failing to timely notify a supervisor or employer if the licensee will not initiate or complete an assignment where the licensee is the sole provider of care
- For the APRN, terminating the nurse–patient relationship without providing reasonable notification to the patient and resources for continuity of care

Source: Vermont Board of Nursing. (2018). *Vermont Board of Nursing position statement on abandonment. (This position statement was last updated in Oct. 2015).* Retrieved April 12, 2018, from https://www.sec.state.vt.us/media/716284/PS-Abandonment-2015-1012.pdf

Report Form for nurses, union or nonunion, to document mandatory or pressured overtime. Similarly, the American Federation of State, County and Municipal Employees (AFSCME) is also working to eliminate mandatory overtime, contending that an increasing prevalence of hospitals that use mandatory overtime do so as a routine staffing solution (AFSCME, 2018). AFSCME makes the following argument: "[P]resumably, hospital administrators believe that the imposition of mandatory overtime will save money by limiting recruitment and benefit expenses. However, multiple studies have shown mandatory overtime to be perhaps the single worst practice to emerge from the era of downsizing and managed care" (para. 1) and that, indeed, it often generates very large costs, even if sometimes unaccounted for, in the form of increased turnover, lower productivity, longer patient stays, and higher rates of treatment errors, which in turn necessitate more extended and costly solutions.

CONCLUSIONS

In the end, the mandatory overtime dilemma, like so many in nursing, comes down to a conflict regarding how best to use limited resources (fiscal and human) to provide safe, quality health care. Most nurses and administrators can agree on two goals: (1) staffing should be at least minimally adequate to assure that all patients receive safe care and (2) nursing staff should not be placed at personal or legal risk to provide that care.

The problem is that the onus is on management to ensure that there is appropriate staffing, and most health care institutions state that there are simply not enough resources to meet the first goal without jeopardizing the second. Clearly, more alternatives such as shift bidding and pay enhancement programs need to be explored. Neither health care administrators nor nurses should have to choose between meeting the needs of patients and meeting the needs of nurses.

The bottom line is that workers should have the right to refuse overtime without fear of repercussion, especially when staffing shortages and mandated overtime are the norm and not the exception. Unfortunately, as long as nursing shortages exist, mandatory overtime will continue to be used as a means of meeting minimum staffing needs.

For Additional Discussion

1. How does the presence of a collective bargaining agreement affect a hospital's ability to require mandatory overtime? How much power do unions have in negotiating this aspect of working conditions?

2. Would passage of a national ban on mandatory overtime tie the hands of hospitals in ensuring that staffing is at least minimally adequate during periods of acute nursing shortages?

3. Does the use of mandatory overtime really save hospitals money in terms of recruitment and benefits?

4. How do the rates of mandatory overtime in nursing compare with those in other professions?

5. Are other nonnursing health care professionals at risk for loss of licensure if they are found guilty of patient abandonment?

6. Are charges of patient abandonment legally and morally appropriate if a nurse works his or her required shift but refuses to stay and work longer?

7. Given the severity and scope of the nursing shortage, what is the likelihood that mandatory staffing will continue to be used for both emergency and routine staffing needs?

References

Academy of Medical-Surgical Nurses. (2018). *Mandatory overtime. (This position statement was updated and combined with a Workplace Advocacy Position Statement on 11/7/2012).* Retrieved April 12, 2018, from https://www.amsn.org/practice-resources/position-statements/archive/mandatory-overtime

American Federation of State, County and Municipal Employees, American Federation of Labor and Congress of Industrial Organizations. (2018). *Worst practices: Mandatory overtime.* Retrieved April 12, 2018, from http://www.afscme.org/news/publications/health-care/solving-the-nursing-shortage/worst-practices-mandatory-overtime

American Federation of Teachers. (n.d.). *Mandatory overtime.* Retrieved April 12, 2018, from http://www.aft.org/health-care/mandatory-overtime

American Nurses Association. (2006). *Position statements: Assuring patient safety: The employers' role in promoting healthy nursing work hours for registered nurses in all roles and settings.* Retrieved April 12, 2018, from https://medcom .uiowa.edu/annsblog/wp-content/uploads/2013/12/ANA-EmployersRole-in-promoting-healthy-work-hours.pdf

American Nurses Association. (2015). *Code of ethics for nurses with interpretive statements.* Silver Springs, MD: Nurse Books.Org.

American Nurses Association. (2017). *Mandatory overtime: Summary of state approaches.* Retrieved July 30, 2017, from Nursing World Website: http://www.nursingworld.org/MainMenuCategories/Policy-Advocacy/State/Legislative-Agenda-Reports/MandatoryOvertime/Mandatory-Over-time-Summary-of-State-Approaches.html

American Nurses Association. (2018a). *Position statement: Addressing nurse fatigue to promote safety and health: Joint responsibilities of registered nurses and employers to reduce risks.* Retrieved April 12, 2018, from https://www.nurs-ingworld.org/practice-policy/nursing-excellence/official-position-statements/

American Nurses Association. (2018b). *Nurses' bill of rights.* Retrieved April 12, 2018, from http://nursingworld.org/NursesBillofRights

Association of Perioperative Registered Nurses. (2014). *AORN Position statement on perioperative safe staffing and on-call practices.* Retrieved July 29, 2017, from https://www.scribd.com/document/317254444/AORN-Position-Statement-on-Perioperative-Safe-Staffing-and-on-Call-Practices

Aveyard, D. (2016, December). How do 12-hour shifts affect ICU nurses? *Kai Tiaki Nursing New Zealand, 22*(11), 34–36.

Bae, S., & Fabry, D. (2014). Assessing the relationships between nurse work hours/overtime and nurse and patient outcomes: Systematic literature review. *Nursing Outlook, 62*(2), 138–156.

Beltempo, M., Blais, R., Lacroix, G., Cabot, M., & Piedboeuf, B. (2017). Association of nursing overtime, nurse staffing, and unit occupancy with health care-associated infections in the NICU. *American Journal of Perinatology, 34*(10), 996–1002.

Chen, J., Davis, K. G., Daraiseh, N. M., Pan, W., & Davis, L. S. (2014). Fatigue and recovery in 12-hour dayshift hospital nurses. *Journal of Nursing Management, 22*(5), 593–603.

Covert, B. (2014, September 2). *The truth about the 40-hour workweek: It's actually 47 hours long.* Think Progress. Retrieved August 12, 2018, from http://thinkprogress.org/economy/2014/09/02/3477937/workweek/

Dawson, S. L. (2007). Taking a cue from the Supreme court. *Nursing Homes: Long Term Care Management, 56*(10), 8–10.

Green, A. (2017, April 24). *Will Congress get rid of mandatory overtime pay?* U.S. News and World Report. Retrieved April 12, 2018, from https://money.usnews.com/money/blogs/outside-voices-careers/articles/2017-04-24/will-congress-get-rid-of-mandatory-overtime-pay

Griffiths, P., Dall'Ora, C., Simon, M., Ball, J., Lindqvist, R., Rafferty, A., & Aiken, L. H. (2014). Nurses' shift length and overtime working in 12 European countries: The association with perceived quality of care and patient safety. *Medical Care, 52*(11), 975–981.

Institute of Medicine. (2004). *Keeping patients safe: Transforming the work environment of nurses.* Washington, DC: The National Academies Press.

Johnson//Becker PLLC, Monheit P.C., and Banville Law. (2017). *Mandatory overtime in nursing.* Retrieved April 12, 2018, from http://wageadvocates.com/faq/is-mandatory-overtime-legal/

Mandatory overtime limitations for nurses. (2014). *The Alaska Nurse, 64*(4), 9.

Marquis, B., & Huston, C. (2017). *Leadership roles and management functions in nursing: Theory and application* (9th ed.). Philadelphia, PA: Wolters Kluwer.

Maryland Board of Registered Nursing. (n.d.). *Abandonment.* Retrieved April 12, 2018, from http://mbon.maryland.gov/Pages/practice-abandonment.aspx

McBrayer, McGinnis, Leslie, & Kirkland, PLLC. (2015, February 2). *What employers can (probably) expect from the FLSA overtime exemption (yet to be) proposed rules.* Retrieved April 12, 2018, from http://www.natlawreview.com/article/what-employers-can-probably-expect-flsa-overtime-exemption-yet-to-be-proposed-rules

Miller, G. E. (2018, January 2). *The U.S. is the most overworked developed nation in the world—When do we draw the line?* Retrieved April 12, 2018, from 20SomethingFinance.com Website: http://20somethingfinance.com/american-hours-worked-productivity-vacation/

National Athletic Trainers Association. (2018). *U.S. Department of Labor overtime exemptions under Fair Labor Standards Act (FLSA) and new rule.* Retrieved April 12, 2018, from https://www.nata.org/advocacy/regulatory/us-dept-of-labor-proposed-salary-and-overtime-protections

Richards, A. M., Harrison Weathers, D., Hassan Barwari, R., & Reith, V. (2016). Is it worth the risk? 12-hour shifts and nurse fatigue. *Nursing News, 40*(2), 18–19.

Sabatino, C. and Newman, C.A. (2015, August). The new status of home care workers under the Fair Labor Standards Act. *Bifocal, 36*(6). Retrieved August 27, 2018 from https://www .americanbar.org/publications/bifocal/vol_36/issue_6_august2015/flsa_rule_change.html

Stimpfel, A. W., Brewer, C. S., & Kovner, C. T. (2015). Scheduling and shift work characteristics associated with risk for occupational injury in newly licensed registered nurses: An observational study. *International Journal of Nursing Studies, 52*(11), 1686–1693.

Thompson, B. J., Stock, M.S., & Banuelas, V.K. (2017, May). Effects of accumulating work shifts on performance-based fatigue using multiple strength measurements in day and night shift nurses and aides. *Human Factors* [serial online]. *59*(3), 346–356. Retrieved from CINAHL Plus with Full Text, Ipswich, MA. Accessed August 27, 2018.

Trossman, S. (2016). Conscientious objection. Reprinted with permission of The American Nurse. *New Mexico Nurse*, *61*(1), 12.

U.S. Chamber of Commerce. (2017, April 5). *Testimony on reviewing H.R. 1180, the Working Families Flexibility Act of 2017*. Retrieved April 12, 2018, from https://www.uschamber.com/testimony/testimony-reviewing-hr-1180-the-working-families-flexibility-act-2017

U.S. Department of Labor. (2018, January). *Final rule: Overtime. Defining and delimiting the exemptions for executive, administrative, professional, outside sales and computer employees under the Fair Labor Standards Act*. Wage and Hour Division. Retrieved April 12, 2018, from https://www.dol.gov/whd/overtime/final2016/

U.S. Department of Labor. (n.d.). *Overtime pay*. Retrieved April 12, 2018, from http://www.dol.gov/dol/topic/wages/overtimepay.htm

Vermont Board of Nursing. (2018). *Vermont board of nursing position statement on abandonment. (This position statement was last updated in October 2015)*. Retrieved April 12, 2018, from https://www.highbeam.com/doc/1G1-389176231.html; https://www.sec.state.vt.us/media/716284/PS-Abandonment-2015-1012.pdf

Wheatley, C. (2017, July/August). Nursing overtime: Should it be regulated? *Nursing Economic$*, *35*(4), 213–217.

Promoting Healthy Work Environments and Civility
Why Is This So Difficult in Nursing?

Charmaine Hockley

CHAPTER OUTLINE

LEARNING OBJECTIVES

The learner will be able to:

1. Identify common factors that have the potential to lead to an unhealthy work environment.

2. Recognize inappropriate workplace behaviors such as incivility and bullying.

3. Identify the impact of incivility and bullying on nurses' work environments including stress and mental illness.

4. Describe a healthy work environment and why having such an environment is important.

5. Discuss the importance of civility in promoting a healthy work environment.

6. Recognize and respond immediately and appropriately to incivility, bullying, and stress.

7. Identify and respond appropriately to mental health problems caused by inappropriate workplace behaviors.

8. Describe the challenges facing nurses to achieve a healthy work environment.

INTRODUCTION

Over the past decade, there has been a strong movement toward creating healthy work environments (HWEs) and a culture of civility. Many studies have reported that health care workers, and in particular nurses, have experienced a higher rate of inappropriate behavior in the workplace than other workers have.

A Health Risk Appraisal conducted by the American Nurses Association (ANA, 2017) provides an illuminating perspective of the realities of professional life in the health workplace. Over a 3-year period, the survey responses from more than 14,000 registered nurses and nursing students provided a national cross section of the health risks they experience in a variety of settings and locations. The summary results show:

- workplace stress was identified as the top work environment health and safety risk, with 82% saying they are at a "significant level of risk for workplace stress."
- up to half had been bullied in some manner in the workplace.
- 25% had been physically assaulted at work by a patient or family member.
- 9% were concerned for their physical safety at work (ANA, 2017, p. 4).

The ANA (2017) Executive Summary further reports:

- 90 percent of respondents are familiar with safety guidelines and policies.
- 80 percent expressed the belief that their employer values their health and safety.
- 78% felt treated with dignity and respect (ANA, 2017, p. 4).

These three comments are a welcome contrast to many other earlier studies into workplace violence and bullying where senior managers were often perceived as the major perpetrators of workplace violence.

A 2015 U.S. study on coworkers as the perpetrator showed that, "[I]n the 199 analyzed incidents, perpetrators were mostly female, full-time workers, and more likely to be patient care associates or nurses" (Hamblin et al., 2016, p. 53). These results may be disappointing, but are not surprising when nurses still remain predominantly female, hold less senior roles in nursing, and have a history of oppression and male dominance. In other words, nursing has engendered a culture in which nurses are powerless and act powerlessly.

> **Consider This** Do you believe that nursing in the 21st century continues to be influenced by its history of oppression and male dominance?

Clearly, promoting a HWE and civility is significant to the safety and well-being of all nurses. The International Council of Nurses (ICN, 2017) suggests that:

> . . . every nurse has the right to work in a healthy and safe environment without risk of injury or illness resulting from that work. Occupational health and safety involves anticipating, recognizing, evaluating and controlling hazards arising in or from the workplace that could impair the health and wellbeing of workers, taking into account the possible impact on the surrounding communities and the general environment. (ICN, 2017)

Although there may be differences in the various international and national HWE definitions, there is a prime and mutual emphasis on the physical, mental, and social well-being of all nurses wherever they may work or the positions they hold. However, there are other critical factors now recognized in contemporary nursing that are important for a HWE. For example, the ANA widened their definition of a HWE to include ". . . one that is safe, empowering and satisfying" (ANA, 2017). It is essential, however, that a HWE has within it a culture of civility. The concept of civility includes terms such as "politeness," "courteousness," and "courtesy," to name a few (Merriam-Webster Thesaurus, n.d.-a).

Through legislation, such as the U.S. Occupational Safety and Health Act (OSH Act, 1970), a wide understanding of the meaning of a safe and healthy workplace has developed and is now part of contemporary professional nursing culture. Nevertheless, there is still the recognized potential for some nurses to work in unhealthy work environments. Furthermore, research has shown that nurses who experience these conditions can live and work in a wide variety of geographical locations and service areas (Natarajan, Muliira, & van der Colff, 2017; Spiri, Brantley, & McGuire, 2017).

Many factors that may contribute to an unhealthy workplace environment, which are discussed later in this chapter, often go unreported, in part because they may not be physical in nature. In addition, these contributing factors may not be acted upon when they are reported and can have a damaging effect on the individual, their colleagues, family and friends, as well as the organization, specifically, and the community, generally.

This chapter briefly recounts the known and well-explored manifestations of an unhealthy work environment—incivility, bullying, stress, mental illness, and workplace violence. It then explores the growing movement to create a more active range of programs designed to address these issues.

Discussion Point

What do HWEs look like to you? From the list below, prioritize what would be important to you in your assessment of a HWE.

- Job satisfaction
- Trust
- Respect
- Flexibility
- Autonomy
- Security
- Effective communication
- Opportunity for promotion
- Time off for study
- Friendship/collegial/professional relationships

Source: Adapted from Pratt, M. (2015). Leading the way: Building the way for building an ethical workplace culture. Ethics and Leadership in the Public Service Conference, Sydney, Australia.

FACTORS THAT CONTRIBUTE TO UNHEALTHY WORK ENVIRONMENTS

There has been a growing awareness of workplace safety and health incidents since the enactment of the OSH Act and the Occupational Safety & Health Administration (OSHA). Much of the earlier reporting from OSHA referred to physical incidents such as workplace injuries and deaths. In recent years, however, OSHA reports on incidents that may be, in part, nonphysical such as psychological and financial harm. A recent amendment to the *Enforcement Procedures and Scheduling for Occupational Exposure to Workplace Violence* (U.S. Department of Labor, OSHA, 2017) demonstrates this.

Workplace issues having the potential to contribute to an unhealthy work environment are, for example, lack of resources and increased workloads. Incidents arising from the workplace may create disruptive behaviors, such as incivility and bullying. Both these behaviors have been associated with stress and mental health concerns.

Incivility

Terms, such as discourteousness, discourtesy, impoliteness, rudeness, surliness, ungraciousness, can define workplace incivility (Merriam-Webster Thesaurus, n.d.-b).

Sometimes incivility is cultivated as an organizational practice to maintain or reinforce psychological toughness. Armed forces, politics, and sporting organizations often use this form of incivility. For example, players use terms such as "sledging" and "trash talk" to explain their behavior on the sports ground to insult an opponent and to gain a psychological advantage (Cambridge Dictionary, n.d.-a, n.d.-b).

However, various studies (Torkelson, Holm, Bäckström, & Schad, 2016; Vagharseyyedin, 2015) have shown that incivility in the workplace, at a lower level, can arise from organizational change and job insecurity, whereas, at a higher level, incivility can appear to be instigated or encouraged. That is, incivility may arise innocently or be intentional. Torkelson et al. (2016) report that intentional incivility ". . . could be reflecting a climate or culture of incivility in the organization, and carry implications for future practice in interventions against workplace incivility as a use of power to control, to punish, or to isolate" (p. 115).

The outcome of a work environment that has a culture of incivility includes the impact on the targets and the witnesses to this behavior. The organization that condones this behavior runs the risk of increased costs because of staff attrition or increased sick leave because of staff experiencing psychological distress and anxiety (Vagharseyyedin, 2015).

Bullying/Mobbing

There is not a universally acceptable definition for workplace bullying. Other terms used interchangeably with bullying are "horizontal violence" and "lateral violence," to name a few. When incivility occurs, the behavior may be more overt, such as being rude, discourteous, or disrespectful, to another person.

Roberts (2015) describes bullying and incivility as "concepts similar to lateral violence that have become increasingly utilized in nursing research and scholarly writing" (p. 36). She considers the difference between bullying and incivility to be that bullying is derived from a power relationship between the perpetrator and the target, whereas incivility is different to bullying because there is no power relationship and it is less intensive and destructive (Roberts, 2015, p. 39). Alternatively, incivility, in comparison to bullying, may indicate socialization issues (Hellebrand, 2018).

Consider This Do you agree with Roberts' (2015) differentiation of bullying and incivility in her statement, earlier? If not, why?

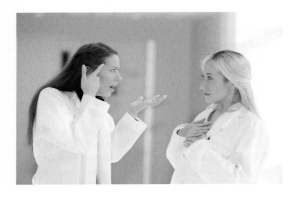

Bullying, however, may begin with behaviors that the target may not even know are occurring. Bullies can gossip, spread rumors, or even blame a person without the target's knowledge. This bullying behavior, which started covertly, may progress to bullying a person, but rarely in front of other people. Only in extreme or obvious cases do bullies, who are generally insecure, show their true self. A bully, for example, may begin by teasing a person, and if the person complains, a bully's response is commonly, "I was only joking." This behavior may escalate over time, however, and eventually the targeted person may withdraw or resign or, if he/she stays, may develop chronic stress and/or mental health issues.

Incivility and bullying behaviors are reported as a cause for burnout in nursing, job dissatisfaction, and attrition (Roberts, 2015, p. 39). This implies that a specific inappropriate behavior (incivility) may occur in parallel with another inappropriate behavior (bullying). It may also imply that one person's inappropriate behavior (incivility) leads to another person retaliating by inappropriate workplace behavior (bullying).

However, what makes bullying standout from the other terms that are used for inappropriate behaviors in the workplace is the emphasis on the length of time this behavior has occurred. Bullying behavior is consistently related to time, such as "persistent," "repeated over time," "recurrent," or "repetitive." It is the repetitive nature of bullying that "some sort of vicious circle of events may exist where bullying leads to mental health problems, which may act to worsen the situation for the target or at least worsen the perception the targets make of their work situation" (Einarsen & Nielsen, 2015, p. 133).

Another identifying factor used in defining bullying is the power imbalance. That is, there is an ongoing misuse of power in workplace relationships, mainly experienced by the targeted person through repeated verbal, physical, and/or social behavior. In most cases, the closer the power relationship, the greater the effect on the targeted person.

Bullying upward is also known as mobbing (Gaudine, Patrick, & Busby, 2017; Karsavuran & Kaya, 2017) and occurs when a group becomes obstructive to a colleague at the same level. However, mobbing behavior is more closely associated with a group who targets an individual at a senior level. In both instances, the group's disruptive behaviors could include blocking decisions, spreading rumors, or uncooperative behavior.

Cyberbullying has also become a major social media issue in the workplace (Bun, 2017; Salvador, 2016; Watts, Wagner, Velasquez, & Behrens, 2017). This behavior provides another avenue to target nurses. Cyberbullying behavior has been described as "fallacious and malicious postings in social networking sites," which leads to nurses fearing their future in nursing (Salvador, 2016, p. 143).

There are many similarities between face-to-face bullying and cyberbullying such as spreading rumors about a nurse. Both forms of bullying can be just as damaging to the targeted person. Unfortunately, what makes cyberbullying different than face-to-face bullying is how intrusive and difficult it is to escape because a nurse can be targeted at any time whether at work or not, day or night. The cyberbully is able to remain anonymous and target the victim through social media, e-mail, or text messages.

The language of cyberbullying has the possibility to minimize the seriousness of this behavior. For instance, stalking is a familiar term and generally understood, and may not be considered bullying. In cyberbullying, the same stalking behavior is considered "trolling," which has the potential to minimize the seriousness of this behavior. Despite the language, cyberbullying and face-to-face bullying can have tragic outcomes.

Discussion Point

Is it possible for a person to be bullied:
- once and suffer long-term physical and/or psychological harm?
- by a group whose deliberate intent is to have the targeted person dismissed?
- by social media in the workplace?

If you agree with these statements, consider how this behavior could be prevented.

Stress

Stress can be defined as "a condition or feeling experienced when a person perceives that demands exceed the personal and social resources the individual is able to mobilize" (American Institute of Stress, 2017, para. 2). A U.S. annual stress survey reported that "most Americans are stressed and a significant proportion feels their coping abilities are inadequate. Further, they report feeling that the stress is affecting their health, both physically and emotionally" (Scott, 2017, para. 1).

> ## Discussion Point
>
> As a nurse, has there been a time when you felt stressed at work? Was it:
> - related to where you were working? or
> - whom you were working with? or
> - other factors that made you feel stressed?

VIOLENCE IN NURSING

Over the years, violence in nursing has often been a difficult concept to grasp, in part because of people's misunderstanding of what the term violence implies, as well as the language used to describe this behavior. The language issues often derive from a reluctance to expand the meaning of violence to being more than a physical act, or it could be the result of an erroneous perception that such things do not happen to nurses. Furthermore, where people consider violence, they often ignore the nonphysical aspects, such as the emotional, financial, and psychological harm, that are experienced by many people who are abused.

Another reason violence in nursing is often misunderstood is the lack of an agreed definition. One possible reason for this misunderstanding is that other terms such as horizontal violence, lateral violence, bullying, and mobbing are used interchangeably when discussing violence in nursing. Although these other terms have slightly different connotations, depending on the context, they all cause harm to another person.

Not having an agreed definition and using different terms to describe violence in nursing often makes meaningful discussion difficult. Furthermore, overlapping factors have the potential to create stressful situations. These situations are caused when

> there is a conflict between job demands on the employee and the amount of control an employee has over meeting these demands. In general, the combination of high demands in a job and a low amount of control over the situation can lead to stress. (Canadian Centre for Occupational Health and Safety, 2017, para. 2)

Employers have a legal, ethical, and human rights responsibility to provide a safe work environment and HWE, free from discrimination. The organization has a duty of care to all their employees and "all employers must comply with the safety and health standards issued and enforced pursuant to the OSH Act 1970." In addition, the Act's General Duty Clause, Section 5(a)(1), "requires employers to provide their workers with a workplace free from recognized hazards that are causing or likely to cause death or serious physical harm." In reference to discrimination, Section 11(c)(1) of the act provides:

> No person shall discharge or in any manner discriminate against any employee because such employee has filed any complaint or instituted or caused to be instituted any proceeding under or related to this Act or has testified or is about to testify in any such proceeding or because of the exercise by such employee on behalf of himself or others of any right afforded by this Act.

Reprisal or discrimination against an employee for reporting an incident or injury related to workplace violence, related to this guidance, to an employer or OSHA would constitute a violation of Section 11(c) of the Act. In addition, 29 CFR 1904.36 provides that Section 11(c) of the Act prohibits discrimination against an employee for reporting a work-related fatality, injury, or illness. Although it is expected that management would know and be responsible for meeting the requirements of the OSH Act, all nurses should also be aware of their responsibility under this Act. It is important for all staff to be aware of current workplace risks and hazards. The Cal/OSHA and NIOSH have identified risk factors that may contribute to violence in the workplace (U.S. Department of Labor, Occupational Safety and Health Administration, 2016, pp. 31–32).

> ## Discussion Point
>
> The following activities increase the risk of violence in the work setting: Employees in contact with the public; employees exchanging money with the public; employees working late or early morning hours; a workplace that is often understaffed.
> Can you add any other activities that might increase the risk of violence in the work setting?
> ***Source:*** *Amended from United States Department of Labor. (2016). DOL guidelines for preventing for healthcare and social service workers (pp. 31–32).*

Here is the conundrum: it is next to impossible to have zero violence in the workplace with or without a respective policy. Therefore, nurses might experience different types of violence, often depending on the location, the service provided, and the perpetrator. In the worst case, violence may occur due to understaffing, remoteness, or misplaced trust. The killing of a nurse in a remote area of South Australia in 2017 led to a State Government Regulation restricting single-nurse stations in remote areas ("Health Practitioner Regulation National Law (South Australia) (Remote Area Attendance) Amendment Act," 2017).

Discussion Point

Identify your state legislation and regulations aimed at protecting nurses from workplace violence.

- Does it specifically cover nurses working alone in rural and remote areas?
- If not, what could you do as an individual, or as a member of a professional association, to raise awareness to have legislation passed to protect them?

Another reason it is difficult to extinguish workplace violence altogether is because what one person considers a harmful experience may not be every person's experience with, or perception about, violence. Such perceptions are unique to that person. Additionally, the types of violence that nurses experience are diverse and complex, which only adds to the difficulty in addressing this issue. Nevertheless, it is possible to categorize the types of violence nurses and nursing students may experience (Box 12.1).

Although the true extent of violence in nursing is considered greater than the statistics indicate, studies show that violence against female nurses is greater than that against male nurses. Compared with the experiences of female nurses, there is a dearth of research into male nurses and their experiences. Studies into violence against men in other contexts tend to focus on rites of initiation of apprentices, college fraternity rites of passage (hazing), and armed service "bastardization" practices. However, the question of whether violence against male nurses is an outcome of the same forces identified in studies into violence against female nurses is open to further research. Because the statistics show that men are often the major perpetrators of violence in society and in the workplace (except possibly for internal violence in nursing—i.e., violence which comes from within the organization), the very fear that some male nurses may experience violence could also create more violent incidents in the workplace, generating a recurring cycle of violence.

Boxes 12.2 and 12.3 expand upon the nonphysical and physical aspects of violence in nursing. Box 12.4 lists the potential factors leading to patient–nurse violence, and Box 12.5 suggests variables that may be predictive of patient–nurse violence.

In addition, nurses working in different locations and settings have different issues to address compared to those

BOX 12.1   Typology of Violence in Nursing

1. Nurse-to-nurse violence (includes nursing students; horizontal violence, lateral violence)
2. Patient-to-nurse violence (including visitors)
3. Organization-to-nurse violence (vertical down violence)
4. External perpetrators (strangers, criminal intent)
5. Third-party violence (other health professionals/family members and significant others as well as other health care workers)
6. Impact of mass trauma or natural disasters on nurses (e.g., terrorism, wars, earthquakes, tornadoes, to name a few)
7. Nurse-to-patient violence
8. Personal violence (e.g., domestic violence, family violence, interpersonal violence)

BOX 12.2   Types of Nonviolence Involving Nurses

- Being uncivil, such as exhibiting rudeness, impoliteness, and/or silence
- Condoning inappropriate behavior by being uncooperative or unsupportive
- Social isolation/social exclusion
- Setting someone up for failure, imposing ideas, taking someone's ideas, undermining, embarrassing someone
- Controlling communication—omitting to tell someone about a meeting
- Increasing unreasonable workloads and timelines
- Exhibiting threatening behavior—making someone feel intimidated, threatened, or fearful
- Spreading rumors, improperly taking credit, assigning blame or fault
- Stalking
- Defaming
- Cyberbullying

BOX 12.3   Types of Violence Involving Nurses (Predominantly by Patients, Families, and Visitors)

Nonphysical
Verbal: For example
- Swearing
- Yelling
- Shouting
- Making threats
- Calling names

Nonverbal: For example
- Invading personal space
- Threatening gestures
- Constant eye contact
- Facial features such as scowling, frowning

Physical
- Hitting/punching/pinching/kicking/scratching/ spitting
- Contact devices such as walking sticks, knives, knuckle dusters, baseball bats, guns, chemical sprays
- Sexual assaults/rape
- Assault
- Homicide

BOX 12.5   Predicting Patient–Nurse Violence

Does the patient
- indicate a heightened level of anxiety or depression?
- have hostile or aggressive body language?
- continually move around (agitation)?
- have a repetitive speech pattern (I want to go home, I want to go home)?
- complain about the provision of services?
- refuse to cooperate?
- display suicidal tendencies or cries for help?
- have rapid breathing, have clenched fists/teeth, appear restless, or talk loudly?
- swear excessively or use sexually explicit language?
- make verbal threats?
- show noncompliance with requests?

Also, a violent person can take their aggression out by using any object near at hand. As well as those outlined in Box 12.3, Box 12.7 expands on objects that may be used as potential weapons or cause property damage through frustration and aggression.

working in a large metropolitan hospital setting. For example, nurses working in homecare, rural and remote nursing, or nurses working alone or on night duty must consider the context in which they are working to determine how best to protect themselves (Box 12.6).

BOX 12.4   Potential Factors Leading to Patient–Nurse Violence

- Patient in a vulnerable state of mind
- Feeling out of control and neglected because of lack of information
- Scared, apprehensive
- Lack of assurance by/in staff
- Lack of privacy
- Negative attitude of staff toward patients
- Certain staff are prone to being assaulted
- Limited time to communicate
- Some nurses appear to have an aggressive approach
- Nurses are increasingly forced to act in controlling ways because of institutional pressures

BOX 12.6   Self-Protective Behaviors

- Have an alarm or monitoring system that requires periodic checking in
- Have a GPS location system turned on at all times on your cell phone or transport
- Policies, procedures, and training should reflect the location and setting nurses work in
- Whether working in a group or individually it is important you are aware of your organization's emergency responses in case of public threats such as terrorist attacks
- There are some aspects of a policy that would be the same wherever you may work, for example, stay calm and don't panic; if you are unable to remove yourself from the situation, attempt to defuse the situation
- There may be some aspects that are different, for example, if a home or community nurse, leave as quickly as possible—say you have to get something for the client from your car
- When working alone have the police emergency number entered on your cell phone speed dial

BOX 12.7   **Potential Weapons/ Damaged Property**

- Furniture, such as chairs, tables
- Syringes, sprays, dangerous liquids, gas/oxygen, fire extinguishers
- Equipment in treatment rooms, scissors, scalpels, chemicals
- Equipment that is sharp or blunt
- Telephone, computers, monitors
- Equipment used by patients—walking sticks, walking frames, cutlery, broken glassware, urinals, bedpans
- Guns

Discussion Point

- Is there a relationship between nurse-to-nurse violence and patient-to-nurse violence and the environment they are in?
- Are nursing students more vulnerable to violence in nursing than other nursing staff?
- What evidence do you have to support your responses?

A U.K. study into workplace violence experienced by nursing students (Tee, Özçetin, & Russell-Westhead, 2016) reported that in the past year 42.2% of students ($n = 657$) on clinical placement had reported bullying/harassment by their colleagues, whereas 30.4% witnessed this behavior. Interestingly, about four times more incidents occurred with qualified nurses (19.6%) being the perpetrator than with preceptor/mentor relationships (5.2%), implying students' clinical placements may have the potential to have a negative impact on their future in nursing. However, the results of this study did not support this proposition. Even though the outcome of these incidents reported that some students wanted to leave the profession (8.8%) or called in absent (3.5%) after these incidents, it is pleasantly surprising that 41.7% had not considered leaving nursing (Tee et al., 2016).

The high price some nurses have paid for workplace violence over many years is shown by the statistics for suicide. A recent report from Public Health England (Ford, 2017) revealed that the "risk of suicide among female nurses is 23% above the national average, while care workers in general are at higher risk, according to latest data revealed" (para. 6). Furthermore, "[B]oth male and female care workers have a risk of suicide that was almost twice the national average" (Ford, 2017, para. 8).

CREATING HEALTHY WORK ENVIRONMENTS

It is possible to create a culture that promotes a HWE. Such a culture is apparent in many organizations such as hospitals, where the private and public face is of mutual respect between staff and their clients. For organizations and institutions to address the primary and secondary effects of an unhealthy work environment and reach the position where a HWE is meaningful requires the efforts of both management and staff, working jointly and as individuals. There are considerations that must be recognized by management to achieve a HWE (Clevenger, 2017) such as the importance of all employees feeling that their contribution will be heard, valued, and that there will be professional and personal satisfaction. In other words, nurses will feel empowered, satisfied, and safe when they are involved from the planning phase.

The organizational action to achieve a HWE is not only to have in place workplace policies, procedures, and programs that eliminate workplace violence but also to include preventative measures. For example, it may require constant vigilance against workplace antisocial activities, such as incivility and bullying, as well as awareness of health issues, such as stress and mental health. These measures are over and above institutional OSHA requirements.

Ensure Civility

Civility is an integral part of a successful HWE. Some may argue that it is not enough for some departments of an organization to have a HWE when other departments do not. Indeed, the modeling of the creation of a HWE should illustrate the various factors and interactions that must be resolved for success. Many organizations (e.g., North Western University, 2017; U.S. Department of Veteran Affairs, 2017) have recognized this by promoting civility and respect in their policies. An excellent example of an organization policy that encourages a culture of civility is from Canada's Ryerson University (2016), which states, "[C]ivility involves treating others with dignity and respect, and acting with regard to other's feelings" (para. 10). In other words, civility is not only the way we speak but also how we behave toward each other. It is an ethical human interaction. For instance, "[C]ivility requires that even the most critical feedback be delivered respectfully, privately, and courteously" (Ryerson University, 2016, para. 12).

To maintain or achieve a culture of civility requires strong leadership at senior management level. Management should not condone any form of incivility and must lead by example. In other words, organizational change starts with management. It may be difficult, but not impossible, to affect a culture change that is ethical in human interactions. It is important that staff know the appropriate policies and act accordingly. For example, all staff should be aware that rudeness is not acceptable behavior. If rudeness occurs, appropriate intervention should be initiated, and if this approach is unsuccessful, then disciplinary action should follow. It is important to remember that it is a nurse's human right to work in a safe and healthy environment.

For an organization to have a HWE, management may have to address a system-wide cultural change in addressing incivility, bullying, and other disruptive behaviors, to avoid resultant stress and mental health issues. However, a total work culture change may be too much to do at one time. Therefore, another approach may be to plan to use one department that has a successful culture of civility as a model for a HWE. This approach would be less threatening, would be more manageable, and may have more success for implementation and evaluation.

Establish Antibullying Cultures

Similar to developing a culture of civility, organizations must also develop an antibullying culture. In recent years, there has been a plethora of literature and conference presentations promoting various strategies to address workplace bullying, including zero bullying behavior in the workplace. However, this may not always be a possible goal to reach without skillful and knowledgeable leadership.

In recent years, there has been a growing awareness about the importance of speaking out about being bullied (Salvador, 2016). In his study, Salvador not only promotes speaking out about bullying but also addressing bullying through education. He proposes that nurses should have training and development that builds "team organization and camaraderie through team building and personality development . . ." (Salvador, 2016, p. 144).

There is another school of thought, however, that promotes the need for a culture of support in the workplace (Copeland & Henry, 2016). They propose that "[I]nvestigative energy can be directed to the role of supportive work environments and strong leadership in managing violence, particularly mitigation of the effects of violence, including compassion fatigue, when it does occur" (Copeland & Henry, 2016, p. 71).

The principles of a *just culture* (Marx, 2001) have recently been revisited in contemporary scholarly literature within the context of the health care system (Dekker & Breakey, 2016; Kennedy, 2016; Usher et al., 2017). Applying the principles of a just culture to minimize disruptive behaviors, such as workplace bullying, may be one solution. It is well recognized that nurses are often reluctant to report bullying behavior because they are concerned about the consequences if they do. If a restorative, just culture has been implemented, as outlined by Dekker and Breakey (2016), the focus would be, in part, on who has been harmed/hurt by this behavior. The outcome of an Australian study by Usher et al. (2017, June) that is particularly relevant to workplace violence, and other inappropriate workplace behaviors, is the need for students to develop skills in questioning decisions and actions of those in authority positions and concerns about disciplinary action, not only when errors are made but also when they see a colleague (or others) being the target of abusive action.

Discussion Point

What would be the advantages and disadvantages of a just culture in addressing incivility and bullying in the organization in which you work?

Promote Stress-Free Work Environments

Organizations should aim to have a healthy, stress-free work environment, or at least to minimize stress factors. However, it may not always be possible to have a stress-free workplace in health care. Hospitals and other complex health care organizations are by their very nature, at times, perceived as stressful. Some departments within these organizations may be more stressful than other departments, for both staff and patients.

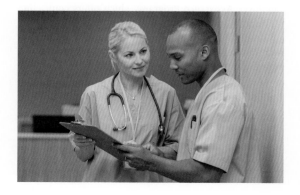

To have a HWE, it is important to address the factors that may contribute to a stressful environment. For example, a 2014 study (Scott, 2017) reported that half of the respondents experienced "irritability or anger" when stressed. This study did not specifically include nurses. However, if a similar study of nurses' response to stress was undertaken the results could possibly find similar results, or even higher.

Various methods have been proposed to manage workplace stress. A one-size-fits-all solution is not viable, so it may be necessary to try different approaches. However, for staff to see that management is working toward a stress-free work environment would have a positive effect. It is important to be aware that not all people respond in the same way to the same stress. In some instances, some people may react immediately, whereas others may have a delayed reaction.

When an individual feels stressed, the body goes through physical and psychological changes. For example, there may be triggers in the workplace that set off a stress response, such as knowing that a nurse is going to work with a particular person. The nurse could have this response even before arriving at work by just the thought of this situation. Furthermore, if the nurse is required to work with this person over time, it is possible that his/her condition could escalate to chronic stress.

Scott (2017) suggests three approaches to respond to stressful situations: self-calming techniques, emotion-focused coping strategies, and solution-focused coping strategies. Scott proposes that by being optimistic, taking action, and good self-care, it is possible to manage a person's stress healthfully without long-term problems.

Nevertheless, it is possible after attempting different stress management strategies that a person may continue to feel stressed. Left untreated, this may lead to chronic stress or mental health problems. If the cause of the stress is unresolved, it may be the time where outside professional help is required. Organizations often have an Employee Assistance Program, which offers counseling services.

Research Fuels the Controversy 12.1 refers to Needham's study showing that aggression and violence in forensic nursing settings contribute to nurses' stress and strain.

Respond to Mental Health Problems Related to Workplace Violence and Incivility

The emphasis on recognizing mental health issues in contemporary work environments is a 21st-century phenomenon. The World Health Organization (WHO, 2018) states, "[M]ental health is an integral and essential component of health" (para. 1). They continue to emphasize that "Mental health and well-being are fundamental to our collective and individual ability as humans to think, emote, interact with each other, earn a living, and enjoy life" (WHO, 2018, para. 3). Taking the broader view, the most important concern of individual, communities, and societies is that the "promotion, protection, and restoration of mental health" (WHO, 2018, para. 3) can be regarded as a vital concern of individuals, communities, and societies throughout the world.

The inappropriate behaviors discussed thus far have as their common aim the disruption of the emotional equilibrium of the targeted nurses, by denying them some part of their needs. The secondary effects of these disempowering activities, if maintained, are often to make these nurses manifest their pain by a range of responses with the potential to develop mental health issues.

Common mental health disorders that nurses may experience because of bullying, incivility, and/or workplace violence include a variety of emotions and feelings such as social isolation, helplessness, despair, panic attacks, anxiety, depression (and other mood disorders), substance use disorders, posttraumatic stress disorder (PTSD), self-harm, and suicide. A 2016 U.S. study into the psychological distress symptoms among registered nurses bullied at work recommends "[T]aking care of oneself emotionally is essential before posttraumatic stress symptoms impede the nurse's ability to perform. Employee Assistance Programs may provide some benefit to these employees" (Berry, Gillespie, Fisher, Gormley, & Haynes, 2016, para. 31).

However, it is important to note that a response or behavior exhibited in the workplace may not have its origin in a workplace incident. A simple example may be the anxiety exhibited by a nurse because of an external situation, such as domestic violence or a custody dispute, but which is exacerbated in an unhealthy work environment.

Consider This
- What should you **not** do when a colleague confides to you that she/he is feeling stressed?
- What does it mean to listen nonjudgmentally?

Discussion Point
- How can an unhealthy work environment affect work and family life?
- What role does the organization play in addressing external mental health issues that impact on a person's work practices?

Research Fuels the Controversy 12.1

Stress and Strain on Forensic Psychiatric Nurses: Violence Just One Part of the Picture

The aim of the study was to assess the psychological impact of forensic psychiatric work on nurses, to establish which psychological variables are associated with this group of nurses.

Source: Needham, I. (2016, October). *Stress and strain on forensic psychiatric nurses: Violence just one part of the picture.* Presented at the International Conference on Violence in the Health Sector—Proceedings of the Fifth International Conference on Violence in the Health Sector Broadening our view—Responding together, Dublin, Ireland.

Study Findings

From the sample of 1,072 forensic and 31 acute psychiatric nurses (47.1% response rate), 57.6% forensic nurses showed low Compassion Satisfaction. The response for high Burnout was 6.4%, and for high Compassion Fatigue the response was 9.9%. Further analysis revealed that the negative psychological impact of forensic psychiatric work is only partially attributable to violent and aggressive behavior such as auto-aggression, sexual harassment, or suicide acts.

The implications of this study are that forensic nurses experience a considerable amount of stress, suggesting psychological risk to the nurses' well-being and possible impairments to patients' care. Furthermore, senior management is advised to be attentive to signs of psychological stress in nurses and to deploy measures to combat stress and strain.

Consider This Incivility and bullying are stressors in the workplace. What are other stressors that maybe as, if not more, stressful?

Namie's (2017) long-term study reported that 40% of the respondents who had been bullied or witnessed bullying considered their health had been affected, whereas the other 60% of respondents reported being uncertain if health was affected or not. The possible reason for this uncertainty is that when targets are bullied over a long period, they may not associate their ill-health with bullying. In other words, "the causal link takes time to be recognized by targets themselves" (Namie, 2017, para. 7).

The results of Einarsen & Nielsen (2015) study into the long-term relationship between exposure to workplace bullying and subsequent mental health in the form of anxiety and depression show that "exposure to workplace bullying to be a significant predictor of mental health problems five years on" (p. 131). Furthermore, their study identified that women were less affected than men, who were more likely to suffer a serious long-term threat to their health and well-being. Mental health treatment and workplace bullying preventative measures were recommended.

Based on these studies (Einarsen & Nielsen, 2015; Namie, 2017), it appears that the long-term effects of bullying in the workplace may not be evident for 5 years or more after its beginning.

Therefore, sometime during a nurse's career there is a high probability that he/she may work with other nurses who have a diagnosed mental illness, such as anxiety, depression, or PTSD, because of being bullied. Lambert (2016) reports, "{D}epression affects 9% of everyday citizens, but 18% of nurses' experience symptoms of depression" (para. 4). She questions that if depression is a common occurrence, "why don't nurses talk about it?" (para. 5). There could be many reasons why nurses may not raise the subject but one reason may be that they are not even aware (or ignore) that they are in the early stages of mental illness or link it to their experience of being bullied.

Consider This How could a nurse provide support and understanding to a colleague, who has confided that he/she is being bullied?

WHY IS CREATING HEALTHY WORK ENVIRONMENTS SO DIFFICULT IN NURSING?

Not only should we ask the question: "Why is creating a healthy work environment so difficult in nursing?" but also ask: "Why has it taken so long?" Phillips (2016) states, "[H]ealth care workplace violence is an underreported, ubiquitous, and persistent problem that has been tolerated and largely ignored" (p. 1661).

It has been over 30 years since Meissner (1986, p. 52) coined the phrase "nurses eat their young," referring to the destructive treatment experienced by new nursing students by educators and nursing administrators. However, after a slow acceptance in the 1990s that violence in nursing was occurring, research has evolved rapidly. Until recently, research has focused on the nature and extent of the various forms of workplace violence. This was, and still is, important work. We now have a good understanding of the nature of violence in nursing and that it is not rare or confined to a single setting but is experienced by nurses in a wide variety of geographical locations and service areas. Research has shown that nurses can be targeted by other nurses or by other health professionals, patients, visitors, or strangers.

However, as Phillips (2016) points out, there are difficulties both in gaining up-to-date statistics on workplace violence and in comparing the studies used to gain these statistics. The major problems with the studies, both governmental and scholarly, are the inconsistencies in instrument design, in defining categories of violence, and the "voluntary retrospective surveys, an approach that risks both selection bias and recall bias" (Phillips, 2016, p. 1662). Nevertheless, as Phillips (2016, p. 1662) notes, "the statistics on the prevalence of workplace violence in the health care setting remains alarming." His conclusion is that there is much to do in this area and that standard legal definitions and better instrument design are essential for effective prevention programs against workplace violence. Furthermore, he claims that "studies showed that after training, nurses had increased confidence and knowledge about risk factors, . . . but existing training does not appear to reduce the rates of workplace violence" (Phillips, 2016, p. 1662).

The difficulties encountered when attempting to minimize disruptive workplace behaviors are not unique to nursing. Therefore, nurses could learn from other disciplines and organizations that have been successful in their methods of improving their work environment.

> **Consider This** Can you change culture without changing management?

Cultural Change Through Change Management

A series of change management models have been implemented over several decades in an effort to create HWEs (e.g., Ashkenas, 2013; Connelly, 2016; Murphy, 2016). Some of these have been successful and others have had their critics (Ashkenas, 2013). Some have been criticized for being too simple and others too complex. Nevertheless, there is a common effect that is recognized—change management, by its very nature, is disruptive.

One of the reasons change management programs fail is because of the lack of clear objectives and inadequate awareness of all the factors required for organizational change. Therefore, the most important factors required for successful change are that the organization has "engagement" and is "change ready" (Bayer, 2016, p. 29). For change management to be effective, "engagement is essential to facilitating lasting meaningful culture change" (Bayer, 2016, p. 29).

Engagement is a term that has both a clinical and a organizational meaning. For example, in a health care focus it means working with the client to move toward clinical goals (Sharp & Polacek, 2016). From an organizational psychology focus "engagement means engaging in the work environment to achieve a sense of fulfilment within the work environment" (Sharp & Polacek, 2016, p. 63).

Bayer (2016) is emphatic that "[E]ffective change happens when an organization and individuals in the organization are 'ready' competency wise for change." The four competencies discussed by Bayer (2016) are "[S]ocial intelligence, cultural competence, systems thinking, and continuous learning . . ." (p. 29). The organization may find it necessary to conduct workshops for all their staff, not only nurses, to be competency ready if there is a need.

Therefore, if there is to be a cultural change in attitude and understanding of violence in nursing, these changes should be strongly supported by the organization. If this is not happening, nurses may feel that they are not adequately prepared, not only to address violence in nursing but also not able to engage with other organizational issues and directives. As Sharp & Polacek (2016) pervasively argue, "[O]ne way that organizational leaders can communicate that they are engaged is to establish a period evaluation program that takes a close look at the work environment and processes" (p. 64).

> ## Discussion Point
>
> The challenge of this statement—Why is creating HWE's so difficult in nursing?—leads to a set of questions:
> - Do nurses want to see change?
> - Are nurses ready for change?
> - Do nurses have the capacity to change?
> - Are nurses ready to unify to protest against workplace violence and bullying?
> - Are nurses prepared to take on the leadership role during the change process?

CONCLUSIONS

There has been a growing interest in organizations working toward a HWE and civility. Many changes, based on research, have already been implemented to improve the work environment. However, nurses' work environments do not remain static. Furthermore, current evidence continues to highlight the need for more research and better understanding of the complexity of both positive and negative workplace behaviors. Nevertheless, research is not the only answer. Education that enables nurses to build resilience and feel empowered is another strategy that requires consideration.

Over 30 years ago, Roberts (1983) wrote the seminal work on oppression in nursing. Since the mid-1980s, there has been a major movement by nurses, through nursing research, scholarship, and personal experiences, to have a significant role in their ongoing cultural change. These changes have come about by determination and tenacity, which are the same characteristics seen in nurses today. Nurses and nursing have benefited from these changes. Raising awareness of disruptive behaviors, the causes, and introducing methods in addressing this phenomenon in the workplace have led nurses to be more insightful regarding workplace relationships. More importantly, these changes have come from within the profession, and in the future, nurses will need to continue to drive the change.

For Additional Discussion

1. What does a HWE and culture mean?

2. What are the characteristics of a HWE?

3. The quality of the cultural socialization process can create or prevent pathologic behavior. Do you agree, and if not, why not?

4. How does an unhealthy work environment affect patient care?

5. Can a workplace with a toxic culture still provide a high standard of health care?

6. Is it possible to have a healthy workplace environment in nursing? If not, why not?

7. Can legislation address all disruptive behaviors such as incivility that lead to stressful situations in nurses' work environments?

8. Which, in your opinion, generally comes first—a stressful situation causing incivility or vice versa?

9. Is it possible for nurses to be immune to influences that affect a HWE?

10. Why is incivility in one department not as disruptive as it is in another department? Alternatively, see this question from a different perspective, such as "Why does one department that has a culture of civility continue to have a disruptive culture?"

11. How should organizations recognize and address the generational differences in the workforce to ensure a HWE with a culture of civility?

References

American Institute of Stress. (2017). *What is stress?* Retrieved May 27, 2018, from https://www.stress.org/daily-life/

American Nurses Association. (2017). *American Nurses Association's (ANA) Health Risk Appraisal (HRA) 2013-2016, Executive Summary, American Nurses Association Health Risk Appraisal Findings* (pp. 1–7). Retrieved May 27, 2018, from https://www.nursingworld.org/~495c56/globalassets/practiceandpolicy/healthy-nurse-healthy-nation/ana-healthriskappraisalsummary_2013-2016.pdf

Ashkenas, R. (2013, April 16). *Change management needs to change*. Harvard Business Review. Retrieved May 27, 2018, from https://hbr.org/2013/04/change-management-needs-to-cha

Bayer, L. (2016). *The 30% solution. How civility at work increases retention, engagement, and profitability*. Melbourne, FL: Motivational Press Inc.

Berry, P., Gillespie, G., Fisher, B., Gormley, D., & Haynes, J. (2016, August 10). Psychological distress and workplace bullying among registered nurses. *The Online Journal of Issues in Nursing, 21*(3), 8. doi:10.3912/OJIN.Vol21No03PPT41

Bun, L. (2017). Cyberbullying. *Journal of Black Studies, 48*(1), 57–73.

Cambridge Dictionary. (n.d.-a). *Sledging.* Retrieved May 27, 2018, from http://dictionary.cambridge.org/us/dictionary/english/sledging

Cambridge Dictionary. (n.d.-b). *Trashtalk.* Retrieved May 27, 2018, from http://dictionary.cambridge.org/dictionary/english/trash-talk

Canadian Centre for Occupational Health and Safety. (2017). *OSH answers fact sheets. Workplace stress—General.* Retrieved May 27, 2018, from http://www.ccohs.ca/oshanswers/psychosocial/stress.html

Clevenger, K. (2017, March 17–19). *Create a healthy work environment with meaningful recognition.* Presented at The Honor Society of Nursing, Sigma Theta Tau International Conference, Creating Healthy Work Environments, Indianapolis, IN.

Connelly, M. (2016, May 26). *The Kurt Lewin change management model.* Change Management Coach. Retrieved May 27, 2018, from http://www.change-management-coach.com/kurt_lewin.html

Copeland, D., & Henry, M. (2016). *Compassion fatigue, compassion satisfaction, perceptions of safety and experiences of violence among emergency department staff.* Presented at the International Conference on Violence in the Health Sector—Proceedings of the Fifth International Conference on Violence in the Health Sector Broadening our view—Responding together, Dublin, Ireland.

Dekker, S. W., & Breakey, H. (2016). 'Just culture': Improving safety by achieving substantive, procedural and restorative justice. *Safety Science, 85,* 187–193. doi:10.1016/j.ssci.2016.01.018

Einarsen, S., & Nielsen, M. B. (2015, February). Workplace bullying as an antecedent of mental health problems: A five-year prospective and representative study. *International Archives of Occupational and Environmental Health, 88*(2), 131–142.

Ford, S. (2017, March 17). *Female nurses at higher risk of suicide than other women.* Nursing Times. Retrieved 27 May, 2018, from https://www.nursingtimes.net/

Gaudine, A. P., Patrick, L. J., & Busby, L. A. (2017, July 21). *Upward violence in nursing: A scoping review of a phenomenon of importance for nursing.* Presented at 28th International Nursing Research Congress, Sigma Theta Tau International, Dublin, Ireland.

Hamblin, L. E., Essenmacher, L., Ager, J., Upfal, M., Luborsky, M., Russell, J., & Arnetz, J. (2016, February). Worker-to-worker violence in hospitals: Perpetrator characteristics and common dyads. *Workplace Health Safety, 64*(2), 51–56.

Health Practitioner Regulation National Law (South Australia) (Remote Area Attendants) Amendment Act 2017. Retrieved 12 December, 2017, from https://www.legislation.sa.gov.au/

Hellebrand, A. M. (2018). No fear: Be proactive to end workplace violence and bullying. *Nephrology Nursing Journal, 45*(1), 11–85.

International Council of Nurses. (2017). *Position statement: Occupational health and safety for nurses.* Retrieved May 27, 2018, from http://www.icn.ch/images/stories/documents/publications/position_statements/ICN_PS_Occupational_health_and_safety.pdf

Karsavuran, S., & Kaya, S. (2017). The relationship between burnout and mobbing among hospital managers. *Nursing Ethics, 24*(3), 337–348.

Kennedy, B. (2016, June). Toward a just culture. *Nursing Management, 47*(6), 13–15.

Lambert, L. (2016, March 1). *Depression in nurses: The unspoken epidemic.* Magazine, Minority and Community Health, Nurse Health, Nursing Stress Management. Retrieved 27 May, 2018, from https://minoritynurse.com/depression-in-nurses-the-unspoken-epidemic/#disqus_thread

Marx, D. (2001). *Patient safety and the "just culture": A primer for health care executives.* New York, NY: Columbia University.

Meissner, J. E. (1986, March). Nurses: Are we eating our young? *Nursing, 16*(3), 51–53.

Merriam-Webster Thesaurus. (n.d.-a). *Civility (Definition).* Retrieved May 23, 2018, from https://www.merriam-webster.com/thesaurus/civility

Merriam-Webster Thesaurus. (n.d.-b). *Incivility (Definition).* Retrieved May 23, 2018, from https://www.merriam-webster.com/thesaurus/incivility

Murphy, M. (2016, May 22). *Stages of successful change management.* Forbes. Retrieved May 27, 2018, from https://www.forbes.com/sites/markmurphy/2016/05/27/3-stages-of-successful-change-management/#6dabcefe61f0

Namie, G. (2017, June). *2017 WBI U.S. Workplace bullying survey.* Workplace Bullying Institute. Retrieved May 27, 2018, from http://www.workplacebullying.org/wbiresearch/wbi-2017-survey

Natarajan, J., Muliira, J. K., & van der Colff, J. (2017). Incidence and perception of nursing students' academic incivility in Oman. *BMC Nursing, 16*(19), 1. doi:10.1186/s12912-017-0213-7

North Western University. (2017). *Staff handbook.* Retrieved May 27, 2018, from http://www.northwestern.edu/hr/policies-forms/policies-procedures/NU_Staff_Handbook.pdf

Phillips, J. P. (2016, April 28). Workplace violence against health care workers in the United States. *The New England Journal of Medicine, 374*(17), 1661–1669.

Roberts, S. (1983). Oppressed group behavior: Implications for nursing. *Advances in Nursing Science, 5*(4), 21–30.

Roberts, S. (2015). Lateral violence. *Nursing Science Quarterly, 28*(1), 36–41.

Ryerson University. (2016). *University administrative policy. Workplace civility and respect policy.* Retrieved May 27, 2018, from http://www.ryerson.ca/policies/board/workcivilitypolicy/

Salvador, J. T. (2016). *Exploring the lived experiences of nurses bullied by their co-worker, patients, and patients significant others in selected hospitals in metro Manila, Philippines.* Presented at the International Conference on Violence in the Health Sector—Proceedings of the Fifth International Conference on Violence in the Health Sector Broadening our view—Responding together, Dublin, Ireland.

Scott, E. (2017). *What coping strategies can help manage stress?* Very Well. Retrieved May 27, 2018, from https://www.very-well.com/what-coping-strategies-are-effective-3144562

Sharp, D., & Polacek, M. (2016). *Applying the process of client engagement to reduce workplace violence in health/social care settings.* Presented at the International Conference on Violence in the Health Sector—Proceedings of the Fifth International Conference on Violence in the Health Sector Broadening our view—Responding together, Dublin, Ireland.

Spiri, C., Brantley, M., & McGuire, M. (2017). Incivility in the workplace: A study of nursing staff in the Military Health System. *Journal of Nursing Education & Practice, 7*(3), 40–46.

Tee, S., Özçetin, Y. S. U., & Russell-Westhead, M. (2016, June). Workplace violence experienced by nursing students: A UK survey. *Nurse Education Today, 41*, 30–35.

Torkelson, E., Holm, K., Bäckström, M., & Schad, E. (2016, April 21). Factors contributing to the perpetration of workplace incivility: The importance of organizational aspects and experiencing incivility from others. *Work Stress, 30*(2), 115–131. doi:10.1080/02678373.2016.1175524

U.S. Department of Labor, Occupational Safety and Health Administration. (2016). *OSHA 3148-06R. Guidelines for preventing workplace violence for healthcare and social service workers.* Retrieved May 27, 2018, from https://www.osha.gov/Publications/osha3148.pdf

U.S. Department of Labor, Occupational Safety and Health Administration. (2017). *Directive number: CPL 02-01-058 Effective Date: 01/10/2017 SUBJECT: Enforcement procedures and scheduling for occupational exposure to workplace violence.* Retrieved May 27, 2018, from https://www.osha.gov/OshDoc/Directive_pdf/CPL_02-01-058.pdf

U.S. Department of Labor, Occupational Safety and Health Administration. (1970). *OSH Act of 1970.* Retrieved May 27, 2018, from https://www.osha.gov/laws-regs/oshact/completeoshact

U.S. Department of Veteran Affairs. (2017). *CREW: Civility, respect, and engagement in the workplace.* Retrieved May 27, 2018, from https://www.va.gov/ncod/crew.asp

U.S. Occupational Safety and Health Act. (1970). *An act.* Retrieved May 27, 2018, from https://www.osha.gov/pls/oshaweb/owadisp.show_document?p_table=oshact&p_id=2743

Usher, K., Woods, C., Parmenter, G., Hutchinson, M., Mannix, J., Power, T., . . . Jackson, D. (2017, June). Self-reported confidence in patient safety knowledge among Australian undergraduate nursing students: A multi-site cross-sectional survey study. *International Journal of Nursing Studies, 71*, 89–96.

Vagharseyyedin, A. S. (2015, March 3). Workplace incivility: A concept analysis. *Contemporary Nurse, 50*(1), 115–125.

Watts, L. K., Wagner, J., Velasquez, B., & Behrens, P. I. (2017, April). Cyberbullying in higher education: A literature review. *Computers in Human Behavior, 69*, 268–274.

World Health Organization. (2018). *Mental health: Strengthening our response. Fact sheet detail.* Geneva, Switzerland: Author. http://www.who.int/news-room/fact-sheets/detail/mental-health-strengthening-our-response%20accessed %2026%20August%202018" http://www.who.int/news-room/fact-sheets/detail/mental-health-strengthening-our-response accessed 26 August 2018 Retrieved 26 August 2018.

The Use of Social Media in Nursing
Pitfalls and Opportunities

Perry M. Gee and Michelle L. Litchman

ADDITIONAL RESOURCES

Visit thePoint® for additional helpful resources
• eBook
• Journal Articles
• WebLinks

CHAPTER OUTLINE

LEARNING OBJECTIVES

The learner will be able to:

1. Define social media and social networking.

2. Identify the different types of platforms used for social media.

3. Analyze how social media can be effectively used by the professional nurse.

4. Explore how patients and caregivers are using social media for self-management support of illness.

5. Identify the challenges nurses may encounter when using social media.

6. Review the standards and guidelines for safe and effective use of social media by the nurse.

INTRODUCTION

What an exciting time to be a nurse! Health care in America is changing—with the focus on patient-centered care, value-driven outcomes, health care reform, and the *democratization* of health information and knowledge, the nurses role is evolving. At the center of this nursing evolution is social media. *Social media* is a method for nurses to share and transmit information as well as knowledge to a far-reaching audience; *social networking* is the process of engaging with that audience using social media. This chapter will focus on the nurses' role with both social media and social networking in practice, administration, education, research, as well as consumers who are using the tools for self-management support and health promotion.

Among all health care consumers and caregivers (including nurses), the use of social media is rapidly on the rise (Box 13.1). Social media is becoming ubiquitous in society and certainly among patients, caregivers, and their health care provider teams. Nurses who are interacting with patients are encountering social media every day, and the nurses' understanding of this phenomenon is imperative for patient teaching and the promotion of health. In fact, social media is starting to play a central role in patient engagement and has potential to improve health outcomes.

BOX 13.1   Social Media Use 2016

- Multiplatform use is on the rise: 56% of online adults now use two or more social media sites, a significant increase from 2013, when it stood at 42% of Internet users.
- Eight out of ten Americans who are Internet users use Facebook; this number continues to increase.
- Over half of Internet-using young adults ages 18–29 (59%) use Instagram. And one-third of all adult Internet users use the platform. Females are more likely than males to use Instagram.
- Nearly 25% of all Internet users use Twitter, especially those with a college education.
- Twenty-five percent of all online adults use LinkedIn. Fifty percent of Internet-using adults who are college graduates use LinkedIn.
- Women dominate Pinterest: 45% of online women now use the platform, compared with 17% of online men.

Source: Greenwood, S., Perrin, A., & Duggan, M. (2016). *Social media update 2016: While Facebook usage and engagement is on the rise, while adoption of other platforms holds steady.* Washington, DC: Pew Research Center.

Patients are using social media to learn about health conditions and treatments, to connect with other patients, to update family members and caregivers, and to communicate with members of the health care team.

> **Consider This** Social media has tremendous power. During the summer of 2017, natural disasters impacted the lives of millions in the United States, the Caribbean, and Mexico. For the first time, social media, specifically Facebook, Snapchat, and Twitter, provided: (1) safety checks for family and first responders; (2) the ability to quickly locate those in need; (3) provide methods for those who required help to reach the proper officials; and (4) facilitated the coordination of the distribution of relief efforts. Using social media saved lives!

Nurses are becoming very savvy users of social media for (1) enhancing their own knowledge; (2) affecting health care policy; (3) promoting of causes and raising money; (4) staying connected with other nurses; (5) participating in professional organizations; (6) informing patients, caregivers, and the public; (7) communicating with patients and colleagues; (8) research; and just to relax and have fun. This chapter will explore the important role of social media for nursing, both now and in the future, and then provide some tools for nurses to successfully navigate this exciting new technology. Pitfalls of social media are discussed as well as how nurses can protect themselves from the drawbacks of participating in this vast new environment. This chapter begins with an overview of different types of social media.

TYPES OF SOCIAL MEDIA AND HOW IT CAN BE USED FOR NURSING

Social media is currently made up of several kinds of platforms. Each platform has unique strengths and it is not unusual to combine different platform types into one social media experience. For instance, a single site may contain both social networking and sharing of media (photos, videos, etc.). There are also multiple forms of social media including social networks, social bookmarking sites, social news, media sharing, microblogging, virtual worlds, wikis, and blogs.

Social Networks

Social networks are supported by software that allows individuals to connect and share with others. Social networks can take several forms and the focus can range from personal relationships to professional relationships and everything in-between. Other names sometimes used for social networks are virtual networks, virtual communities, or online communities. Note the use of the term "community"; this social media platform gives others access to communities or groups of people outside their geographic boundaries. This access may promote engagement with a nurse in a rural area who wants to have a relationship with other nurses who have similar interests. These online communities may also provide a supportive environment for a person with a chronic illness who can learn about self-care management activities.

The most used social network is Facebook. Facebook currently has over 2.2 billion active users worldwide; 1.45 billion people log into Facebook every day! Even without access to a personal computer, people worldwide use Facebook every day using a smartphone. A smartphone or mobile phone is a cellular telephone with expanded capabilities like e-mail, calendar functions, and access to the Internet using browser software. People in very remote parts of the earth are using smartphones for networking, accessing health care information, and social networking on sites like Facebook or Instagram. People with similar interests can use Facebook *groups* or *pages* to communicate and engage with peers. There are currently over 620 million individual groups on Facebook and many of those groups are devoted to nursing interests or health care.

To illustrate, nurses in the most remote counties in far Northern California have developed a group to network and stay connected to the current issues in nursing care using a Facebook group. This group was easy to develop, taking 5 minutes or less to build. The group is free to join and members were invited by word of mouth and through e-mail. As of today the group is very active and has almost 500 members. Members of the *Northern California Professional Nurse Network* (https://www.facebook.com/groups/101668026599850/) have used the group to find jobs, to get advice on furthering education, to share best practices, and to promote community health initiatives. Most nursing organizations have groups or pages in Facebook to communicate and share information with members and people who are interested in the groups. To illustrate, simply check out the American Association of Critical-Care Nurses page at www.Facebook.com/aacnface.

Social networking groups in Facebook can be open to the public or "closed" and only open by invitation. The regulation and access to these groups is controlled by the group or page administrator through settings in the software application. Patients or health care consumers also use social networking groups in Facebook. For example, www.Facebook.com/groups/100425715503/ is a Facebook group where caregivers of children with severe food allergies and asthma can go to get health information that may impact their children. Social networking is one of the most powerful and used components of social media and can be important for the professional nurse and the patient.

> ### Discussion Point
>
> It is common for nursing students to set up private Facebook groups for discussion of school-related issues. If negative postings appear in the group about curriculum, faculty, or clinical sites, what can be done to keep the discussion from getting out-of-hand or becoming inappropriate?

Social Bookmarking Sites

Bookmarking sites are a way nurses can search, organize, individualize, and comment with lists of Internet bookmarks or links to Web pages of interest. There are several popular social bookmarking sites including Digg.com, Reddit, and Stumbleupon. Stumbleupon has a great listing of pages organized for nursing (www.stumbleupon.com/interest/nursing). Individuals can go to social bookmarking sites and comment on individual links and even critique a site. This may provide a valuable tool for nurses to rapidly find sites important to their areas of interest or the needs of their patients.

Social News

Similar to social bookmarking, *Social news* has user posted story links on the Internet that are organized, posted, and voted upon, with the most popular news links appearing at the top of the list. The social news site Reddit (www.reddit.com) helps users find top relevant news articles in nursing by going to the site and performing a search on the word "nursing." Conducting this type of search yields top news stories voted to be of interest to nursing. Social news sites are another good method for nurses to rapidly stay apprised about what is happening in the world of nursing and health care.

Media Sharing

Media Sharing is a platform where users can share photos and/or videos and these sites may also have user profiles and other social components. YouTube is the most used form of media sharing. In addition to sharing videos, users can log in, comment, or vote on the videos and see a profile of the person who posted the video. YouTube has over 1 billion users and every day hundreds of millions of videos are

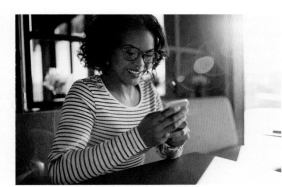

and patients. Twitter users tweet out messages that are limited to 280 characters or less (an increase from the 140 characters limit from prior to 2017). In addition to messages, users can send out photos, links to websites, and links to other media like videos. Users have a Twitter "handle" or name that starts with the @ symbol. For example, the University of Utah College of Nursing has a handle of @ UofUNursing. Hashtags are used in microblogs like Twitter to bring conversations about the same topic together so people can view the topics and compare ideas. A hashtag is preceded by the pound or "#" sign and the word or phrases are listed without spaces following this symbol. So if one wanted to start a conversation about homecare nursing, a hashtag "#homecarenursing" could be created to keep the conversation together in one easily searched location. Tweet chats are focused conversations online and typically include four or more questions to generate a dialogue on a specific topic. Engaging in a tweet chat can be exciting and allows for increased perspective based on differences in geographic location, culture, health care stakeholder role, and other factors. #WeNurses is a nursing-specific tweet chat and #HCLDR is an interdisciplinary health care leader–specific tweet chat. Both occur weekly with a worldwide following.

Virtual Worlds

Virtual worlds are computer-generated simulated settings where the user can manipulate the elements of the environment and interact in the environment using an avatar. Users may be able to interact with others in the environment, learn in the environment, and even purchase goods and services in the environment. Nursing has successfully used virtual worlds to educate nursing students in public health and even a simulated birthing center. The University of Delaware has the Te Wāhi Whānau—the birthplace in SecondLife, which is an example of a virtual setting where nurses can simulate a training experience working as a nurse in a birthing center. A video clip of this virtual center can be seen at http://youtu.be/Kw-KL-lCesE.

uploaded to YouTube. There are thousands of good videos related to nursing and health care on YouTube that are free to view and provide a great opportunity for educating nurses. For example, the nurse educator Michael Linares has a YouTube channel (www.YouTube.com/results?search_query=simple+nursing) called Simple Nursing where there are dozens of educational videos geared for nursing students as well as seasoned nurses who need a refresher on nearly any clinical topic. Nurse educators can create videos related to any subject area, upload that video to YouTube, and send a link to students who can access the video from any computer or smartphone worldwide. Nurses may also want to take advantage of these educational videos when illustrating treatments or procedures to patients and/or their caregivers. Media sharing is a great way to stay current in nursing and to visually share knowledge with others, including patients.

> ### Discussion Point
> What is the responsibility of the nurse who observes a YouTube or other media-sharing site that contains a video of a nursing procedure that would be considered unsafe or even potentially dangerous to patients?

Microblogging

Microblogging is a social media platform where users can post short comments and links to their "wall" and where others can view or follow the comments. Twitter (Twitter.com) is far and away the most popular microblogging site on the Internet. There are over 600 million Twitter users worldwide and people send out over 500 million "Tweets" (comments on Twitter) every day. Thousands of nurses have Twitter accounts and so do schools of nursing, nursing organizations, hospitals, governmental health organizations,

Wikis

A *Wiki* allows multiple users to post Internet-based content, modify content, and create online communities. The largest and most popular Wiki is of course Wikipedia (www.wikipedia.org). Wikipedia is essentially a Web-based encyclopedia that is dynamic and has an open structure that can be authored or corrected by users. Wikihealth.com is a wiki site devoted to health care and wellness issues and might be a good site for nurses and patients to access when looking for health resources. Although there is excellent content throughout Wikipedia, because of its open source nature, the nurse must carefully evaluate the clinical and evidence-based content to assure its accuracy and currency.

Blogs

Blogs (or Weblogs) are a place where individuals can write comments or forums about the topic of their choice. Typically users are focused on one specific topic area, for example, public health nursing. Blogs may also promote discussion or engagement and can be developed for free using many software platforms; WordPress is one example (wordpress.org). There are many excellent nursing blogs where professionals may go and observe and interact with nurses who choose to post comments.

A well-known and award-winning nursing blog is RT-Connections (blog.rtconnections.com). Dr. Renee Thompson has developed a blog devoted to professional nursing subjects and highlights current and future nursing issues. She is especially passionate about the problem of nurse bullying and frequently "blogs" about solutions for this troublesome condition. Keith Carson is another well-known nurse blogger. He is the cohost of RN FM Radio, which is an online radio station devoted to the field of nursing, and Nurse Keith has a blog called the Digital Doorway where he posts comments weekly about issues important to the nursing profession (digitaldoorway.blogspot.com). Nurses also pen blogs to support patients and caregivers. For example, Dr. Rita Jablonski, nurse practitioner and researcher, writes Make Dementia your B*tch (https://makedementiayour-bitch.com) focused on providing expert help for caregivers supporting individuals with various types of dementia.

> **Consider This** Blogging can be an easy, immediate, and free way for nurses to share their important messages. Have you ever thought about writing or hosting a blog? Or being a guest blog contributor?

SOCIAL MEDIA USE BY PATIENTS (HOW NURSES CAN SUPPORT PATIENTS)

Like nurses, health care consumers (patients and/or caregivers) are rapidly adopting social media. With all the different types of social media available to patients, Nyongesa, Munguti, Omondi, and Mokua (2014) suggest that there is an opportunity for nurses to provide guidance. When nurses have a strong understanding of the social media tools available, they can then educate patients and caregivers in their

selection and use. For instance, a new model for chronic illness self-managed support has been developed utilizing social media and other eHealth tools. The Enhanced Chronic Care Model (eCCM) augments the traditional supportive "community" for a person with chronic illness by providing an "eCommunity" or online community using social networking (Gee, Greenwood, Paterniti, Ward, & Miller, 2015). The eCCM also promotes the role of nurses and providers in helping patients choose a social network and to train them on effective participation in the group that will help promote self-management goals.

> **Discussion Point**
> Are there appropriate times for the nurse to use social media in the clinical setting? When would it be inappropriate?

Patients are already quite active using technology for self-management support, and in fact about 80% of adults have sought health information on the Internet (Fox & Duggan, 2013). Patients are already seeking and sharing health information on the Internet through blogs, wikis, microblogging, media sharing, and social networking. Some health care providers have concerns about patients going online to consult "Dr. Google" because of accuracy concerns. One in three American adults is going online to figure out a health condition. Of those, only 18% of individuals who self-diagnosed based on their online search were disproved by a medical provider (Fox & Duggan, 2013). Although inaccurate information can be found online, nurses can help patients identify trustworthy sources of online information.

The Rise of the e-Patient

There is a new and powerful movement of engaged patients using social media to seek care and help others with their illness. People who are empowered, engaged, educated, and informed are sometimes known as *e-Patients* (Gee et al., 2012). e-Patients are consumers of health care for those affected by illness and who actively use social media. e-Patients may include care partners in addition to patients themselves. e-Patients (1) seek out the most current evidence for care; (2) engage peers who are affected by illness for care advice and knowledge; and (3) use the *collaborative wisdom* provided by a social network of others who are also ill (Gee et al., 2012; Greenwood, 2015; Litchman, Edelman, & Donaldson, 2018; Litchman, Rothwell, & Edelman, 2017). e-Patients are experts at using social media to manage complex health conditions and nurses can learn from their success (Fox, 2008). With both patients and providers using social media, the opportunity exists to better coordinate care and collaborate together using the collective wisdom of both the provider world and the patient community (Gee et al., 2012; Timimi, 2013). At this time most of the research related to patients using social media has been descriptive, and there have only been a small number of randomized controlled trials (Hamm et al., 2013). The opportunity exists for more rigorous research and for research focusing on health outcomes (Korda & Itani, 2013).

> **Consider This** Stanford Medicine X is an annual conference that is augmented by the use of social media to engage all stakeholders in health care. Patients are at the forefront of educating health care providers and industry leaders from their point of view. Kim Vlasnik, a person living with type 1 diabetes, shared her story about the importance of having a peer community.
>
> A video of her talk can be found here: https://www.youtube.com/watch?v=HwilZ8TnZJw

Facebook has been used extensively by patients wanting to connect with others for help, advice, and social support. For instance, people with diabetes are using the Facebook platform for asking questions about their condition, for the sharing of information, and for other health promotion activities (Greene, Choudhry, Kilabuk, & Shrank, 2011; Litchman et al., 2017; Litchman et al., 2018). The informed e-patient may arrive at the health care setting with substantial knowledge about their own health condition, possibly even more than the nurse or other members of the provider team. The challenge for the nurse is to find a way to evaluate the e-patient's knowledge and then to work together as a proactive team member with the patient to meet the individual's health care goals.

Given the propensity of adolescents, young adults, to use social media and the rise of older adults in social media use, greater opportunities exist for health care professionals to use these sites to educate the e-patients of the future. Research by Hausmann, Touloumtzis, White, Colbert, and Gooding (2017) supports this idea (Research Fuels the Controversy 13.1).

Research Fuels the Controversy 13.1

Social Media and Health Care for Adolescents and Young Adults

Adolescents and younger adults are the most active groups of social media users. This group of individuals is also the fastest adopters of wireless and mobile technologies, for example, mobile phones or smartphones. This is also a time in a person's life when many life-long health habits are formulated. Social media may have an impact on the health choices of the adolescent or younger adult. This was a cross-sectional study of adolescents and younger adults exploring how they use social media for obtaining health information and communication with the health care team.

Source: Hausmann, J. S., Touloumtzis, C., White, M. T., Colbert, J. A., & Gooding, H. C. (2017). Adolescent and young adult use of social media for health and its implications. *Journal of Adolescent Health, 60*(6), 714–719. doi:10.1016/j.jadohealth.2016.12.025

Study Findings

This research paper focused on how adolescents and young adults use social media to share their own health information, to learn about health information, and to communicate with health care providers. The study was in the form of a survey administered to a convenience sample of 204 people age 12 and older. The study participants were all either English- or Spanish-speaking patients at a large children's health clinic in the Boston area. Among the participants, 51% had posted online about their health conditions in the past 6 months. The conditions they reported included acute conditions, chronic illness, and sexual health. Some were looking for others who have similar health issues for support and advice, whereas others looked for treatment options. Some mentioned it was "fun" to share their personal health information. Females shared more of their own health information than males. Participants who were between 12 and 14 years of age used social media more than the other age groups but at the same time were less likely to share their own personal health information. The most common platforms for information sharing were Facebook, Instagram, and Twitter. Study participants who rated their health as "poor" were more likely to share health-related information on social media. This study has a relatively small sample size but points to several potential areas for future research.

Virtual Health Communities That Are Consumer Centered

Many patients all over the world are using social media, specifically social networking, in the form of a virtual on-line community, to find information and support for their health conditions. Many people with rare diseases have historically been isolated and have had very limited access to pertinent health information. Now, these same people with rare conditions can find support for their health using social media (Litchman et al., 2018; Litchman, Gabel, Head, & Gee, 2017). To illustrate, a site devoted to the parents of children with clubfoot can seek information and communicate with the parents and caregivers of children who have the same condition (Oprescu, Campo, Lowe, Andsager, & Morcuende, 2013). Similarly, people with rare forms of cancer can find specialty provider contact and self-care information, as well as social support from others with the same condition on several sites, such as *PatientsLikeMe* (www.patientslikeme.com) or *Inspire* (www.inspire.com).

People with diabetes have created a supportive virtual community through their engagement with the Diabetes Social Media Advocacy (#DSMA) tweet chat. #DSMA is a 1-hour weekly tweet chat that was initiated by Cherise Shockley, a person living with diabetes, in 2012. During this tweet chat, a moderator poses diabetes-related questions and participants (patients, health care providers, advocacy organizations, etc.) respond to the questions and with each other. #DSMA tweet chats have identified how individuals with diabetes want to age successfully, which has included using forms of social media into old age (Litchman, Snyder, Edelman, Wawrzynski & Gee, in press). On World Diabetes Day, #DSMA hosts a 24-hour tweet chat, resulting in a global conversation and community around diabetes. In their recent paper, Betton and Tomlinson (2013) found that people with mental illness can feel less isolated and provide peer support for one another with the use of social networking for engagement. There is no end to the types of health conditions or demographic makeup of people who can be helped with virtual health communities.

Discussion Point

Is there a role for the professional nurse in virtual health communities or would nurses' involvement in the group change the dynamics?

What about the nurse who is also a patient and wants to join a virtual health community? What should we disclose?

Patients are also participating in research regarding their condition using social media. The social networking site *PatientsLikeMe* (www.patientslikeme.com) is a location where patients and caregivers can join groups of others with the same conditions. The community also ranks the best treatments for specific conditions and allows users to participate in research about things like symptom management should they choose to partake. The *Society of Participatory Medicine* (participatorymedicine.org) is a place where patients, providers, and health researchers can come together using social media to explore treatment options and support health conditions using the collective wisdom of the group.

The Nurse's Role

Nurses who use social media, either for personal or for professional reasons, need to understand the elements of digital citizenship. Digital citizens encompass the norms of appropriate and responsible technology use. Nurses should not post information about patients, or anything that could be linked to patients. Further, nurses should not provide medical advice online. Social media has the power to transform how the public views the nursing profession. Nurses should be mindful of how their social media presence not only reflects themselves, but also the profession as a whole.

To help patients traverse the world of these new Web-based platforms, nurses can become familiar with some of the major social media outlets for patients and steer them to those resources. Nurses should develop the skills to educate patients and caregivers on the use of social media. Nurses should routinely assess if their patients are good candidates for using social media to support their health conditions, then develop an education plan around these assessment findings (Box 13.2).

Nurses must also consider if their patients have access to broadband technologies that support the social media tools being discussed. A *digital divide* is the situation where consumers do not have access to the Internet or social media tools. The older adult, the poor, the rural, and some underrepresented groups have less access to the broadband Internet technology and have fewer computers in their homes (Chou, Hunt, Beckjord, Moser, & Hesse, 2009). People who live in rural areas make up the majority of those who have not accessed the Internet for the past year. Additionally, the majority of Americans who do not use or have access to the Internet live in rural areas; for example, 68% of those living on rural American Indian lands do not have Broadband access (Stenberg et al., 2009; Tveten, 2016). Recent research indicates the digital divide is closing to some degree now that the Internet can be accessed on mobile phones (Anderson, 2015).

BOX 13.2	Potential Patient Education Topics Related to Social Media

- The pros and cons of using social media
- How to choose an appropriate social media for specific health conditions
- The type of hardware, software, and networking needed to participate in social media
- How to join a social network
- How to navigate the individual sites
- How to maintain one's privacy on social media
- How to verify if information is credible
- How to protect one's self from scams
- How to formulate a message in a blog or microblog
- How to ask for help from an online community

Discussion Point

Should nurses routinely include assessment of social media use and broadband Internet access when taking a history and physical?

Consider This Nurses are excellent at troubleshooting very complicated and potentially life-threatening health care–related technologies, for example, IV pumps, cardiac and hemodynamic monitors, defibrillators, pacemakers. Should nurses be trained to troubleshoot basic home-networking and broadband systems used in the patient's home?

Cell phones, smartphones, tablet computers, and other mobile devices are ways individuals affected by a digital divide are gaining access to the Internet and the health care system. In fact nearly six out of every seven of the inhabitants of planet Earth have a cellular or mobile phone (Pricewaterhouse Coopers, 2012). African and Hispanic Americans and those with lower incomes highly rely on smartphones for online access (Pew Internet Research, 2018). These numbers show it is possible to provide mobile access to social media even though patients may not have home computers with traditional Internet access. Older Americans are also adopting mobile technologies at a rapid pace. Nearly 85% of those over age 65 now use a cell phone and 46% own a smartphone; this number is up 24% since the year 2013 (Pew Internet Research, 2018). Nurses should advocate for broadband or Internet access for their patients and make it part of the assessment process to evaluate Web access and individuals' ability to obtain these services.

PITFALLS OF SOCIAL MEDIA AND NURSING

Social media may prove to be a major factor in encouraging patient engagement and in improving health care. However, social media can also be unpredictable, dangerous, and harmful if not used correctly. As nurses we must advocate and protect our patients as they use social media. As professionals, it is imperative for nurses to follow ethical and professional standards as we use this new media platform.

Social media can literally expose nurses and/or their patients to access of billions of individuals on the Internet. Although this open access may offer endless opportunities, it can also open people to serious breaches in privacy and exposure to Internet predators and criminals who take advantage of users of the medium. One problem with social media is that the environment allows users to remain anonymous (Korda & Itani, 2013). The nurse or patient may believe they are interacting with a highly trained professional or a caring friend and find the individuals are not who they say they are. Patients may encounter a social media environment that reports to offer a "cure" for their conditions. Further, nurses may find a group of "experts" who claim to have new standards for nursing care, such as not vaccinating according to the Centers for Disease Control (CDC) guidelines. Your profile on social media sites, such as LinkedIn, may be used for an unsolicited invitation to provide a presentation at a conference or sit on an editorial board that isn't legitimate. Social media sites and unsolicited invitations need to be carefully analyzed to determine if they are legitimate. This analysis may be an excellent opportunity for the professional nurse to act in an advocacy and education role for their patients.

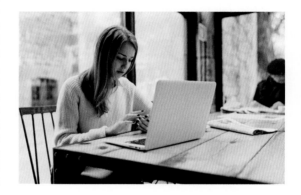

Nurses, from students to veteran professionals, have been negatively impacted by the interaction with social media. Many times the nurse has just unintentionally revealed personally identifiable patient information or revealed patient information in an environment they believed was safe and private. The privacy laws of the Health Insurance Portability and Accountability Act (HIPAA) equally apply to the world of social media. As a case in point, a young nursing student was being romantically pursued by one of her patients in the hospital. Later in the shift the patient was discharged and somehow managed to pass a note expressing his affections to the student. Disturbed by the letter the student wanted to share the note with her classmates in a "private" social media platform. The student scanned a digital image of the note and posted the document to the group; unfortunately, the image of the note also contained the patient's full name. Within hours of the image being posted in the "private" Web location it somehow ended up on a public Facebook page where the patient saw the note and reported the HIPAA infraction to the hospital. The hospital, nursing school, and individual nursing student all suffered serious consequences because of this unintentional breach by the student. This story highlights many concerns with social media, starting first with the notion that just because something says it is private does not mean it will remain private. As a rule, assume anything you post in social media can and will be viewed by all. This is an especially important rule for the nurse to follow.

Discussion Point

What should the nurse do if they witness a posting with identifiable patient information on a social media site? What if they live in a different community or even state?

Nurses can face personal liability for inappropriate use of social media. In fact according to the National Council of State Boards of Nursing (NCSBN) the majority of states have sanctioned nurses because of complaints of social media abuse (National Council of State Boards of Nursing, 2011). The majority of the infractions are due to nurses violating privacy laws and exposing identifiable patient information. The NCSBN has been working with the American Nurses Association and has developed a comprehensive whitepaper highlighting the appropriate and inappropriate use of social media by the professional nurse (www.ncsbn.org/Social_Media.pdf; Boxes 13.3 and 13.4).

BOX 13.3   National Council of State Boards of Nursing Implications for Inappropriate Use of Social Media

Instances of inappropriate use of social and electronic media may be reported to the Board of Nursing (BON). The laws outlining the basis for disciplinary action by the BON vary between jurisdictions. Depending on the laws of a jurisdiction, the BON may investigate reports of inappropriate disclosures on social media by a nurse on the grounds of:

- Unprofessional conduct
- Unethical conduct
- Moral turpitude
- Mismanagement of patient records
- Revealing a privileged communication
- Breach of confidentiality

If the allegations are found to be true, the nurse may face disciplinary action by the BON, including a reprimand or sanction, assessment of a monetary fine, or temporary or permanent loss of licensure.

Source: National Council of State Boards of Nursing. (2011). *White paper: A nurse's guide to the use of social media.* Chicago, IL: Author.

BOX 13.4   American Nurses Association's Principles for Social Networking

1. Nurses must not transmit or place online individually identifiable patient information.
2. Nurses must observe ethically prescribed professional patient–nurse boundaries.
3. Nurses should understand that patients, colleagues, institutions, and employers may view postings.
4. Nurses should take advantage of privacy settings and seek to separate personal and professional information online.
5. Nurses should bring content that could harm a patient's privacy, rights, or welfare to the attention of appropriate authorities.
6. Nurses should participate in developing institutional policies governing online conduct.

Source: American Nurses Association. (2011). *ANA's principles for social networking and the nurse.* Silver Spring, MD: Author.

The literature suggests avoiding the invitation of patients to be "friends" in social media sites. Although some health care providers are known to interact with patients using social media, the standard practice at this time is to keep personal and professional use of these platforms separated by clear boundaries (Barry & Hardiker, 2012). Nurse practitioners and other healthcare providers may want to resist the temptation to accept patients as "friends" on social media sites. The act of becoming friends with patients may violate organization policies and violate the boundaries of the nurse-patient relationship (Ventola, 2014). Patients may use social media to give the nurse practitioner bad scores for quality of care, length of the visit, cleanliness of the office, friendliness of the office staff, and even what the nurse is wearing. One disgruntled patient can use social media to cause significant damage to the nurse's reputation of ability to recruit new patients. This concern holds true for health care businesses or even hospitals. It is prudent for practitioners and health care businesses to routinely examine their Web presence for negative comments from customers.

Discussion Point

Is there ever a time the nurse or other health care provider would want to be social media "friends" with one or more of their patients?

Consider This Page West, R.N., senior vice president and chief nursing executive officer at San Francisco–based Dignity Health, is challenging her team to find creative ways to communicate with their nearly 20,000 nurses: "As a nurse leader it is important to communicate with our nurses in a way that is meaningful for them; social media may be that instrument." How might nurse leaders use social media to communicate with their staff?

Nurse leaders with a high local or national profile need to realize that participation in social media may be great for the promotion of a cause; however, it may also open the individual to personal scrutiny. Recently the nurse leader of a large health care professional organization was viciously and personally attacked for several days in the microblog *Twitter* for a personal photo that was found on a public social media site. The photo was of the professionally dressed and physically fit nurse leader holding a cake that had been presented at a party. This photo was then attached to a tweet and exposed to the Internet to degrade the leader and identify the leader as a hypocrite who was promoting unhealthy eating. The innocent photo caused several days of grief and inhibited the nurse leader from promoting the intended national health agenda. Nurse leaders who use social media on a large scale may need to develop a "thick skin" and prepare to occasionally be attacked using the Internet platform (Marshall, 2015).

In addition, more and more employers are looking at social media as part of the hiring process. In a survey completed in 2017, 70% of employers were using social media sites to screen for potential employees (Nauen, 2017). For nursing leadership positions, using the Internet is commonplace for human resource specialists, recruiters, or hiring managers to review a candidate's profile in the social media professional site *LinkedIn* (www.LinkedIn.com). The professional nurse will want to carefully use online platforms and consider steps to evaluate and tidy up their current social media presence. Strategies for keeping a positive social media image and avoiding problems with social media are shown in Boxes 13.5 and 13.6.

SOCIAL MEDIA IN PROFESSIONAL NURSING PRACTICE

Although the social media environment does contain some risks, carefully utilized Web-based platforms can potentially enhance practice, education, and research. Nurses will need to carefully consider their use of social media as a tool and develop knowledge and expertise in its implementation.

Social Media in Nursing Practice

Clinically practicing nurses need to be familiar with these new media so they can incorporate these tools into their practice. In public and population health, social media has a strong presence in surveillance of disease. Public health experts have used social media and an analysis of the content of consumer's messages in social networking and blogs to identify the rising incidence in diabetes (Eggleston & Weitzman, 2014). At an even more detailed level, algorithms have been developed and used to identify the differences between "chatter" about the flu and actual incidence of the flu (Broniatowski, Paul, & Dredze, 2013). Both Google and the CDC evaluate Internet searches and social media comments to accurately track to detect outbreaks and incidence of the flu at state and national levels (www.google.org/flutrends/us/#US). Photosurveillance techniques have been used to identify if individuals with diabetes are using their continuous glucose monitors as recommended by the Food and Drug Administration (Litchman & Woodruff, 2017).

BOX 13.5   Keeping a Positive Social Media Image

Five tips for nurse job seekers to keep a positive image online:

1. **Clean up digital dirt before you begin your job search.** Remove any photos, content, and links that can work against you in an employer's eyes.
2. **Consider creating your own professional group** on sites like Facebook or LinkedIn. It's a great way to establish relationships with leaders, recruiters, and potential referrals.
3. **Keep gripes offline.** Keep the content you post focused on positive things, whether it's related to professional or personal information. Make sure to highlight specific accomplishments inside and outside of work.
4. **Be selective about whom you accept as friends.** Don't forget others can see your friends when they search for you. Monitor comments made by others and consider using the "block comments" feature. Even better, set your profile to "private" so only designated friends can view it.
5. **If you're still employed, don't mention your job search** in your Tweets or status updates. There are multiple examples of people who have gotten fired as a result of doing this. In addition, a potential employer might assume that if you're willing to search for a new job on your current company's time, why wouldn't you do so on theirs?

Source: Haefner, R. (2009). *More employers screening candidates via social networking sites: Five tips for creating a positive online image.* Retrieved October 7, 2017, from https://www.careerbuilder.com/share/aboutus/pressreleasesdetail.aspx?ed=12%2F31%2F2009&id=pr519&sd=8%2F19%2F2009

BOX 13.6   How to Avoid Problems Using Social Media

It is important to recognize that instances of inappropriate use of social media can and do occur, but with awareness and caution, nurses can avoid inadvertently disclosing confidential or private information about patients.

The following guidelines are intended to minimize the risks of using social media:

- First and foremost, nurses must recognize that they have an ethical and legal obligation to maintain patient privacy and confidentiality at all times.
- Nurses are strictly prohibited from transmitting by way of any electronic media any patient-related image. In addition, nurses are restricted from transmitting any information that may be reasonably anticipated to violate patient rights to confidentiality or privacy, or otherwise degrade or embarrass the patient.
- Do not share, post, or otherwise disseminate any information, including images, about a patient or information gained in the nurse–patient relationship with anyone unless there is a patient care–related need to disclose the information or other legal obligation to do so.
- Do not identify patients by name or post or publish information that may lead to the identification of a patient. Limiting access to postings through privacy settings is not sufficient to ensure privacy.
- Do not refer to patients in a disparaging manner, even if the patient is not identified.
- Do not take photos or videos of patients on personal devices, including cell phones. Follow employer policies for taking photographs or video of patients for treatment or other legitimate purposes using employer-provided devices.
- Maintain professional boundaries in the use of electronic media. Like in-person relationships, the nurse has the obligation to establish, communicate, and enforce professional boundaries with patients in the online environment. Use caution when having online social contact with patients or former patients. Online contact with patients or former patients blurs the distinction between a professional and personal relationship. The fact that a patient may initiate contact with the nurse does not permit the nurse to engage in a personal relationship with the patient.
- Consult employer policies or an appropriate leader within the organization for guidance regarding work-related postings.
- Promptly report any identified breach of confidentiality or privacy.
- Be aware of and comply with employer policies regarding use of employer-owned computers, cameras, and other electronic devices and use of personal devices in the workplace.
- Do not make disparaging remarks about employers or coworkers. Do not make threatening, harassing, profane, obscene, sexually explicit, racially derogatory, homophobic, or other offensive comments.
- Do not post content or otherwise speak on behalf of the employer unless authorized to do so and follow all applicable policies of the employer.

Source: National Council of State Boards of Nursing. (2011). *White paper: A nurse's guide to the use of social media.* Chicago, IL: Author.

In addition to surveillance, nurses can use social media to promote self-management for patients with chronic illness. For instance, a person with pulmonary fibrosis can be steered to a social network to meet others with the same condition for social support on the self-management of their condition. An online health community has been shown to increase empowerment, self-management, and social support among chronically ill adults (Barak, Boniel-Nissim, & Suler, 2008; Litchman et al., 2017; Shaw & Johnson, 2011; van Uden-Kraan, Drossaert, Taal, Seydel, & van de Laar, 2009). The opportunity exists for nurses working with patients and caregivers of people with chronic illness to guide them in using social media for engagement and support. Nurses who work with those with chronic illness may want to begin to explore health issue–specific social media resources, evaluate the offerings, catalog a list of resources, and make those resources available to patients.

Discussion Point

If the nurse were asked by a patient or caregiver "what would be some good social media resources" for the person with a specific condition, where would the nurse go to find these tools?

To help the nurse who is new to using social media, the American Nurses Association (2011) maintains a Web site that is a *Social Networking Principles Took Kit* where one can find a variety of resources for the nurse (https://www.nursingworld.org/practice-policy/nursing-excellence/social-networking-Principles/). Nurses who are part of the policy development process in their organization may want to inform themselves on social media issues and generate unit-based or facility policies to guide nurses new to the organization.

Social Media in Nursing Education

Social media provides an excellent platform for training nurses, patients, and other providers (Lipp, Davis, Peter, & Davies, 2014). Nurses in the large academic medical center or in the very remote part of the country can have access to the exact same clinical reference materials. For the practicing clinical nurse, there are thousands of videos devoted to nursing skills and the management of illness. Nurse educators can use YouTube to store and distribute videos to students or the nursing profession in general. Nurse educators can explore the available videos for a specific skill or management of a particular condition and share that content with students without having to take the time to research and develop the content. Students can learn from a variety of nurses and see care accomplished using a range of different methods. One caution, faculty and educators need to

carefully review the available audio and video contents to be sure the materials are safe, appropriate, and evidence based.

Faculty or nurse researchers can use the free online media tool SurveyMonkey (www.surveymonkey.com) for education in the classroom, scheduling of meetings, or obtaining survey results (Drake & Leander, 2013). Faculty or their nurse educators can use microblogging hashtags to keep topics grouped and organize their online classroom content (Schmitt, Sims-Giddens, & Booth, 2012). Social media tools like blogs, microblogs, wiki pages, and virtual worlds offer a wide variety of methods for students to interact with their local cohort or with students literally anywhere on the planet.

Consider This Social media is a way to be "present" and even participate at a professional conference or symposium without even attending. During the 2013 Stanford Medicine X, a conference that is devoted to patients, health care providers, researchers, designers, and technologists who are interested in technology, social media, and health promotion, 3,576 individual conference participants sent out nearly 8,900 Tweets (microblogs) per day and totaled over 27,000 conversations for the entire conference. The Tweets were real-time, informing interested persons all over the globe (medicinex.stanford.edu). The 2016 and 2017 Stanford Medicine X conference has highlighted several nurses as keynote and breakout session presenters.

Social Media in Nursing Research

To date, there has been paucity of significant research in social media and nursing. However, a Twitter analysis of the public perception of the nursing profession following the wrongful arrest of registered nurse, Alex Wubbels, was conducted. In this case, a video and multiple new articles of the arrest were circulated on social media, including Twitter. A tweet analysis indicated that the public perceived Alex Wubbels, and the nursing profession at large, as being trustworthy (Litchman, Tay, & Guo, 2018), which is consistent with the last 16 Gallup Polls (Brenan, 2017). Nurses who are highlighted in the media may support recruitment, retention, and professionalism within the nursing profession; thus, it is important to understand the role you play online.

The opportunity exists to examine how social media can be used to augment health care and professional nursing, and how nurses can support patients and their use of social media (Grajales, Sheps, Ho, Novak-Lauscher, & Eysenbach, 2014). Chretien and Kind (2013) suggest that the use of social media by nurses can help facilitate a faster transition of research evidence into clinical practice. We are starting to see patients participating in the research process using social media with the surveillance of hypoglycemia among members of an online community and with research available to members of the site *PatientsLikeMe* (Weitzman, Kelemen, Quinn, Eggleston, & Mandl, 2013). And last, social media sites afford the nurse researcher opportunities to connect with colleagues with similar nursing research interests using sites like *ResearchGate* (www.researchgate.net/home.Home.html) where scientists can share ideas and research literature.

CONCLUSIONS

If properly harnessed, social media is a powerful tool for professional nursing practice and patient support. Nurses need to add an understanding of these new web-based platforms to their knowledge base, and nursing education is duty-bound to deliberately add social media at all levels of curriculum. As part of the patient advocate role, nurses must learn these tools and be prepared to guide

patients who are new to social media and those who are experienced in using these platforms. We can also keep in mind that millions of health care consumers and/or their caregivers are already using social media effectively, and as nurses we can take this occasion to learn about this dynamic platform from our patients. We must also note that an opportunity exists for nurses to conduct research with all forms of social media and that we can use this platform to rapidly disseminate new evidence to the nursing domain.

Social media does come with inherent risks for both nurses and patients. Nurses must review the ANA *Scope and Standards of Practice* (www.nursingworld.org/scope-andstandardsofpractice) and *Code of Ethics for Nurses* (www.nursingworld.org/codeofethics) resources and critically apply this content to the use of social media. The rules are the same; however, the reach and magnitude of the consequences of poor decisions are greatly amplified. Social media comes with pitfalls and opportunities for both nurses and patients. Now is the opportunity for nursing to embrace this new and exciting platform and use the social media tools to improve our profession and the health of our communities.

For Additional Discussion

1. What are three components of social media, and how can they be used by the professional nurse?

2. How might social media be used to promote the nursing profession? Give some examples.

3. How do the HIPAA requirements apply to the various types of social media? Are there differences in the legal consequences for a social media breach of confidentiality?

4. What are some examples of using social media for the person with a chronic illness? What is the nurses' role?

5. What is the digital divide and how can we as nurses assess the impact of the digital divide related to social media use by our patients?

6. Can you describe two resources available for nurses to explore when considering the implementation of social media projects or interventions?

7. As our population ages what are some considerations for social media use in the older adult?

References

American Nurses Association. (2011). *ANA's principles for social networking and the nurse.* Silver Spring, MD: Author. Retrieved from https://www.nursingworld.org/~4af4f2/globalassets/docs/ana/ethics/social-networking.pdf

Anderson. M. (2015, October). *Technology device ownership. Pew Research Center.* Available at: http://www.pewinternet.org/2015/10/29/technology-device-ownership-2015

Barak, A., Boniel-Nissim, M., & Suler, J. (2008). Fostering empowerment in online support groups. *Computers in Human Behavior, 24*(5), 1867–1883.

Barry, J., & Hardiker, N. R. (2012). Advancing nursing practice through social media: A global perspective. *Online Journal of Issues in Nursing, 17*(3), 1–11.

Betton, V., & Tomlinson, V. (2013). *Benefits of social media for nurses and service users.* Retrieved February 1, 2015, from http://www.nursingtimes.net/nursing-practice/specialisms/educators/benefits-of-social-media-for-nurses-and-service-users/5060041.article

Brenan, M. (2017). *Nurses keep healthy lead as most honest, ethical profession.* Gallup. Retrieved from http://news.gallup.com/poll/224639/nurses-keep-healthy-lead-honest-ethical-profession.aspx

Broniatowski, D. A., Paul, M. J., & Dredze, M. (2013). National and local influenza surveillance through Twitter: An analysis of the 2012–2013 influenza epidemic. *PLoS One, 8*(12), e83672. doi:10.1371/journal.pone.0083672

Chou, W. Y., Hunt, Y. M., Beckjord, E. B., Moser, R. P., & Hesse, B. W. (2009). Social media use in the United States: Implications for health communication. *Journal of Medical Internet Research, 11*(4), e48. doi:10.2196/jmir.1249

Chretien, K. C., & Kind, T. (2013). Social media and clinical care: Ethical, professional, and social implications. *Circulation, 127*(13), 1413–1421. doi:10.1161/CIRCULATIONAHA.112.128017

Drake, M. A., & Leander, S. A. (2013). Nursing students and Ning: Using social networking to teach public health/community nursing in 11 baccalaureate nursing programs. *Nursing Education Perspectives, 34*(4), 270–272.

Eggleston, E. M., & Weitzman, E. R. (2014). Innovative uses of electronic health records and social media for public health surveillance. *Current Diabetes Reports, 14*(3), 468. doi:10.1007/s11892-013-0468-7

Fox, S. (2008). *The engaged e-patient population: People turn to the Internet for health information when the stakes are high and the connection fast.* Washington, DC: Pew Research Center.

Fox, S., & Duggan, M. (2013). *Health online 2013.* Washington, DC: Pew Internet & American Life Project.

Gee, P. M., Greenwood, D. A., Kim, K. K., Perez, S. L., Staggers, N., & Devon, H. A. (2012). Exploration of the e-patient phenomenon in nursing informatics. *Nursing Outlook, 60*(4), e9–e16. doi:10.1016/j.outlook.2011.11.005

Gee, P. M., Greenwood, D. A., Paterniti, D. A., Ward, D., & Miller, L. M. (2015). The e-health enhanced chronic care model: A theory derivation approach. *Journal of Medical Internet Research, 17*(4), e86. doi:10.2196/jmir.4067

Grajales, F. J., III, Sheps, S., Ho, K., Novak-Lauscher, H., & Eysenbach, G. (2014). Social media: A review and tutorial of applications in medicine and health care. *Journal of Medical Internet Research, 16*(2), e13. doi:10.2196/jmir.2912

Greene, J. A., Choudhry, N. K., Kilabuk, E., & Shrank, W. H. (2011). Online social networking by patients with diabetes: A qualitative evaluation of communication with Facebook. *Journal of General Internal Medicine, 26*(3), 287–292. doi:10.1007/s11606-010-1526-3

Greenwood, D. A. (2015). *Collaborative wisdom: Remote monitoring technology facilitates e-patient and diabetes educator engagement.* Paper presented at the American Telemedicine Association 20th Annual Meeting, Los Angeles, CA.

Hamm, M. P., Chisholm, A., Shulhan, J., Milne, A., Scott, S. D., Given, L. M., & Hartling, L. (2013). Social media use among

patients and caregivers: A scoping review. *BMJ Open, 3*(5). doi:10.1136/bmjopen-2013-002819

Hausmann, J. S., Touloumtzis, C., White, M. T., Colbert, J. A., & Gooding, H. C. (2017). Adolescent and young adult use of social media for health and its implications. *Journal of Adolescent Health, 60*(6), 714–719. doi:10.1016/j.jadohealth.2016.12.025

Korda, H., & Itani, Z. (2013). Harnessing social media for health promotion and behavior change. *Health Promotion Practice, 14*(1), 15–23. doi:10.1177/1524839911405850

Lipp, A., Davis, R. E., Peter, R., & Davies, J. S. (2014). The use of social media among health care professionals within an online postgraduate diabetes diploma course. *Practical Diabetes, 31*(1), 14a–17a.

Litchman, M. L., & Woodruff, W. (2017, August). *Photosurveillance of non-FDA approved activity in the diabetes online community.* 4th Annual Meeting of the American Association of Diabetes Educators, Indianapolis, IN.

Litchman, M. L., Edelman, L. S., & Donaldson, G. W. (2018). Effect of diabetes online community engagement on health indicators: Cross-sectional study. *Journal of Medical Internet Research Diabetes, 3*(2), e8.

Litchman, M. L., Gabel, H., Head, R., & Gee, P. (2017, August). *The power of "me too": An analysis of peer health in the diabetes online community.* 44th Annual Meeting of the American Association of Diabetes Educators, Indianapolis, IN.

Litchman, M. L., Rothwell, E., & Edelman, L. S. (2017). The diabetes online community: Older adults supporting self-care through peer health. *Patient Education and Counseling.* doi:10.1016/j.pec/2017.08.023

Litchman ML, Snider C, Edelman LS, Wawrzynski SE, Gee PM. (2018). Diabetes online community user perceptions of successful aging with diabetes: Analysis of a# DSMA tweet chat. *JMIR Aging,* 1(1):e10176.

Litchman, M. L., Tay, D. L., & Guo, J. (2018). *Public perceptions of nursing following a high profile nurse arrest.* Conference Paper, Western Institute of Nursing's 51st Annual Communicating Nursing Research Conference, Spokane, WA.

Marshall, K. (2015). *Embrace your online nemesis.* Retrieved from Vitae, The Chronicle of Higher Education Website: https://chroniclevitae.com/news/895-embrace-your-online-nemesis?cid=VTEVPMSED1

National Council of State Boards of Nursing. (2011). *White paper: A nurse's guide to the use of social media.* Chicago, IL: Author.

Nauen, R. (2017). *Number of employers using social media to screen candidates at all-time high, finds latest career builder study.* Retrieved October 2, 2017, from http://press.careerbuilder.com/2017-06-15-Number-of-Employers-Using-Social-Media-to-Screen-Candidates-at-All-Time-High-Finds-Latest-CareerBuilder-Study

Nyongesa, H., Munguti, C., Omondi, C., & Mokua, W. (2014). Harnessing the power of social media in optimizing health outcomes. *The Pan African Medical Journal, 18,* 290. doi:10.11604/pamj.2014.18.290.4634

Oprescu, F., Campo, S., Lowe, J., Andsager, J., & Morcuende, J. A. (2013). Online information exchanges for parents of children with a rare health condition: Key findings from an online support community. *Journal of Medical Internet Research, 15*(1), e16. doi:10.2196/jmir.2423

Pew Internet Research. (2018, February 5). *Mobile fact sheet.* Washington, DC: Pew Internet & American Life Project. Retrieved from http://www.pewinternet.org/fact-sheet/mobile

Pricewaterhouse Coopers. (2012). *Emerging mHealth: Paths for growth.* New York, NY: Author.

Schmitt, T. L., Sims-Giddens, S. S., & Booth, R. G. (2012). Social media use in nursing. *The Online Journal of Issues in Nursing, 17*(3), 1–13. doi:10.3912/OJIN.Vol17No03Man02

Schroeder, D. G., Hix, B., Dean, D., Fiordelisi, V., & Thorpe, K. (2011). *Improving the health of Hispanics using mobile technology: A roadmap to reach and impact America's fastest growing population.* Roswell, GA: HolaDoctor & 3CInteractive.

Shaw, R. J., & Johnson, C. M. (2011). Health information seeking and social media use on the Internet among people with diabetes. *Online Journal of Public Health Informatics, 3*(1). doi:10.5210/ojphi.v3i1.3561

Stenberg, P., Morehart, M., Vogel, S., Cromartie, J., Breneman, V., & Brown, D. (2009). *Broadband Internet's value for rural America (Economic Research Service, Trans.).* Washington, DC: United States Department of Agriculture.

Timimi, F. K. (2013). The shape of digital engagement: Health care and social media. *The Journal of Ambulatory Care Management, 36*(3), 187–192. doi:10.1097/JAC.0b013e3182965512

Tveten, J. (2016). *On American Indian reservations, challenges perpetuate the digital divide: After mild improvements, American Indian reservations still suffer from "digital divide".* Retrieved October 8, 2017, from https://arstechnica.com/information-technology/2016/01/on-american-indian-reservations-challenges-perpetuate-the-digital-divide/

van Uden-Kraan, C. F., Drossaert, C. H., Taal, E., Seydel, E. R., & van de Laar, M. A. (2009). Participation in online patient support groups endorses patients' empowerment. *Patient Education and Counseling, 74*(1), 61–69. doi:10.1016/j.pec.2008.07.044

Ventola, C. L. (2014). Social Media and Health Care Professionals: Benefits, Risks, and Best Practices. *Pharmacy and Therapeutics, 39*(7), 491–520.

Weitzman, E. R., Kelemen, S., Quinn, M., Eggleston, E. M., & Mandl, K. D. (2013). Participatory surveillance of hypoglycemia and harms in an online social network. *JAMA Internal Medicine, 173*(5), 345–351. doi:10.1001/jamainternmed.2013.2512

Medical Errors
An Ongoing Threat to Quality Health Care

Carol J. Huston

CHAPTER OUTLINE

LEARNING OBJECTIVES

The learner will be able to:

1. Differentiate among the terms medical error, medication error, and adverse event.

2. Describe highly publicized patient cases from the mid- to the late 1990s as well as seminal research studies that brought national attention to the problem of medical errors in the United States.

3. Identify current research studies examining the scope, common causes, and financial/human costs of medical errors in the United States.

4. Summarize key findings of the 1999 Institute of Medicine (IOM) report *To Err Is Human*, as well as the multipronged approach identified by the IOM to address the problem of medical errors in the United States.

5. Identify national committees and groups formed as a result of governmental or legislative intervention to address the problem of medical errors.

6. Describe the intent and impact of Medicare's Pay for Performance initiatives, as well as Medicare's 2008

decision to no longer reimburse health care providers for care needed as the result of "never events" or other preventable errors.

7. Differentiate between workplaces that emphasize a "culture of blame" and those that seek to provide a "just culture" or a "culture of safety management."

8. Identify the meaning of a Six Sigma error failure rate and determine how error rates in health care compare with other industries such as banking and the airlines.

9. Analyze the effect of the medical liability system on systematic efforts to uncover and learn from mistakes that are made in health care.

10. Differentiate among the three evidence-based standards identified by Leapfrog as having the

greatest potential to reduce medical errors: computerized physician order entry, evidence-based hospital referral, and intensive care unit physician staffing.

11. Track current federal and state legislative efforts that encourage the voluntary reporting of health care errors by affording confidentiality protections for such reports.

12. Review current research to determine whether organizational, governmental, and national efforts to reduce the incidence of medical errors in the United States have resulted in desired outcomes.

13. Reflect on the likelihood that he or she would self-report his or her medical errors to his or her employer, as well as to the involved patients and families.

INTRODUCTION

Quality health care has emerged as a critically important yet underachieved goal. Among the most significant threats to achieving quality health care are the scope and prevalence of medical errors. Indeed, preventable medical errors are reported to be the third highest cause of death in the United States, following heart disease and cancer, claiming the lives of somewhere between 250,000 and 440,000 Americans every year (Sipherd, 2018). Similarly, a recent study in Canada found that 1 out of every 18 patients in Canadian hospitals—138,000 patients—experienced a harmful event that was potentially preventable. Of those patients, 30,000 faced more than one preventable harmful event (Schadenberg, 2017).

Indeed, Kliff (2015) points out that medical errors kill more people than car crashes or new disease outbreaks. They also kill more people annually than breast cancer, AIDS, plane crashes, or drug overdoses. "Those left dead as a result of their medical care could fill an average-sized Major League Baseball stadium—sometimes twice over" (Kliff, 2015, p. 2). Kliff goes on to note that "something like 2 to 3 percent of people who go into the hospital are going to have some pretty severe harm as a result" and "Australian studies suggest the rate might be as high as 12 percent. The harder you look, and the more you study the issue, the more errors you find" (p. 2).

> **Consider This** In Minnesota alone, in 2014, 98 patients were seriously injured and another 13 patients died as a result of medical errors. Falls, pressure ulcers, and wrong-site surgeries declined, but other errors increased, including incorrectly placed catheters and feeding tubes.
>
> On 20 occasions, facilities lost irreplaceable patient lab specimens including colon polyps, placentas, and gallbladders (Benson, 2015).

Surprisingly though, the problem of medical errors did not receive nationwide attention in the United States until several highly publicized cases between the late 1990s and early 2000s. One such case involved Betsy Lehman, a *Boston Globe* reporter, who died following chemotherapy administration errors. The news media jumped on the story because it demonstrated repeated widespread communication and dispensing errors, despite multiple safeguards in place to keep them from happening.

Libby Zion's case occurred about this same time. Zion, an 18-year-old, died 8 hours after entering a New York emergency department with seemingly minor complaints of fever and earache. Her death from drug interactions brought attention both to the all-too-narrow range between effective and toxic doses of some drugs and the danger of drug–drug interactions, even when all drugs are administered in doses that are considered safe when administered individually. The case also brought attention to the lack of supervision of residents and interns in the United States, as well as the excessive work hours forced on them and the errors that occur as a result.

There was also the story of Willie King, a diabetic man from Tampa, Florida, who had the wrong leg amputated. This case, which became known as the "wrong leg" case, captured the collective dread of wrong-site surgery, but it is a medical error that occurs too frequently because of the symmetry of the human body.

Finally, there was the story of Lewis Blackman, a healthy, gifted 15-year-old, who slowly bled to death after undergoing a minor surgical procedure at a major university medical center. Despite multiple warning signs, those caring for him repeatedly missed signs and symptoms that he was bleeding internally from a perforated ulcer.

Discussion Point

Were medical errors historically just considered an unavoidable consequence of health care? If so, did this reduce incentives to address the problem?

Perhaps, it was the clustering of these high-profile cases that made Americans stop and look at the problem of medical errors, or maybe it was just time to do so. The result was that an unprecedented number of seminal research studies delving into medical errors were undertaken over the past 20 years to discover how many errors were occurring, what was causing them, and what their financial and human costs were.

The results have been disconcerting, to say the least. Most studies have highlighted multiple concerns about quality of care, including high rates of provider-induced injury, unnecessary care, and inappropriate care. Many studies found the number of errors in health care to be unacceptably high. The seminal study of this time, *To Err Is Human*, published in 1999 by the National Academy of Medicine (NAM; formerly the Institute of Medicine [IOM]), a congressionally chartered independent organization, provided evidence that the public was highly vulnerable to human error in U.S. health care institutions, an arena in which many thought they were safe.

In addition, unlike most health care research, which generally receives little if any national press, medical error research findings in the late 1990s were published and analyzed in almost every media forum in the country. Consumers were barraged with study findings suggesting that the quality of health care was inadequate and that medical errors were a significant problem leading to increased morbidity and mortality.

Discussion Point

Do you believe that error disclosure rates differ between nurses and physicians? If so, which professional group do you believe might be more likely to disclose errors and why?

As a result, consumers, providers, and legislators stepped forward to voice their concerns and to demand, at a minimum, a safer health care system. The government listened and directed providers to reexamine how quality health care was provided, measured, and monitored so that cultures of safety could be developed in all health care organizations.

This chapter examines seminal and current research on medical errors, medication errors, and adverse events, as well as the directives that emerged from their findings. Mechanisms for achieving four goals put forth by the IOM as part of *To Err Is Human* are identified. Finally, strategies for creating a culture of safety management in health care are identified, as are the challenges of changing a system that all too often focuses on individual errors rather than on the need to make system-wide changes.

DEFINING TERMS: MEDICAL ERRORS, MEDICATION ERRORS, AND ADVERSE EVENTS

In reviewing the literature on medical errors, medication errors, and adverse events in health care, it is helpful to first define common terms. *Medical errors* are defined by the *Encyclopedia of Surgery* (2018) as adverse events that could be prevented given the current state of medical knowledge. In addition, the Quality Interagency Coordination (QuIC) Task Force suggests that medical errors are "the failure of a planned action to be completed as intended or the use of a wrong plan to achieve an aim. Errors can include problems in practice, products, procedures, and systems" (Encyclopedia of Surgery, 2018, para. 3).

Medication errors are the most common type of medical error and are a significant cause of preventable adverse events. *Medication errors* are defined by the National Coordinating Council for Medication Error Reporting and Prevention (NCC MERP) as follows:

> *Any preventable event that may cause or lead to inappropriate medication use or patient harm while the medication is in the control of the health care professional, patient, or consumer. Such events may be related to professional practice, health care products, procedures, and systems, including prescribing; order communication;*

product labeling, packaging, and nomenclature; compounding; dispensing; distribution; administration; education; monitoring; and use. (U.S. Food & Drug Administration, 2018, para. 4)

The U.S. Food and Drug Administration (FDA) estimates that 1.3 million people are injured by medication errors annually in the United States (Hayes, 2017). In a recent study, the medications most frequently associated with serious medical outcomes included those commonly taken by individuals over age 50. These included cardiovascular medications used for high blood pressure; analgesic pain relievers (e.g., acetaminophen and opioids); and hormones, primarily insulin and sulfonylurea, which are used in the treatment of diabetes. Cardiovascular medications and pain relievers were responsible for two-thirds of the deaths included in the study (Hayes, 2017).

Finally, *adverse events* are defined as adverse changes in health that occur as a result of treatment. When medications are involved, these are known as *adverse drug events.*

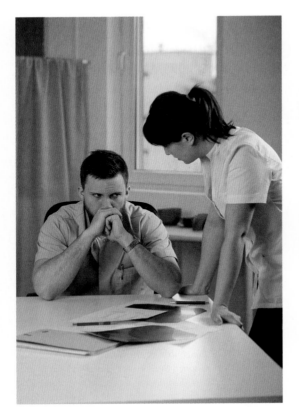

SEMINAL RESEARCH ON MEDICAL ERRORS: 1990 TO 2000

The last decade of the 20th century was marked by a rapid increase in research on medical errors. One of the earliest large-scale studies suggesting that medical errors were a significant problem in health care was published by Brennan et al. (1991) in *The New England Journal of Medicine.* This benchmark study involved more than 30,000 hospitalized patients in New York State. Nearly 5 of every 100 patients suffered an adverse event caused by a medical error of omission or commission. Of these adverse events, approximately one in four involved negligence. The overwhelming majority of iatrogenic occurrences, however, resulted from organization, system, or process failures. This study, extrapolated to the national population, suggested that 1.3 million people were injured each year in hospitals; of that number, 180,000 would die from those injuries. Providing additional cause for alarm, the report suggested that most of those injuries were actually preventable.

Leape et al. (1991) also reported that drug complications represented 19% of these adverse events and that 45% of these adverse events were caused by medical errors. In this study, 30% of the individuals with drug-related injuries died.

In another study, Leape (1994) reported that the average intensive care unit (ICU) patient experienced almost two errors per day. One of five of these errors was potentially serious or fatal. In fact, this translates into a level of proficiency of approximately 99%, which seems reasonable. However, if performance levels of 99.9%—substantially better than those found in the ICU by Leape—were applied to the airline and banking industries, it would equate to two dangerous landings per day at Chicago's O'Hare International Airport, or 32,000 checks deducted hourly from the wrong account (Leape, 1994).

> **Consider This** The safety record in health care is a far cry from the enviable record of the similarly complex aviation industry.

Another seminal study in the late 1990s involving medical errors was completed by Thomas et al. (1999). Their research, based on a chart review of 14,732 medical records from 28 hospitals in Colorado and Utah, found that 265 of 459 (57%) adverse events were preventable. The total cost of adverse events was US$661,889,000, with preventable adverse events costing an additional US$308,382,000. In addition, the study estimated the national costs of all preventable adverse events to be just under US$17 billion (in 1996 dollars). A follow-up study just 12 years later, suggested the cost of medical errors to be closer to $1 trillion annually (Goedert, 2012).

To Err Is Human

Many of the studies done in the 1990s laid the foundation for what is perhaps the best known and largest study ever done on the quality of health care: *To Err Is Human* (Kohn, Corrigan, & Donaldson, 2000). This report, which represented a compilation of more than 30 studies completed by the NAM (formerly IOM), found the following:

- At least 44,000 Americans die each year as a result of medical errors, and the number may be as high as 98,000.

- Even when using the lower estimate, deaths because of medical errors could be considered the eighth leading cause of death in 1999.

- More people die in a given year as a result of medical errors than from motor vehicle accidents, breast cancer, or AIDS.

The IOM study also examined the types of errors that were occurring. Many of the adverse events were associated with the use of pharmaceutical agents and were potentially preventable. Medication errors alone, both in and out of the hospital, were estimated to account for more than 7,000 deaths in 1993, and one of every 854 inpatient hospital deaths was the result of a medication error. Children experienced harmful medication errors three times more often than adults (5.7% of medication orders for pediatric patients), and the rate was higher yet for neonates in the neonatal ICU. In addition, ICU patients suffered more life-threatening medication errors than any other patient population.

> *Consider This* Pediatric patients are at even greater risk for medication errors than the general population because of weight-based dosing calculations and the misreading of decimal points.

Within a short time of the IOM report's release, some people began to question the numbers, asking whether the problem of medical errors could be as serious as it seemed. The first study to reliably confirm the IOM figures was a 2004 study by the health care ratings company Health-Grades (2004). This study looked at 3 years of Medicare data in all 50 states and Washington, DC, and reported that approximately 1.14 million patient safety incidents (PSIs) occurred among the 37 million hospitalizations in the Medicare population for the study period. The most commonly occurring PSIs were failure to rescue, decubitus ulcer, and postoperative sepsis.

Of the total 323,993 deaths among Medicare patients who developed one or more PSIs, 263,864, or 81%, of these deaths were directly attributable to the incidents (Health-Grades, 2004). In addition, one in every four Medicare patients who were hospitalized from 2000 to 2002 and experienced a PSI died. Perhaps most startling, however, was the conclusion that the United States loses more lives to PSIs every 6 months than it did in the entire Vietnam War. This also equates to three fully loaded jumbo jets crashing every other day for the last 5 years. Finally, the study noted that if the Centers for Disease Control and Prevention's annual list of leading causes of death included medical errors, it would show up as number six, ahead of diabetes, pneumonia, Alzheimer's disease, and renal disease (HealthGrades, 2004).

Additional reports since that time have repeatedly confirmed that the figures suggested in *To Err Is Human* were underreported. Indeed, recent study findings released by Patient Safety America suggested that up to 400,000 patients die each year as the result of medical errors (MacDonald, 2013). The lead researcher concluded that

> There was much debate after the IOM report about the accuracy of its estimates. In a sense, it does not matter whether the deaths of 100,000, 200,000 or 400,000 Americans each year are associated with preventable adverse events in hospitals. Any of the estimates demand assertive action on the part of providers, legislators and people who will one day become patients. (MacDonald, 2013, para. 6)

Discussion Point

Is the U.S. public aware of the prevalence of medical errors? If not, what could be done to galvanize them to take action?

The Response to the National Academy of Medicine (Institute of Medicine) Report

Within weeks of the release of *To Err Is Human*, the Senate held its first hearings on the issue, and additional hearings were conducted by committees of both the House of Representatives and the Senate. Local, state, and national leaders, as well as private and public sector leaders, took immediate action. The significance of the report as a catalyst for change cannot be overstated.

That said, however, it is important to note that the problems of medical errors and patient safety were not completely unrecognized before *To Err Is Human* was published.

Perhaps the most significant aspect of the study was that it summarized the high human cost of medical errors in language that was understandable by the public. In addition, previously, an assumption was made that most patient injuries were the result of negligence, incompetence, or corporate greed. The report indicated, however, that errors are simply a part of the human condition and that the health care system needed to be redesigned so that fewer errors would occur.

Because of these findings, the NAM (IOM) recommended a national goal of reducing the number of medical errors by 50% over 5 years (Kohn et al., 2000). To that end, it outlined a four-pronged approach to reducing medical mistakes nationwide (Box 14.1). The strategies needed to achieve this national goal and attend to each of the four approaches are numerous, however, and only a few are detailed in this chapter.

WORKING TO ACHIEVE THE NATIONAL INSTITUTE OF MEDICINE (IOM) GOALS

The first of the four-pronged approach to reducing medical errors was to "establish a national focus to create leadership, research, tools, and protocols to enhance the knowledge base about safety" (Kohn et al., 2000, p. 6). The second was to "raise standards and expectations for improvements in safety through the actions of oversight organizations, group purchasers, and professional groups" (Kohn et al., 2000, p. 6). Work to achieve both of these goals began almost immediately after the IOM report was published.

BOX 14.1   **The Institute of Medicine's Four-Pronged Approach to Reducing Medical Mistakes Nationwide**

- Establish a national focus to create leadership, research, tools, and protocols to enhance the knowledge base about safety.
- Identify and learn from medical errors through both mandatory and voluntary reporting systems.
- Raise standards and expectations for improvements in safety through the actions of oversight organizations, group purchasers, and professional groups.
- Implement safe practices at the delivery level.

Source: Kohn, L. T., Corrigan, J. M., & Donaldson, M. S. (Eds.). (2000). *Executive summary. In To err is human: Building a safer health system* (pp. 1–6). Retrieved August 27, 2017, from https://www.nap.edu/read/9728/chapter/2

Indeed, a number of national committees and groups were formed as a result of governmental or legislative intervention. Some of the committees, groups, and legislative efforts spearheading the task to reduce medical errors are outlined here.

Quality Interagency Coordination Task Force

The QuIC Task Force was established by former President Bill Clinton in 1998 to coordinate federal agencies that provided health care services. In December 1999, the task force began to evaluate the IOM recommendations and develop strategies for identifying threats to patient safety and reducing medical errors.

The final report, *Doing What Counts for Patient Safety: Federal Actions to Reduce Medical Errors and Their Impact*, was delivered to the president in February 2000. The report proposed taking strong action on all of the IOM recommendations to reduce errors, implementing a system of public accountability, developing a robust knowledge base about medical errors, and changing the culture in health care organizations to promote the recognition of errors and improvement in patient safety.

The National Forum for Health Care Quality Measurement and Reporting

Consistent with the QuIC's recommendations, the National Forum for Health Care Quality Measurement and Reporting was launched by former Vice President Al Gore in 2000. Known as the National Quality Forum (NQF, 2018a), it is a broad-based, private, not-for-profit body that establishes standard quality measurement tools to help people better ensure the delivery of quality services. The mission of the NQF is to lead collaboration to improve health and health care quality through measurement (para. 1).

Since its inception, the NQF has endorsed hundreds of performance measures and practices, and many more are either in the early stages of development or moving through the NQF endorsement process. NQF was also the first to create a list of 27 *serious reportable events* (SREs), a list that has grown to 29 as of 2018 (NQF, 2018b; Box 14.2).

In addition, the NQF board of directors approved expansion of their mission in 2008 to include working in partnership with other leadership organizations to establish national priorities and goals for performance measurement and public reporting. The first draft of their core set of national priorities was created in 2008. The National Quality

BOX 14.2   **Serious Reportable Events in Health Care**

1. Surgical or invasive procedure events
   - Surgery or other invasive procedure performed on the wrong site
   - Surgery or other invasive procedure performed on the wrong patient
   - Wrong surgical or other invasive procedure performed on a patient
   - Unintended retention of a foreign object in a patient after surgery or other invasive procedure
   - Intraoperative or immediately postoperative/postprocedure death in an American Society of Anesthesiologists Class 1 patient
2. Product or device events
   - Patient death or serious injury associated with the use of contaminated drugs, devices, or biologics provided by the health care setting
   - Patient death or serious injury associated with the use or function of a device in patient care, in which the device is used or functions other than as intended
   - Patient death or serious injury associated with intravascular air embolism that occurs while being cared for in a health care setting
3. Patient protection events
   - Discharge or release of a patient/resident of any age, who is unable to make decisions, to other than an authorized person
   - Patient death or serious injury associated with patient elopement (disappearance)
   - Patient suicide, attempted suicide, or self-harm that results in serious injury, while being cared for in a health care setting
4. Care management events
   - Patient death or serious injury associated with a medication error (e.g., errors involving the wrong drug, wrong dose, wrong patient, wrong time, wrong rate, wrong preparation, or wrong route of administration)
   - Patient death or serious injury associated with unsafe administration of blood products
   - Maternal death or serious injury associated with labor or delivery in a low-risk pregnancy while being cared for in a health care setting
   - (NEW) Death or serious injury of a neonate associated with labor or delivery in a low-risk pregnancy
   - Patient death or serious injury associated with a fall while being cared for in a health care setting
   - Any Stage 3, Stage 4, and unstageable pressure ulcers acquired after admission/presentation to a health care setting
   - Artificial insemination with the wrong donor sperm or wrong egg
   - (NEW) Patient death or serious injury resulting from the irretrievable loss of an irreplaceable biologic specimen
   - (NEW) Patient death or serious injury resulting from failure to follow up or communicate laboratory, pathology, or radiology test results
5. Environmental events
   - Patient or staff death or serious injury associated with an electric shock in the course of a patient care process in a health care setting
   - Any incident in which systems designated for oxygen or other gas to be delivered to a patient contains no gas, the wrong gas, or is contaminated by toxic substances
   - Patient or staff death or serious injury associated with a burn incurred from any source in the course of a patient care process in a health care setting
   - Patient death or serious injury associated with the use of physical restraints or bedrails while being cared for in a health care setting
6. Radiologic events
   - (NEW) Death or serious injury of a patient or staff associated with the introduction of a metallic object into the magnetic resonance imaging area
7. Potential criminal events
   - Any instance of care ordered by or provided by someone impersonating a physician, nurse, pharmacist, or other licensed health care provider
   - Abduction of a patient/resident of any age
   - Sexual abuse/assault on a patient or staff member within or on the grounds of a health care setting
   - Death or serious injury of a patient or staff member resulting from a physical assault (i.e., battery) that occurs within or on the grounds of a health care setting

Source: National Quality Forum. (2018a). *NQF's mission and vision.* Retrieved May 29, 2018, from http://www.qualityforum.org/about_nqf/mission_and_vision; National Quality Forum. (2018b). *List of SREs.* Retrieved May 29, 2018, from http://www.qualityforum.org/Topics/SREs/List_of_SREs.aspx

BOX 14.3   **The National Quality Strategy (2017): Aims, Priorities, and Levers**

Aims

These aims guide and assess local, state, and national efforts to improve health and the quality of health care.
* *Better Care*: Improve the overall quality, by making health care more patient-centered, reliable, accessible, and safe.
* *Healthy People/Healthy Communities*: Improve the health of the U.S. population by supporting proven interventions to address behavioral, social, and environmental determinants of health in addition to delivering higher-quality care.
* *Affordable Care:* Reduce the cost of quality health care for individuals, families, employers, and government.

Priorities

The National Quality Strategy focuses on six priorities:
1. Making care safer by reducing harm caused in the delivery of care.
2. Ensuring that each person and family is engaged as partners in their care.
3. Promoting effective communication and coordination of care.
4. Promoting the most effective prevention and treatment practices for the leading causes of mortality, starting with cardiovascular disease.
5. Working with communities to promote wide use of best practices to enable healthy living.
6. Making quality care more affordable for individuals, families, employers, and governments by developing and spreading new health care delivery models.

Levers

Each of the nine National Quality Strategy levers represents a core business function, resource, and/or action that stakeholders can use to align to the strategy.
* *Public Reporting*: Compare treatment results, costs, and patient experience for consumers.
* *Learning and Technical Assistance*: Foster learning environments that offer training, resources, tools, and guidance to help organizations achieve quality improvement goals.
* *Certification, Accreditation, and Regulation*: Adopt or adhere to approaches to meet safety and quality standards.
* *Consumer Incentives and Benefit Designs*: Help consumers adopt healthy behaviors and make informed decisions.
* *Payment*: Reward and incentivize providers to deliver high-quality, patient-centered care.
* *Health Information Technology*: Improve communication, transparency, and efficiency for better coordinated health and health care.
* *Innovation and Diffusion*: Foster innovation in health care quality improvement, and facilitate rapid adoption within and across organizations and communities.
* *Workforce Development*: Invest in people to prepare the next generation of health care professionals and support lifelong learning for providers.

Source: National Quality Strategy. (2017). *About the National Quality Strategy (NQS)*. Retrieved May 29, 2018, from https://www.ahrq.gov/workingforquality/about/index.html#aims

Strategy as of 2018 in terms of aims, priorities, and levers is shown in Box 14.3.

Finally, the NQF was identified as the consensus-based entity for implementation of the Affordable Care Act (ACA), which launched in late 2011, including convening a multistakeholder group to provide annual input to the Department of Health and Human Services on the development of a National Quality Strategy (NQF, 2018c). The resultant National Priorities Partnership includes representatives from 52 major national organizations representing public and private sector stakeholder groups in a forum that balances the interests of consumers, purchasers, health plans, clinicians, providers, communities, states, and suppliers (NQF, 2018c).

The National Patient Safety Foundation

The National Patient Safety Foundation (NPSF) was also formed in response to the IOM report. The mission of the NPSF, as amended in 2003, is to partner with patients and families, the health care community, and key stakeholders to advance patient safety and health care workforce safety and disseminate strategies to prevent harm (Institute for Healthcare Improvement/National Patient Safety Foundation [IHI/NPSF], 2018).

In 2017, the NPSF merged with the Institute for Healthcare Improvement (IHI), which had been established in the late 1980s by Donald Berwick. The IHI is an independent not-for-profit organization focused on improvement capability; person- and family-centered care; patient safety; quality, cost, and value; and the triple aim for populations—improve care, improve population health, and reduce costs per capita (IHI/NPSF, 2018). During the annual National Forum on Quality Improvement in Health Care conference, the IHI highlights evidence-based best practices in an effort to more rapidly translate research into practice. In addition, the group maintains disciplined research and development processes and prototyping projects to pursue health care quality improvements.

The Joint Commission

New organizations were not the only ones that responded to the recommendations of the IOM. The Joint Commission, in existence since 1951, accredits hospitals, long-term care facilities, psychiatric facilities, ambulatory care programs, and home health operations.

The Joint Commission's National Patient Safety Goals, implemented in January 2003, set forth clear, evidence-based recommendations to focus health care organizations on significant documented safety problems. These goals are updated annually for ambulatory care settings, behavioral health settings, hospitals, home care disease-specific care, laboratories, home-based care, and office-based surgery. The goals for hospitals in 2018 are shown in Box 14.4.

The Joint Commission also maintains one of the nation's most comprehensive databases of sentinel (serious adverse) events by health care professionals and their underlying causes. A *sentinel event* is defined by the Joint Commission (2017) as "a Patient Safety Event (not primarily related to the natural course of the patient's illness or underlying condition), that results in either death, permanent harm, or severe temporary harm and intervention required to sustain

life" (para. 2). Such events are called *sentinel* because they signal the need for immediate investigation and response. Information from the Joint Commission sentinel database is regularly shared with accredited organizations to help them take appropriate steps to prevent medical errors.

Another Joint Commission priority is the development of a *root cause analysis* with a plan of correction for the errors that do occur. The Joint Commission's (2017) Sentinel Event Policy provides that organizations that are either voluntarily reporting a sentinel event or responding to the Joint Commission's inquiry about a sentinel event submit their related root cause analysis and action plan electronically to the Joint Commission whenever such events occur. The sentinel event data are then reviewed, and recommendations are made. The Joint Commission defends the confidentiality of the information, if necessary, in court.

Similarly, some organizations use a *failure mode and effects analysis* to examine all possible failures in a design—including sequencing of events, actual and potential risk, points of vulnerability, and areas for improvement (American Society for Quality, 2018).

> **Consider This** National legislation designed to keep such error analyses confidential is a critical but still-unrealized step. This discourages error reporting.

Centers for Medicare and Medicaid Services

The Centers for Medicare and Medicaid Services (CMS), formerly the Health Care Financing Administration, also plays an active role in setting standards and measuring quality of health care. With the introduction of the Medicare Quality Initiatives in November 2001, a new era of public reporting on quality began. These diverse initiatives encouraged the public reporting of quality measures for nursing homes, home health agencies, hospitals, and kidney dialysis facilities. These data are then made available to consumers on the Medicare website to assist them in making health care choices or decisions.

Medicare also established *pay for performance* (P4P), also known as *quality-based purchasing*, in the middle of the first decade of the 21st century. Because research conducted in the past decade has suggested little relationship between quality of care provided and the cost of that care, P4P initiatives were created to align payment and quality incentives and to reduce costs through improved quality and efficiency.

As part of P4P, the Physician Quality Reporting Initiative (PQRI), which was launched in 2007, allowed for

---

BOX 14.4 **Joint Commission 2018 National Patient Safety Goals for Hospitals**

1. Identify patients correctly.
2. Improve staff communication.
3. Use medicines safely.
4. Use alarms safely.
5. Prevent infection.
6. Identify patient safety risks.
7. Prevent mistakes in surgery.

Source: Joint Commission. (2018). *2018 National patient safety goals.* Retrieved May 29, 2018, from https://www.joint commission.org/assets/1/6/2018_HAP_NPSG_goals_final.pdf

payments to eligible professionals who satisfactorily reported quality information to Medicare on at least 3 of 74 individual quality measures on 80% of the cases from July 1, 2007 through December 31, 2007. Those who met the criteria for submitting quality data were eligible to earn a lump-sum incentive payment equivalent to 1.5% of their total estimated allowable charges for Medicare Part B Physician Fee Schedule (American Academy of Orthopaedic Surgeons [AAOS], 1995–2018).

The Medicare Improvements for Patients and Providers Act of 2008 made the PQRI program permanent, with incentive payments increased to 2.0% and authorized through 2010. There were 153 individual quality measures and 7 measure groups for reporting under the program in 2009. For 2010, there were 175 individual measures and 13 measure groups (AAOS, 1995–2018).

With the introduction of the ACA in 2011, the PQRI was changed to the *Physician Quality Reporting System* (PQRS), and incentive payments of 1.0% were established for successfully reporting the then 190 individual PQRS measures. An additional 0.5% incentive payment was possible for providers who qualified for or maintained board certification status, participated in maintenance of certification program, and successfully completed a qualified maintenance of certification program practice assessment (AAOS, 1995–2018).

The PQRS program, however, ended at the end of 2016, transitioning to the *Merit-based Incentive Payment System* (MIPS) under the Quality Payment Program (2018). As of 2017, providers who billed Medicare more than US$30,000 in Part B-allowed charges per year and provided care for more than 100 Medicare patients per year must participate in one of two tracks in the Quality Payment Program; the MIPS or *Alternative Payment Models* (APMs). Providers participating in an APM may be eligible for a 5% incentive payment in 2019 if they sent in data about the care they provided and how the practice used technology in 2017 by March 31, 2018. Providers in MIPs will receive a negative 4% payment adjustment if those data were not submitted by the March 2018 deadline (Quality Payment Program, 2018). Thus, PQRS transitioned from incentive payments to penalty charges if quality data are not submitted.

Discussion Point

Should it be necessary to pay health care professionals bonuses to submit quality information? Do you believe incentives or penalty charges are a stronger motivation for provider data submission?

Also, as part of the ACA, the CMS has now instituted hospital *value-based purchasing* (VBP). In this program, participating hospitals are paid for inpatient acute care services based on the quality of care, not just quantity of the services they provide. The program uses the hospital quality data reporting infrastructure developed for the Hospital Inpatient Quality Reporting Program, which was authorized by Section 501(b) of the Medicare Prescription Drug, Improvement, and Modernization Act of 2003 (Centers for Medicare and Medicaid Services [CMS], 2017).

The Hospital VBP Program was funded in 2018 by reducing participating hospitals' base operating Medicare Diagnosis Related Groups payments by 2%. Any leftover funds are redistributed to hospitals based on their *Total Performance Scores*. It is possible for a hospital to earn back a value-based incentive payment percentage that is less than, equal to, or more than the applicable reduction for that fiscal year (CMS, 2017).

In addition, to reduce the number of preventable medical errors, including *never events* (errors that should never happen, such as removing the wrong limb in surgery, leaving a foreign object inside a patient during surgery, or sending a baby home with the wrong parents), Medicare announced that effective October 1, 2008, it would no longer pay for care that was required as a result of eight specific preventable errors or never events identified by the NQF. Medicaid followed suit in 2011. Private insurance companies are following suit. These new policies require hospitals to maintain meticulous documentation about what conditions are present on admission to differentiate between preexisting conditions and those that are acquired during the hospital stay.

Also, in 2011, the medical errors list was further updated and expanded to cover 29 events that fall under seven categories and the name never events was changed to SREs (Torrey, 2016; Box 14.5).

BOX 14.5 **The National Quality Forum's Seven Categories of Serious Reportable Events**

1. Surgical or invasive procedure events
2. Product or device events
3. Patient protection events
4. Care management events
5. Environmental events
6. Radiologic events
7. Potential criminal events

Source: Torrey, T. (2016, January 2). *Medical errors, adverse events and the National Quality Forum.* Very Well. Retrieved May 29, 2018, from https://www.verywell.com/medical-errors-list-2615322

Discussion Point

Should public or private insurance plans refuse to pay for care that is extended as a result of medical errors?

Quality and Safety Education for Nurses Project

The Quality and Safety Education for Nurses (QSEN) project (funded by Robert Wood Johnson Foundation) began in 2005 with the goal of preparing future nurses who will have the knowledge, skills, and attitudes (KSAs) necessary to continuously improve the quality and safety of the health care systems within which they work (QSEN Institute, 2018). When nurses have these KSAs, they are better able to identify potential errors and intervene before errors occur.

HEALTH CARE REPORT CARDS

In response to the demand for objective measures of quality, including the number and type of medical errors, many health plans, health care providers, employer purchasing groups, consumer information organizations, and state governments have begun to formulate health care quality report cards. Most states have laws requiring providers to report some type of data. The Agency for Healthcare Research and Quality is also exploring the development of a report card for the nation's health care delivery system, and the National Committee for Quality Assurance's Health Plan Report Card lets an individual create a health plan report card online. In addition, CMS released a proposed rule in June 2011 that would make Medicare information regarding provider cost and quality available to certain organizations.

It is important to remember, however, that many report cards do not contain information about the quality of care rendered by specific clinics, group practices, or physicians in a health plan's network. In addition, most report cards focus on service utilization data and patient satisfaction ratings and have minimal data regarding medical errors. Critics of health care report cards also point out that health

plans may receive conflicting ratings on different report cards. This results from using different performance measures, as well as how each report card pools and evaluates individual factors. Report cards might also not be readily accessible or might be difficult for the average consumer to understand. Still, there is no doubt that consumers want more access to meaningful quality-of-care information and it is apparent that such data, which have long been kept secret, are now becoming public.

CREATING A CULTURE OF SAFETY MANAGEMENT

In response to public forces and professional concerns, patient safety has become one of the nation's most pressing challenges and a mandate for every health care organization. Indeed, the final recommendation of the IOM report was to implement safe practices at the delivery level. The strategies that have been recommended to achieve this goal are overwhelming both in scope and quantity.

Strategies discussed in this chapter include the "Six Sigma" approach (a customer-based management philosophy) to error management; the mandatory/voluntary reporting of errors; attempts to increase confidentiality of reporting to reduce the fear of legal liability for reporting errors that do occur; the Leapfrog recommendations; the use of bar coding; a change in organizational cultures from that of "individual blame" to error identification and system modification; and the development of patient safety solutions by the World Health Organization's (WHO) World Alliance for Patient Safety.

A Six Sigma Approach

One approach that has been taken to create a culture of safety management at the institutional level has been the implementation of the "Six Sigma" approach. *Sigma* is a statistical measurement that reflects how well a product or process is performing. Higher sigma values indicate better performance. Historically, the health care industry has been comfortable striving for three-sigma processes (all data points fall within three standard deviations) in terms of health care quality instead of six. This is one reason why health care has more errors than the banking and airline industries, in which achieving Six Sigma is the expectation. Organizations aim for this lofty target by carefully applying Six Sigma methodology to every aspect of a product or process.

Discussion Point

Should the health care industry be willing to accept higher error rates than the banking or airline industries? Why or why not? Is the public willing to do so?

Discussion Point

Is a Six Sigma failure rate a reasonable goal for all health care organizations? Should some health care organizations be expected to have higher failure (defect) rates than others? What variables might affect an organization's ability to achieve this goal?

Mandatory Reporting of Errors

The third prong of the IOM's four-pronged approach to creating a safer health care system was "to identify and learn from medical errors through both mandatory and voluntary reporting systems" (Kohn et al., 2000, p. 6). To accomplish this, the IOM report recommended developing a mandatory reporting system for medical errors and adverse events at both the state and national levels.

State mandates for reporting medical errors and adverse events have been slow to materialize, although as of 2018, a total of 25 states required hospitals and/or other medical facilities to report serious medical errors (Lockwood, 2018) and some states also have reporting mandates that apply only to specific types of error, such as hospital-acquired infections. It is important to note that the IOM report did suggest, in addition to mandatory reporting, that more options be created for limited voluntary reporting systems in all 50 states. The IOM also recommended that more research be conducted on how best to develop voluntary reporting systems that complement proposed mandatory reporting systems.

Increased mandatory and voluntary reporting must also occur at the institutional level, as well as by individual providers. As a result, the IOM report suggested that mandatory adverse event reporting should initially be required of hospitals and eventually of other institutional and ambulatory care delivery facilities. This was the impetus for the subsequent Joint Commission action for sentinel event reporting as part of the accreditation process.

Yet, even when error rates are reported, there is some question as to the accuracy of the reported data. Many hospitals rely on incident reporting as their key quality and safety measure, despite widespread acknowledgment that many errors go unreported (Macquarie University, 2015). Indeed, a recent comparative study of two hospitals in Australia found no relationship between the number of reported medication incidents and the "actual" rate of prescribing and medication administration errors observed (Macquarie University, 2015). The hospital with the higher number of incident reports had lower "actual" prescribing errors and vice versa. Thus, in this instance, the higher number of medication incidents actually reported reflected a lower patient risk.

It is difficult, however, to enforce greater disclosure and reporting at the individual provider level. Ethical and professional guidelines suggest that providers have a responsibility to disclose medical errors. Yet, the literature continues to suggest that this does not happen because of a fear of legal suits or disciplinary measures by employers. The ironic part is that full disclosure after errors occur often reduces the likelihood of legal suit or the extent of patient retribution.

Discussion Point

Do you believe the majority of medical errors are reported? Why or why not?

Perhaps, this failure to disclose medical errors is a major contributor to the disconnect that exists between consumers' perceptions of the quality of their health care and the actual quality provided. Even consumers who are aware of medical error statistics often report that they believe medical errors to be a problem but believe that such errors will not happen to them because they trust and believe in their health care provider.

Discussion Point

Do you consider the care you receive from your primary care provider to be of a high quality? Are your perceptions subjective, or do you have objective data to back up your impression? Have you actively searched for such data on your primary care provider?

Legal Liability and Medical Error Reporting

If quality health care is to be achieved, the medical liability system and our litigious society must be recognized as potential barriers to systematic efforts to uncover and learn from mistakes that are made in health care.

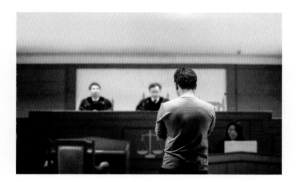

One recommendation of the IOM panel was to encourage learning about safety from cross-institutional reporting systems for errors. This reporting is inhibited by fears that such data will be discovered in liability lawsuits.

Discussion Point

Have you ever encouraged a family member, friend, or colleague to seek compensation for medical errors? If so, do you think this was the most appropriate means of redress?

The provision of stronger confidentiality protections likely would improve the voluntary sharing of data. In 2002, the Patient Safety Improvement Act was introduced in the House of Representatives. This bill provided legal protections for medical error reporting, stating that error information voluntarily submitted to patient safety organizations could not be subpoenaed or used in legal discovery. It also generally required that the information be treated as confidential. After multiple revisions, the final legislation, called the Patient Safety and Quality Improvement Act of 2005, was signed into law by former President George W. Bush in July 2005.

Federal legislation has also been proposed to protect the voluntary reporting of ordinary injuries and "near misses"—errors that did not cause harm this time but easily could the next time. This would be like what is done in aviation, in which near misses are confidentially reported and can be analyzed by anyone.

Discussion Point

Given the known incidence of medical errors and adverse events that result in patient injury and the challenges inherent in tracking errors that have already been made, how difficult will it be to track "near misses?" What resources would be needed to accomplish this goal?

Leapfrog Group

The Leapfrog Group is a conglomeration of non–health care *Fortune 500* leaders dedicated to reducing preventable medical mistakes and improving the quality and affordability of health care (Leapfrog Group, 2018a). The group has advised the health care industry that big leaps in patient safety and customer value can occur if specific evidence-based standards are implemented, including (1) computerized physician (or prescriber) order entry (CPOE), (2) evidence-based hospital referral (EHR), and (3) ICU physician staffing (IPS).

CPOE is a promising technology that allows physicians to enter orders into a computer instead of handwriting them. Studies have also shown that CPOE reduces length of stay; reduces repeat tests; reduces turnaround times for laboratory, pharmacy, and radiology requests; and delivers cost savings (Leapfrog Group, 2018c). Indeed, a study led by David Bates, M.D., Chief of General Medicine at Boston's Brigham and Women's Hospital, demonstrated that CPOE reduced error rates by 55%—from 10.7 to 4.9 per 1,000 patient days ("Preventing Medication Errors in Hospitals," 2016). In addition, rates of serious medication errors fell by 88% in a subsequent study by the same group. The researchers concluded that implementation of CPOE systems at all nonrural U.S. hospitals could prevent 3 million adverse drug events each year.

To verify, however, that hospital CPOE systems stay up-to-date with changes in available medications and in recordkeeping systems, Leapfrog developed an evaluation tool in collaboration with leading academic researchers. Hospitals enter simulated patient data into their system and are then given a list of orders—some containing a potentially harmful or even fatal error—to run through their CPOE system. Results of the 2015 data are shown in Research Fuels the Controversy 14.1.

EHR involves making sure that patients with high-risk conditions are treated at hospitals whose characteristics are associated with better outcomes. Indeed, HealthGrades analysis found that patients treated in one of HealthGrades 2017 100 Best Hospitals had, on average, a 27.1% lower risk of dying than if they were cared for in hospitals that did not receive the designation (Gooch & Punke, 2017). If all hospitals, as a group, performed similarly to the 100 Best Hospitals, on average, 179,438 lives could potentially have been saved.

IPS considers the level of training of ICU medical personnel. Evidence suggests that quality of care in hospital ICUs is strongly influenced by whether "intensivists" (those familiar with ICU complications) are providing care and how the staff is organized (Leapfrog Group, 2018b). "Mortality rates are significantly lower in hospitals with

---

Research Fuels the Controversy 14.1

A computerized physician (or prescriber) order entry (CPOE) evaluation tool developed by Leapfrog in collaboration with leading academic researchers allows hospitals to enter simulated patient data into their system, including potentially harmful or even fatal errors. This tool is the only known system in the United States that allows hospitals to test how well their CPOE systems are detecting prescribing errors.

Source: *Preventing medication errors in hospitals.* (2016). Cast Light Health Inc. Retrieved May 29, 2018, from http://www.leapfroggroup.org/sites/default/files/Files/Leapfrog-Castlight%20Medication%20Safety%20Report.pdf

Study Findings

On the 2015 Leapfrog Hospital Survey, hospitals' CPOE systems failed to flag 39% of all potentially harmful drug orders, or nearly two out of every five orders. The systems also missed 13% of potentially fatal orders. If administered to actual patients, all of these orders had the potential to cause injury or even death. The most common unflagged errors related to medications or dosage. Hospitals' ability to correctly flag potential errors has improved only slightly (1% point) from 2014. The study concluded that without accelerated improvement, patients will continue to receive medications or dosages that increase their risk of injury or death.

ICUs managed exclusively by board-certified intensivists. Research has shown that hospitals staffing their ICUs with doctors specializing in critical care medicine can reduce ICU mortality by as much as 40%" (Leapfrog Group, 2018b).

Bar Coding Medications

In addition, Leapfrog has endorsed the use of bar coding to reduce point-of-care medication errors. Per a FDA rule adopted in April 2004, all prescription and over-the-counter medications used in hospitals must contain a national drug code number. The FDA suggested that a bar code system, coupled with a CPOE system, would greatly enhance the ability of all health care workers to follow the "five rights" of medication administration—that the *right* person receives the *right* drug, in the *right* dose, via the *right* route, at the *right* administration time.

In addition, the Joint Commission originally proposed in its 2005 National Patient Safety Goals and Requirements that accredited organizations would have to implement bar code technology to identify patients and match them to their medications or other treatments by January 2007. Because of implementation concerns, especially in terms of costs, this proposal was abandoned by the Joint Commission in July 2004.

It is noteworthy, however, that although bar code medication administration (BCMA) increases the likelihood of the right patient, receiving the right medication, at the right dose, at the right time, errors still occur. In 2018, the Pennsylvania Patient Safety Authority identified a statewide increase of near-miss BCMA events over a 12-year period (2005–2016), occurring at each point of the medication management process ("Barcode Medication Errors," 2018).

Sometimes, it was the result of bar code scans of the wrong patient, apparently the result of workarounds that staff employed to pursue better efficiency. At other times, a difficulty accessing records resulted in wrong patient selections and a lack of internet connectivity led to additional staff workarounds.

Patient Safety Solutions

Recognizing that health care errors affect at least one in every 10 patients around the world, the WHO's World Alliance for Patient Safety and the Collaborating Centre packaged nine effective solutions, called *patient safety solutions*, to reduce such errors. A patient safety solution was defined as any system design or intervention that has demonstrated the ability to prevent or mitigate patient harm stemming from the processes of health care and is based on interventions and actions that have reduced problems related to patient safety in some countries (World Health Organization [WHO], 2017). The priority program areas related to patient safety in 2015 are shown in Box 14.6.

In 2017 the WHO initiated its third Global Patient Safety Challenge: *Medication Without Harm*, to address a number of issues related to medication safety. The Challenge focuses on improving medication safety by strengthening the systems for reducing medication errors and avoidable medication-related harm, with the goal to reduce the level of severe, avoidable harm related to medications by 50% over 5 years, globally (WHO, 2018). Countries are requested to prioritize taking action on medication safety, designate leaders to drive action, and devise their own tailored programs centered on local priorities. WHO will provide support to countries for developing national programs, instigating large-scale international research, providing

BOX 14.6   World Health Organization's Global Patient Safety Challenges (2015)

1. *Clean Care Is Safer Care* (focuses on health care–associated infection and hand hygiene in health care)
2. *Safe Surgery Saves Lives* (prioritizes the use of surgery checklists at three phases of an operation: before the induction of anesthesia ["sign in"], before the incision of the skin ["time out"], and before the patient leaves the operating room ["sign out"])
3. *Patients for Patient Safety* (builds a paneled, global network of patients and patient organizations to champion patient safety)
4. *Research for Patient Safety* (undertakes global prevalence studies of adverse effects and is developing a rapid assessment tool for use in developing countries)
5. *International Patient Safety Classification* (aims to define, harmonize, and group patient safety concepts into an internationally agreed classification)
6. *Reporting and Learning* (aims to generate best practice guidelines for existing and new reporting systems, and facilitate early learning from information available)
7. *Solutions for Patient Safety* (interventions and actions that prevent patient safety problems recurring and thus reduce risk to patients)
8. *The High 5s initiative* (spreads best practice for change in organizational, team, and clinical practices to improve patient safety)
9. *Technology for Patient Safety* (focuses on the opportunities to harness new technologies to improve patient safety)
10. *Knowledge Management* (works with Member States and partners to gather and share knowledge on patient safety developments globally)
11. *Eliminating Central Line–Associated Bloodstream Infections*
12. *Education for Safer Care* (develops a curricular guide for medical students as well as other resources)
13. *Safety Prize* (international award for excellence in the field of patient safety that will act as a driver for change and improvement)
14. *Medical Checklists*

Source: World Health Organization (2018). *Medication without harm: WHO's third global patient safety challenge.* Retrieved August 28, 2018 from http://www.who.int/patientsafety/medication-safety/en/

guidance, and developing practical tools for front-line health workers and for patients (WHO, 2018).

> **Consider This** WHO (2018) notes that globally, the cost associated with medication errors is US$42 billion each year, almost 1% of global expenditure on health.

Promoting Just Cultures

Perhaps though, the most significant change that must occur before a nationwide culture of safety management can exist is that organizational cultures must be created that remove blame from the individual and instead focus on how the organization can be modified to reduce the likelihood of such errors occurring in the future. Cultures where voluntary reporting is encouraged and constructive feedback is given to those who self-report are often called *just cultures*. Just cultures will be needed to encourage voluntary reporting and reduce the prevalence of errors. Just cultures exhibit "giving constructive feedback and critical analysis in skillful ways, during assessments based on facts, and having respect for the complexity of the situation." This type of intervention encourages people to reveal the errors they have made so that the organization can learn from them.

A paper published by Vapiwala and Han calls for better education and training of physicians regarding the psychological challenges that coincide with errors and error disclosure (Penn Medicine News, 2017). Vapiwala suggested, "We must transform the culture of error disclosure in the medical community from one that is often punitive to one that is restorative and supportive. And to do that, we must tend to the psychological challenges that medical professionals wrestle with when they face the possibility of disclosing an error" (Penn Medicine News, 2017, para. 3). The paper concludes that the primary change will need to be cultural, not just among trainees, but at every level of medical practice, in order to successfully pivot away from the current stigma related to error disclosure.

Clearly, a punitive approach to medical errors is not productive, and errors will not be reported if workers fear the consequences. Employees and patients need to feel comfortable and without fear of personal risk in reporting hazards that can affect patient safety.

Consider This Ignoring the problem of medical errors, denying their existence, or blaming the individuals involved in the processes do nothing to eliminate the underlying problems.

CONCLUSIONS

Medical errors are not the only indicator of quality of care. They are, however, a pervasive problem in the current health care system and one of the greatest threats to quality health care. Nurses are uniquely positioned to identify, interrupt, and correct medical errors and to minimize preventable adverse outcomes. Only recently, however, have their error recovery strategies been described.

Efforts to reduce medical errors, however, over the last decade have not resulted in the achievement of desired outcomes. There is a plethora of current studies that suggest that the health care system continues to be riddled with errors and that patient and worker safety is compromised. Yet, movement toward the IOM goals is occurring. It is likely that there has never been another time when the public, providers, and government have worked together so closely to achieve a shared health care goal.

Much, however, remains to be done. Sustained public interest will be needed to create the momentum necessary to systematically change the health care system in a way that reduces patients' vulnerability to medical errors. In addition, although there has been a great deal of talk about using a systems approach to address the problem of medical errors, there has not been much discussion regarding exactly how this integration is to be accomplished. The bottom line is that significant and continuous reform of the health care system will be needed before the problem of medical errors shows any resolution.

For Additional Discussion

1. If cost containment and quality goals conflict, which do you think will take precedence in health care organizations today?

2. Why do so many providers, despite stated dissatisfaction levels, state that they feel helpless about reducing medical errors and improving the quality of health care?

3. Why have quality control efforts in health care organizations evolved primarily from external requirements and not as voluntary monitoring efforts?

4. Where does individual provider responsibility and accountability begin and end in a culture in which medical errors are recognized as being a failure of the system?

5. How common is it that medical error documentation is used against employees as part of the performance appraisal process? If so, does this discourage reporting?

6. Does the average consumer have access to and an accurate understanding of health care report cards?

7. Given that most individuals can quickly identify medical errors that have happened to them, a friend, or a family member, why does the U.S. public seem so reluctant to accept that medical errors constitute a threat to the quality of their health care?

8. Has your fear of legal liability ever influenced your decision to report a medical error?

References

American Academy of Orthopaedic Surgeons. (1995–2018). *Physician quality reporting system (PQRS)*. Retrieved May 29, 2018, from https://www.aaos.org/AAOSNow/2014/Jun/advocacy/advocacy6/?ssopc=1

American Society for Quality. (2018). *Quality tools: Failure mode effects analysis (FMEA)*. Retrieved May 29, 2018, from http://asq.org/learn-about-quality/process-analysis-tools/overview/fmea.html

Barcode medication errors reported for analysis. (2018). Relias. Retrieved May 29, 2018, from https://www.ahcmedia.com/articles/142072-barcode-medication-errors-reported-for-analysis

Benson, L. (2015, February 26). *Minnesota struggles to reduce medical errors.* MPR News. Retrieved May 29, 2018, from http://www.mprnews.org/story/2015/02/26/medical-errors

Brennan, T. A., Leape, L. L., Laird, N. M., Hebert, L., Localio, A. R., Lawthers, A. G., . . . Hiatt, H. H. (1991). Incidence of adverse events and negligence in hospitalized patients: Results of the Harvard Medical Practice Study 1. *The New England Journal of Medicine, 324*(6), 370–376.

Centers for Medicare and Medicaid Services. (2017, October 31). *Hospital value-based purchasing.* Retrieved May 29, 2018, from https://www.cms.gov/Medicare/Quality-Initiatives-Patient-Assessment-Instruments/Hospital QualityInits/Hospital-Value-Based-Purchasing-.html

Encyclopedia of Surgery. (2018). *Medical errors: Introduction and definitions.* Advameg. Retrieved May 29, 2018, from http://www.surgeryencyclopedia.com/La-Pa/Medical-Errors.html

Goedert, J. (2012, October 19). *Study pegs cost of medical errors near $1 trillion annually.* Health Data Management. Retrieved May 29, 2018, from https://www.healthdata management.com/news/study-pegs-cost-of-medical-errors-near-1-trillion-annually

Gooch, K., & Punke, H. (2017, February 21). *Healthgrades names 2017 best hospitals: 5 things to know.* Retrieved May 29, 2018, from http://www.beckershospitalreview.com/rankings-and-ratings/healthgrades-names-2017-best-hospitals-5-things-to-know.html

Hayes, K. (2017, July 24). *Medication errors more than double.* AARP. Retrieved September 4, 2017, from http://www.aarp.org/health/drugs-supplements/info-2017/medication-errors-rise-fd.html

HealthGrades. (2004, July). *HealthGrades quality study: Patient safety in American hospitals.* Retrieved September 4, 2017, from http://www.providersedge.com/ehdocs/ehr_articles/Patient_Safety_in_American_Hospitals-2004.pdf

Institute for Healthcare Improvement/National Patient Safety Foundation. (2018). *About. IHI/NPSF.* Retrieved May 29, 2018, from http://www.npsf.org/?page=aboutus

Joint Commission. (2017). *Sentinel event policy and procedures.* Retrieved May 29, 2018, from https://www.jointcommission.org/sentinel_event_policy_and_procedures

Kliff, S. (2015, January 29). *Medical errors in America kill more people than AIDS or drug overdoses. Here's why.* Retrieved May 29, 2018, from http://www.vox.com/2015/1/29/7878731/medical-errors-statistics

Kohn, L. T., Corrigan, J. M., & Donaldson, M. S. (Eds.). (2000). *Executive summary. In To err is human: Building a safer health system* (pp. 1–6). Retrieved May 29, 2018, from https://www.nap.edu/read/9728/chapter/2

Leape, L. L. (1994). Error in medicine. *Journal of the American Medical Association, 272*(23), 1851–1857.

Leape, L. L., Brennan, T. A., Laird, N., Lawthers, A. G., Localio, A. R., Barnes, B. A., . . . Hiatt, H. (1991). The nature of adverse events in hospitalized patients: Results of the Harvard Medical Practice Study II. *New England Journal of Medicine, 324*(6), 377–384.

Leapfrog Group. (2018a). *About Leapfrog.* Retrieved May 29, 2018, from http://www.leapfroggroup.org/about

Leapfrog Group. (2018b). *ICU physician staffing.* Retrieved May 29, 2018, from http://www.leapfroggroup.org/ratings-reports/icu-physician-staffing

Leapfrog Group. (2018c). *Computerized physician order entry.* Retrieved May 29, 2018, from http://www.leapfroggroup.org/ratings-reports/computerized-physician-order-entry

Lockwood, W. (2018). *Prevention of medical errors and medication errors.* Retrieved May 29, 2018, from http://www.rn.org/courses/coursematerial-135.pdf

MacDonald, I. (2013, September 20). *Hospital medical errors now the third leading cause of death in the U.S.: New study highlights the fact that estimates in 'To Err is Human' report were low.* Fierce Healthcare. Retrieved May 29, 2018, from http://www.fiercehealthcare.com/story/hospital-medical-errors-third-leading-cause-death-dispute-to-err-is-human-report/2013-09-20

Macquarie University. (2015, March 23). *Medication error reporting not indicative of patient safety.* Retrieved May 29, 2018, from Medical Xpress Website: http://medicalxpress.com/news/2015-03-medication-error-indicative-patient-safety.html

National Quality Forum. (2018a). *NQF's mission and vision.* Retrieved May 29, 2018, from http://www.qualityforum.org/about_nqf/mission_and_vision

National Quality Forum. (2018b). *List of SREs.* Retrieved May 29, 2018, from http://www.qualityforum.org/Topics/SREs/List_of_SREs.aspx

National Quality Forum. (2018c). *NQF national priorities partnership.* Retrieved May 29, 2018, from http://www.qualityforum.org/Show_Content.aspx?id=59894

National Quality Strategy. (2017). *About the National Quality Strategy (NQS).* Retrieved August 28, 2017, from https://www.ahrq.gov/workingforquality/about/index.html#aims

Penn Medicine News. (2017, May 19). *To curb medical errors, physicians must be better trained to admit mistakes.* Retrieved May 29, 2018, from https://www.pennmedicine.org/news/news-releases/2017/may/to-curb-medical-errors-physicians-must-be-better-trained-to-admit-mistakes

Preventing medication errors in hospitals. (2016). Cast Light Health Inc. Retrieved May 29, 2018, from http://www.leapfroggroup.org/sites/default/files/Files/Leapfrog-Castlight%20Medication%20Safety%20Report.pdf

QSEN Institute. (2018). *Project overview. The evolution of the Quality and Safety Education for Nurses (QSEN) initiative.* Retrieved May 29, 2018, from http://qsen.org/about-qsen/project-overview

Quality Payment Program. (2018). *APMS overview.* Department of Health and Human Services. Retrieved May 29, 2018, from https://qpp.cms.gov/apms/overview

Schadenberg, A. (2017, August 24). *Medical errors now third leading cause of death. This should concern you about assisted suicide.* LifeNews.com. Retrieved May 29, 2018, from http://www.lifenews.com/2017/08/24/medical-errors-now-third-leading-cause-of-death-this-should-concern-you-about-assisted-suicide

Sipherd, R. (2018, February 22). *The third-leading cause of death in US most doctors don't want you to know about.* CNBC. Retrieved May 29, 2018, from https://www.cnbc.com/2018/02/22/medical-errors-third-leading-cause-of-death-in-america.html

Thomas, E. J., Studdert, D. M., Newhouse, J. P., Zbar, B. I. W., Howard, K. M., Williams, E. J., & Brennan, T. A. (1999). Costs of medical injuries in Colorado and Utah in 1992. *Inquiry, 36*(3), 255–264.

Torrey, T. (2016, January 2). *Medical errors, adverse events and the National Quality Forum.* Very Well. Retrieved May 29, 2018, from https://www.verywell.com/medical-errors-list-2615322

U. S. Food & Drug Administration. (2018, May 25). *Medication errors related to drugs.* Retrieved May 29, 2018, from https://www.fda.gov/Drugs/DrugSafety/MedicationErrors/default.htm

World Health Organization. (2015). *World alliance for patient safety.* Retrieved March 22, 2015, from http://www.who.int/patientsafety/worldalliance/en

World Health Organization. (2017). *Patient safety: Making healthcare safer.* Retrieved May 29, 2018, from http://apps.who.int/iris/bitstream/10665/255507/1/WHO-HIS-SDS-2017.11-eng.pdf?ua=1

World Health Organization. (2018). *Medication without harm: WHO's third global patient safety challenge.* Retrieved May 29, 2018, from http://www.who.int/patientsafety/medication-safety/en

Collective Bargaining and the Professional Nurse

Carol J. Huston

ADDITIONAL RESOURCES

Visit thePoint® for additional helpful resources
- eBook
- Journal Articles
- WebLinks

CHAPTER OUTLINE

LEARNING OBJECTIVES

The learner will be able to:

1. Explore possible motivations behind nurses' decisions to join or not join unions.

2. Identify major U.S. legislation that has affected the ability of nurses to unionize over time.

3. Describe the shifting balance of power between unions and management in the United States over the last century and analyze the power balance that currently exists between the two entities.

4. Identify the largest unions representing health care employees, and nurses in particular.

5. Investigate the current status of rulings by the National Labor Relations Board and the courts regarding the definition of "supervisor" in nursing and the effect those rulings have on the eligibility of nurses for protection under the National Labor Relations Act.

6. Delineate common union organizing strategies as well as specific steps for starting a union.

7. Debate the potential conflicts inherent in having the American Nurses Association serve as both a professional association for all nurses and a collective bargaining agent.

8. Explore the impact management has on creating a work environment that eliminates or reduces the need for unionization.

9. Reflect on whether going on strike can be viewed as an ethically appropriate action for professional nurses.

10. Explore his or her beliefs about whether belonging to unions, a practice historically reserved for blue-collar workers, undermines nursing's quest for increased recognition as a profession.

INTRODUCTION

There is likely no greater dichotomy than stereotypical images of gentle nurse angels of mercy and images of angry nurses in picket lines waving strike placards at passersby. Although both the images are stereotypical, they are at the heart of the debate about whether nursing, long recognized as a caring and altruistic profession, should be a part of collective bargaining efforts to improve working conditions.

Collective bargaining involves activities occurring between organized labor and management that concern employee relationships. Such activities include negotiation of formal labor agreements and day-to-day interactions between unions and management. A *labor union* (hereafter referred to as a *union*) is an organization of workers, often in a trade or profession, formed to protect their rights and interests and improve their economic status and working conditions through collective bargaining with employers.

Many nurses have strong feelings about unions and collective bargaining activities. Often these feelings have to do with their exposure to unions while growing up. Many nurses from working-class families were raised in a cultural milieu that promoted unionization. Other nurses know little about unions and know only what they have seen portrayed in the media. Some nurses, however, have been actively involved in collective bargaining in their place of employment and have emerged from the experience with either positive or negative impressions or a combination thereof.

Despite this tension, collective bargaining and unions are very much a part of many nurses' lived experiences. Union activity tends to change in response to workforce excesses and shortages. For decades, employment demand for nurses has increased and decreased periodically. High demand for nurses is tied directly to a healthy national economy, and, historically, this has been correlated with increased union activity. Similarly, when nursing vacancy rates are low, union membership and activity tend to decline.

The Department for Professional Employees (2018) notes that as of 2014, 17% of registered nurses (RNs) and 10.7% of licensed practical nurses (LPNs)/licensed vocational nurses (LVNs) were union members, a number that has shrunk several percentage points over the past decade. Still, health care workers represent a large portion of all workers holding union representation elections; more than one in six of the 1,835 National Labor Relations Board (NLRB) union representation elections held in 2010 were held among workers in the health care and social assistance industries (Department for Professional Employees, 2018).

Similarly, OR Manager ("Be Constructive," 2015) suggests that approximately 21% of hospitals in the United States in 2012 had a unionized nursing staff but noted that percentage may increase as an unintended consequence of health care reform. The issues driving nurses to pursue unionization, however, continue to exist. Increased nursing workloads and a feeling that management does not care are significant factors encouraging increased union activity during the second decade of the 21st century.

This chapter explores the historical development of unions in the United States, particularly in nursing. The motivations behind nurses' decisions to join or not join unions are explored, and the unions that represent the majority of nurses are described. Union organizing strategies are presented, as are specific steps for starting a union. Emphasis is given to the importance of management creating a work environment that eliminates or reduces the need for unionization in the first place. The chapter concludes with a discussion of the definition of "supervisor" in nursing, types of labor union–management relationships, and whether striking can be viewed as an ethically appropriate action for professional nurses.

HISTORICAL PERSPECTIVE OF UNIONIZATION IN THE UNITED STATES

Unions have been present in the United States since the 1790s. Skilled craftsmen formed early unions to protect themselves from wage cuts during the highly competitive era of industrialization. Strikes were rare, and when they did occur, they were short and peaceful. This changed in the early 1800s, with strike activity increasing during economic prosperity and declining during less prosperous economic times. By the mid- to late 1800s, the labor movement began to more closely resemble what we see today. Unions started negotiating with employers, addressing not only wages but also work rules, hours, and grievances, thus arbitrating contracts between employees and employers.

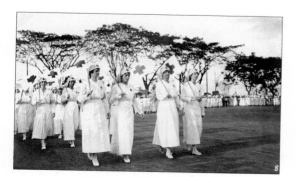

By the 1930s, and after 4 years of the Great Depression, repressive management was the norm, and tensions were high between workers and their employers. There were no legal protections for workers, no overtime compensation, no child labor laws, and no health or safety regulations. Workers attempted to form unions to improve working conditions, but business owners responded by blacklisting organizers and using force to prevent strikes (Franklin D. Roosevelt Presidential Library and Museum, 1935).

President Franklin Roosevelt attempted to intervene by promoting the National Industrial Recovery Act, but he was forced to take an even bolder stand alongside labor when the Supreme Court ruled that act unconstitutional. Roosevelt promoted the National Labor Relations Act (NLRA), also known as the Wagner Act after New York Senator Robert Wagner, which was enacted in 1935. This act gave workers the right to form unions and bargain collectively with their employers (Box 15.1). It also provided for the creation of the NLRB to oversee union certification, arrange meetings with unions and employers, and investigate violations of the law (Franklin D. Roosevelt Presidential Library and Museum, 1935).

With this rapid shift in power from management to labor, labor–management relationships were turbulent throughout the 1930s and 1940s. History books are filled with battles, strikes, mass picketing scenes, and brutal treatment by both management and employees. The balance of power, however, fell to labor unions.

Because of this, it was necessary to pass additional federal legislation to restore what was perceived to be a balance of power with management. Passed in 1947, the Taft–Hartley Labor Act, also known as the Labor–Management Relations Act, retained the provisions under the Wagner Act that guaranteed employees the right to collective bargaining but added the provision that employees had the right to refrain from taking part in unions ("closed shops" were illegal; Box 15.2). In addition, the act permitted unions to form only if approved by a majority of the employees. It also forbade *jurisdictional strikes* ("an illegal strike about which trade union should have the right to represent a particular group of employees in an organization") ("Jurisdictional Strike," 2018), secondary boycotts, and unions from contributing to political campaigns.

Discussion Point

The Taft–Hartley Labor Act also required union leaders to affirm they were not supporters of the Communist Party. Why was this requirement a part of the act and how did it mesh with the culture of the time?

BOX 15.1   **Unfair Management Practices Identified in the Wagner Act (1935)**

1. To interfere with, restrain, or coerce employees in a manner that interferes with their rights as outlined under the act. Examples of these activities are spying on union gatherings, threatening employees with job loss, or threatening to close down a company if the union organizes
2. To interfere with the formation of any labor organization or to give financial assistance to a labor organization
3. To discriminate with regard to hiring, tenure, and so on to discourage union membership
4. To discharge or discriminate against an employee who filed charges or testified before the National Labor Relations Board
5. To refuse to bargain in good faith

BOX 15.2   **Unfair Labor Union Practices Identified in the Taft–Hartley Amendment (1947)**

1. Requiring a self-employed person or an employer to join a union
2. Forcing an employer to cease doing business with another person. This placed a ban on secondary boycotts, which were then prevalent
3. Forcing an employer to bargain with one union when another union has already been certified as the bargaining agent
4. Forcing the employer to assign certain work to members of one union rather than another
5. Charging excessive or discriminatory initiation fees
6. Causing or attempting to cause an employer to pay for unnecessary services

Eventually, federal legislation such as the Fair Labor Standards Act (1938), the Occupational Safety and Health Act (1970), and the Equal Employment Opportunity Act (1972) were passed, providing federal protection for workers. These acts were important in the history of unions because unions no longer had to be the primary source of security for workers. As a result, there has been little growth of unions in the private and blue-collar sectors since membership peaked in the 1950s.

To counteract these dwindling numbers, several major unions merged, and new affiliations were formed. In addition, new organizing tactics were developed. Nowhere is this turnaround more apparent than in the health care industry.

HISTORICAL PERSPECTIVE OF UNIONIZATION IN NURSING

Collective bargaining was slow in coming to the health care industry for many reasons. Until labor laws were amended, unionization of health care workers was illegal. In addition, nursing's long history as a service commodity further delayed labor organization in health care settings.

Discussion Point

Is it appropriate for nurses to organize into collective bargaining units, something historically reserved for blue-collar workers?

Initial collective bargaining in nursing took place in government or public organizations as a result of Executive Order 10988 issued by former President John Kennedy. This 1962 order lifted restrictions that prevented public employees from organizing. As a result, city, county, and district hospitals and health care agencies joined collective bargaining in the 1960s.

In 1974, Congress amended the Wagner Act, extending national labor laws to private nonprofit hospitals, nursing homes, health clinics, health maintenance organizations, and other health care institutions. These amendments opened the door to much union activity for professions and the public employee sector. Indeed, a review of union membership figures shows that since 1960, most collective bargaining activity in the United States has occurred in the public and professional sectors of industry, most notably among faculty at institutions of higher education, teachers at primary and secondary levels, and physicians.

Discussion Point

Why is white-collar union membership growing when the private and blue-collar sectors are not? Have societal norms altered perceptions regarding the appropriateness of unionization in white-collar industries?

From 1962 through 1989, there were slow but steady increases in the numbers of nurses represented by collective bargaining agents. In 1989, the NLRB ruled that nurses could form separate bargaining units, and union activity increased. However, the American Hospital Association immediately sued the American Nurses Association (ANA), and the ruling was put on hold until 1991 when the Supreme Court upheld the 1989 decision by the NLRB. A summary of the legislation affecting the development of unionization in nursing is shown in Table 15.1.

TABLE 15.1	**Labor Legislation**	
Year	**Legislation**	**Effect**
1935	National Labor Relations Act/Wagner Act	Gave unions many rights in organizing; resulted in rapid union growth
1947	Taft–Hartley Amendment	Returned some power to management; resulted in a more equal balance of power between unions and management
1962	Executive Order 10988 (President John Kennedy)	Amended the 1935 Wagner Act to allow public employees to join unions
1974	Amendments to the Wagner Act	Allowed workers in nonprofit organizations to join unions
1989	National Labor Relations Board ruling	Allowed nurses to form separate bargaining units

UNIONS REPRESENTING NURSES

Various unions represent nurses and other health care workers. The *California Nurses Association* (CNA)/*National Nurses Organizing Committee* joined with two other nurses' unions (*United American Nurses* [UAN] and the *Massachusetts Nurses Association*) to create a new 150,000+ member advocacy association known as *National Nurses United* (NNU) in 2009. Although all three unions maintained their separate identities, the merger did give these members a greater national voice.

The *Service Employees International Union* (SEIU, 2018a) is another large union in the health care industry, representing more than 1.5 million nurses, LPNs, doctors, lab technicians, nursing home workers, and home care workers; of these, 85,000 RNs in 21 states are united in the Nurse Alliance of SEIU Healthcare. In addition, the National Federation of Nurses (NFN) merged with the American Federation of Teachers (AFT) in February 2013, making AFT another large union.

Also in 2013, the National Union of Healthcare Workers (NUHW), which formed in 2009 when SEIU took control of California local United Healthcare Workers West, affiliated with CNA. Like NNU, this is a strategic alliance, and not a merger. Such alliances are becoming increasingly commonplace as unions recognize that increased negotiating power comes with greater membership.

Some of the other unions that represent nurses include the ANA, which had 172,107 members as of 2016 (about 7% of nurses; Center for Union Facts, 2018); the National Union of Hospital and Health Care Employees of the Retail, Wholesale and Department Store Union; the American Federation of Labor–Congress of Industrial Organizations (AFL-CIO); the United Steelworkers of America; the American Federation of Government Employees, AFL-CIO; the American Federation of State, County, and Municipal Employees, AFL-CIO; the International Brotherhood of Teamsters; the American Federation of State, County, and Municipal Employees, which operates mostly in the public sector; the "24/7 Frontline Service Alliance"; and the United Auto Workers.

Union representation also varies by state. The states with the most unions organizing for all industries, including health care, are New York, California, Pennsylvania, Michigan, and Illinois. Among states for 2016 to 2017, New York had the highest union membership rate (23.6%), whereas South Carolina continued to have the lowest (1.6%; Bureau of Labor Statistics, 2018).

Discussion Point

Is it appropriate for RNs to be represented by non-nursing unions? Why would nurses seek out non-nursing unions for representation?

MOTIVATORS TO JOIN UNIONS

Knowing that human behavior is goal directed, it is important to examine what personal goals union membership fulfills. Nurse-managers often tell each other that health care institutions differ from other types of industrial organizations. This is really a myth because most nurses work in large and impersonal organizations, just like workers in other industries.

> ***Consider This*** People are motivated to join or reject unions because of many needs and values.

Deciding whether to join a union is a personal and often complex decision because there are typically many influencing factors. Both choices can be justified, however, so both driving and restraining forces for union membership are presented here.

There are six primary motivations for joining a union (Box 15.3). The first is to increase the power of the individual. Employees know that singly they are much more dispensable. Because a large group of employees is generally less dispensable, nurses greatly increase their bargaining power and reduce their vulnerability by joining a union. Hagedorn, Paras, Greenwich, and Hagopian (2016) concur, suggesting that unions promote well-being by encouraging democratic participation and a sense of community among workers, among other benefits (Research Fuels the Controversy 15.1).

> ***Consider This*** The rapid downsizing and restructuring of the 1990s left many nurses feeling that management did not listen to them or care about their needs. This discontentment provides a fertile ground for union organizers because unions thrive in a climate that perceives the organizational philosophy to be insensitive to the worker.

BOX 15.3   Reasons Nurses Join Unions

1. To increase the power of the individual
2. To achieve wage advantages
3. To increase their input into organizational decision making
4. To eliminate discrimination and favoritism
5. Because they are required to do so as part of employment (closed shop)
6. To satisfy a social need to be accepted
7. Because they believe it will improve patient outcomes and quality of care

Research Fuels the Controversy 15.1

Union Representation and Public Health Outcomes

Public health practitioners have not typically viewed unions as partners in promoting public health, nor have they explored contract negotiations as a way to ensure health protections. This cross-sectional, mixed-methods study identified specific mechanisms that link labor union representation and public health outcomes. The primary unit of analysis was the negotiated contract between management and labor for a variety of unions in the Puget Sound region of Washington State.

Source: Hagedorn, J., Paras, C. A., Greenwich, H., & Hagopian, A. (2016). The role of labor unions in creating working conditions that promote public health. *American Journal of Public Health, 106*(6), 989–995. doi:10.2105/AJPH.2016.303138

Study Findings

The research found that unions generate higher prevailing wages in a community and that almost all union contracts included retirement or pensions. Most contracts also included paid annual leave, paid rest periods, and bereavement leave. In addition, most contracts explicitly required employee training before the assignment of work and some contracts included compensation for providing mentorship to encourage more senior employees to provide support to new employees or employees taking on new roles. Most contracts also guided how health and safety regulations are communicated to workers, including written and verbal forms.

The researchers concluded that these findings suggest that union contract language advances many of the social determinants of health, including income, security, time off, access to health care, workplace safety culture, training and mentorship, predictable scheduling to ensure time with friends and family, democratic participation, and engagement with management.

This is a particularly strong motivating force for nurses when jobs are scarce and nurses feel vulnerable. Indeed, during the massive downsizing and restructuring of the 1990s, collective bargaining priorities shifted from wages and benefits to job security. This focus shifted again to worker safety when the first U.S. Ebola patient died in Fall 2014 in Dallas ("Be Constructive," 2015). Union leaders argued that hospitals were not providing nurses with adequate training and protective equipment to care for infected patients. The protests succeeded in focusing public awareness on Ebola readiness and safety.

Indeed, Weinstock and Failey (2014) argue that unions, joined at times by worker advocacy groups (e.g., Public Citizen and the American Public Health Association), have played a critical role in strengthening worker safety and health protections. They have sought to improve standards that protect workers by participating in the rulemaking process, through written comments and involvement in hearings; lobbying decision makers; petitioning the Department of Labor; and defending improved standards in court. Their efforts have culminated in more stringent exposure standards, access to information about the presence of potentially hazardous toxic chemicals, and improved access to personal protective equipment, further improving working conditions.

A second reason for joining unions is economics. In some organizations, pay is neither fair nor competitive, and most economists agree that joining a union is typically an effective means of raising one's pay. Indeed, the median weekly earnings of nonunion workers ($829) were only 80% of the earnings of union members ($1041) in 2016 to 2017 (Bureau of Labor Statistics, 2018).

In addition, 92% of union employees in the United States had access to health care benefits in 2009, as compared with only 68% of nonunion workers, and companies with 30% or more unionized workers were five times as likely to have their entire family health insurance premium paid for, in comparison to companies with no unionized workers (SEIU, 2018b). Hagedorn et al. (2016) agree, noting that labor union contracts create higher wage and benefit standards, working hour limits, and workplace hazards protections for employees.

Another reason nurses join unions is to communicate their aims, feelings, complaints, and ideas to others. The desire to have input into organizational decision making is a strong motivator for people to join unions. A feeling of powerlessness or the perception that administration does not care about employees is one of the most common reasons for seeking unionization.

> **Consider This** Although unions historically focused heavily on wage negotiations, current issues that nurses deem just as or more important are nonmonetary, such as guidelines for staffing, float provisions, shared decision making, and scheduling.

In addition, nurses join unions because they want to eliminate discrimination and favoritism. Unions emphasize equality and fairness. This might be an especially strong motivator for members of groups that have experienced discrimination, such as women and minorities.

The fourth primary motivation for joining a union stems from the social need to be accepted. Sometimes, this social need results from family or peer pressure. Because many working-class families have a long history of strong union ties, children are frequently raised in a cultural milieu that promotes unionization.

Another reason nurses join unions is that the union contract dictates that all nurses belong to the union. This has been a big driving force among blue-collar workers. However, the *closed shop*, or requirement that all employees belong to a union, has never prevailed in the health care industry. Most health care unions have *open shops*, allowing nurses to choose whether they want to join the union. Employees who do not want to join the union do not have to pay union dues, but typically, they must pay what is known as *fair share*. Fair share is usually only a small percentage of the union dues that members pay.

A case currently under consideration by the Supreme Court—Janus v. AFSCME Council 31—however, could negate the ability of public sector unions to collect fair share fees from workers (Johnson, 2018). If the court determines that fair share fees are unconstitutional, the entire U.S. public sector would essentially be a "right-to-work" zone–meaning employees could no longer be required to pay anything to the unions that bargain on their behalf (Johnson, 2018).

Finally, some nurses join unions because they believe that patient outcomes are better in unionized organizations because of better staffing and supervised management practices.

MOTIVATORS TO NOT JOIN UNIONS

Just as there are many reasons to join unions, there are also many reasons nurses reject unions, including societal and cultural factors (Box 15.4). Many people distrust unions because they believe that they promote the welfare state and oppose the U.S. system of free enterprise. Other individuals reject unions because they feel a need to demonstrate that they can get ahead on their own merits.

In addition, some professional employees reject unions for reasons that deal with class and education. They argue that unions were appropriate for the blue-collar worker but not for the university professor, physician, or engineer. Nurses rejecting unions on this basis are usually driven by a need to demonstrate their individualism and social status.

| BOX 15.4 | Reasons Nurses Do Not Join Unions |

1. The belief that unions promote the welfare state and oppose the U.S. system of free enterprise
2. The need to demonstrate individualism
3. The belief that unionization allows for mediocrity and substandard practice
4. The belief that professionals should not unionize
5. Identification with management's viewpoint
6. Fear of employer reprisal
7. Fear of lost income associated with a strike or walkout

Other employees identify with management and thus frequently adopt its viewpoint toward unions. These nurses, therefore, reject unions because their values more closely align with management than with workers.

In addition, although most employees are protected under the NLRA, some nurses reject unions because of fears of employer reprisal. Nurses who reject unions on this basis could be said to be motivated most of all by a need for job security.

Finally, some employees reject unions because they fear losing income associated with a strike or walkout. Strikes and walkouts are a reality of unionization; however, they are heavily regulated by law (striking is discussed later in this chapter).

Once managers understand the needs and driving forces behind nurses' decisions to join or reject unions, they can begin to address them. Organizations with unfair management policies are more likely to become unionized. It is certainly then within managerial power to eliminate some of the needs staff feel for joining unions.

Managers can encourage feelings of power by allowing subordinates to have input into decisions that will affect their work. Managers also can listen to ideas, complaints, and feelings and take steps to ensure that favoritism and discrimination are not part of their management style. In addition, managers can strengthen the drives and needs that make nurses reject unions. By building a team effort, sharing ideas and future plans from upper management with the staff, and encouraging individualism in employees, managers can facilitate identification of the worker with management.

When nurses begin showing signs of job dissatisfaction (frustration, stress, perceived powerlessness), they are sending a wake-up call to nursing management. Leaders must be alert to employment practices that are unfair or insensitive to employee needs and intervene appropriately before such issues lead to unionization. However, organizations offering liberal benefit packages and fair management practices may still experience union activity if certain social and cultural factors are present. If union activity does occur, managers must be aware of specific employee and management rights so that the NLRA is not violated by either managers or employees.

ELIGIBILITY FOR UNION MEMBERSHIP

The NLRA defines a supervisor as

> *any individual having authority, in the interest of the employer, to hire, transfer, suspend, lay off, recall, promote, discharge, assign, reward, or discipline other employees, or responsibly to direct them, or to adjust their grievances, or effectively to recommend such action, if in connection with the foregoing the exercise of such authority is not of a merely routine or clerical nature, but requires the use of independent judgment.* (National Labor Relations Board [NLRB], n.d., para. 17)

Up until two decades ago, only *supervisors* in nursing were considered managers and, as such, they were prohibited from joining unions. However, a 2006 NLRB ruling deemed that *charge nurses* might also be considered supervisors because they are responsible for the coordination and provision of patient care throughout a unit. Even part-time charge nurses were so labeled. This finding has been contested legally since that time and several interpretations have occurred. Reinterpretations by the NLRB are expected in the future.

In addition, the definition of supervisor in nursing came into question with several administrative and court rulings in the early 1990s. These rulings came about as a result of a case involving four LPNs/LVNs employed at Heartland Nursing Home in Urbana, Ohio. During late 1988 and early 1989, these LPNs complained to management about what they thought were disparate enforcement of the absentee policy; short staffing; low wages for nurses' aides; an unreasonable switching of prescription business from one pharmacy to another, which increased the nurses' paperwork; and management's failure to communicate with employees (Justia, 2018). Despite assurances from the vice president for operations that they would not be harassed for bringing their concerns to headquarters' attention, three of the LPNs were terminated (they believed) as a result of their actions.

In response to what they perceived to be illegal termination, the LPNs filed for protection under the NLRA. The NLRB ruled that because the LPNs had responsibility to ensure adequate staffing, to make daily work assignments, to monitor the aides' work to ensure proper performance, to

counsel and discipline aides, to resolve aides' problems and grievances, to evaluate aides' performances, and to report to management, they should be classified as "supervisors," thereby making them ineligible for protection under the NLRA.

On appeal, the administrative law judge (ALJ) disagreed, concluding that the nurses were not supervisors and that the nurses' supervisory work did not equate to responsibly directing the aides *in the interest of the employer*, noting that the nurses' focus is on the well-being of the residents rather than on the employer.

In another turnabout, the U.S. Court of Appeals for the Sixth Circuit then reversed the decision of the ALJ, arguing that the NLRB's test for determining the supervisory status of nurses was inconsistent with the statute and that the interest of the patient and the interest of the employer were not mutually exclusive. The court said that, in fact, the interests of the patient are the employer's business, and argued that the welfare of the patient was no less the object and concern of the employer than it was of the nurses. The court also argued that the statutory dichotomy the NLRB first created was no more justified in the health care field than it would be in any other business in which supervisory duties are necessary to the production of goods or the provision of services (Justia, 2018).

The court further stated that it was up to Congress to carve out an exception for the health care field, including nurses, should Congress not wish for such nurses to be considered supervisors. The court reminded the NLRB that the courts, and not the board, bear the final responsibility for interpreting the law. After concluding that the board's test was inconsistent with the statute, the court found that the four LPNs involved in this case were indeed supervisors and ineligible for protection under the NLRA (Justia, 2018).

This same interpretation, at least for full-time charge nurses, was used in another landmark court case in September 2006 to determine whether charge nurses, both permanent and rotating, at Oakwood Healthcare Inc. were "supervisors" within the meaning of the NLRA, and thus could be excluded from a unit of nurses represented by a union. Upholding the definition that supervisors "assign" and "responsibly direct" employees as well as exercise "independent judgment," the NLRB concluded that 12 permanent charge nurses employed by Oakwood Healthcare were supervisors. Rotating charge nurses were not, if this role was less than 10% to 15% of their work time (Law Room, 2018).

The Oakwood case has set precedence and figured in numerous subsequent decisions in both health care and industrial settings, although there have been only minimal further rulings addressing the charge nurse/supervisor status. For example, in 2016, the NLRB ruled that nurses who supervise and assign other hospital staff are not statutory supervisors and that a position expressly created to be supervisory is not necessarily supervisory (Becker & Green, 2017). Hence, the *Oakwood* ruling is still in effect today, specifying that nurses, on average, with less than 10% to 15% (equal to about one shift per pay period) of their total work time as charge nurse are considered staff nurses, whereas nurses working more than 15% of their professional time as charge nurses are considered supervisors (Law Room, 2018).

> **Discussion Point**
>
> Would the NLRB's definition of supervisor affect charge nurses' eligibility for union membership at the facility in which you work?

ORGANIZING A UNION AND SEEKING REPRESENTATION

Unions use a variety of tactics when organizing health care workers (Box 15.5). The first step in seeking union representation is determining that adequate levels of desire for unionization exist. The NLRB requires that at least 30% of employees sign an interest card before an election for unionization can be held. Most collective bargaining agents, however, require 60% to 70% of the employees to sign interest cards before they begin an organizing campaign. Union representatives are generally careful to keep a campaign secret until they are ready to file a petition for election. They do this so that they can build momentum without interference from the employer.

After enough interest cards have been signed, the organization must hold an election. At that time, all employees

> **BOX 15.5** **Union Organizing Strategies**
>
> 1. Meetings (both group and one-on-one)
> 2. Leaflets and brochures
> 3. Pressure on the hospital corporation through media and community contacts
> 4. Political pressure of regional legislators and local lawmakers
> 5. Corporate campaign strategies
> 6. Activism of local employees
> 7. Using lawsuits
> 8. Bringing pressure from financiers
> 9. Technology

of the same classification, such as RNs, vote on whether they desire unionization. A choice in every such election is *no representation*, which means that the voters do not want a union. During the election, 50% plus one of the petitioned units must vote before the union can be recognized. Unions can also be decertified by a process like that of certification. *Decertification* can occur when at least 30% of the eligible employees in the bargaining unit initiate a petition asking to no longer be represented by the union.

There are important differences, however, between organizing in a health care facility and in other types of organizations. Generally, the solicitation and distribution of union literature are banned entirely in immediate patient care areas. Managers should never, however, independently attempt to deal with union organizing activity. They should always seek assistance and guidance from higher-level management and the personnel department. The entire list of rights for management and labor during the organizing and establishment phases of unionization is beyond the scope of this book.

Throughout the years, Congress has amended various labor acts and laws in the attempt to balance power between management and labor. At times, the balance of power has shifted to management or labor, but Congress eventually enacts laws that attempt to restore what it judges to be the balance. The manager must ensure that the rights of management and employees are protected.

LABOR–MANAGEMENT RELATIONSHIPS

In the last 30 years, employers and unions have substantially improved their relationships. Although evidence is growing that contemporary management has come to accept the reality that unions are here to stay, businesses in the United States are still less comfortable with unions than their counterparts in many other countries. Likewise, unions have come to accept the fact that there are times when organizations are not healthy enough to survive aggressive union demands.

> ***Consider This*** It is possible to create a climate in which labor and management can work together to accomplish mutual goals.

Once management is faced with dealing with a collective bargaining unit, it has a choice of either accepting or opposing the union. It may actively oppose the union by using various union-busting techniques, or it may more subtly oppose the union by attempting to discredit it and win employee trust. *Acceptance* also may run along a continuum. The company may accept the union with reluctance and suspicion. Although they know that the union has legitimate rights, managers often believe they must continually guard against the union encroaching further into traditional management territory.

There is also the type of union acceptance known as *accommodation*. As is increasingly common, accommodation is characterized by management's full acceptance of the union, with both union and management showing mutual respect. When these conditions exist, labor and management can establish mutual goals, especially in the areas of safety, cost reduction, efficiency, waste elimination, and improvement of working conditions. Such cooperation represents the most mature and advanced type of labor–management relationships.

The bottom line is that the attitudes and the philosophies of the leaders in management and the union determine what type of relationship develops between the two parties in any given organization. When dealing with unions, managers must be flexible. It is critical that they do not ignore issues or try to overwhelm others with power. The rational approach to problem solving must be used.

It is also important to remember that employees have a right to participate in union organizing under the NLRA, and managers must not interfere with this right. Prohibited managerial activities include threatening employees, interrogating employees, promising employees rewards for cessation of union activity, and spying on employees. However, if management picks up early clues of union activity, the organization may be able to take legitimate steps that will discourage unionization of its employees.

Discussion Point

When unions are present in the workplace, what should be the relationship between them and management? What is accomplished by having a competitive or hostile relationship?

AMERICAN NURSES ASSOCIATION AND COLLECTIVE BARGAINING

One difficult union issue faced by nurse-managers is the dual role of their professional organization, the ANA. The NLRB recognizes the ANA, at most state levels, as a collective bargaining agent. The use of state associations as bargaining agents is divisive among U.S. nurses. Some nurse-managers believe that they have been disenfranchised

by their professional organization. Other managers recognize the conflicts inherent in attempting to sit on both sides of the bargaining table. Even for members who feel that the issue presents no real dilemma, there appears to be some conflict in loyalty.

Discussion Point

If you are a student, do you belong to the state student nurses association? If you are an RN, have you joined your state nurses association?

This conflict has manifested itself in the recent splitting away of state nurses' associations from the parent ANA organization. Since California RNs broke from the ANA in 1995 over dissatisfaction with the control held by nurses in managerial positions in hospitals, other states have also disaffiliated, including Massachusetts, Maine, New York, and Pennsylvania. In addition, many nurse unions, including the absorbed NFN, split off from the ANA as a result (Moberg, 2013).

In 1999, the ANA responded by establishing, then spinning off, the UAN as a parallel association of state collective bargaining organizations. NFN consisted of some of the UAN groups that did not want to join with NNU, but then the New York State Nurses Association left NFN. Moberg questions whether new mergers will lead to more cooperation among the sometimes-rancorous nursing unions—or to more progress in organizing a field that is growing faster than its union membership.

There are no easy solutions to the dilemma created by the dual role held by the ANA. Clarifying issues begin with the manager examining the motivation of nurses to participate in collective bargaining. The manager must at least try to hear and understand the employees' points of view.

Discussion Point

The ANA acts as both a professional association for RNs and a collective bargaining agent. To some nurses, this dual purpose poses a conflict in loyalty. Should the ANA—the recognized professional association for nurses in the United States—also be a collective bargaining agent?

NURSES AND STRIKES

The NLRA states in part that employees shall have the right to engage in "other concerted activities" for the purpose of collective bargaining or other mutual aid or protection (application of the NLRB, n.d.). The phrase "other concerted

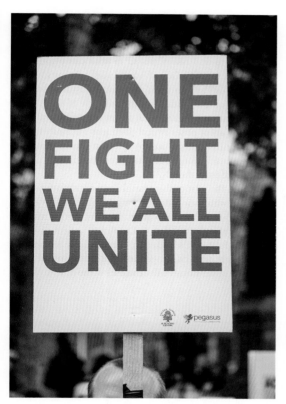

The controversy over whether nurses should strike is long-standing, and is likely at the heart of why so many individuals fear union activity. Critics of nurses having the ability to strike suggest that it is unethical because it leaves patients without care providers. McGrath (2017) concurs, suggesting that at first glance, strikes do cause harm to the general public because they rarely achieve instantaneous results. However, she suggests that it may be necessary as a result of slow-moving and seemingly ineffective previous policies that have created a significant loss of trust.

Unions argue that strikes must be supported because they are used only as a last resort and after careful consideration of every factor. Indeed, the ANA has held consistently for 50+ years that nurses not only have a right to strike but also have a professional responsibility and ethical duty to do so if it means maintaining work conditions conducive to providing high-quality care. The issue of striking then continues to divide the nursing profession. Ironically, both proponents and opponents of strikes in nursing argue that they aim for the same goal: safe patient care.

McGrath (2017) suggests that strikes may be ethically justified in three circumstances. The first occurs when one fully understands the policy being contested and still feels the conclusion or action is unjust. The second is when the employer has remained indifferent to other forms of negotiation and the third is when the employee is willing to undergo personal inconveniences in the face of achieving justice.

Mason (2018, para. 3) adds to the discussion of strike ethics in her assertion that for a strike to be justified, the cause must be realistic. Mason argues that there is no point in striking for something that cannot be obtained but cautions that determining what is unrealistic is not always easy. "There was a time when votes for women seemed unrealistic. . . and twenty years ago, marriage equality might have seemed an unrealistic goal."

In addition to the moral dilemmas related to the decision to strike, nurses must also determine how they feel about crossing the picket line should a strike occur. Nurses do have a choice not to participate in strikes or to cross picket lines when strikes occur. They risk derision by their peers in doing so, however, because strikebreakers, commonly known as "scabs," are viewed as taking management's side on the issue and may never be fully accepted by their peers after the strike action has ended.

activities" refers to "the right to effectively communicate with one another regarding self-organization at the jobsite" (para. 8).

The law then gives union members time to work together to determine whether strikes are necessary to achieve desired goals. Such strikes, however, are not allowed without giving the employer and the Federal Mediation and Conciliation Service 10 days' notice of the intent to strike. In doing so, the facility should have a reasonable amount of time to stop admitting patients, transfer existing patients to other facilities, and reduce medical procedures that require nurse-intensive labor. Problems occur when management continues to admit new patients or maintains normal operations.

Discussion Point

Can strikes, walkouts, "blue flu epidemics," and picket lines be considered ethical actions if nurses believe that they are the only ways in which they can improve working conditions or ensure safe patient care?

Consider This Not everyone will agree on the ethical nature of every individual strike but their very existence gives a voice to the overlooked and provides a springboard from which equality may leap. Once regulated, they play an important role in bridging the gap between conflicted parties and encouraging open lines of communication and negotiation (McGrath, 2017, para. 11).

CONCLUSIONS

The question of whether nurses should participate in collective bargaining has been around since legislation made such organization possible. Advocates on both sides of the issues present earnest, well-reasoned arguments to support their positions. McGrath (2017) suggests there is no doubt about the value unions provide to society; however, harsh economic times call into moral question the scope to which they can and should enforce their power.

Clearly, nurses working in unionized organizations appear to have some economic advantage, and their individual vulnerability to arbitrary action on the part of their employer is reduced. Yet nursing's long-standing struggle to be recognized as a profession underscores concerns that the profession's involvement in collective bargaining associations, historically reserved for blue-collar industries, may undermine this goal. In addition, some nurses think that union activities draw attention away from patients and patient-related activities. Union advocates argue the opposite—that improving pay, benefits, and working conditions ultimately leads to improved patient care.

There are also issues related to who can belong to a union, what the definition of "supervisor" is in nursing, and whether strikes and walkouts are ethically justified for nursing professionals. In addition, the dual role of the ANA as both the national organization for nurses and a collective bargaining agent poses ethical dilemmas for many nurses. Even unionized nurses cannot agree on the intensity and direction their unions should take, resulting in state unions breaking off from the ANA.

Finally, the relationships health care organizations have developed with their collective bargaining agents vary from direct opposition to collaboration. The effect of that relationship on working conditions and quality of patient care cannot be overstated. Unionization, then, is likely to continue to be fraught with challenges and will be one of the most passionate issues nurses will debate for some time to come.

For Additional Discussion

1. Does the presence of unions increase the likelihood that management will be fairer and more consistent with employees?

2. Can the need for unionization be eliminated simply by management being more attentive to worker needs and being willing to provide employees with reasonable working conditions and a voice in decision making?

3. Would you be willing to cross a picket line to work during an authorized strike?

4. Are there other ways nurses can increase their group power other than by unions? If so, are they as effective?

5. Some state unions are choosing to break off from the ANA. Does this further fragment nursing's collective power in the political arena by diminishing group size, or does it increase the broad-based support of nursing issues?

6. Do you believe that the current nursing shortage will accelerate the rate of unionization in nursing?

7. How does a nursing shortage affect a union's power in negotiating wages, benefits, and working conditions?

References

Be constructive, not combative, with union staff. (2015). *OR Manager, 31*(1), 24–26.

Becker, E., & Green, P. C. (2017, January 9). *NLRB on track to continue pro-union rulings in 2017*. Retrieved September 10, 2017, from http://www.healthemploymentandlabor.com/2017/01/09/nlrb-on-track-to-continue-pro-union-rulings-in-2017/

Bureau of Labor Statistics. (2018, January 19). *Economic news release. Union members summary*. Retrieved May 17, 2018, from https://www.bls.gov/news.release/union2.nr0.htm

Business Dictionary. (2018). *Jurisdictional strike [Definition]*. Web Finance, Inc. Retrieved May 17, 2018, from http://www.businessdictionary.com/definition/jurisdictional-strike.html

Center for Union Facts. (2018). *American Nurses Association.* Retrieved May 17, 2018, from https://www.unionfacts.com/union/American_Nurses_Association

Department for Professional Employees, American Federation of Labor and Congress of Industrial Organizations. (2018). *Fact sheet 2015. Nursing: A profile of the profession.* Retrieved May 17, 2018, from http://dpeaflcio.org/programs-publications/issue-fact-sheets/nursing-a-profile-of-the-profession

Franklin D., Roosevelt Presidential Library and Museum. (1935, July 4). *Our documents: National Labor Relations Act (The Wagner Act).* Retrieved September 7, 2017, from http://docs.fdrlibrary.marist.edu/odnlra.html

Hagedorn, J., Paras, C. A., Greenwich, H., & Hagopian, A. (2016, June). The role of labor unions in creating working conditions that promote public health. *American Journal of Public Health, 106*(6), 989–995. doi:10.2105/AJPH.2016.303138

Johnson, J. (2018, February 22). *Nurses rally in defense of unions as Supreme Court prepares to hear 'biggest threat to organized labor in years.'* Retrieved May 17, 2018, from https://www.commondreams.org/news/2018/02/22/nurses-rally-defense-unions-supreme-court-prepares-hear-biggest-threat-organized

Justia. (2018). *Health Care & Retirement Corporation of America, petitioner/cross-respondent, v. National Labor Relations Board, Respondent/cross-petitioner, 987 F.2d 1256 (6th Cir. 1993).* Retrieved May 17, 2018, from https://law.justia.com/cases/federal/appellate-courts/F2/987/1256/240885/

Law Room. (2018). *Supervisors defined.* Retrieved May 17, 2018, from https://answers.lawroom.com/story.aspx?STID=1517

Mason, E. (2018, April 3). *On striking, and the recognition that ethics are a collective affair.* Open Democracy UK. Retrieved May 16, 2018, from https://www.opendemocracy.net/uk/elinor-mason/on-striking-and-recognition-that-ethics-are-collective-affair

McGrath, A. (2017, April 24). *Is striking ethically justifiable?* Retrieved May 17, 2018, from http://www.universityobserver.ie/comment/is-striking-ethically-justifiable/

Moberg, D. (2013, February 20). *Are mergers the answer for fractious nurses unions?* In These Times. Retrieved September 7, 2017, from http://inthesetimes.com/working/entry/14631/are_mergers_the_answer_for_nurses_unions

National Labor Relations Board. (n.d.). *National Labor Relations Act.* Retrieved May 18, 2018, from https://www.nlrb.gov/resources/national-labor-relations-act

Service Employees International Union. (2018a). *Healthcare.* Retrieved May 17, 2018, from http://www.seiu.org/healthcare

Service Employees International Union. (2018b). *The union advantage: Facts and figures.* SEIU Local 105. Retrieved May 17, 2018, from http://www.seiu105.org/the-union-advantage

Weinstock, D., & Failey, T. (2014). The labor movement's role in gaining federal safety and health standards to protect America's workers. *New Solutions: A Journal of Environmental and Occupational Health Policy, 24*(3), 409–434. doi:10.2190/NS.24.3.k

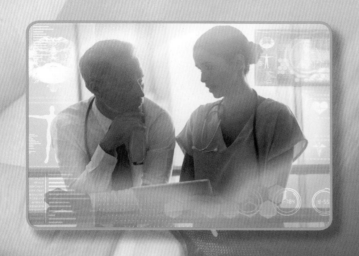

4

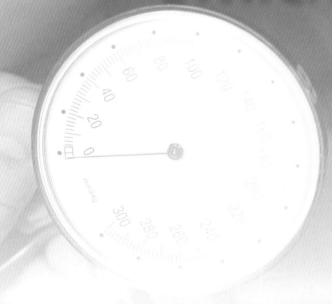

LEGAL AND
ETHICAL ISSUES

Whistle-Blowing in Nursing

Carol J. Huston

ADDITIONAL RESOURCES

Visit thePoint° for additional helpful resources
- eBook
- Journal Articles
- WebLinks

CHAPTER OUTLINE

LEARNING OBJECTIVES

The learner will be able to:

1. Define whistle-blowing and differentiate between internal and external whistle-blowing.

2. Identify conditions that should be met before whistle-blowing occurs, as well as situations in which whistle-blowing is clearly indicated.

3. Examine how cultural background may affect a nurse's willingness to blow the whistle on unsafe practices.

4. Identify risks and retaliatory consequences frequently experienced by whistle-blowers because of their actions.

5. Explore why reactions to whistle-blowers are often mixed and why the courage to speak out is something we honor more often in theory than in fact.

6. Differentiate among the consequentialist, deontologic, and utilitarian viewpoints regarding the purposes of whistle-blowing.

7. Analyze how whistle-blowing could be considered a failure of organizational ethics.

8. Delineate strategies to create an organizational climate that both discourages the need for whistle-blowing and supports the whistle-blower when it is necessary for him or her to come forward.

9. Identify strategies that whistle-blowers should use to reduce their likelihood of retaliation as well as legal liablity.

10. Analyze existing and proposed federal and state legal protections for whistle-blowers.

11. Identify the process used by a whistle-blower to file a *qui tam* or whistle-blower lawsuit under the False Claims Act and the potential benefits of doing so.

12. Reflect on his or her willingness to assume the personal risks associated with whistle-blowing, should the need arise.

INTRODUCTION

Enron and the artificial manipulation of energy prices . . . Martha Stewart and insider trading . . . WorldCom and accounting fraud . . . Bridgestone and Firestone tires . . . Dow Corning and silicone breast implants . . . Morgan Stanley and overcharging customers . . . long patient wait times at the Veteran's Administration (VA) . . . fraudulent bank loans by Wells Fargo . . . and artificial home price inflation. These high-profile cases, involving some degree of ethical malfeasance, have led the U.S. public to an increased sense of moral awareness about what is right and what is wrong. In addition, these cases have all come to the attention of the public as the result of *whistle-blowing*.

Dictionary.com ("Whistleblowing," 2018) suggests whistle-blowing occurs when a person informs on another or makes public disclosure of corruption or wrongdoing. Similarly, the Free Online Dictionary ("Whistleblower," 2003–2018) defines a whistle-blower as "an informant who exposes wrongdoing within an organization in the hope of stopping it" (para. 3).

> **Consider This** Virtually all definitions of whistle-blowing suggest the importance of advocating for others who may be harmed.

It is generally accepted that there are two types of whistle-blowing: internal and external. *Internal whistle-blowing* typically involves reporting concerns up the chain of command within an organization in the hope that whatever the problem is, it will be resolved. *External whistle-blowing* involves reporting concerns outside the organization and, in particular, to the media. In many cases, whistle-blowing becomes external only if inadequate action is taken at the organizational level to address the concerns of the whistle-blower. In some cases, however, whistle-blowing becomes external in an effort to embarrass an organization publicly or to seek financial redress.

> **Discussion Point**
> Is it ever appropriate to whistle-blow externally before attempting to resolve the problem internally?

In an era of transparency in quality reporting, declining reimbursements, and the ongoing pressure to remain fiscally solvent, the risk of fraud, misrepresentation, and ethical malfeasance in health care organizations has never been

higher. As a result, the need for whistle-blowing has also likely never been greater.

This chapter explores the effect of "groupthink" on the likelihood that whistle-blowers will come forward. In addition, it presents select cases of whistle-blowing. Personal risks associated with whistle-blowing are described, as are the mixed feelings many individuals hold about whistle-blowing. Whistle-blowing is also explored as a failure of organizational ethics, and strategies are identified to create an organizational climate that both discourages the need for whistle-blowing and supports the whistle-blower when it is necessary for him or her to come forward. Finally, legal protections (or the lack thereof) for whistle-blowing are discussed.

> **Consider This** "To see what is right, and not do it, is want of courage, or of principles."
> —Confucius

GROUPTHINK AND WHISTLE-BLOWING

Being a whistle-blower takes great courage and self-conviction because it requires the whistle-blower to avoid *groupthink*—an inappropriate conformity to group norms. Going outside group norms often carries significant personal and professional risks. Unfortunately, these risks are more common than not, because whistle-blowers may be viewed as disloyal rather than as courageous. For example, Colvin (2002) recounted how Sherron Watkins, an accountant, first blew the whistle on Enron's complex "special-purpose entities." She detailed them in a memo to Chief Executive Officer Ken Lay, her boss's boss's boss. She understood that something wrong was going on—something everyone else seemed to think was perfectly okay—and that public revelation would be disastrous.

What Colvin argued was most important in this scandal was that Watkins had access to the same facts as did many other people inside Enron, yet, somehow, she was able to escape the groupthink that ensnared her colleagues. Soon after writing the memo, she identified herself as its author and met with Mr. Lay. When her memo eventually became public, the wrongness of what happened was apparent even internally (Colvin, 2002).

Colvin recounts a similar story at WorldCom, where Cynthia Cooper, another internal auditor, saw something that did not look right and took matters into her own hands. In this case, Cooper began investigating some of the company's capital expenditures and discovered bookkeeping entries that would eventually uncover what is likely the largest accounting fraud in U.S. history.

Faced with disturbing facts, Cooper discussed her findings with the company's controller and with Scott Sullivan, the chief financial officer. Sullivan tried to explain to her why costs that had previously been expensed were suddenly being capitalized. Then he asked her to stop the audit, which was being conducted early, and to put it off until the third quarter. She did not. Instead, she continued—and immediately went over her boss's head and called the chairman of the board's audit committee. He arranged to meet with her and the company's new auditor, KPMG. Two weeks later, WorldCom announced that it would restate earnings by US$3.9 billion—the largest restatement ever.

Again, Colvin (2002) suggested that the importance of Cooper's refusal to postpone her audit, as Sullivan had asked, is even greater than it may appear. Facts uncovered about the company, combined with the memo Sullivan wrote to the board in a last-ditch attempt to defend himself, show that if Cooper had "been a good soldier," the whole problem might have been concealed forever.

A similarly unsettling case was reported by Smith (2008), who profiled corporate whistle-blower Dana de Windt, a stockbroker at the financial services firm of Morgan Stanley. de Windt complained to government regulators that the company was cheating brokerage clients, having overcharged brokerage customers on 2,800 purchases of US$59 million of bonds. de Windt repeatedly confronted his bosses with "questions tucked inside a thick, three-ring binder" for more than 4 years, and management's response was simply for "him to get over it" (para. 5). Finally, de Windt reported the situation to regulators, and in August 2007, Morgan Stanley settled the resulting complaint brought by the U.S. Securities and Exchange Commission (SEC) by paying a $6.1 million fine.

> **Consider This**　Although the U.S. public wants corruption and unethical behavior to be unveiled, the individual reporting such behavior is often looked on with distrust and considered to be disloyal.

In another case, whistle-blower Jeffrey Sterling, an ex-CIA officer, was convicted of exposing a dubious covert operation without presenting clear-cut evidence that he did, something Solomon (2015) calls "a chilling message to others" (para. 1). Solomon alleges that prosecutors were trying to vindicate *Operation Merlin*, 9 years after a book by James Risen reported that it "may have been one of the most reckless operations in the modern history of the CIA." "That bestselling book, *State of War*, seemed to leave an indelible

stain on Operation Merlin while soiling the CIA's image as a reasonably competent outfit" (Solomon, 2015, para. 2).

Interestingly, journalist Risen was beyond the reach of the law, but Sterling, as a CIA employee, was not. Sterling had gone through channels in 2003 to warn Senate Intelligence Committee about Operation Merlin, and he was later indicted for allegedly giving Risen classified information about it. "For CIA officials, the prosecution wasn't only to punish Sterling and frighten potential whistle-blowers; it was also about payback, rewriting history and assisting with a PR comeback for the operation as well as the agency" (Solomon, 2015, para. 1). Sterling emerged from prison in early 2018 after serving most of a 42-month sentence. "Like his trial, his release drew little media attention, but his case has important implications for all Americans at a critical time in US history" ("Jeffrey Sterling is Free," 2018, para. 1).

An even more recent case of whistle-blowing malfeasance involved Wells Fargo Bank. Lewis (2017a) notes that the bank reportedly put heavy pressure on employees to meet sales quotas, and accounts were opened without authorization for customers who were charged fees for accounts they "knew nothing about." Lewis notes that that this corruption occurred despite more than 700 whistle-blower complaints to the Comptroller of the Currency, the federal banking regulator, before the scandal finally broke. The Comptroller neither "investigated the root cause" nor forced Wells Fargo to probe it. Indeed, Wells Fargo responded to internal ethics complaints from employees by firing them (Lewis, 2017a). Senator Elizabeth Warren suggested the possibility that a system operated by the Financial Industry Regulatory Authority to promote integrity may actually have perversely enabled whistle-blower blacklisting (Lewis, 2017a).

Perhaps the most frightening aspect of all these cases is that the responses to the whistle-blower are not unique. Many organizations are aware of problem situations but choose to ignore them until a crisis occurs or the problem becomes public.

Some nurses take comfort in thinking that nursing is different and that any moral professional would report substandard care. The reality, however, is often very different, and many professionals are torn between what they believe they should do and what they actually do. "When surveyed, over 99% of all nurses understood that reporting unethical practices was part of their obligations as nurses. However, less than 45% of surveyed nurses strongly believed they would have the courage to do so" (IV Infusion Home, 2015). This is particularly disconcerting, because those who bear witness are required to overcome groupthink despite their moral distress. This is a primary reason why so many whistle-blowers delay reporting their concerns outside the organization.

This willingness to speak out requires even greater courage when the whistle-blower lacks official power and status. For example, research by Fagan, Parker, and Jackson (2016) of student nurses suggests that "speaking up" is a complex and challenging social practice that requires negotiation in complicated cultural and organizational circumstances. Nursing students' transient position in the workplace (learners and visitors to a clinical organization) and their role and position of subservience often negatively influence their self-perception of the value of their contribution, and their confidence to speak up (see Research Fuels the Controversy 16.1).

Discussion Point

Why is speaking out often honored more in theory than in fact?

Discussion Point

In the United States, there is some evidence that the events of September 11, 2001, have made people more public spirited and more inclined to blow the whistle. Do you think this inclination is driven more by fear or by a desire to promote public good?

EXAMPLES OF WHISTLE-BLOWING IN NURSING

Complaints about unsafe staffing and unlicensed assistive personnel performing nursing tasks outside their scope of practice are fairly common. In addition, some nurses claim that they have been told to participate in illegal or unethical activities such as fraudulently altering medical records, falsifying insurance claims, and covering up the failure to meet mandated staffing ratios. A review of the literature reveals multiple case studies of whistle-blowing by nurses.

Mason (2011) shared the story of two nurses, Anne Mitchell and Vicki Galle, who blew the whistle on a physician for a variety of charges, including unprofessional conduct, via what they thought was a confidential report to the state board for medicine. Instead of the physician being investigated, the nurses found themselves the target of unprofessional conduct charges brought by the local sheriff and county attorney, who were friends and business associates of the reported physician. In the end, the nurses, who had a combined 47 years of experience at the hospital, were fired. The charges for Galle and Mitchell were eventually dropped, and the sheriff, county attorney, and hospital administrator were indicted for retaliating against the whistle-blowers. Each faced six counts, including misuse of official information and retaliation, which are third-degree felonies (Sack, 2011). The nurses sued the county and settled for a shared $750,000 (Sack, 2011).

Research Fuels the Controversy 16.1

Students Speaking Up

'Speaking up' in clinical situations through questions or statements of opinion or information with appropriate persistence is a vital communication skill for nursing students, and doing so is linked to patient safety. Most of the research done on "speaking up" has focused on the registered or experienced practitioners. To better understand the position and experiences of student nurses who speak up, a concept analysis was completed of literature published between 1970 and 2015 from MEDLINE, CINHAL, PUBMED, and SCOPUS. One of the search terms was whistle-blowing.

Source: Fagan, A., Parker, V., & Jackson, D. (2016, October). A concept analysis of undergraduate nursing students speaking up for patient safety in the patient care environment. *Journal of Advanced Nursing, 72*(10), 2346–2357. doi:10.1111/jan.13028

Study Findings

There is evidence to suggest that nurses do not always speak up. Nor do students who often feel powerless in their position, ignored by physicians and at times invisible. Students are mindful of their safety responsibilities, yet many articulate a fear of potential professional consequences for speaking up, including being negatively labelled.

The willingness of nursing students to speak up is influenced by individual and contextual factors that differ from those influencing more experienced colleagues. Motivators and barriers to voicing concerns include moral and ethical beliefs, willingness and confidence to speak up in the workplace. Students' subordinate and often vulnerable position creates additional tensions and challenges that impact their decisions and actions.

For students to speak up, sound clinical knowledge, commitment to patient safety, "speaking up" skills and confidence along with good supervision and support in the clinical environment are required. In addition, a just culture must be in place to enable students to be confident that speaking up will not bring about the risk of punishment or burden.

Rohner (2015) wrote about a more recent case in Cape Dorset, Nunavut, Canada, following the "preventable" death of a 3-month-old baby in 2012. The Government of Nunavut's policies and procedures for nurses state that nurses must examine sick children less than 1 year old when a parent contacts them after normal working hours. Gwen Slade, the whistle-blower nurse, alleges that another nurse told the mother not to bring the baby into the health center (to bathe the infant instead) and that the accused nurse faced numerous complaints that coworkers and members of the public had filed against her. The territory's health minister ordered an immediate independent review, but this had not begun nearly 3 months later. In the meantime, the accused nurse was promoted to acting nurse-in-charge despite restrictions being placed on her license by the Registered Nurses Association of the Northwest Territories and Nunavut.

In addition, Slade said she was suspended for speaking out against what she believed to be misdiagnoses and irresponsible behavior by a coworker. An investigation ensued, and Slade was eventually cleared of any wrongdoing. Slade suggests, however, that she continues to suffer the consequences of speaking out and that she has not been able to find work in Nunavut as a nurse since the alleged incidents. Slade also suggests that the investigation into her own conduct prevented her from getting two teaching jobs in Ontario and that she is only months away from losing her farm, her dream. Slade suggests that she is the victim of an extraordinary abuse of power, which has brought pain, devastation, and destruction to someone who did nothing wrong.

Clearly, patient advocacy has a central role in nursing. So too does professional advocacy, through which nurses are committed to improving the practice of nursing and maintaining the integrity of the health care profession. Both advocacy roles suggest that the nurse is accountable for ensuring that at least minimum standards are met. Both of these cases depict nurses who believed that they were acting honorably in the role of patient advocate. Yet all suffered negative consequences, including job loss. Unfortunately, this is more common than not.

> **Consider This** Advocacy is the foundation and essence of nursing, and nurses have a responsibility to promote human advocacy (Marquis & Huston, 2017).

It is important, however, to remember that whistle-blowing should never be considered the first solution to ethically troubling behavior. Indeed, it should be considered only after other prescribed avenues of solving problems have been attempted. This is true, however, only if patients' lives are not at stake. In those cases, immediate action must be taken.

In addition, the employee should typically go up the chain of command in reporting his or her concerns. This process, however, must be modified when the immediate supervisor is the source of the problem. In such a case, the employee might need to skip that level to see that the problem is addressed. Indeed, Foose, Penman, and Petry (2015) noted that most would rather raise the issue internally to their manager than take it outside. Thus, companies generally get the opportunity to resolve issues internally—the question is whether they will take this opportunity or miss it.

There are other general guidelines for blowing the whistle that should also be followed, including carefully documenting all attempts to address the problem and being sure to report facts and not personal interpretations. These guidelines, as well as others, are presented in Box 16.1.

CULTURAL BACKGROUND AND WHISTLE-BLOWING

For some minority nurses, cultural issues further complicate whether a decision is made to blow the whistle and, if so, how it should be done. It has been observed that "nurses with certain cultural backgrounds—for example, some Asians, Filipinos, and Africans—may be more reluctant to blow the whistle because they've been raised to respect a clear chain of command and hierarchy" (Minority Nurse Staff, 2013, para. 11). Indeed, a recent Middlesex University survey on staff members of the National Health Service (NHS) revealed that British health care staff are more likely to raise concerns than their Asian and black counterparts in the sector, indicating the significance of ethnicity as a predictor for whistle-blowing ("Staff Surveys Reveal," 2017).

The same goes for nurses whose first language is not English. According to Winifred Carson, nurse practice counsel for the American Nurses Association (ANA), "They fear problems related to communication—whether they accurately communicate the magnitude of the problem and whether not speaking English as a first language would be used against them if they continue to challenge authority" (Minority Nurse Staff, 2013, para. 13).

In addition, "reporting incidents of wrongdoing in the workplace is always a risky business—but for minority nurses who blow the whistle, the stakes are even higher" (Minority Nurse Staff, 2013, para. 1). That's because minority nurses are more apt to be retaliated against, especially if they are working in nonminority settings.

BOX 16.1   **Guidelines for Blowing the Whistle**

- Stay calm and think about the risks and outcomes before you act.
- Know your legal rights, because laws protecting whistle-blowers vary by state.
- First, make sure that there really is a problem. Check resources such as the medical library, the Internet, and institutional policy manuals to be sure.
- Seek validation from colleagues that there is a problem, but do not get swayed by groupthink into not doing anything if you should.
- Follow the chain of command in reporting your concerns, whenever possible.
- Confront those accused of the wrongdoing as a group whenever possible.
- Present just the evidence; leave the interpretation of facts to others. Remember that there may be an innocent or good explanation for what is occurring.
- Use internal mechanisms within your organization.
- If internal mechanisms do not work, use external mechanisms.
- Private groups, such as The Joint Commission or the National Committee for Quality Assurance, do not confer protection. You must report to a state or national regulator.
- Although it is not required by every regulatory agency, it is a good rule of thumb to put your complaint in writing.
- Document carefully the problem that you have seen and the steps that you have taken to see that it is addressed.
- Do not lose your temper, even if those who learn of your actions attempt to provoke you.
- Do not expect thanks for your efforts.

Source: American Nurses Association. (2017). *Things to know about whistle blowing.* Retrieved May 29, 2018, from https://www .nursingworld.org/practice-policy/workforce/things-to-know-about-whistle-blowing; Minority Nurse Staff. (2013). *What color is your whistle?* Retrieved May 29, 2018, from http://minoritynurse.com/what-color-is-your-whistle

THE PERSONAL RISKS OF WHISTLE-BLOWING

Being a whistle-blower is not without risks. Indeed, it is filled with risks. Unfortunately, most whistle-blowers set out believing that their actions will be welcomed, only to discover that the problems raised go much deeper than they imagined, and the personal consequences can be overwhelming. Such consequences include negative reactions from coworkers, losing one's job, and, in the extreme, legal retaliation. In many cases, whistle-blowers are fired from their jobs, especially those who are termed *at-will* employees.

Lewis (2017a, para. 7) agrees, noting that "the experiences of numerous whistleblowers show that reporting wrongdoing internally is a risky endeavor even when federal laws appear to offer whistle-blower protection. Court remedies are frequently out of reach for whistleblowers with no source of income. For this reason, many concerned workers choose to report problems anonymously, although staying anonymous is increasingly difficult as surveillance by industry and government continues to grow."

Minority Nurse Staff (2013) concurs, noting an Australian survey of 95 nurses that suggested that there were severe repercussions for the 70 nurses who reported incidents of misconduct but few professional consequences for the 25 nurses who remained silent: "Fourteen percent

of the whistle-blowers reported being treated as traitors, 16% received professional reprisals in the form of threats, 14% were rejected by peers, 11% were reprimanded, 9% were referred to a psychiatrist and 7% were pressured to resign" (para. 6).

> *Consider This* Whistle-blowers are still often considered to be traitors, snitches, and tattletales.

Peters et al.'s (2011) interviews with Australian nurses whose actions had been affirmed by whistle-blowers or who were whistle-blowers themselves also suggested that whistle-blowing brought about negative effects in virtually every aspect of their lives. The nurses shared such problems as tremendous and chronic distress, acute anxiety, flashbacks, nightmares, and disturbing thoughts. Peters et al. concluded that many nurse whistle-blowers were not prepared for the impact on their personal, emotional, physical, and professional welfare.

Similarly, Lewis (2017b) shared the story of Oregon whistle-blower Vikki Mata, who reported that officials improperly diverted to state coffers federal funds intended to provide health care for uninsured children via the Healthy Kids Program. An audit Mata requested confirmed her allegation that state officials overstated the number of uninsured children in the state and that those inflated numbers allowed authorities to improperly claim additional federal funds, thus reducing the money available to aid qualified children. The state later returned $4.5 million dollars to the federal program, where it was again available for its intended purpose thanks to Vikki Mata. Unfortunately, Mata lost her job in the process and was unable to cover the expense of an appeal herself.

Lewis (2017b, para. 4) notes that Mata's case highlights a flaw in our justice system. "Unlike other witnesses, whistleblowers often must take alleged wrongdoers to court on their own dime. Absurdly, the welfare of millions of people may rely on how much a whistle-blower has in his savings account. It's a great incentive for employers to evade accountability by firing whistle-blowers and crippling them financially. Americans protect their own interests when they help whistle-blowers overcome obstacles imposed by employers and the justice system."

> **Consider This** There isn't an employee in your organization who doesn't gauge the potential for retaliation when considering raising an issue (Foose et al., 2015).

Not all whistle-blowing, however, results in repercussions from employers. For example, in late 2014, Anderson Cooper featured the story of Nurse Briana Aguirre who spoke out about the treatment of Ebola patient Thomas Duncan and others at Texas Presbyterian Hospital, where she worked (Cable News Network [CNN], 2014). Ms. Aguirre described chaos, a lack of training, confusing protocols from the Centers for Disease Control (CDC), and unnecessary risks that she says nurses were exposed to on the job. She also claimed that 2 weeks into the hospital's Ebola crisis, nurses like her did not have the same level of protection as sanitation workers at the hospital. Although Ms. Aguirre expressed concerns about recrimination for openly sharing her concerns, the hospital responded that "Her employment status is the same today as it was yesterday. We would welcome the opportunity to learn more about her observations when she is willing" (CNN, 2014, para. 4).

It is imperative then that nurses working on the frontline be encouraged to speak up and that they be supported in their actions to do so. For example, nursing departments within hospitals should provide their nurses with an ethics committee chaired by a nurse with experience in bioethical issues (not one who has a vested interest in promoting administrative or hierarchical constraints). Nurse managers should promote the values inherent in patient advocacy, and the organization should openly support individuals

who are willing to take the risk of being a whistle-blower. The reality is that if an employee is willing to go to the trouble and risk the repercussions of blowing the whistle, those concerns should be taken seriously and investigated.

> **Consider This** The motive of most whistle-blowers is advocacy, not troublemaking.

More research, however, is being conducted on the motivation behind whistle-blowing. Recent research conducted by Guthrie and Taylor at North Carolina State University (2015) and Bucknell University suggests that strong, reliable antiretaliation policies can encourage employees to notify internal authorities of possible wrongdoing, but that offering monetary incentives does not necessarily influence whistle-blowing behavior—or at least not right away. However, when monetary incentives increase, so too does the incidence of whistle-blowing.

The bottom line, though, is that whistle-blowers should never assume that doing the right thing will result in a financial incentive or protect them from retaliation. Instead, potential whistle-blowers should determine their legal duty for reporting and carefully research the specifics of their protection under the law. In addition, they should try to report anonymously when possible. Moreover, they must be prepared to defend their claims. In addition, prospective whistle-blowers should always at least try to solve problems internally before going public. When that is impossible and there is a clear indication of serious harm, they must document their actions and go public. They should also seek support and counsel before taking any steps.

> **BOX 16.2   Pros and Cons of Whistle-Blowing**
>
> **Pros**
> - Protects patients
> - Improves quality of care
> - Meets professional expectations and standards
> - Satisfies ethical duty
> - Brings problems out into the open
> - Provides validation of concerns and moral rightness
>
> **Cons**
> - Poses personal and professional risks
> - Casts doubt on motives
> - Leads to possible job loss or employer retaliation
> - Is typically a tiring, anxiety-producing, and often frustrating experience

Clearly, whistle-blowers often face both social- and work-related retaliation, and at times this retaliation can be severe and life altering. Yet it must be noted that at least some self-satisfaction and pride must come with the recognition that unethical behavior has been exposed and that at least the potential for correction is possible because of the whistle-blower's actions. Box 16.2 summarizes some of the pros and cons of whistle-blowing.

ETHICAL DIMENSIONS OF WHISTLE-BLOWING

Ethical organizations practice in such a way that patients and workers are protected from harm. Sometimes, however, health care organizations fail to provide accountability for the safety and welfare of their patients and workers. Nurses or other employees then feel compelled to take action against the wrongdoing in an effort to fulfill their professional obligations.

Whistle-blowing, however, can create considerable moral distress for nurses as they weigh the consequences of their actions against the duties of their profession. In other words, they must weigh a consequentialist view based on utilitarianism with their professional duty and values, which is founded more in a deontologic framework.

Clearly, nurses are bound to the role of patient advocacy by ethical codes of conduct. The problem is that nurses also have professional commitments to their employer and to other health care professionals, and this loyalty to the employer can be misplaced when it leads to patient harm. The end result all too often, then, is a conflict between principles and duty. This tension between loyalty to employer and the need to protect patients is a major reason so many nurses delay in blowing the whistle.

A compelling argument can be made, however, for the precedence of the nurse's duty to the patient over his or her duty to the employer. Indeed, nurses must always remember that their primary professional responsibility is to their patients, not to their employers. As such, the need to uphold the rights of others, to promote fairness, and to provide for the greater good becomes paramount.

Discussion Point

Can you think of a situation in which you have been involved in which utilitarianism (the greater good) would support not blowing the whistle on unethical behavior?

Consider This   A whistle-blower must blow the whistle for the right reason for it to be a moral action.

McKee (2013) suggests that justice and fidelity are other ethical principles that must be examined when considering the ethics of whistle-blowing. McKee argues that society could not function if individuals routinely broke their agreements. Employees of all types owe fidelity to their employers, if not to a professional code of conduct. At times, however, claims of justice may supersede the claims of fidelity, and one's professional duty sometimes includes a legal and moral duty to report violations, especially if they are being covered up.

The ANA *Code of Ethics for Nurses with Interpretive Statements* may also provide guidance for nurses who are considering becoming a whistle-blower. Provision 3 of the *Code of Ethics* states that the nurse "promotes, advocates for, and strives to protect the health, safety, and rights of the patient" (American Nurses Association [ANA], 2015, p. 9). In addition, Section 3.5 states:

> *When incompetent, unethical, illegal, or impaired practice is not corrected and continues to jeopardize patient well-being and safety, nurses must report the problem to appropriate external authorities such as practice committees or professional organizations, licensing boards, and regulatory or quality assurance agencies. Some situations are sufficiently egregious as to warrant the notification and involvement of all groups and/or law enforcement.* (ANA, 2015, p. 12)

Ethical codes of conduct from Canada, the United Kingdom, Australia, and Japan mandate similar action. Such ethical codes bind nurses to the role of patient advocacy and compel them to take action when the rights or safety of patients is jeopardized. The bottom line is that although whistle-blowing can result in negative consequences for both the employing institution and the whistle-blower, nurses must uphold a professional standard and protect their patients.

LEGAL PROTECTION FOR WHISTLE-BLOWERS

There is no universal legal protection for whistle-blowers; however, under the 1st and 14th Amendments to the U.S. Constitution, state and local government officials are prohibited from retaliating against whistle-blowers. In addition, although they do not fall under the category of "whistle-blower" protections, the laws protecting individual employees from mistreatment in the workplace, such as Title VII of the Civil Rights Act or the Fair Labor Standards Act, also protect employees from retaliation for asserting their rights under those laws. For example, it is illegal to terminate an employee for reporting sexual harassment or for challenging an employer's failure to pay overtime (Joseph & Kirschenbaum, LLP, 2018).

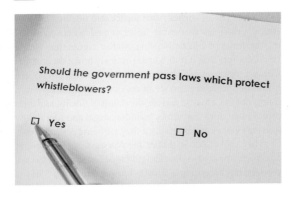

In addition, in 2017, President Donald Trump signed an Executive Order establishing an Office of Accountability and Whistleblower Protection (OAWP), to be led by a Special Assistant to the Secretary ("Trump Creates Office," 2017). This office was charged with working closely with relevant VA components to ensure swift and effective resolution of veterans' complaints of wrongdoing at the VA and to "ensure adequate investigation and correction of wrongdoing throughout the VA." The Office would also protect employees who lawfully disclose wrongdoing from retaliation.

Still, recent reports suggest that some VA whistle-blowers continue to be intimidated, bullied, and threatened with physical violence as they report wrongdoing in their agencies (Diaz, 2018). Reporting wrongdoing through official VA channels like the OAWP can take months, and complaints often go back to the employee's supervisors at work—even when anonymity is supposedly guaranteed (Diaz, 2018).

The False Claims Act

Some whistle-blower legislation has been enacted at the federal level, however, to encourage people to report wrongdoings. One such piece of legislation is the False Claims Act (FCA), originally a Civil War statute, which encourages whistle-blowers to come forward regarding fraud committed against the federal government and to file a lawsuit seeking lost monies in the government's name.

The individual would file a *qui tam* or whistle-blower lawsuit and provide knowledge that a person defrauded the government. Qui tam lawsuits are brought by a citizen, known as a "relator" or whistle-blower, against a company, person, or entity that he or she believes is cheating the federal or state government in some way (WhistleblowerLaws, 2016). Since the *qui tam* suit is brought in the name of the whistle-blower on behalf of the government, the government

may actually join the case and litigate alongside the whistle-blower's lawyers. These FCAs or "*qui tam* laws" exist at the federal level. An individual who successfully pursues a *qui tam* action is entitled to a bounty that ranges between 15% and 30% of the government's recovery (The Employment Law Group, 2018). Indeed, since January 2009, the government has recovered almost $20 billion through the FCA for health care fraud and has paid hundreds of millions of dollars in rewards to whistle-blowers (Khurana Law Firm, 2017).

For example, a whistle-blower may have knowledge of a colleague inappropriately billing Medicare or Medicaid. The FCA provides protection for government whistle-blowers, thereby prohibiting employers from punishing employees who report the fraud or assist in the investigation of the fraud. If the whistle-blower is dismissed or discriminated against in any way as a result of the lawsuit, the whistle-blower can file a claim against that employer for unlawful retaliation.

To have a case brought to trial under federal law, the whistle-blower must first exhaust his or her internal chain of command and then file a complaint with the Department of Health and Human Services (DHHS). If the DHHS decides that the complaint is valid, the government proceeds with litigation against the employer, and the whistle-blower receives a percentage of the damages awarded. The case discussed earlier in this chapter involving the two nurses in Missouri who alleged nursing home abuse and fraud was a FCA *qui tam* lawsuit.

Schmitt (2014) details the story of a strip mall with two dozen or so health care businesses listed on the building's directory. Yet when visited by the U.S. DHHS, the offices were empty, despite one of the businesses billing Medicare for $2.2 million in 3 months in 2007. Schmitt also details the story of a Los Angeles doctor charged with conspiracy in connection with a $33-million scheme in which he allegedly signed prescriptions and other documents for medically unnecessary home health services, hospice service, and durable medical equipment. The prescriptions were then allegedly used by supply companies and other firms to bilk Medicare.

Similarly, Richey (2014) noted that in a nationwide takedown by Medicare Fraud Strike Force operations, 90 people, including 27 doctors, nurses, and other medical professionals, were charged for their alleged participation in fraud schemes involving approximately $260 million in false billings to Medicare. The defendants were charged with various health care fraud-related crimes, including submitting claims to Medicare for treatments that were either not provided or not necessary, recruiters paying kickbacks to get Medicare billing numbers of patients so that providers could submit fraudulent bills to Medicare, supplying motorized wheelchairs that were not needed, and conspiring to bill Medicare for medically unnecessary home health services.

More recently, Phoenix-based Banner Health was required to pay more than $18 million as part of an FCA lawsuit to settle whistle-blower claims that they admitted patients who could have been treated less expensively at outpatient facilities (Alltucker, 2018). The settlement resolves a complaint brought forth by a former Banner Health employee who claimed one dozen hospitals in Arizona and Colorado overcharged Medicare for brief, inpatient procedures that should have been billed on a less costly outpatient basis. The employee who filed the claim was paid $3.3 million as part of the FCA settlement (Alltucker, 2018).

Because the FCA has been fairly effective in detecting fraud at the federal level, some state versions of the FCA have also passed, although the federal laws contained with the FCA may not be exactly duplicated by state governments (The Employment Law Group, 2018). Under these state laws, whistle-blowers can file lawsuits seeking lost monies in the state or local government's name and share in the proceeds. As of 2016, False Claims Acts or "*qui tam* laws" had been adopted by 29 states, the District of Columbia, the city of New York, and the city of Chicago, although a number of other states are considering the introduction of such legislation (WhistleblowerLaws, 2016).

There are some state legal protections for whistle-blowers as well. Although some state laws prohibit retaliation, the standards for proving retaliation vary. Employees in most states increase their likelihood of whistle-blower protection under general statutes or common law if they meet criteria similar to those established at the federal level: (1) They must be acting in good faith that the employer or its employees are breaking the law in some way, (2) they must complain about that violation either to the employer or to an outside agency, (3) they must refuse to be a party to the violation, and (4) they should be willing to assist in any official investigations of the violation.

Discussion Point

What whistle-blowing protections, if any, exist in the state where you live? Is any legislation pending?

Other Federal Legislation Related to Whistle-Blowing

Another piece of legislation, the *Whistleblower Protection Act of 1989*, protects federal employees who disclose government fraud, abuse, and waste. The *Whistleblower Protection Enhancement Act of 2007* extended the *Whistleblower Protection Act of 1989* to federal employees who specialize in national security issues. In addition, the *Paul*

Revere Freedom to Warn Act protects federal employee whistle-blowers who speak out about abuse, harassment, and unethical behavior in the workplace.

The National Labor Relations Act might protect employees in the private sector from retaliation when employees act as a group to modify working conditions or ask for better wages. The best protection for employees who work for publicly traded companies or companies that are required to file certain reports with the SEC in the United States at this time, however, is likely the *Sarbanes–Oxley Act of 2002* (further amended by the *Dodd–Frank Wall Street Reform and Consumer Protection Act* in 2010). This act dramatically redesigned federal regulation of public company corporate governance and reporting obligations and provided some protection for whistle-blowers who report fraud in publicly traded companies to the proper authorities (Joseph & Kirschenbaum, LLP, 2017).

Employees in these companies who experience retaliation for whistle-blowing have 180 days to file a written complaint with OSHA. If the evidence supports an employee's claim of retaliation and a settlement cannot be reached, OSHA will issue an order requiring the employer to reinstate the employee, pay back wages, and restore benefits (Occupational Safety and Health Administration [OSHA], n.d., para. 7). After OSHA issues its final ruling, either party may request a full hearing before an administrative law judge of the Department of Labor. That decision can then be appealed to the Department's Administrative Review Board for final review.

The SEC has awarded more than $262 million to 53 whistle-blowers since issuing its first award in 2012 ("SEC Announces," 2018). In March 2018, it announced its highest-ever Dodd–Frank whistle-blower awards, with two whistle-blowers sharing a nearly $50-million award and a third whistle-blower receiving more than $33 million. The previous high was a $30-million award in 2014 ("SEC Announces," 2018).

In late 2018, the Supreme Court, however, will rule on whether whistle-blower protections under the Dodd–Frank Act should apply only to people who report misconduct directly to the SEC (Kelly, 2018). That is, people who report misconduct internally would not be protected from retaliation. This places increased pressure on company compliance programs to ensure their monitoring, reporting, and investigation policies, procedures, and practices are in a position to sufficiently incentivize and encourage employees to report securities law violations internally (Giampetruzzi, Montes, & Baker, 2018).

WHISTLE-BLOWING AS AN INTERNATIONAL ISSUE

Whistle-blowing cases involving nurses are not limited to the United States. In November 2014, the SEC issued its Annual Report to Congress on the Dodd-Frank Whistleblower

Program. The report notes that during 2014, the Commission received submissions from individuals in all 50 states, as well as from individuals in 60 countries (Foose et al., 2015). The highest numbers of international reports came from the UK, Canada, Australia, China, and India, with the most coming from the UK (70 reports). After a lengthy study by a commission formed by the Bank of England and the U.K. Financial Conduct Authority, the commission rejected U.S.-style "bounties" for individuals who report financial crimes to government authorities (Foose et al., 2015).

The lack of protection for whistle-blowers, then, is a global problem, and mounting pressure exists internationally to adopt whistle-blower protection laws to reduce the risk of retaliation to whistle-blowers. Federal law in Canada (enacted in 2004) with section 425.1 of the Criminal Code prohibits employers from retaliating or threatening to take action against employees who provide information to law enforcement officials, and the Public Servants Disclosure Protection Act has protected whistle-blowers in the federal public sector since 2007 (The State of Whistleblowing, 2016). Yet legal experts suggest these laws are still too limited to fully protect whistle-blowers.

In early 2017, recognizing the role of the nurse as patient advocate and the lack of support and legislative frameworks, the NHS published draft regulations to give legal protection to NHS whistle-blowers (Glasper, 2017; Watson & O'Connor, 2017). These plans augment the legal steps whistle-blowers can take if they seek re-employment in the NHS and believe that a potential employer has discriminated against them because they are suspected of blowing the whistle in exposing aspects of poor care.

> ### Discussion Point
> Would international adoption of legislation similar to the FCA increase the likelihood that whistle-blowers will both come forward and be protected from recrimination globally?

CONCLUSIONS

Nurses as health care professionals have a responsibility to uncover, openly discuss, and condemn shortcuts that threaten the clients they serve. Clearly, however, there has been a collective silence in many such cases. The reality is that whistle-blowing offers no guarantee that the situation will change, or the problem will improve, and the literature is replete with horror stories regarding negative consequences endured by whistle-blowers. The whistle-blower cannot even trust that other health care professionals with similar belief systems about advocacy will value their efforts because the public's feelings about whistle-blowers are so mixed. In addition, state laws vary, and protections for the nongovernment employee whistle-blower are often limited.

For all these reasons, it takes tremendous courage to come forward as a whistle-blower. It also takes a tremendous sense of what is right and what is wrong, as well as a commitment to follow a problem through until an acceptable level of resolution is reached. Whistle-blowers are heroes and should be treated as such; their courage is nothing short of exceptional. How unfortunate that we frequently do not treat them that way.

For Additional Discussion

1. Why do Americans have a "love–hate" relationship with whistle-blowers? Is this dichotomy prevalent in other countries as well?

2. Which is greater for you personally—your duty to your patients, your duty to your employer, or your duty to yourself? How do you sort out what you should do when these duties are in conflict?

3. Do you believe that most whistle-blowing must be external before appropriate action is taken?

4. Should whistle-blowers receive compensation under the FCA?

5. Would you be willing to bear the risks of becoming a whistle-blower?

6. Do you believe that there is more, less, or the same amount of whistle-blowing in health care as in other types of industries?

7. Can you identify a whistle-blowing situation in which it might be appropriate to go outside the chain of command in reporting concerns about organizational practice?

References

Alltucker, K. (2018, April 12). *Banner Health settles whistle-blower case for $18 million.* Retrieved May 29, 2018, from https://www.azcentral.com/story/money/business/health/2018/04/12/banner-health-settles-whistleblower-case-18-million/511848002

American Nurses Association. (2015). *Code of ethics for nurses with interpretive statements.* Silver Spring, MD: Author.

Cable News Network. (2014, October 16). *Whistleblower nurse: I would do anything and everything not to be a patient there.* Anderson Cooper 360°. Retrieved May 29, 2018, from http://ac360.blogs.cnn.com/2014/10/16/whistleblower-nurse-i-would-do-anything-and-everything-not-to-be-a-patient-there

Colvin, G. (2002). Wonder women of whistleblowing. *Fortune, 146*(3). Retrieved February 20, 2015, from http://money.cnn.com/magazines/fortune/fortune_archive/2002/08/12/327047/index.htm

Diaz, A. (2018). *VA whistleblowers, under threat, seek help from the outside.* Retrieved May 28, 2018, from http://www.foxnews.com/us/2018/04/10/va-whistleblowers-under-threat-seek-help-from-outside.html

Dictionary.com. (2018). *Whistleblowing [Definition].* Retrieved May 29, 2018, from http://dictionary.reference.com/browse/whistleblowing?s=t

Fagan, A., Parker, V., & Jackson, D. (2016, October). A concept analysis of undergraduate nursing students speaking up for patient safety in the patient care environment. *Journal of Advanced Nursing, 72*(10), 2346–2357. doi:10.1111/jan.13028

Foose, A., Penman, C., & Petry, E. (2015). *2015 trends: #8 top whistleblowing priorities for compliance professionals.* Sausalito, CA: JD Supra. Retrieved May 28, 2018, from http://www.jdsupra.com/legalnews/2015-trends-8-top-whistleblowing-prior-00132

Giampetruzzi, G., Montes, J., & Baker, J. (2018, April 19). *In light of digital realty and the largest ever Dodd-Frank Whistleblower award, whistleblower risks are up and company compliance programs are under pressure.* Paul Hastings. Retrieved May 29, 2018, from https://www.paulhastings.com/publications-items/details/?id=e3d88c6a-2334-6428-811c-ff00004cbded

Glasper, A. (2017). Protecting whistleblowers against discrimination in the NHS. *British Journal of Nursing, 26*(9), 522–523.

IV Infusion Home. (2015, February 22). *Whistleblowing and nursing practice* [Web log post]. Retrieved May 29, 2018, from https://ivinfusion.wordpress.com/2015/02/22/whistleblowing-and-nursing-practice

Jeffrey Sterling is free—but are we? (2018, February 1). Whistleblowing Today. Retrieved May 29, 2018, from http://whistleblowingtoday.org

Joseph & Kirschenbaum, LLP. (2018). *Whistleblower and Sarbanes-Oxley claims.* New York, NY: Author. Retrieved May 29, 2018, from http://www.jhllp.com/lawyer-attorney-1324989.html

Kelly, M. (2018, January 8). *Whistleblower risks at the Supreme Court.* Retrieved May 29, 2018, from https://www.navexglobal.com/blog/article/whistleblower-risks-at-the-supreme-court

Khurana Law Firm. (2017). *Medicare whistleblower center.* Retrieved May 29, 2018, from http://www.medicarewhistleblowercenter.com

Lewis, L. (2017a). *Regulator ignored 700 Wells Fargo whistleblower complaints.* Whistleblowing Today. Retrieved May 29, 2018, from http://whistleblowingtoday.org/2017/05/regulator-ignored-700-wells-fargo-whistleblower-complaints

Lewis, L. (2017b). *Child health whistleblower Vikki Mata appeals for donations.* Whistleblowing Today. Retrieved May 29, 2018, from http://whistleblowingtoday.org/2017/01/child-health-whistleblower-vikki-mata-appeals-for-donations

Marquis, B., & Huston, C. (2017). *Leadership roles and management functions in nursing* (9th ed.). Philadelphia, PA: Wolters Kluwer.

Mason, D. J. (2011, January 14). *Public officials indicted in RN whistleblowing case* [Web log post]. Retrieved May 29, 2018, from http://www.healthmediapolicy.com/2011/01/14/public-officials-indicted-in-rn-whistleblowing-case

McKee, C. (2013, September 23). *Whistleblower ethics.* America Press. Retrieved May 29, 2018, from http://www.americamagazine.org/issue/whistleblower-ethics

Minority Nurse Staff. (2013). *What color is your whistle?* Retrieved May 29, 2018, from http://minoritynurse.com/what-color-is-your-whistle

North Carolina State University. (2015, March 2). *Protections, not money, can boost internal corporate whistleblowing.* Science Daily. Retrieved May 29, 2018, from https://www.sciencedaily.com/releases/2015/03/150302091701.htm

Occupational Safety and Health Administration. (n.d.). *OSHA fact sheet: Filing whistleblower complaints under the Sarbanes-Oxley Act.* Retrieved May 29, 2018, from http://www.osha.gov/Publications/osha-factsheet-sox-act.pdf

Peters, K., Luck, L., Hutchinson, M., Wilkes, L., Andrew, S., & Jackson, D. (2011). The emotional sequelae of whistleblowing: Findings from a qualitative study. *Journal of Clinical Nursing, 20*(19/20), 2907–2914.

Richey, W. (2014, May 13). *Medicare fraud: Feds charge 90-plus people for $260 million in false claims.* Retrieved May 29, 2018, from https://www.csmonitor.com/USA/Justice/2014/0513/Medicare-fraud-Feds-charge-90-plus-people-for-260-million-in-false-claims

Rohner, T. (2015, February 6). *Whistle-blowing nurse wants action on Nunavut nursing scandal.* Nunatsiaq Online. Retrieved May 29, 2018, from http://www.nunatsiaqonline.ca/stories/article/65674whistle-blowing_nurse_wants_action_on_nunavut_nursing_scandal

Sack, K. (2011, January 14). *Sheriff charged in Texas whistle-blowing case.* The New York Times. Retrieved May 29, 2018, from http://www.nytimes.com/2011/01/15/us/15nurses.html?_r=1

Schmitt, R. (2014, November). Medicare Special Report: Inside the Medicare strike force. *AARP Bulletin, 55*(9), 10–12.

SEC announces its largest-ever whistleblower awards. (2018, March 19). Retrieved May 29, 2018, from https://www.sec.gov/news/press-release/2018-44

Smith, R. (2008, May 24). A Morgan Stanley crusader: Bond-pricing issues prompt one broker's inside investigation. *The Wall Street Journal* (Eastern edition, p. B1). Retrieved May 29, 2018, from http://online.wsj.com/article/SB121158398445518845.html

Solomon, N. (2015, February 4). *Convicting Sterling to chill whistleblowing.* Consoritumnews.com. Retrieved May 29, 2018, from https://consortiumnews.com/2015/02/04/convicting-sterling-to-chill-whistleblowing

Staff surveys reveal link between ethnicity. (2017, February). *Nursing Management—UK, 23*(9), 7.

The Employment Law Group. (2018). *Do you need a whistleblower rewards attorney?* Retrieved May 29, 2018, from https://www.employmentlawgroup.com/what-we-do/whistleblower-protection-rewards/how-our-attorneys-help-whistleblowers/?utm_campaign=Bing%20Whistleblower%20Law&_SR=Bing&_AC=Whistleblower%20Law&_AG=Whistleblower%20Law&_kk=Federal%20%2Bwhistleblower%20Law&_ph=1-888-387-3057&mm_campaign=8f347e770d565c22a9c780b9d17bed34&keyword=Federal%20%2Bwhistleblower%20Law&utm_source=Bing&utm_medium=CPC

The Free Online Dictionary. (2003–2018). *Whistleblower [Definition].* Retrieved May 29, 2018, from http://www.thefreedictionary.com/whistleblower

The State of Whistleblowing. (2016, Summer). *Canadian Journal of Medical Laboratory Science, 78*(2), 25–27.

Trump creates Office of Whistleblower Protection at Veterans Administration. (2017, April 30). Retrieved May 29, 2018, from http://whistleblowingtoday.org

Watson, C. L., & O'Connor, T. (2017). Legislating for advocacy: The case of whistleblowing. *Nursing Ethics, 24*(3), 305–312. doi:10.1177/0969733015600911

WhistleblowerLaws. (2016). *What is a qui tam?* Guttman, Buschner & Brooks PLLC. Retrieved May 29, 2018, from http://www.whistleblowerlaws.com/what-is-qui-tam

Impaired Nursing Practice
Is Progress Being Made?

Jennifer Lillibridge

CHAPTER OUTLINE

LEARNING OBJECTIVES

The learner will be able to:

1. Examine the prevalence of substance abuse in the nursing profession.

2. Describe early risk factors that result in an increased risk for chemical addiction in the nursing profession.

3. Identify links between national nursing policies about impaired practice and local implementation of strategies to address the problem.

4. Describe challenges and barriers nurses face when confronting and/or helping an impaired colleague.

5. Explore the concept of drug diversion and how nurses and managers can prevent or detect drug diversion in the workplace.

6. Examine the role of nursing education in the prevention of impaired nursing practice.

7. Examine the role nurse leaders in the workplace hold in preventing impaired nursing practice.

8. Explore reasons nurses with substance abuse problems often fail to receive the same caring attitude or approach from their peers that is extended to other individuals who misuse drugs and alcohol.

9. Identify State Board of Nursing reporting requirements for nurses suspected of chemical dependency or of diverting drugs for personal use.

10. Describe typical components of a state diversion program, as well as a "return to work" agreement, for a chemically impaired nurse.

11. Identify the driving forces that compelled most State Boards of Nursing in the United States to move from mandatory disciplinary action for impaired nurses to diversion program treatment.

12. Reflect on personal feelings regarding the extent to which a State Board of Nursing has the right and/or responsibility to invade the impaired nurse's privacy to ensure recovery is ongoing.

INTRODUCTION

"Helping the impaired nurse is difficult but not impossible. The choices for action are varied. The only choice that is clearly wrong is to do nothing". (A 2001 NCSBN report cited by the Colorado Board of Nursing, 2003). Definitions of impaired practice vary, but most include that professional judgment is impaired because of the effects of drugs or alcohol (or mental illness), and this compromises patient safety. A position statement of the Canadian Nurses Association states that "problematic" substance use by nurses occurs when "the effects or aftereffects of substance use impair their work performance to the extent that expected standards of professional practice are not met" (Ross, Berry, Smye, & Golder, 2017, para. 1).

The problem of impaired nursing practice has plagued nursing for decades; however, it continues to remain poorly understood, underresearched (Ross et al., 2017), and underreported. Nutty (2016) suggests the "stigma of addiction" (p. 6) prevents many nurses from self-reporting and seeking treatment, whereas Cares, Pace, Denious, and Crane (2015) cite fear, humiliation, and concerns of punitive measures as a barrier to nurses seeking treatment.

A discussion about impaired nursing practice often raises more questions than it answers. Two key issues surround impaired nursing practice. The first is concern for patient safety. The second is concern for the health of the impaired nurse. With denial common, the problem can go without detection or treatment for years. Typically, if nurses gain access to substances from work, patient harm can occur through drug diversion. Examples of drug diversion include substitution, removal of medication without orders, frequent medication overrides, salvaging from waste, and reduced or skipped dose of medications (Relias Media, 2017; New, 2014). Patient safety is also compromised when nurses are impaired because of alcohol or substances obtained from outside the workplace. Supervisory actions to protect patients are shown in Box 17.1.

Without wanting to discount the individual nurse with a substance use problem, patient safety has been at the forefront of national considerations about professional nursing practice and the future of nursing since the seminal publication by the Institute of Medicine, *To Error Is Human* (1999), and has been reinforced repeatedly in the literature (Cares et al., 2015; Kunyk, 2015; Ross et al., 2017). Given this agenda, it seems critical that preventing impaired practice and dealing with it proactively when it does happen should be inclusive in all discussions about patient safety. Kunyk (2015, p. 54) states: "If active and hidden, SUD [substance use disorder] presents threats to patient safety, the health of nurses with these disorders and to the professional image of nursing."

PREVALENCE OF THE PROBLEM

Estimates on the prevalence of substance use disorder in the nursing profession are varied; efforts to quantify the prevalence are fraught with problems. It has been suggested that the difficulty may be due in part to the fact that self-disclosure is reduced because of the stigma, shame, and denial (Kunyk, 2015). Cares et al. (2015) suggest that another barrier when estimating prevalence rests with the differing approaches used to garner prevalence information, which makes it difficult to draw meaningful conclusions.

Estimates often state that prevalence mirrors statistics from the general population. The American Nurses Association's (ANA) estimate of 6% to 8% is dated (and the basis of this estimate is unclear); the NCSBN reports other estimates of between 10% and 15% (NCSBN, 2018). Kunyk's (2015) study in Canada supports the suggestion that the prevalence of substance use disorder in nursing is similar to that in the general population. Cares et al. (2015) report that use of nonmedical prescription drug use among nurses is higher than in the general population, whereas alcohol and drug use disorders are less. The difficulty in using the general population as a benchmark for nurses' use of substances is that the National Institute on Drug Abuse (2015) does not report an overarching statistic of drug abuse. What is reported reflects specific areas of drug use; for example, according to 2015 statistics, illicit drug use by the general population was 9.4%. This does not take into account the nonmedical use of drugs when nurses divert medication from the workplace.

Previously, it has been suggested that prevalence is not as important as patterns of substance use among health professionals, such as physicians and nurses. Although examining patterns may still be important, the critical consideration must be the performance of the nurse and

BOX 17.1	**Three Supervisory Actions to Protect Patients**	
Check in Early	**Correct Early**	**Contain the Risk**
Follow routine procedures	Investigate further	Escort nurse from practice setting immediately
Conduct check-in meetings	Document the facts	Follow policy for fitness evaluation
Observe and assess nurse performance	Request on-demand meeting when indicated	Request alcohol and drug screen
Document safe practice	Follow disciplinary procedures if warranted	Document the facts
Submit routine written reports	Report a compliance issue immediately	Submit incident report

Source: O'Neill, C., & Cadiz, D. (2014). Worksite monitors protect patients from unsafe nursing practices. *Journal of Nursing Regulation, 5*(2), 22.

whether the nurse is making safe, appropriate decisions in the provision of quality patient care.

> **Consider This**   Given current estimates of impaired nursing practice, it is likely that 1 out of every 10 nurses you work with will struggle with a substance use problem.

OVERVIEW OF THE LITERATURE

Although gaps about many issues related to impaired practice continue to exist, research on this persistent problem is emerging. Kunyk (2015) investigated the prevalence of substance use disorder in nurses and impaired nursing practice, including nurse health, in a disciplinary jurisdiction in Canada. Underreporting, which has been identified as a significant problem with impaired practice, was also found in Kunyk's study. Over 95% of self-identified impaired nurses were currently employed and unknown to their employers as having a substance use problem. This finding highlights the critical nature of substance use disorder as impaired nurses continue to put patients and themselves at risk.

Cook (2013) conducted a study to examine whether nurses could trust their recovering (from substance use) colleagues in direct care. Cook discovered that nurses were willing to trust recovering nurses and found strong agreement that they should be able to return to work in health care. Although a small study, this finding might suggest a change in perceptions of nurses generally that previously were thought to not take care of their own.

A recent joint position statement of the Emergency Nurses Association and the International Nurses Society on Addictions (Strobbe & Crowley, 2017) focuses on four distinct areas: (1) the importance of education about substances including alcohol (includes policies and procedures), with the goal of ensuring "safe, supportive, drug-free workplaces" (p. 105); (2) the availability of alternative to discipline (ATD) programs with suitable return to work goals; (3) considering drug diversion as a symptom of problematic substance use; and (4) the risks related to use of substances, impaired practice, and drug diversion are understood by both nurses and nursing students. Critical to item four is that nurses (and students) understand their role and the process to report suspected or actual concerns. Although this position statement emerges from the specialty of emergency nursing, these goals apply to all areas of nursing practice.

Boulton and Nosek (2014) investigated the perceptions of nursing students and substance abusing nurses. They found that students generally had positive perceptions of nurses with a substance use problem and that these perceptions were reinforced with education. A nonstatistically significant finding supported previous research that nursing education falls short of effectively preparing nurses to identify and respond supportively to an impaired colleague. Participants also believed that even after exposure to an educational program on the topic, they would not be able to recognize or support an impaired nurse. The authors suggest this might be indicative of the reluctance of the profession to deal with the problem.

More recent studies were found with the subpopulation of nursing students and use of substances, including alcohol. The aims of a photovoice study by McCulloh Nair, Nemeth, Sommers, Newman, and Amella (2016) were twofold. The first was to explore "students' perceptions of the risk and protective factors associated with alcohol behaviors among themselves and their peers" (p. 12). The second aim focused on students' knowledge and the influence of substance use policies. McCulloh et al. found stress and environmental influences were risk factors as were lack of addiction education and nursing school expectations. Protective factors included influence from peers, perceived reputation, and nursing program policies.

The existence of substance abuse policies related to nursing students in the United States was examined in a descriptive scoping study conducted by McCulloh Nair, Nemeth, Sommers, and Newman (2015). Their findings include inconsistencies in several important areas: prelicensure requirements, education on substance use disorder in nursing, obligation of faculty to report impaired practice, disciplinary actions toward students found to abuse substances, and the limited accessibility of ATD programs for students. Although acknowledging difficulty with implementation, McCulloh et al. suggest a national uniformity of policy regarding nursing students with problematic substance use. This might go a long way toward ensuring students who had problems with substances in nursing school enter the profession as safe, healthy practitioners.

Boulton and O'Connell (2017) investigated perceived faculty support, stress, and substance misuse in nursing students. Although the response rate for this cross-sectional survey was low (9.95%), findings warrant discussion. It is not surprising that students were found to experience a moderate level of stress and may use substances in order to cope with that stress; the risk of using substances increased with increased levels of stress. Although faculty support was seen as a protective factor, students experienced only moderate levels of faculty support. Perhaps most importantly are conclusions highlighting the importance of recognizing problematic substance use in nursing students as it has been found repeatedly that nurses often identify using substances as students.

A common thread in the literature about impaired nursing practice is that awareness and education need to begin in schools of nursing, yet there is limited documentation of specific content and specific outcomes. Stewart and Mueller (2018) report on the initiation of an education strategy in two prelicensure programs (BSN and MN) to "improve nursing students' knowledge, skills, and attitudes about SUD among nurses" (p. 132). Assignments were tailored to online and classroom environments and included readings, video viewing, lecture, and the completion of a case study. Moderated peer discussion of the case study was included, with an estimated time for module completion of 6 to 9 hours. Outcomes were assessed using a quiz and the

Perception of Nursing Impairment Inventory (PNII), which was given as a pre- and posttest. Both groups of students showed improvement in mean scores of the PNII; however, only two factors were statistically significant ("orientation of need to know" and "perception of recognizability"). Especially important is the finding of recognizability as this highlights students' perceived confidence in identifying an impaired peer, which many studies have found is one component of underreporting. Considering the long-term impact to decrease the prevalence of impaired nurses and improve return to work processes, the authors highlight the importance of viewing the issue longitudinally, for example, what impact will this learning have on these students as practicing nurses? Stewart and Mueller recommend that all schools of nursing consider the importance of adding content about "the prevention and awareness of SUD among nurses into their curricula" (p. 135).

Ross et al. (2017) conducted a critical integrative literature review to gain knowledge about the influence of structural factors in a nurse's workplace environment as they related to problematic substance use. Their findings include an overwhelming burden on "individual culpability and failing" (p. 1) that dominates the literature. In addition, they found a gap in published literature that explored the impact of structural factors as a driving force in nurses' problematic substance use (Research Fuels the Controversy 17.1).

Although there is no consistent theme in recent literature on substance use disorder among nurses, nursing students, and health care professionals generally, it is encouraging to note that research is being conducted and that the topic remains active. However, without comprehensive empirically based research, there is limited help for the profession to move closer toward prevention, recognition, management, and resolution of the problem, if indeed resolution is even possible.

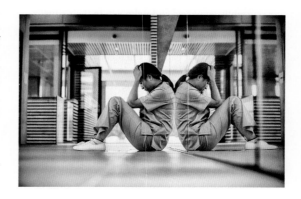

Research Fuels the Controversy 17.1

A Critical Review of Knowledge on Nurses with Problematic Substance Use: The Need to Move From Individual Blame to Awareness of Structural Factors

Source: Ross, C. A., Berry, N. S., Smye, V., & Goldner, E. M. (2017). A critical review of knowledge on nurses with problematic substance use: The need to move from individual blame to awareness of structural factors. *Nursing Inquiry, 25*(4). doi:10.1111/nin.12215

Study Findings

Initially the authors of this review about nurses with problematic substance use found the literature was predominately focused on the individual in terms of risk factors. As the review shifted to literature about policy and treatment approaches, they found a predominant "focus on the culpability, shortcomings, and correction of individuals" (p. 2). Pursuant to this initial finding they noted a lack of critical scholarly inquiry into structural influences that might contribute to a nurse's substance use. The term "structural factors" refers to both micro- and macrolevels of the "physical, social, economic, and policy environments that shape individuals' risk" (p. 2) as related to problematic substance use. The review was organized around contributing factors, policies, and professional nursing culture.

Contributory Factors

Access: The literature was both exclusionary and overemphasized access as a chief contributor toward substance use. This focus (which they found to be unsubstantiated) meant there was limited investigation into less explored aspects of other, perhaps significant structural stressors.

Stress: The stress caused by working conditions seemed to be accepted as the reality of health care and therefore was not measured as an important structural factor for consideration in terms of the policy environment. A superficial treatment of structural stressors was noted in the literature and blame was reallocated back to individual nurses. In other words, nurses do not cope with or have a "correct" attitude toward the challenges they face in the workplace.

Attitudes: Attitudes toward nurses' use of medications was also focused on the individual in that problematic substance use arose from "faulty attitudes and poor choices" (p. 4) of individual nurses. It was proposed that the notion of cultural logic and the risk environmental model may better explain and drive risk behaviors. In the conclusion on attitudes, Ross et al. state,

> Nowhere in this review were works found that endorsed any educational initiatives geared toward targeting structural factors, such as capacity-building education aimed to empower nurses with the knowledge and skills necessary to advocate for improving the working conditions that increase their vulnerability to substance-related harms (p. 5)

Policies for Treatment of Nurses With Problematic Substance Use

This aspect of the literature review addressed treatment from an historical perspective, from initial punitive measures (still in effect in some states) to alternative to discipline (ATD) approaches (with proven successes). Although ATD approaches are more progressive than discipline, Ross et al. believe they have substantial limitations in that the focus was on individual factors and health manifestations. Ross et al. propose that the insistent focus at policy level on the individual both "reflects and perpetuates existing structural inequities situated in sociocultural norms within the professional nursing culture that marginalize and stigmatize nurses with problematic substance use" (p. 5).

Professional Nursing Culture

Stigma and negative attitudes toward nurses with problematic substance use persist in nursing despite efforts of ATD programs that offer support and return to work policies. However, there was a small body of evidence that highlighted the value of peer support and that peer education has resulted in positive structural interventions.

The authors conclude that individual failing and culpability is a very narrow view of nurses with problematic substance use and that changes to structural factors in working conditions and education to intensify peer support are critical recommendations. The other essential area to be addressed is "actively engaging policy-makers, employers and professional bodies in creating safe, healthy workplaces for nurses" (p. 6).

Discussion Point

Why hasn't more nursing research been conducted that explores the experiences and perspectives of nurses with a substance use disorder?

Identifying Early Risk Factors for Substance Abuse

The very nature of the work of nurses seems to be challenged when risk factors are considered. Nurses have constant access to narcotics, and fatigue seems to come with the job, no matter what shift is worked. It is difficult to avoid job strain in the current health care environment, which is in the middle of the worst nursing shortage ever reported. Despite the difficulties inherent in the practice setting today, many nurses do work hard to get experience and increase knowledge so they can become specialists, only to find this, too, can put them at higher risk of turning to drugs or alcohol when coping is difficult. These issues highlight the complexity of the problem for the profession, requiring that all nurses become more aware of how to prevent it from occurring.

Discussion Point

Workplace risk factors for nurses include access, stress, lack of education, and attitude. Whose responsibility is it to address these issues?

Darbo and Malliarakis (2012) analyzed specific risk factors that affect nurses. They identified them as specialty, gender, and workplace, as well as the more general risk factors that apply to everyone. Unique to the article is the discussion of what is termed "protective factors" that would assist nurses to avoid destructive coping that leads to a substance use disorder as well as to recover from an existing problem. Identification of risk factors has been presented in previous literature; the more interesting component of the article is discussion of the protective factors. Workplace protective factors include work satisfaction, workplace social support, and workplace constraints regarding use. Identifying these areas highlights the importance of the role of the workplace and employers in the prevention and support for nurses with a substance use problem and those nurses who might be at risk.

Although risk factors on the surface seem critical to addressing problematic substance use in nurses, perhaps the focus should expand to identifying the behavior(s) or cue(s) to assist with early detection in individual nurses. This expansion might also help to address the barriers to seeking assistance. One aim of an investigation by Cares et al. (2015)

was to identify early detection behaviors and barriers to seeking treatment by nurses who use substances. The authors surveyed nurses who had participated in a peer assistance program in one state. Behavior cues, such as changes in physical condition, pain medication discrepancies, absenteeism, increase in wastage of drugs, missing doses, and barriers to self-report, such as fear, embarrassment, confidentiality concerns, and loss of license, were among the findings. One important conclusion reached was that participants (just over one-third) thought that their impairment was so obvious that a peer or their employer could have recognized it sooner. This finding highlights the importance of education and awareness practices that could assist nurses to identify behavior cues of problematic substance use.

National: Impaired Practice Position and Policies

For policies to be in place at the local level, it is imperative that there be support from leading national nursing organizations about impaired practice. The ANA (2015) position about impaired practice can be found on its website under the recently updated Code of Ethics with Interpretative Statements, 3.6 Patient Protection and Impaired Practice. The ANA supports treatment as opposed to discipline and a process that facilitates reentry of the recovered nurse back into practice (ANA, 2015).

The American Association of Colleges of Nursing (AACN, 1998) focuses on policy development in nursing education. Their policy was written in 1994 and updated in 1998. The AACN's policy can be found on its website. The policy has guidelines for prevention and management of substance abuse in the nursing education community. There are specific features that address the issue for students, faculty, and staff. Critical to successful policy development is attention to confidentiality and legal perspectives. From the perspective of process and content, the necessary areas are identification, intervention, evaluation, treatment, and reentry into practice. The AACN is in agreement with the ANA regarding the importance of treatment over a reasonable time frame and a process for successful reentry into practice.

The NCSBN (2018) published *Substance Use Disorder in Nursing*, and the manual can be found on their website. The purpose of the *Substance Use Disorder in Nursing* manual "is to provide practical and evidence-based guidelines for evaluating, treating and managing nurses with a substance use disorder" (NCSBN, 2011, p. 16). The NCSBN has also more recently published several brochures (NCSBN, 2014) and videos (NCSBN, 2013) on the topic that serve as "quick guides" for nurses to read and view. As with the AACN and the ANA, the NCSBN supports early detection and treatment of the impaired nurse, with the goal of returning a recovered nurse to work. National nursing organizations support ATD programs in the treatment of substance use disorder in nursing.

Local: Impaired Practice Policies in the Workplace

In keeping with the position at the national level, it is imperative that health care organizations and educational institutions have a policy in place about impaired practice that clearly identifies the process to be followed if problematic substance use is suspected. A commitment to a drug- and alcohol-free educational setting or workplace environment is critical to policy development. Although not specifically a policy, Leverence (2015) proposes that discussion about impaired practice begins during the hiring process. Leverence suggests that at this time, expectations about a drug-free workplace should be raised and medication administration prac tices should be discussed (including drug diversion prevention/waste protocols). Reviewing information about identifying an impaired colleague and hospital guidelines for reporting should also be included during the hiring interview.

Nurses Reporting an Impaired Colleague—Issues and Ethics

It is a difficult and often traumatic experience for a nurse to report an impaired colleague. The important considerations are that patients are not harmed, the nurse is helped, and the provider is protected. It is the responsibility of every nurse to be aware of reporting requirements when a colleague is suspected of problematic substance use or of diverting drugs for personal use. No uniform agreement exists among the states as to what those reporting requirements are. Information regarding reporting requirements can be found from each State Board of Nursing, which often can be easily accessed via its website. Before a nurse can be reported or referred to a treatment program, there must be recognition that the nurse needs help. It might not be easy to recognize that a nurse is impaired or suspect drug diversion. This has been addressed in the literature as an area in which nurses lack knowledge and skills, making them uncomfortable to act.

> *Consider This*   Considering your nursing education, practice experience, and workplace support, how comfortable do you feel about recognizing and reporting an impaired colleague?

In theory, reporting an impaired nurse seems like a decision that would be easy to make. The position of the ANA (2015) is clear: It is the ethical and legal duty of a nurse to advocate for public safety, their colleagues, and the profession. This means simply that it is a nurse's job to protect the patient from harm; if that means reporting an impaired colleague that is what one must do. In practice, however, the situation is anything but clear.

Research conducted with both nurses and physicians suggests that although both groups of professionals understand the need for reporting an impaired colleague, most do not report (Bettinardi-Angres & Bologeorges, 2011; DesRoches et al., 2011). Previous literature suggests there is a "code of silence" about impaired practice. However, these studies suggest there are also other reasons responsible for a lack of peer reporting.

In the DesRoches et al. (2011) study, the main reason physicians did not report seemed to be that they thought someone else was dealing with the problem. However, Bettinardi-Angres and Bologeorges (2011) found that the reasons were more complex. These authors identified barriers such as lack of general knowledge of substance abuse in the workplace, lack of a clear protocol or process for reporting or intervening, and lack of compassion in the workplace for peers. They also found that the word *confrontation* itself was a barrier to reporting and that perhaps more compassionate terminology would help, such as assisting a nurse, addressing a problem, and so forth.

Cook (2013) examined direct care nurses' ability to trust nurses in recovery from substance use disorders reentering the workplace. Although other research has highlighted the reluctance of nurses to report an impaired colleague, this small quantitative study found that most nurses would report a nurse colleague that was impaired in a variety of circumstances including alcohol, illegal drugs, prescription medication, and drug diversion. Nearly 75% of nurses had worked with an impaired colleague in their career. Although nurses were willing to work with nurses recovering from alcohol (96%) or drug addiction (90%), they were less likely to trust a nurse who had diverted medication from patients (61%). The majority of nurses thought their recovering colleagues should be allowed to return to work in health care.

An important implication of Cook's (2013) study is that most nurses wanted to help nurses in recovery but were not knowledgeable about substance use disorder generally, how to help a colleague, or find support about treatment programs. Other studies about the specific concept of trust could not be found, but further investigation in this area might improve understanding about how to better educate nurses about substance use disorder in the profession as well as providing support for nurses in recovery when they return to work. Although the removal of all barriers might not be realistic, Cook's findings that nurses were willing to report an impaired colleague suggest that some barriers might be lessening.

Drug Diversion

Identifying and investigating drug diversion is a current topic in health care literature and is critical to consider when examining impaired nursing practice. The American Society of Health-System Pharmacists (ASHP) advocates that best practices to detect and prevent drug diversion be in place in all health care facilities. In 2017, the ASHP published guidelines on preventing diversion of controlled substances. The ASHP challenges organizations to establish a controlled substance policy that not only discourages diversion but "strengthens accountability, rapidly identifies suspected diversion and responds to known or suspected diversion incidents" (p. 328). This organization also recognizes the ongoing process this requires, including continual review and improvement with robust organizational oversight. Although these guidelines focus mainly on the role of pharmacists in prevention and investigation of drug diversion, nursing cannot be complacent in its role in these processes.

New (2016a, 2016b, 2016c), a specialist in controlled substance security and regulatory compliance, highlights the complexity of harm that drug diversion causes to the patient when they are given less than a prescribed medication, receive substandard care by an impaired nurse, or contract an infection when there is medication tampering (Centers for Disease Control and Prevention, 2017). Harm is also extended to peers who cover for the impaired nurse or make up for errors committed. New discusses the rise in medication tampering, indicating the most effective way to prevent tampering is to make it difficult to divert. New (2016c) also emphasizes the importance of internal reporting, irrespective of the quantity. Finally, New (2014) stresses the importance of all health care facilities to have in place comprehensive preemployment screening, drug security, and diversion-risk rounds, and a clear policy in place for investigation of drug diversion if it is suspected.

Wright (2013) examined factors that contribute to drug diversion that have been identified elsewhere, such as increases in workload, mandatory overtime, floating to unfamiliar units, fatigue, and medical issues requiring the need for prescription pain medication. A common factor identified in the literature is the easy access nurses have to controlled substances. Other issues identified that contribute to the problem are the reluctance of nurses to believe that a trusted colleague is diverting drugs. Wright highlights the importance of professional awareness in recognizing and combating drug diversion and presents eight strategies to identify and detect drug diversion. Although identification and detection are critical, only one of the eight strategies focuses on education programs about stress management and coping techniques that might prevent drug diversion before it occurs.

Investigated by a medical center were three dimensions related to workplace access that influenced diverting behaviors. These included "perceived availability of controlled substances, frequency of administration, and the degree of workplace control" (Rohman, 2012, p. 29). Following a lengthy process of trial and error, the facility adopted a drug diversion surveillance program that included a public safety officer, the director of public safety, director of pharmacy, and appropriate nurse leaders. This process identified nurses who were diverting drugs. An unexpected outcome of this process was an increased awareness of direct care nurses about appropriate policies and procedures for medication administration that were not being followed.

There exist regulatory and legal risks to employers as well as negative publicity to the community when the effects of drug diversion are made public (Brummond et al., 2017). The significance of education for all health care workers cannot be overlooked, as many may not be aware of the serious nature of the problem.

Boulton and Nosek (2014) suggest that nursing students are not taught how to recognize an impaired colleague or what to do about it if they did. For nurse educators, are students being taught how to keep themselves healthy as they deal with the often traumatic nature of nursing? If not, this means the new generation of nursing graduates may not have the necessary tools to help address this serious problem. If schools of nursing do not consider this content a critical component of the curriculum, how is the problem ever going to be satisfactorily addressed? What are health care facilities doing to prevent or discourage drug diversion prior to it occurring? For nurse leaders, are nurses working in a toxic environment that is fraught with short staffing, trauma, and stress that can all contribute to a nurse turning to drug diversion as a way to cope? The challenge then becomes not only putting in place surveillance programs to detect and investigate drug diversion but also putting in place mechanisms to support a population of nurses that are increasingly being taxed to their limit so that they remain healthy and their patients remain safe. Box 17.2 lists some of the common methods of drug diversion.

BOX 17.2   **Common Methods of Diversion**

- Removal of medication when a patient does not need it
- Removal of medication for a discharged patient
- Removal of a duplicate dose
- Removal of fentanyl patches
- Removal of medication without an order
- Removal under a colleague's sign-on
- Substitution of a noncontrolled substance for a controlled substance
- Theft of patient medications brought from home
- Failure to waste when indicated
- Frequent wasting of entire doses

Source: New, K. (2014). Preventing, detecting, and investigating drug diversion in health care facilities. *Journal of Nursing Regulation, 5*(1), 18–23.

Discussion Point

You suspect that a coworker/friend is diverting drugs for personal use. You find yourself covering up for her because you know that she is depressed, exhausted, and having family problems. Your supervisor makes a casual comment with similar suspicions. Your first instinct is to make excuses for your friend; what would you do?

Consider This   Most addiction specialists and the American Medical Association view addiction as a chronic medical illness and argue that it should be approached in an analogous way to, say, diabetes or asthma.

Alternative to Discipline Programs

The current state of programs and resources to assist nurses with substance use disorders was collated by Eisenhut (2016). Eleven states had no program in place, one had a voluntary disciplinary alternative program, and the remaining 38 had some form of peer assistance or ATD program in place. The first treatment program offered in the United States was the Intervention Project for Nurses (IPN, 2016) in Florida in 1983. The IPN has a comprehensive website offering information about the history of the program, including frequently asked questions and available services.

California also offers a diversion program; information is available from the California Board of Registered Nursing (CBRN, 2016). Established in 1985, its goal is to "protect the public by early identification of impaired registered nurses and by providing these nurses access to appropriate intervention programs and treatment services" (para. 2). Impaired nurses can be self-referred or can be referred by family, coworkers, or the board. All licensed registered nurses residing in California are eligible to enter the program, but they must agree to enter the program voluntarily. Since 1985, more than 1,900 nurses have successfully completed the diversion program in California. Requirements for completion include "a change in lifestyle that supports continuing recovery and [having] a minimum of 24 consecutive months of clean, random, body-fluid tests" (para. 8). Law protects confidentiality of participants, and nurses who successfully complete the program have their records regarding chemical impairment destroyed.

A different approach is followed in the Texas Peer Assistance Program (TPAPN, n.d.) for Nurses. This program offers services to nurses suffering from chemical dependency, as well as from anxiety and other mental health disorders. It requires abstinence, maintains confidentiality, is strictly voluntary, and is independent of the state licensing board. Information from the TPAPN website includes how and when to make referrals, how the program works, and important links to services and organizations.

Consider This   Although the majority of states lean toward treatment rather than discipline for substance use problems, some nurses still attach a stigma and think that impaired nurses should be punished and not allowed to return to work.

The Recovered Nurse: Reentry Into Practice

When a nurse has completed a treatment or rehabilitation program and is ready to return to work, he or she typically encounters a number of issues. These issues include whether the nurse's practice is limited or restricted in some way, how long the nursing board has a right to invade the nurse's privacy to ensure that recovery is ongoing, where organizational responsibility ends, and who bears the cost if the nurse does not return to work at full capacity. Although maintaining confidentiality of the returning nurse might be a goal, the question remains how this would play out in practice if a nurse has restricted access to narcotics (Box 17.3).

BOX 17.3 **Issues to Consider When the Recovered Nurse Returns to Work**

- Should the nurse returning to work following re-habilitation have his or her practice limited or restricted in some way, such as no exposure to the drug of choice or no access to controlled substances for a period of time?
- How long does the board of nursing have a right to invade the privacy of a recovered nurse?
- Where does the organizational responsibility end?
- Who bears the cost if the recovered nurse is not able to return to work at full capacity?
- Can confidentiality be maintained?
- Should the nurse be allowed to work in stressful practice areas?
- Should the nurse initially be allowed to work full-time?

Although many anecdotal or discussion articles were found on the topic of what constitutes a disciplinary or treatment approach to impaired practice, limited information was found that addressed the concerns of reentry of the impaired nurse to the practice setting.

Matthias-Anderson and Yurkovich (2016) examined the work reentry process of nurses following the completion of a substance use disorder treatment program. Findings from this experiential perspective identified internal and external facilitators and barriers to work reentry. A common internal barrier to reentry by study participants was the negative impact of stigma toward both patients and nurses with substance use disorder. Lack of education was a common external barrier finding. Both these areas are often discussed in the literature but the question needs to be asked and answered as to what strategies need to be employed to change this. The authors conclude that "stressful work environments and a workplace culture that stigmatizes patients with SUDs [substance use disorders] led to nurses internally feeling shame and hiding their own issues regarding SUDs, resulting in not accessing help in a timely manner" (p. 32). The literature analysis by Ross et al. (2017) that addresses the structural factors that contribute to the creation of a stressful work environment may be a first step in resolution.

Employers often require the completion of a return to work agreement or contract between the nurse and the organization. O'Neill and Cadiz (2014) propose that the monitoring of a recovered nurse requires two agreements, one between the nurse and the external body, such as a disciplinary board or ATD program. The second agreement is

with the employer and may be in the form of an individualized contract with the nurse. This document would outline the terms and conditions in which the nurse can return to direct care.

Despite a lack of standardized guidelines, there are some general considerations that should be taken into account when a recovered nurse returns to work. To protect patient safety, practice restrictions may be in place for a varying time, depending on the length of the program and whether it was treatment based or disciplinary action occurred. It is important that staff nurses realize the commitment of the recovering nurse to reestablish his or her career and continue in the profession.

Some State Boards of Nursing have detailed documents about return to work processes. One such state is Massachusetts, which has supported impaired nurses for 30 years with a peer assistance program (Mallia, 2015). The Massachusetts Nurses Association (2011) developed a guidebook of interventions and resources about impaired nursing practice that provides detailed information about topics such as how to assist a nurse with a substance use problem, an algorithm for that process, available resources, legal considerations, and a sample return to work agreement.

Most Board of Registered Nursing websites offer little information about the reentry process. Instead, they focus primarily on what should be done if someone suspects an impaired colleague, how to report it, the treatment or disciplinary action once impairment is identified, and the specific aspects of each program. A question that is left unanswered is how long the board follows a recovered nurse in terms of random drug testing. Some hospitals or health care agencies already do random drug testing, so the question of invasion of privacy has in some instances already been dealt with.

Discussion Point

You just came from a staff meeting at which the nurse-manager informed everyone that a recovered nurse would begin working on the unit in a few weeks. Some nurses had the attitude that the nurse not be allowed back to work because he or she could not be trusted. How would you respond to your colleagues?

Research Dissemination—Is It Happening?

Although there are some new research findings to disseminate, it is important to consider whether the profession and education community are applying/using the available findings. Issues have been raised about student problematic substance use. If you work in an educational setting or interact with students in your workplace, do you know what policies are in place if a student is suspected of impaired practice? Does your educational institution have an ATD program or approach? More important, what is being done in the educational community to address the issue of alcohol and substance use by students that might be affecting their performance in the clinical setting? Is impaired nursing practice part of the nursing curricula? If not, why not? As suggested by the AACN (1998), it is critical that policies regarding impaired practice be clear and in place in the educational community and that all faculty and students be aware of the content of the policy.

The literature clearly supports that impaired practice policies should be in place in every health care setting. However, anecdotal evidence suggests that many nurses in clinical practice have no knowledge of such policies and would not know what to do if they suspected a colleague was impaired. Impaired practice policies, including drug diversion prevention, should be introduced during hospital orientation for new employees and during annual renewal of hospital safety procedures. This would highlight the issue for everyone and put the problem clearly in the spotlight, especially if barriers (such as stigma and fear) to reporting an impaired colleague and prevalence of the problem were discussed. Nurses should be allowed to ask questions so that they are clear about the process of reporting and so that a nurse who is using substances irresponsibly knows where to go for help.

HOW CAN WE STOP LOSING NURSES TO SUBSTANCE ABUSE?

Preventative health care is finally receiving much needed attention in the media and in practice. Insurance companies are increasingly paying for prevention and screening procedures, yet many areas of health care still lag behind what would be ideal for preventative practices. The issue of preventing substance use disorder is no exception to this situation. How can nurses individually and as a profession help to prevent the cycle of nurse addiction from starting?

Some of the risk factors for substance abuse that have been identified are difficult to modify. Nurses will always have easy access to narcotics, do shift work, and suffer from fatigue. The ongoing stress that has worked its way into clinical settings due to the nursing shortage seems a long way from dissipating. What, then, can be done to diminish the effects of these factors so that nurses do not turn to substances as an inappropriate coping mechanism? The impact of structural factors that influence substance use has been

raised in recent literature. What is being done to identify and address this issue?

Perhaps one avenue is to more fully explore the experiences of nurses who do not turn to substances. Do nurses who use self-care strategies to cope with a stressful work environment and to prevent burnout also use those same strategies to avoid harmful substance use? Perhaps this information about how nurses cope with difficulties of the workplace when they do not turn to drugs or alcohol will contribute to prevention.

Where does the education about substance abuse begin? Student nurses need not only to be made aware of the risks of substance abuse but also to be self-aware about their attitudes and beliefs regarding those who do abuse substances, whether those people are patients or colleagues. Nursing school is an incredibly stressful time for students. Not only could appropriate education in nursing school help prevent the onset of substance abuse, it might also allow students to explore their feelings and beliefs about impaired practice. This increased self-awareness might help students have empathy toward impaired nurses and encourage them to take the appropriate steps to assist a nurse or fellow student in getting help.

Nursing is going through a very tumultuous time. The nursing shortage is never far from the minds of most nurses as they struggle on a daily basis with low staffing levels and a stressed work setting. How this stress is channeled can lead a nurse to have positive or negative coping strategies. What are hospitals doing to acknowledge and diffuse this stress? Are nurses too stressed to seek counsel from each other when they have a particularly bad day? Are nurses debriefing with each other or at home so they can let go of the often traumatic nature of work and move forward? Nurses and nurse-managers need to answer these questions for their particular work settings to know whether they are doing enough for themselves, their colleagues, and their staff.

CONCLUSIONS

Losing one nurse to substance abuse is losing one nurse too many. We are a profession known for its caring nature toward others, yet often we fail to care for ourselves. The harmful coping strategies that lead to substance abuse can begin even before nursing school. Educating our students may help us to increase awareness about this ever-present problem. If new graduates can bring current evidence-based information to their nursing practice and be self-aware about their attitudes, beliefs, and coping strategies, then perhaps they can come armed with more positive strategies to help them when times get tough.

Do we teach our students, new graduates, and seasoned nurses to ask for help when they need it, or do we expect them to "do it all?" All nurses who suspect an impaired colleague need to take action as they have an ethical, regulatory, and legal obligation in the interest of patient safety (ANA, 2015). If all nurses are aware of the problem of substance use disorder and take the initiative to intervene when they suspect a colleague of impaired practice, we are one step closer to decreasing the incidence of substance abuse in the nursing profession.

Finally, responsibility rests not just with individual nurses. Educators must accept the challenge to teach students about impaired practice and how to recognize it when they see it and in addition to assist them to develop positive coping strategies so they don't turn to substances to deal with stress. Employers must also accept the challenge to create a safe work environment that supports nurses to deal with stress successfully, to know employees so that confrontation can occur early, to increase awareness about substance abuse so that nurses are not afraid to ask for help, to support nurses if they do suspect drug diversion or an impaired colleague, to ensure that an impaired practice policy is in place, and lastly to provide a process that facilitates reentry into practice following recovery.

For Additional Discussion

1. Explore your attitudes and beliefs about impaired nursing practice. How would you treat a colleague suspected of diverting drugs for personal use? Would you trust a recovered nurse returning to work?

2. What kind of peer support exists in your work setting? How do staff debrief from stressful situations?

3. Should recovered nurses who return to work have a limited practice? If so, for how long, and with what types of limitations? How does this affect the workload of other nurses?

4. What practices are in place in your work setting that could deter a nurse from diverting drugs for personal use?

5. Have you known a colleague who was caught diverting drugs for personal use? If so, how was it handled? Did the nurse seek treatment and return to work? Could it have been managed better?

6. You are a nurse-manager for an intensive care unit and have been asked to talk to student nurses about impaired practice. What key points would you make?

7. Does your workplace have an impaired practice policy in place? If so, have you read it and was it discussed during your initial hospital orientation? Is it discussed annually? If not, what might you do to ensure that one is in place?

References

American Association of Colleges of Nursing. (1998). *Policy and guidelines for prevention and management of substance abuse in the nursing education community.* Retrieved from http://www.aacnnursing.org/News-Information/Position-Statements-White-Papers/

American Nurses Association. (2015). *Code of ethics for nurses with interpretive statements.* Silver Spring, MD: Nursesbooks.org.

Bettinardi-Angres, K., & Bologeorges, S. (2011). Addressing chemically dependent colleagues. *Journal of Nursing Regulation, 2*(2), 10–15.

Boulton, M., & O'Connell, K. A. (2017). Nursing students' perceived faculty support, stress, and substance misuse. *Journal of Nursing Education, 56*(7), 404–411.

Boulton, M. A., & Nosek, L. J. (2014). How do nursing students perceive substance abusing nurses? *Archives of Psychiatric Nursing, 28*, 29–34.

Brummond, P., Chen, D. F., Churchill, W. W., Clark, J. S., Dillon, K. R., Dumitru, D., . . . Smith, J. S. (2017). ASHP guidelines on preventing diversion of controlled substances. *American Journal of Health-System Pharmacists, 74*(5), 325–339.

California Board of Registered Nursing. (2016). *What is the intervention program?* Retrieved from http://www.rn.ca.gov/intervention/whatisint.shtml

Cares, A., Pace, E., Denious, J., & Crane, L. A. (2015). Substance use and mental illness among nurses: Workplace warning signs and barriers to seeking assistance. *Substance Abuse, 36*, 59–66.

Centers for Disease Control and Prevention. (2017). *Risks of healthcare-associated infections from drug diversion.* Retrieved from https://www.cdc.gov/injectionsafety/drug-diversion/index.html

Colorado Board of Nursing (2003). *Resource manual: The impaired nurse.* Retrieved Sept. 4, 2018 from http://www.diversionspecialists.com/wpcontent/uploads/reg52202im72003internet.pdf

Cook, L. M. (2013, March). Can nurses trust nurses in recovery reentering the workplace? *Nursing, 43*(3), 21–24.

Darbo, N., & Malliarakis, K. D. (2012). Substance abuse: Risk factors and protective factors. *Journal of Nursing Regulation, 3*(1), 44–48.

DesRoches, C. M., Rao, S. R., Fromson, R. J., Iezzoni, L., Vogeli, C., & Campbell, E. G. (2011). Physicians' perceptions, preparedness for reporting, and experiences related to impaired and incompetent colleagues. *Journal of the American Medical Association, 304*(2), 187–193.

Eisenhut, B. (2016). Programs and resources to assist nurses with substance use disorders. *Journal of Addictions Nursing, 27*(1), 53–55.

Institute of Medicine. (1999). *To error is human: Building a safer health system.* Retrieved from https://www.nap.edu/catalog/9728/to-err-is-human-building-a-safer-health-system

Intervention Project for Nurses. (2016). *IPN history.* Retrieved from https://ipnfl.org/about

Kunyk, D. (2015). Substance use disorders among registered nurses: Prevalence, risks and perceptions in a disciplinary jurisdiction. *Journal of Nursing Management, 23*, 54–64. doi:10.1111/jonm.12081

Leverence, K. (2015, December). Tackling the taboo of substance abuse among nurses. *ONS Connect, 30*(4), 64.

Mallia, C. (2015). Over 30 years of support to nurses with impaired practice. *Journal of Addictions Nursing, 26*(1), 53–54.

Massachusetts Nurses Association. (2011). *Impaired practice in nursing: A guidebook for interventions and resources.* Canton, MA: Author. Retrieved from http://www.mass-nurses.org/files/file/Nursing-Resources/Nursing-Practice/Impaired_Practice.pdf

Matthias-Anderson, D., & Yurkovich, E. (2016). Work re-entry for RNs after substance use disorder treatment: Implications for the nursing profession. *Journal of Nursing Regulation, 7*(3), 26–32.

McCulloh Nair, J., Nemeth, L. S., Sommers, M., & Newman, S. (2015). Substance abuse policy among nursing students. *Journal of Addictions Nursing, 26*(4), 166–174.

McCulloh Nair, J., Nemeth, L. S., Sommers, M., Newman, S., & Amella, E. (2016). Alcohol use, misuse, and abuse among nursing students. *Journal of Addictions Nursing, 27*(1), 12–23.

National Council of State Boards of Nursing. (2001). *Chemical dependency handbook for nurse managers.* Retrieved from https://www.ncsbn.org/chem_dep_handbook_intro_ch1.pdf

National Council of State Boards of Nursing. (2018a). *Substance use disorder in nursing.* Retrieved from https://www.ncsbn.org/substance-use-in-nursing.htm

National Council of State Boards of Nursing. (2011). *Substance use disorder in nursing: A resource manual and guidelines for alternative and disciplinary monitoring programs.* Retrieved from https://www.ncsbn.org/SUDN_11.pdf

National Council of State Boards of Nursing. (2013). *Substance use disorder in nursing (video).* Retrieved from https://www.ncsbn.org/333.htm

National Council of State Boards of Nursing. (2014). *A nurse manager's guide to substance use disorder in nursing (brochure).* Retrieved from https://www.ncsbn.org/3692.htm

National Institute on Drug Abuse. (2015). *Nationwide trends.* Retrieved from https://www.drugabuse.gov/publications/drugfacts/nationwide-trends

New, K. (2014). Preventing, detecting, and investigating drug diversion in health care facilities. *Journal of Nursing Regulation, 5*(1), 18–25.

New, K. (2016a). *Recognizing drug diversion in health care facilities.* Retrieved from http://www.diversionspecialists.com/wp-content/uploads/Signs-of-diversion-brochure-multi-color-3.pdf

New, K. (2016b). *Considerations when tampering occurs.* Association of Healthcare Internal Auditors, Fall. Retrieved from http://www.diversionspecialists.com/wp-content/uploads/Considerations-When-Tampering-Occurs.pdf

New, K. (2016c). *We have confirmed diversion: Now what?* Association of Healthcare Internal Auditors, Summer. Retrieved from http://www.diversionspecialists.com/wp-content/uploads/ControlledSubstanceSecurity-WeHaveConfirmedDiversion-NowWhatbyKimNew-2.pdf

Nutty, A. (2016, August/September). Nursing and substance use disorder: An occupational hazard. *Alaska Nurse, 67*(4), 6–7.

O'Neill, C., & Cadiz, D. (2014). Worksite monitors protect patients from unsafe nursing practices. *Journal of Nursing Regulation, 5*(2), 22.

Relias Media. (2017). *For addicted nurses, a way back to the bedside.* Retrieved from https://www.reliasmedia.com/articles/139690-for-addicted-nurses-a-way-back-to-the-bedside

Rohman, C. (2012). Roads to recovery: Drug diversion surveillance programs. *Nursing Management, 43*(3), 28–31.

Ross, C. A., Berry, N. S., Smye, V., & Goldner, E. M. (2017). A critical review of knowledge on nurses with problematic substance use: The need to move from individual blame to awareness of structural factors. *Nursing Inquiry, 25*(4). doi:10.1111/nin.12215

Stewart, D. M., & Mueller, C. A. (2018). Substance use disorder among nurses: A curriculum improvement initiative. *Nurse Educator, 43*(3), 132–135.

Strobbe, S., & Crowley, M. (2017). Substance use among nurses and nursing students. *Journal of Addictions Nursing, 28*(2), 104–106.

Texas Nurses Association. (n.d.). *Texas peer assistance program for nurses.* Retrieved from http://www.texasnurses.org/?page=TPAPN

Wright, R. L. (2013). Drug diversion in nursing practice: A call for professional accountability to recognize and respond. *Journal of the Association of Occupational Health Professionals in Healthcare, 33*(1), 27–30.

Academic Integrity in Nursing Education
Is It Declining?

George C. Pittman

LEARNING OBJECTIVES

The learner will be able to:

1. Identify types of cheating common in nursing programs.
2. Identify variables that contribute to integrity failures.
3. Discuss possible reasons for academic dishonesty.
4. Discuss consequences of a lack of academic integrity in nursing programs.
5. Identify methods/strategies to ensure academic integrity and decrease cheating.
6. Analyze conditions that promote academic integrity or that promote cheating.
7. Discuss barriers to self-reporting cheating or reporting others for cheating.
8. Reflect on his or her individual willingness to report other students for cheating.

INTRODUCTION

Loschiavo (2015) suggests that cheating in college has occurred since the inception of higher education and that much of this cheating appears to take shape in high school, with 64% of 24,000 students at 70 high schools admitting to cheating on a test, 58% admitting to plagiarism, and 95% saying they participated in some form of cheating, whether it was on a test, plagiarism, or copying homework. Data from another large national study indicated that 51% of high school students admit that they have cheated during a test ("Why Students at Prestigious High Schools," 2018).

The cell phone appears to be a cheating vector for many of these teenagers, with one out of three students in grades 7 through 12 admitting they used their cell phones to cheat on tests and 65% saying other kids in their schools are using their cell phones to cheat ("The Latest Ways That Kids Cheat on Exams," 2009). In addition, more than half the cheaters said they texted or used their cell phones to call friends to warn them of pop quizzes, and only half of the students believed that using their cell phones to cheat during tests was a serious offense.

Equally disconcerting, Buchmann (2014) suggests that about 75% of college students admit to cheating, and that probably even more than three-quarters of college students have done something against the rules to improve their grades. "With an increasingly competitive atmosphere and a culture that some say is more accepting of cheating than it was in past generations, cheating has sadly become a somewhat expected phenomenon at universities across the country" (Buchmann, 2014, para. 2). For example, the number of students caught cheating at Russell Group universities rose 40% between 2014–2015 and 2016–2017 (Lodhia, 2018).

Indeed, in recent months, cases of cheating, including large-scale cheating at elite colleges, have become front-page headlines. For example, Buchmann (2014) notes that in May 2012, a teaching fellow for a government class at Harvard started noticing similarities between students' final exams that shouldn't have been there. The professor brought the case forward, and it was discovered that approximately 125 students—nearly half the entire lecture class—had been cheating. Buchmann (2014) concluded "that if students at Harvard—the most prestigious school in the world—can be caught cheating in large numbers, it's safe to assume that cheating happens on every campus much more often than we would like to think" (para. 1).

Similarly, in 2017, students at the prestigious Stuyvesant High School in New York were caught sharing answers to Spanish assignments via a Facebook group. This followed a highly publicized incident that occurred at Stuyvesant several years before, when students were caught cheating on a language examination via text messaging ("Why Students at Prestigious High Schools," 2018).

Statistics are similar in online courses. Morgan (2018) suggests that 30% of all online test takers bring an unpermitted resource (class notes, scratch paper, a calculator, or another unauthorized element) to their exam. This means that without proctor supervision, almost 600,000 items would have gone unnoticed before an exam in 2017 alone.

> **Consider This** "It's no secret that students cheat" (Online Degree Programs, 2012). Indeed, research increasingly suggests that cheating from middle school through college is epidemic.

> **Discussion Point**
>
> Does a legacy of cheating exist in academe today? Are cheating cultures accepted or even condoned in contemporary secondary and collegiate settings?

CHEATING IN NURSING EDUCATION

Nurses are viewed as among the most trustworthy, ethical, and honest professionals in American society. From 1999 to 2016, *Gallup* polls found between 79% and 85% of respondents viewed the honesty and ethical standards of nurses as high to very high (Gallup, 2016). It would seem to follow, then, that nursing students would exhibit high or very high ethical standards. The comment of a student who participated in a longitudinal study on academic dishonesty illustrated this view: "I think that . . . the type of people who

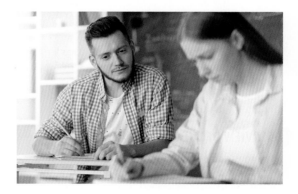

choose to go into nursing . . . results in less cheating than in other disciplines" (McCabe, 2009). Unfortunately, the data don't support this assumption.

Cheating is a concern in any academic discipline. It is of particular concern to nursing educators because nurses hold the well-being and health of their patients in their hands. Lapses of integrity can have grave consequences for patients. It follows, then, that nursing educators and leaders must inculcate the highest standards of honesty and integrity in students to create a culture of trustworthiness in the nurses who graduate from their programs. Although there isn't a great deal of data that define the link between academic integrity and professional integrity, there is some evidence, beyond the intuitive, that there is a correlation.

Lapses in academic integrity can take many forms. Cheating in the classroom can include copying answers from another's exam sheet, offering answers to exam questions to another student, soliciting answers to exam questions from students who have already taken the exam, collaborating with other students on assignments when collaboration is not allowed, quoting without appropriate attribution, using disallowed materials to get answers on exams or quizzes, or any of a myriad of practices that pass another's work as one's own. It can also include downloading papers from the Internet, taking photos of tests and posting them online, hiring someone to take their online tests, purchasing an instructor's version of a book to get copies of tests and answers, and faking test scores or letters of recommendation for employers or academic pursuits.

In the clinical setting, dishonest practices include recording vital signs that weren't actually taken or recorded accurately, reporting medications as given that were not administered, reporting patient/client responses to treatment that weren't observed, attempting procedures without adequate knowledge or asking for guidance from the instructor, breaking sterile technique without reporting it or replacing contaminated items, and discussing protected client information in public places or with nonmedical personnel (McCrink, 2010).

Discussion Point

Do you believe that students who lack academic integrity are more likely to demonstrate the same behaviors in clinical practice?

OVERVIEW OF THE LITERATURE

Numerous studies of nursing students' academic misconduct have been published in the past 30 years. Two of the earliest studies were by Hilbert in 1985, with a follow-up

study in 1987. Other studies that documented academic dishonesty among nursing students were conducted by Bailey (2001), Beasley (2014), Gaberson (1997), Krueger (2014), McCabe (2009), McCrink (2010), Sheer (1989), Stonecypher and Willson (2014), and Woith, Jenkins, and Kerber (2012). These studies, and others, indicate that nursing students engage in a wide variety of dishonest academic practices in both the classroom and clinical settings. More than just documenting the size of the problem, these studies examined the attitudes among nursing students that caused them to engage in these behaviors as well as the strategies that may be employed to deter such behavior. These studies also suggest that students engage in a variety of rationalizations to explain their misconduct such as time constraints, unfair course assignments, and the unrealistic expectations of nursing faculty, among others (McCrink, 2010).

Prevalence of the Problem in Nursing

The question of whether academic dishonesty is rising among nursing students may not be answerable. However, there is considerable evidence that such behavior is common. McCrink (2010) studied nursing students in two associate degree nursing programs in the northeastern United States (193 respondents) and found a mean score of 21.58 (range 19–95, SD 3.46) for frequency of self-reported misconduct. Krueger (2014) found that 216 of 334 (64.7%) participants admitted to engaging in some form of academic dishonesty in the classroom setting and that 181 of 335 (54%) engaged in academic dishonesty in the clinical setting.

Similarly disconcerting data were noted in a study by McCabe (2009) that involved nursing students from 12 schools. A request to participate was sent to 6,290 students, and 1,057 responses were received (a return of 16.8%). He found that more than half of the undergraduate students and almost half of the graduate students self-reported engaging in one or more of 16 behaviors identified as classroom cheating.

Clearly, there is cause for concern. Moreover, because all these studies involved self-reporting of academic dishonesty, there is likely considerable underreporting. As one of McCabe's (2009) participants put it, "I think that you may have difficulty generating accurate statistics. I don't think that people who cheat are willing to give out that information." In an article in the *British Journal of Nursing*, Glasper reported that 1,700 nursing students of a population of 64,000 student nurses (2.6%) over a 3-year period had been found guilty of cheating (Glasper, 2016). Although it might seem that British nursing students are more honest than American nursing students, it's important to note that Glasper was writing about nursing students convicted of cheating, while McCrink, Krueger, and McCabe studied nursing students who self-reported cheating by themselves or their peers, without necessarily being caught and found guilty.

There also seems to be a correlation between self-reported cheating in the classroom and self-reported cheating in the clinical setting. Krueger (2014) found a statistically significant correlation between the two behaviors ($r = 0.42$, $p < 0.01$). This correlation suggests that students who cheat in the classroom are likely to cheat in the clinical setting as well.

McCrink's (2010) data recorded the most common self-reported behaviors of academic dishonesty as discussing clients in public or with nonmedical personnel (35.3%), paraphrasing material without appropriate attribution (35.2%), working collaboratively when it was not allowed (24.3%), obtaining test questions from other students (21.8%), and recording vital signs that were not taken or recorded accurately (13%; Box 18.1). Moreover, 8.8% of McCrink's (2010) respondents reported recording client treatments that were neither performed nor observed, 6.7% reported they'd recorded client responses to treatment they hadn't observed, and 2.1% reported they'd recorded administration of medications that had not been administered.

Discussion Point

What do you believe is driving these significant numbers of self-reported academic dishonesty? Is it a quest for a higher grade? For recognition of success? Is it driven by more intrinsic or extrinsic factors?

Another finding by Krueger (2014) was also disturbing. In her study of 335 participants in two associate degree nursing programs in the Midwest, 329 participants (98.2%) believed that plagiarism occurs at their college, and 97 participants (28.9%) reported witnessing another student cheating. Further, 291 of 329 participants (88.4%) said they'd never reported an incident of cheating, and 74 of 332 (22.3%) believed that the typical student would never report an incident of cheating they observed. In a recent student survey of graduating students in the author's nursing program, graduating students rated the academic integrity of their classmates at a mean of 3.58, the lowest score of the questions related to how these students viewed their classmates. Students who had reported cheating to the faculty were extremely reluctant to name the students they'd observed cheating. This, of course, makes taking action against the perpetrators even more difficult. Another consequence of this reluctance is that a policy to assure academic integrity by catching and punishing offenders is almost certain to fail.

Why Do Students Cheat?

Many researchers have explored the question of why students cheat, and the responses are varied. Running out of the time needed to complete an assignment correctly or to study for an exam adequately is the most common reason students give for cheating (Colorado State University [CSU], 1993–2015). A second reason students give for cheating is not having fully understood the material or assignment at hand. In addition, sloppy note-taking leads to unintentional plagiarism, which is often treated just as seriously as intentional plagiarism (CSU, 1993–2015).

Woith et al. (2012) found that student participants identified competition among students for grades as fostering an environment conducive to cheating. Buchmann (2014) suggests that competitive pressures placed on children at a very young age carry on with them through high school and college. With so much pressure to stand out as the smartest

---

BOX 18.1   **Commonly Self-Reported Types of Academic Dishonesty by Nursing Students**

- Discussing clients in public places or with nonmedical personnel
- Paraphrasing material without appropriate attribution
- Working collaboratively on assignments or tests when it was not allowed
- Obtaining test questions from other students
- Recording vital signs that were not taken or recorded accurately
- Recording client treatments that were neither performed nor observed
- Recording administration of medications that had not been administered
- Reporting patient/client responses to treatment that weren't observed
- Attempting procedures without adequate knowledge or asking the instructor for guidance
- Breaking sterile technique without reporting it or replacing contaminated items

in a class, some students may give in to the opportunity to succeed at the price of integrity.

Another reason cited by participants as pressures that led to cheating were the time constraints related to acquiring a vast amount of knowledge in the short period offered by nursing programs (typically, approximately 2 years). Krueger (2014) found that participants in her study who worked more than 40 hours per week rated academic dishonesty as more ethical than participants who worked 1 to 10 hours per week.

Institutional apathy has also been identified as a reason why students cheat (Buchmann, 2014). Students may cheat when they do not see the academic environment as one that deserves their honesty. "Just like cheating at Monopoly is easier to justify than tax evasion, if students don't believe their university deserves high standards then they may see no reason to follow all the rules about grading. Lack of respect for the collegiate institution may also prevent students from reporting instances of dishonesty they see around them" (Buchmann, 2014, para. 8).

Buchmann (2014) suggests that self-interest is also a factor in why people cheat and that this factor appears to encompass all cheating. Students who cheat hope to see a return on their investment of time and resources in college, and watching someone else make a better grade can be painful. "With only his or herself in mind, cheating is hard not to justify when someone can get away with it" (Buchmann, 2014, para. 10).

Lodhia (2018) agrees, noting that tuition fees and the stress of securing a job mean that some students are fixated on exam results, rather than intellectual development. "For students, the pressure to succeed has never been greater due to the increased cost attached to learning as well as the seeming necessity for students to get jobs as soon as they graduate. Both of these factors have led to an environment where results and grades are more important than scholarship and intellectual development and ultimately undermine the entire purpose of universities" (Lodhia, 2018, para. 2).

Reasons that students identify as compelling them to cheat are provided in Box 18.2.

Learning theory also offers insight into the development of a culture of cheating. As Krueger (2014) found in her study, students who witness other students engaging in academically dishonest behavior or who believe their peers are cheating are, themselves, more likely to cheat. The study of Woith et al. (2012) had this same observation. This was one of the situational conditions related to cheating that Krueger (2014) identified for her study. The other two were consequences and enforcement of academic dishonesty policies, and the students' personal beliefs and values

---

BOX 18.2 **Why Students May Feel Compelled to Cheat**

- Procrastination on assignments and studying
- Time constraints
- Not fully understanding the material or assignment at hand
- Sloppy note-taking, leading to unintentional plagiarism
- Competition for grades or success
- Ambiguous attitudes among students about what qualifies as cheating
- Institutional apathy
- Self-interest

Source: Buchmann, B. (2014, February 20). *Cheating in college: Where it happens, why students do it and how to stop it.* The Huffington Post. Retrieved May 28, 2015, from http://www.huffingtonpost.com/uloop/cheating-in-college-where_b_4826136.html; Colorado State University. (1993–2015). *Why do students cheat?* Retrieved June 10, 2018, from https://tilt.colostate.edu/integrity/resourcesFaculty/whyDoStudents.cfm

---

related to cheating and academic honesty. Krueger's study found that students generally perceived that the risk of being caught was high and the consequences severe. Krueger also found a significant negative correlation between a commitment to integrity and the occurrence of dishonest behaviors. In other words, students who valued integrity highly cheated less. These findings suggest some possible approaches to deterring cheating.

Simola (2017) uses the discipline of behavioral ethics to propose several steps to prevent academic dishonesty. In her discussion of students' perceptions of sanctioning systems, or punishment, she makes the observation that the use of punishment or sanctions for academic dishonesty may induce students to use a calculative decision-making process rather than an ethical one. In this model, the student focuses on the probability and cost of getting caught, rather than on the ethical question of whether academic dishonesty is right or wrong (Simola, 2017).

Student Attitudes Regarding Academic Dishonesty

There seems to be some disagreement among nursing students as to what constitutes academic dishonesty, and even more disagreement as to the seriousness of the conduct described. Most students in McCrink's (2010) study agreed that reporting vital signs that aren't taken is highly or severely unethical. Similarly, falsely reporting medication administration, recording responses to treatment that weren't observed, failure to report an error or incident that involved a client/patient, and coming to the clinical setting under the influence of alcohol or drugs were all viewed as highly unethical or severely unethical by these same students. However, 21.6% of the participants felt that working with another student when it wasn't allowed wasn't unethical or only slightly unethical. Sixteen percent of students felt the same way about getting answers from another student.

McCabe also noted that students tended to engage more readily in behaviors they viewed as less serious (McCabe, 2009). Such a result might be expected, but the question remains as to why students who rate behaviors as very unethical still engage in those behaviors. Similarly, how are we to reconcile the observation that most nursing students in the various studies felt the likelihood of, and penalties for, getting caught cheating were very high with the large number of students who self-report engaging in these behaviors (McCabe, 2009; McCrink, 2010; Woith et al., 2012)? In some cases, students reported that they didn't know that their actions constituted unethical conduct or cheating (Beasley, 2014; Bezek, 2014; McCrink, 2010).

> ***Consider This***   Loschiavo (2015) notes that cheating "can be an intentional, calculated decision in order to get ahead. Often, it is motivated by the path to success that they see around them—people cheating without incurring any real consequences. Students then come to believe that dishonest behavior is rewarded and often do not hesitate to engage in it" (para. 8).

FERTILE GROUND FOR CHEATING?

Nursing school may be a breeding ground for academic dishonesty, despite nursing students' generally wide acceptance that trust, honesty, and fairness are essential to the formation of the therapeutic relationships that are foundational to practice. Although nursing educators and leaders, and even nursing students, may disagree as to whether the factors that promote cheating are actually causes or rationalizations for bad behavior, or just excuses for moral laxity, if we are to deter academic dishonesty we must understand and acknowledge the context within which it occurs. Without question, many of the reasons, cited by students,

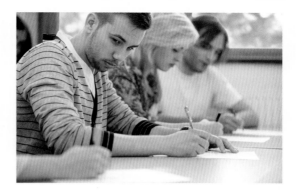

for cheating exist in nursing programs in abundance: time constraints, large body of knowledge to assimilate in a short time, significant culture challenge for many students, great pressure for grades, and so on.

Since the first studies of cheating by nursing students in the mid-1980s, the use of Internet-based research and sources, electronic media, electronic submission of papers and exams, online management of courses, complete with quizzes, exams, and various assignments completed online, has made the burden of detecting and deterring academic dishonesty even more difficult.

As McCabe (2009) observed, nursing students are exposed to the same influences as students in other disciplines. Opportunities for cheating have certainly increased with the increased use of electronic technologies, but there is little evidence that the actual number of students cheating has increased as a result (McCabe, 2009). The ease with which students can access material is certainly a time saver, a valuable incentive in nursing programs (McCabe, 2009). In McCabe's (2009) study, more than a third of nursing students reported "copying a few sentences from a Web source without citing it." Among the questions raised by this finding is whether students are ignorant of appropriate citation of sources, seduced by the ease of such plagiarism, or whether there is some other explanation for such widespread cheating (Research Fuels the Controversy 18.1).

Interestingly, participants in two of the studies (McCrink, 2010; Woith et al., 2012) rejected the neutralization statements (rationales) for academic dishonesty and recognized the correlation between public/patient safety and academic integrity. This finding may offer insight into ways that both faculty and students may cooperate to decrease the incidence of cheating in both the classroom and clinical settings.

Research Fuels the Controversy 18.1

What Can Stop Student Academic Dishonesty?

This study explored the responses of 298 students who had been caught cheating and were assigned to a remediation class to answer the question "What, if anything, would have stopped you from committing your act of academic dishonesty?"

Source: Beasley, E. M. (2014). Students reported for cheating explain what they think would have stopped them. *Ethics & Behavior, 24*(3), 229–252. doi:10.1080/10508422.2013.845533

Study Findings

The researcher analyzed the responses and found several themes. Students said they were ignorant of what constituted academic dishonesty and were ignorant of the consequences and/or seriousness of those violations; students deflected blame, usually by saying the instructor could have done something differently; students felt they didn't have sufficient time, resources, and/or skills to get the desired result, but didn't take responsibility for this lack of time, resources, or skills.

Students also felt they did not manage their time appropriately and did take responsibility for the poor time management; some said a bad grade was not an option; and some cited peer behavior as a contributing factor. Beasley concluded that many of the students in his study believed that having better information about what constituted academic dishonesty and the penalties for such behavior would have inhibited them. In addition, students cited ideas consistent with neutralization and strain theories and felt that lack of time was a major factor in ultimately leading them to cheat (Beasley, 2014).

WHAT SHOULD THE CONSEQUENCES BE FOR CHEATING?

Both Krueger (2014) and McCabe (2009) report that students who observe their classmates engaging in academic dishonesty are more prone to engage in such activity themselves. Clearly, academic dishonesty must be confronted and addressed so that a culture of cheating is not allowed to exist, much less condoned.

> **Consider This** According to the Boston Globe, cheating is no more prevalent today than it was 50 years ago (Buchmann, 2014).

Given that the number of students who admit to cheating has remained constant since it was first measured in 1963, whatever is being done to stop cheating today clearly isn't working (Buchmann, 2014). What, then, should the consequences be for cheating? Clearly, consequences can range from no action to disciplinary expulsion (Box 18.3). Finding an appropriate balance between an excessively punitive culture that allows for no exceptions and an apathetic attitude that actually encourages cheating may be more difficult than one would expect. Expulsion and formal disciplinary actions clearly affect a student's future as well as career choice. Perhaps even more importantly, and

not often addressed, is the fact that students who cheat their way through their education may be missing critical information they need to safely perform in their chosen career

BOX 18.3   Common Consequences of Academic Misconduct

- No action
- Warning or written reprimand
- General disciplinary probation
- Disciplinary probation with loss of good standing
- Discretionary sanctions such as:
  - Educational programs
  - Restorative justice assignments
- Grading penalties such as:
  - An "F" on the assignment or exam
  - Failure in the class
  - Reduced grade
  - Academic Misconduct or "AM" noted on transcript
- Loss of Repeat/Delete privilege
- Disciplinary suspension
- Disciplinary expulsion
- Revocation of admission or degree
- Withholding of degree

Source: Colorado State University. (1993–2015). *Why do students cheat?* Retrieved May 28, 2015, from https://tilt. colostate.edu/integrity/resourcesFaculty/whyDoStudents.cfm

path. Certainly, this is the case in nursing, and allowing students who cheat to earn professional degrees clearly places patients at risk.

> **Consider This**   Some students cheat because they believe that grades and test scores are the only thing that really matter, not mastery of the content.

> **Discussion Point**
> Who carries the responsibility for assuring academic integrity in nursing programs, students or faculty? Support your choice.

HOW CAN ACADEMIC INTEGRITY BE FOSTERED?

Nursing students and faculty, alike, recognize the importance of academic integrity as fostering the kind of ethical behavior essential to nursing care (McCrink, 2010; Woith et al., 2012). Given the positive correlation between academic misconduct in the classroom and unethical behavior in the clinical setting, classroom and clinical faculty as well as nursing leaders must be alert to instances of cheating in both arenas.

The approach to fostering academic integrity, however, must not be just reactive (negative sanctions when punishment is discovered). It must be proactive and include establishing an ethical culture, using professional standards as a guide for ethical behavior, establishing clear guidelines and expectations, increasing faculty supervision, fostering self-discipline, implementing honor codes, teaching students about research and appropriate citation, and providing mentoring and support. The importance of student participation (buy in) cannot be overemphasized. A study by Robinson and Glanzer (2017) used McCabe et al.'s model to analyze students' perceptions of academic integrity in general and at their institution. The researchers found that students consistently focused on the negative, punitive aspects of the system and ignored the positive messaging about academic integrity. As a result, they lacked the most important ingredient for an atmosphere that promotes academic integrity: the commitment to values such as mutual trust, respect, and supportiveness (Robinson & Glanzer, 2017).

Establishing an Ethical Culture

Ethical conduct and its role in establishing trustworthiness and a caring, therapeutic relationship among nursing students, nurses, and clients must be a central focus of students, faculty, and professional nurses. The establishment of a culture of ethical behavior and trustworthiness in nursing programs, however, must be a joint endeavor between faculty and students. Without significant participation, "buy in" by students, faculty efforts to stop cheating are likely to fail. As Krueger (2014) and other researchers point out, if the perceptions among students that they are likely to get caught cheating and the consequences for cheating are quite severe don't deter cheating, a punitive approach alone seems unlikely to solve the problem. Nevertheless, faculty, students, and the institution must be resolute that academic dishonesty will not be tolerated.

If the development of a culture of cheating is a result of socialization as Krueger (2014) and Woith et al. (2012) suggest, then one avenue toward reversing that course would be to socialize student nurses into a culture of caring, trustworthiness, and accountability. An emphasis on the importance of these attributes to the professional nurse should come early and be repeated often during the course of a student's progression through a nursing program. This socialization would involve teaching and role modeling ethical behavior and integrity. Educators also need to establish the relevance of the work they assign and endeavor to help students manage their time better in order to deal with the increasing complexity and amount of knowledge required of the professional nurse (Woith et al., 2012).

Miron (2016) studied predictors for behaving with academic integrity among nursing students in Canada. She found that attitude, subjective norms, and perceived behavioral control were the strongest predictors for ethical behavior. Her study recommended such strategies as case-based pedagogy, simulation, and instructors finding ways to help students identify and engage in ethical behavior (planned, real-time clinical conferences, for example) as ways to help create an environment of academic integrity.

Using Professional Standards as a Guide for Ethical Behavior

McCrink (2010), Krueger (2014), and Woith et al. (2012) agree that faculty play a central role in helping students incorporate such exemplars as the American Nurses Association (ANA) Code of Ethics (2015) into their interactions with patients. Faculty must also provide clear guidelines and expectations for ethical behavior and model such behavior. In addition, they must help students identify and discuss lapses of ethical conduct they encounter in the clinical setting by both students and professional nurses. Student peer leaders can be helpful in modeling and promoting accountability and trustworthiness (Beasley, 2014; Woith et al., 2012).

The observation of Robinson and Glanzer (2017) that students largely situate responsibility for academic integrity on their teachers and administrators overseeing the system rather than on their student peers seems to support Simola's notion that the more practical approach to achieving academic integrity may lie in such actions as: helping students clarify the meaning and types of academic dishonesty; making clear the ethical nature of decisions surrounding academic integrity and its relationship to the ethical norms of nursing; fostering ethical values within courses and classes; and having students sign an honesty pledge before testing, rather than afterward (Simola, 2017). One more suggestion that fits very well with the ethical standards of nursing is that faculty and peers actively encourage and educate students about the importance of seeking help and support early if students are feeling overwhelmed (Simola, 2017).

Indeed, Buchmann (2014) suggests that because cultural ideas may influence the prevalence of cheating, the best long-term solution may be to take a societal approach. Instead of seeing cheating as something that can't be done, students must come to recognize that it should not be done. Faculty have a clear responsibility to model ethical behavior. Not only should clinical standards and expectations regarding original work, allowed collaboration, and so on be crystal clear, but faculty must also be sure to credit sources in lectures, assignments, and so on.

Establishing Clear Guidelines and Expectations

Buchmann (2014) suggests that many students lack understanding of what constitutes cheating because they may not have fully read or comprehended their student rules. This lack of understanding may lead students to cheat by accident or in a way that isn't known to be called cheating. In addition, "ambiguous attitudes among students about what qualifies as cheating may cause more academic dishonesty than intended by students. While most students will call plagiarism cheating, many of them will define plagiarism in a way that allows them to indirectly copy the work of others" (Buchmann, 2014, para. 6).

In addition, faculty should revisit the parameters and expectations of ethical conduct frequently, rather than only at the beginning of the program. Clear delineation of the types of activities that are approved for collaborative work and of those that require individual work would eliminate the rationalization that students didn't realize they weren't to work together. Faculty and students should work together to establish the policies that govern behavior in the academic and clinical settings (Stonecypher & Willson, 2014).

Faculty should also encourage discussions regarding ethical dilemmas associated with academic integrity. This is particularly important in the clinical setting when students may be exposed to unethical conduct by the staff nurses they are working with. Clinical instructors should be very clear about their expectations for ethical conduct and the consequences for failing to report errors in an appropriate manner.

Increasing Faculty Supervision

The quality of faculty supervision in test taking can be either a deterrent or a promoter of academic dishonesty. Indeed, Buchmann (2014) suggests that tightening the rules on classroom behavior during exams seems like the most obvious and readily available solution to reducing academic dishonesty. He goes on to detail extensive efforts made by universities to record everything suspicious, efforts made to prevent students from photographing a test, and not allowing students to chew gum because it provides a way to hide that they're talking into a hidden microphone.

Similarly, more faculty are requiring online students to take exams under the supervision of a proctor. Indeed, research demonstrates that students taking online unproctored exams perform better than when they sit for exams before a proctor enforcing the closed-book exam rules (Winneg, n.d.). In other words, more students cheat when taking exams unproctored, online at home.

Unfortunately, the Internet is filled with strategies students can use to individually or collaboratively cheat, including "the long-sleeved shirt method" (students write important information on their arms for an exam and then roll up their sleeves when instructor is not looking); the "buddy system" (students sit near a student they believe will do well on the test, and that student holds up their exam sheet as if reflecting on their answers so that the other person can copy); "the telephone scam" (students are allowed to use the calculator on their phone for exams, but actually use the telephone to text answers to other students or search online); "the distraction method" (one student distracts the instructor so that other students can exchange answers); using crib notes written on band-aids, Kleenex, gum wrappers, and other commonly used innocuous items; and "sign language" (using a series of coughs, Morse code, hand or foot tapping, or other nonverbal cues to let another student know which answer is the correct one), to name just a few.

An attentive instructor may be able to detect some of these strategies, but it is equally clear that the sophistication and skill of academic cheaters is continuing to increase. Using multiple test proctors may be a useful strategy in increasing the degree of faculty supervision.

But new technology is unfolding that includes smart watches, smart pens, and Google glasses to help students cheat (Vandoorne, 2014). Some new devices are almost impossible to see—such as "invisible" Bluetooth earpieces. They work with a tiny microphone, which is synced to a Bluetooth cell phone and enable questions, whispered from exam rooms, to be answered from someone outside the room. Such wearable technology will only make it more difficult for instructors to spot cheating when it is occurring.

Discussion Point

Can observant teachers detect academic dishonesty or are cheating strategies so sophisticated or well practiced that being caught is unlikely?

Discussion Point

Is collaborative cheating typically instigated by a few people and others simply follow, or do you believe academic dishonesty is simply more common than most people would like to admit?

Using Test Security or Plagiarism Assessment Tools

Some instructors have begun computerized adaptive testing (CAT) to address cheating concerns. CAT uses an algorithm to choose test items based on the students' strengths and weaknesses (Bleiberg & West, 2013). Every student takes a different test when using CAT, which decreases the number of items tests have in common. Students take the test online, eliminating inappropriately administered testing accommodations and making it difficult for students to share answers.

In addition, plagiarism assessment tools such as Turnitin.com and SafeAssign have become commonplace. These sites have millions of catalogued articles, papers, and webpages to determine what percentage of student papers are original work and what percentage is the work of others.

Instructors are also using webcams to monitor students taking tests offsite and increasingly requiring some type of biometric sign-in to make sure that the student taking the test is the same student taking the course. (The 2008 Higher Education Opportunity Act contains a requirement that schools offering distance learning programs have a system in place to authenticate the identity of their online students.) More computers are being recessed into desktops so that students who attempt to photograph screens are more obvious. In addition, some schools have begun using jamming devices to block the use of cell phones during testing.

Fostering Self-Discipline

A focus on quality improvement rather than a punitive approach to each mistake may encourage students to report errors rather than hiding them. Frank discussion between clinical faculty and students about the problems students observe can help inculcate an attitude of vigilance regarding their own personal practice.

Faculty should also emphasize the findings of the Institute of Medicine's (2004) report linking errors with outcomes in discussions with students regarding academic integrity. Although the evidence that students who cheat become nurses who cheat in the workplace is sketchy, it seems intuitively true, and student respondents in several of the studies cited noted the link (McCabe, 2009; McCrink, 2010; Woith et al., 2012). Instructors should continually discuss with students the importance of the data they're collecting, the procedures they perform, and the dependence of patients' well-being on their honesty and ethical behavior (Krueger, 2014).

Implementing Honor Codes

An academic honor code is a set of rules or expectations that govern an academic community and is based on ideals that define honorable behavior within that community. An honor code's utility depends on the notion that members of the community can be trusted to act with honor. Infractions of the honor code are enforced with various sanctions, including expulsion from the program or institution (Wikipedia, the Free Encyclopedia, 2015). Honor codes may be quite complex, listing various types of infractions, or they may be quite brief: a statement that the student who has signed the honor code pledges that all work is his or her own and that he or she has received no disallowed assistance.

Woith et al. (2012) and Krueger (2014) both noted that earlier researchers had found that schools that had formal honor codes reported fewer instances of student cheating. It may be that the formalization and discussion of these codes not only lay clear guidelines for student behavior but also cause students to actively consider their behavior in the context of the fundamental principles of the nursing profession. Stonecypher and Willson (2014) note that honor codes are effective if students understand the expectations of the code. Honor codes place the responsibility for academic integrity on the student and must be written with clear, easy-to-understand expectations and steps that guide students, faculty, and administrators (Stonecypher & Willson, 2014).

A common feature of honor codes is a "no tolerance" policy that obligates students to report infractions of academic honesty. Others may opt for a policy that allows a student to first confront another student about violations and encourage the accused to self-report before the formal reporting obligation is in force (Wikipedia, 2015). Failure to report a violation is generally considered a violation.

Discussion Point

Would you report one of your classmates for academic dishonesty?

What factors would influence your decision? How does tolerance of academic dishonesty affect the culture of integrity in the nursing program?

Teaching Students About Research and Appropriate Citation

Loschiavo (2015) suggests that one reason students cheat is that they are unprepared for college-level work. He suggests that the reason many students plagiarize is that they were never taught how to write a research paper. He also suggests that students are not being taught how to paraphrase and instead are just expected to cut and paste from the articles they read on the Internet.

In addition, Loschiavo suggests that some students don't have any confidence in their own ideas, so when given the chance to write a paper in which they must share their own thoughts, they simply go to the Internet and use others' words or ideas, thinking they are worth more than their own. Or students think that the author's words were so eloquent that they are afraid of their ability to interpret what has been read and to translate it into their own words.

Educators might help students with these deficiencies by requiring submission of intermediate steps (summaries, rough drafts, etc.) before deadline for finished papers and assignments. Students might also benefit from a course on research and writing during nursing school. Such a course could also help students learn how to evaluate other research papers and articles in their quest for evidence-based practice.

Providing Mentoring and Support

Loschiavo (2015) suggests that some students cheat because they don't know how to manage their time and thus underestimate how long assignments or studying will take them. They then panic and take shortcuts. In addition, he suggests that some students cheat as a cry for help, subconsciously wishing to be caught so they can share what is going on in their lives with someone they believe may be able to help. He suggests then that faculty should always ask questions about why students made the choices they did.

CONCLUSIONS

Unethical conduct and cheating in both the classroom and the clinical setting are a serious concern for nursing faculty, nursing leaders, and students. Recognition and amelioration of some of the factors in nursing programs that may encourage student dishonesty are critical. Because integrity and trustworthiness are foundations of good nursing practice, faculty must be prepared to help students develop and incorporate these values. As McCabe (2009) put it, "Nursing schools, as the gateway to a profession whose members are assumed to have a strong professional identity that is built on integrity and a desire to serve should assume some responsibility for developing these standards among future members of its profession" (p. 622).

Creating a culture of honesty and accountability is crucial to this end and has been shown to deter cheating. Both Stonecypher and Willson (2014) and McCrink (2010) noted that student attitudes toward ethical standards of behavior made the strongest contribution to an ethic of caring and honesty. As one of McCabe's faculty respondents put it, "We have to help students learn that being a student with integrity is a critical part of their socialization into the role of professional health care provider with responsibility for life and death decisions" (McCabe, 2009, p. 620).

For Additional Discussion

1. Which is more important to you—building a culture of integrity in the nursing program and the profession, or loyalty to your classmates or coworkers? How do you handle conflicts between these two values?

2. Do you support the development and use of honor codes in nursing programs? What should an honor code for nursing school look like?

3. Do you believe there is a culture of cheating in your nursing program? What do you do personally to promote academic integrity?

4. What do you think is the relationship between academic integrity and professional integrity? Is a student who cheats in nursing school more likely to cheat in the professional realm? Would you want a nurse who cheated in nursing school caring for someone you cared about?

5. What steps would you recommend to build a culture of strict academic integrity in your nursing program?

References

American Nurses Association. (2015). *Code of ethics for nurses.* Retrieved June 10, 2018, from American Nurses Association Website: https://www.nursingworld.org/coe-view-only

Bailey, P. A. (2001). Academic misconduct: Responses from deans and nurse educators. *Journal of Nursing Education, 40*(3), 124–131.

Beasley, E. M. (2014). Students reported for cheating explain what they think would have stopped them. *Ethics & Behavior, 24*(3), 229–252. doi:10.1080/10508422.2013.845533

Bezek, S. M. (2014). Who is taking care of you? A study of the correlation of academic and professional dishonesty. *Dissertation Abstracts International: Section A. Humanities and Social Sciences,* 114. (Publication No. 3630808)

Bleiberg, J., & West, D. (2013, August 20). *How technology can stop cheating.* The Huffington Post. Retrieved June 10, 2018, from http://www.huffingtonpost.com/darrell-west/how-technology-can-stop-c_b_3784392.html

Buchmann, B. (2014, February 20). *Cheating in college: Where it happens, why students do it and how to stop it.* The Huffington Post. Retrieved June 10, 2018, from http://www.huffingtonpost.com/uloop/cheating-in-college-where_b_4826136.html

Colorado State University. (1993–2015). *Why do students cheat?* Retrieved June 10, 2018, from https://tilt.colostate.edu/integrity/resourcesFaculty/whyDoStudents.cfm

Gaberson, K. B. (1997, July–September). Academic dishonesty among nursing students. *Nursing Forum, 32*(3), 14–20.

Gallup. (2016, December). *Honesty/ethics in professions.* Retrieved June 10, 2018, from http://www.gallup.com/poll/1654/honesty-ethics-professions.aspx

Glasper, A. (2016, July). Does cheating by students undermine the integrity of the nursing profession? *British Journal of Nursing, 25*(16), 932–933.

Hilbert, G. A. (1985, July–August). Involvement of nursing students in unethical classroom and clinical behaviors. *Journal of Professional Nursing, 1*(4), 230–234.

Institute of Medicine. (2004). *Keeping patients safe: Transforming the work environment of nurses.* Washington, DC: National Academic Press.

Krueger, L. (2014, February). Academic dishonesty among nursing students. *Journal of Nursing Education, 53*(2), 77–87.

Lodhia, D. (2018, May 1). *More university students are cheating—But it's not because they're lazy.* Guardian News. Retrieved June 10, 2018, from https://www.theguardian.com/education/2018/may/01/university-students-cheating-tuition-fees-jobs-exams

Loschiavo, C. (2015, May 19). *Why do students cheat? Listen to this dean's words.* The Conversation. Retrieved June 10, 2018, from http://theconversation.com/why-do-students-cheat-listen-to-this-deans-words-40295

McCabe, D. L. (2009, November). Academic dishonesty in nursing schools: An empirical investigation. *Journal of Nursing Education, 48*(11), 614–623.

McCrink, A. (2010). Academic misconduct in nursing students: Behaviors attitudes rationalizations and cultural identity. *Journal of Nursing Education, 49*(11), 653–659.

Miron, J. B. (2016). *Academic integrity and senior nursing undergraduate clinical practice.* Retrieved June 10, 2018, from https://qspace.library.queensu.ca/handle/1974/14708

Morgan, J. (2018, February 14). *How students cheat online, and why stopping them matters.* Inside Higher Ed. Retrieved June 10, 2018, from https://www.insidehighered.com/digital-learning/views/2018/02/14/creative-cheating-online-learning-and-importance-academic

Online Degree Programs. (2012). *7 Most common ways students cheat.* Retrieved June 10, 2018, from http://www.onlinedegreeprograms.com/blog/2012/7-most-common-ways-students-cheat

Robinson, J., & Glanzer, P. (2017, Summer). Building a culture of academic integrity: What students perceive and need. *College Student Journal, 51*(2), 209–221.

Sheer, B. L. (1989). *The relationships among socialization, empathy, autonomy and unethical student behaviors in baccalaureate nursing students* (Unpublished doctoral dissertation). Widener University School of Nursing, Chester, PA. Retrieved June 10, 2018, https://www.google.com/search?q=Sheer%2C+B.L.+%281989%29.+The+relationships+among+socialization%2C+empathy%2C+autonomy+and+unethical+student+behaviors+in+baccalaureate+nursing+students.&ie=utf-8&oe=utf-8&client=firefox-b-1-ab

Simola, S. (2017). Managing for academic integrity in higher education: Insights from behavioral ethics. *Scholarship of Teaching and Learning in Psychology, 3*(1), 43–57.

Stonecypher, K., & Willson, P. (2014, May). Academic policies and practices to deter cheating in nursing education. *Nursing Education Perspectives, 35*(3), 167–179.

The Conversation. (2018, February 15). *Why students at prestigious high schools still cheat on exams.* Retrieved June 10, 2018, from https://theconversation.com/why-students-at-prestigious-high-schools-still-cheat-on-exams-91041

The latest ways that kids cheat on exams. (2009). Retrieved June 10, 2018, from http://www.cbsnews.com/news/the-latest-ways-that-kids-cheat-on-exams

Vandoorne, S. (2014, June 19). *From smartwatch and smartpen. . . to smartcheat?* CNN. Retrieved June 10, 2018, from http://www.cnn.com/2014/06/19/business/high-tech-cheating/index.html

Wikipedia, the Free Encyclopedia. (2015, May 28). *Academic honor code.* Retrieved June 10, 2018, from http://en.wikipedia.org/w/index.php?title=Academic_honor_code&oldid=664372276

Winneg, D. (n.d.). *Students will cheat—So, deal with it!* [Web log post]. Software Secure. Retrieved June 10, 2018, from http://www.softwaresecure.com/students-will-cheat-so-deal-with-it

Woith, W., Jenkins, S. D., & Kerber, C. (2012, October). Perceptions of academic integrity among nursing students. *Nursing Forum, 47*(4), 253–259.

Technology in Health Care
Opportunities, Limitations, and Challenges
Carol J. Huston

LEARNING OBJECTIVES

The learner will be able to:

1. Describe emerging applications for biomechatronics in health care.

2. Reflect on the degree to which technologically sophisticated, emotion-sensing, mental service robots will replace professional caregivers in the future.

3. Discuss how biometric technology can increase the likelihood that access to health care information is both targeted and appropriate.

4. Detail how point-of-care bar coding is implemented and the potential benefits/limitations of its use.

5. Explore the effect of computerized physician/prescriber order entry on the reduction of medication errors and adverse drug events, as well as barriers to implementation of its use.

6. Identify resistance to change and cost barriers to the implementation of electronic health records (EHRs) despite government pressure to develop this technology.

7. Identify how clinical decision support systems can both improve existing care processes and provide a means for high-quality clinical decision making.

8. Describe the perils inherent in having consumers independently seek out and interpret genomic testing without the support of a primary care provider.

9. Identify how EHRs, telehealth, and point-of-care testing can be used to overcome geography-of-care issues.

10. Analyze how the Internet has changed the relationship between providers and patients in terms of the power of information in health care decision making.

11. Engage in futuristic thinking regarding how technology may further alter 21st-century health care and health care provider roles.

12. Assess personal strengths and weaknesses in terms of technology skill development.

13. Identify strategies to optimally integrate the use of technology with the human element, as part of the art of nursing.

14. Identify the nurse's role and responsibility in ensuring the ethical use of technology in patient care.

INTRODUCTION

Andersen and Rasmussen (2015) suggest that society is transformed whenever new technologies emerge that change our means of production and ability to communicate. They also suggest that the rapid technological developments of the past century—in biotechnology, information technology, nanotechnology, and artificial intelligence (AI)—hold promise to do the same for our current, postindustrial world. There are few venues where this is more obvious than in health care.

Technology has already dramatically transformed health care, shaping both consumer and provider expectations. Indeed, D'Onfro (2018) suggests that people have begun viewing health care with the same expectations they would have for other consumer products, including on-demand access and transparent pricing and that technology companies, from start-ups to top firms, have started to fill those gaps and provide solutions. For example, Apple is testing a product that will let users keep their medical records on their iPhones and start-ups like Oscar Health, which processes insurance claims, and Cedar, which provides simplified health care billing, are also working to address "pain points" across the health care space (D'Onfro, 2018, para. 5).

With these advances in technology, however, have come new opportunities, limitations, and challenges. Technology can cut costs, improve patient outcomes, streamline workflow, and improve information accessibility. It can also be costly, require almost limitless ongoing training, and continually bring about new ethical dilemmas, including the need to ensure the "human element" is not lost in patient care. Determining what technology should be developed and how it should be used in an era of limited resources, with vulnerable populations, raises multiple ethical questions.

Wadhwa (2014) agrees, suggesting, that with the pace of technology growth, we have not been able to come to grips with what is ethical, let alone determine what laws or rules should be in place. Gabr (n.d.) also agrees, suggesting that the ethical consequences associated with technological change must be further examined so that some institutionalization of health ethics can be created. In doing so, new, sensitive, reliable indicators as well as a vigilance system could be developed to monitor inequalities in health care and the abuse or neglect of human rights related to technology use.

> **Consider This** Technology is like a rolling freight train—it's very difficult to stop it and even more dangerous to get in the way.

This chapter addresses only a few of the technology advances shaping 21st-century health care. Biometrics, point-of-care testing (POCT), and computerized data access/entry are presented as technological approaches for improving documentation and knowledge acquisition. Electronic health records (EHRs) and telehealth are recognized as strategies for overcoming geography-of-care issues, and computerized physician/provider order entry (CPOE) and clinical decision support (CDS) systems are discussed both as strategies for improving existing care processes and promoting high-quality clinical decision making. The Internet's effect on both patients and providers is also examined, including the concept of "expert patient" and the resultant need for health care providers trained in consumer health informatics. In addition, genetics/genomics is highlighted as a preventive, diagnostic, and treatment tool for precision medicine, although many ethical issues associated with its use need further exploration.

Finally, the chapter argues that the "human element" is the art of nursing and that this should not be lost in the quest to develop and use emerging technologies. Huston (2013) suggests it is nurses who need to be actively involved in determining how best to use technology to supplement, not eliminate, professional nursing care. Questions related to the ethical use of technology should be reviewed by ethics committees prior to technology implementation but nurses should have a voice in that conversation. Roy Simpson, vice president and CNO at Cerner Corp., a major EHR vendor, agrees, noting that "Too often, nurses are not at the table because they are not the user that drives the organization's revenue" (Robert Wood Johnson Foundation [RWJF], 2016d, p. 8). But Simpson argues that it is the insufficient attention to clinical workflows—the actual sequence of different tasks—before installing new technologies that prevents them from operating efficiently and is a major contributor to clinician dissatisfaction.

SELECT TECHNOLOGY ADVANCES IN HEALTH CARE

Biomechatronics

Biomechatronics, which creates machines that replicate or mimic how the body works, will continue to increase in prominence in the future. This interdisciplinary field encompasses biology, neurosciences, mechanics, electronics, and robotics to create devices that interact with human muscle, skeleton, and nervous systems to establish or restore human motor or nervous system function (Freudenrich, 2018).

In addition, applied biomechatronics uses mathematical models that, when applied to engineering principles and techniques in the medical field, can be used in assistive devices that work with bodily signals. The use of data in the kinematic and kinetic analysis of the human body, including musculoskeletal kinetics and joints and their relationship to the central nervous system (CNS), underscores the complexity of how the skeletal and muscular system work together to allow movement controlled by the CNS (Ulloa, 2018).

Future biomechatronics applications are innumerable and will likely include such things as functional stimulation of paralyzed limbs, pancreas pacemakers for diabetics, wireless active capsule endoscopy, and mentally controlled electronic muscle stimulators for patients with brain injuries.

Robotics

Surgical Robotics

The use of surgical robotics in health care is becoming commonplace. Indeed, the robot-assisted surgery market is expected to grow steadily into 2023 and potentially beyond (Matthews, 2017). The first robotic-assisted surgery actually dates to the mid-1980s when a robot was used to place a needle for brain biopsy using computed tomographic guidance. Robotic-assisted heart bypass surgery followed in the late 1990s, and the first unmanned robotic surgery took place in May 2006 in Italy. Several years later, engineers at Duke University, using novel three-dimensional technology and a basic AI program, guided the actions of a rudimentary tabletop robot to perform surgery. The engineers suggested this technology would eventually allow robots to perform surgery on patients in dangerous situations or in remote locations, such as on the battlefield or in space, with minimal or no human guidance.

In addition, similar technology began making certain contemporary medical procedures safer for patients. For example, robots are now performing cataract surgery. With femtosecond laser surgery, a laser light can be fired at a target, reducing stress on the retina and other delicate tissues of the eye during cataract extraction. Because this is computer controlled rather than performed with manual surgical tools, greater surgical precision is possible and patient safety is increased (Segre, 2018). Major surgeries that used to leave scars and kept patients in the hospital for several days have turned into fairly minor procedures (Abate, 2016).

For example, a small controlled study on the use of robotic-guided spine surgery indicated that relative risk for a complication was 5.3 times higher in fluoro-guided surgeries compared to robotic guidance; and that the relative risk for revision surgery was 7.1 times higher for a fluoro-guided surgery compared to the robotic-guided cases. In addition, patients experienced a 78% decrease in exposure to radiation with robotic surgery (Kite-Powell, 2017).

Surgical robotics are not, however, cheap. Lee (2014) notes that the average robotic system costs between $1.5 million and $2 million. In addition, volumes must be large enough to produce a viable financial return within 6 years (the average life of the technology). This is in addition to the ongoing maintenance, special instrumentation, and disposable equipment costs to maintain such a system and does not include the annual service contracts that cost an additional $100,000 to $170,000. In addition, each procedure costs between $3,000 and $6,000 more than a laparoscopic operation because of the need for single-use tools (Abate, 2016).

Questions have also been raised about whether need is driving surgical robotics or whether the introduction of such robotics is creating a need where one did not exist before. For example, one study showed that after Wisconsin hospitals acquired robotic surgery technology, the number of prostate removals performed, doubled within 3 months. In contrast, the number of prostate surgeries stayed the same at hospitals that did not purchase the $2 million technology ("Do Robots Drive Up Prostate Surgeries?" 2011). One must question whether surgeons at hospitals with robots are recommending this surgery because the outcomes (potential reductions in incontinence and impotence) are better or whether the new technology is simply more exciting than alternative treatments like radiation or "watchful waiting" ("Do Robots Drive Up Prostate Surgeries?" 2011).

Also disconcerting, Kite-Powell (2017) reported that University of Stanford researchers compared patient outcomes and hospital stay for robotic versus free hand surgery on 24,000 patients undergoing laparoscopic surgery for kidney cancer. The study found no statistical difference in outcome or length of hospital stay, but the robotic-assisted surgeries cost more and had a higher probability of prolonged operative time. Indeed, over the 13-year period of the study, robotic surgeries cost on average $2,700 more per patient.

Similarly, Kirkner (2017) notes that although robot-assisted operations for inguinal hernia repair (IHR) and cholecystectomy have grown steadily in recent years, research suggests these procedures can be done equally well by traditional operations at a fraction of the cost. In a study of 1,248 cholecystectomies and 723 initial IHRs from 2007 to 2016, there were no differences in 30-day readmission rates or 30-day mortality between patients who had robotic-assisted surgery and those who had traditional surgery techniques. In addition, robotic procedures required longer operative times—a risk in and of itself. This makes it difficult to justify the additional $60 billion ambulatory surgery centers will spend on overhead costs and reduced efficiencies for robotic surgery for IHR and cholecystectomies over the next year years (Kirkner, 2017).

In the end, many argue that robotic surgery hasn't improved patient outcomes as dramatically as the first wave of minimally invasive surgery did (Abate, 2016). The ECRI Institute, a nonprofit organization that synthesizes data on medical procedures, drugs, and devices to support hospitals and doctors in creating quality protocols, has analyzed more than 4,000 studies on robotic surgery. Conclusions suggest "the evidence isn't strong enough to determine whether or not a robot is better than traditional minimally invasive surgery, but the evidence does indicate that it's better compared to open surgery, however,—more evidence from higher quality studies may change this conclusion" (Abate, 2016, para. 5).

Robots in Diagnostics

In addition, robots are increasingly being used in diagnostics because their accuracy typically exceeds that of human caregivers. For example, robotics and, more specifically, AI programs like IBM Watson can help interpret medical imaging more efficiently and accurately than basic human visual inspection (Matthews, 2017). AI or basic machine learning program is also better able to find patterns and make more accurate diagnoses than ever before.

AI, machine learning, and predictive algorithms could also help speed up the long and often tedious process of drug discovery (Matthews, 2017). "Imagine if researchers could input the kind of medicine they're trying to make and the kind of symptoms they're trying to treat into a computer and let it do the rest. With robotics, that may someday be possible" (Matthews, 2017, para. 8).

Robots as Direct Care Providers

Robots are also being developed to provide direct patient care. In fact, robots are already being used as caregivers, particularly for the elderly. This is especially true in Japan,

known as the "Robot Kingdom," as a result of a burgeoning elderly population and a low birth rate, which has resulted in a severe shortage of caregivers. Indeed, Japan's Ministry of Economy, Trade and Industry expects the robotic service industry to skyrocket to nearly $4 billion annually by 2035 in Japan—25 times its level in 2017 (Tarantola, 2017).

Robot caregivers are often divided into two categories: *physical service* and *mental service* robots. The former are designed to help with basic care tasks such as serving and fetching (already commercially produced) or bathing or carrying people (not yet in commercial production). Serving robots can ferry food and drinks from the kitchen and keep elderly patients stimulated by playing memory games (Tarantola, 2017). These robots can also remind people to take their pills, track their health, and automatically answer incoming calls from family and doctors. In addition, robotic walkers now exist that can obtain information about the environment through sensors, cameras, obstacle recognition systems, and software and guide elderly users to paths that minimize the chances of stumbling and falls (European Commission, 2015).

Mental service robots are also being commercially produced and have been in use for some time. One of the best known is *Paro*, a sophisticated, interactive robot designed to help people relax and reduce their stress levels. The robot, which as of 2017 was the eighth generation of a design that has been in use since 2003, is shaped like a baby harp seal and can remember its name and change its behavior depending on how it is treated. It is being used extensively in homes for elderly people and with autistic children worldwide. It was also used extensively in Japan after recent earthquakes and tsunamis to provide emotional support to survivors. Research by Bidin, Lokmanb, Mohdc, and Tsuchiyad (2017) suggests it may be used soon in Malaysia as well to address the health care needs of a growing elderly population (Research Fuels the Controversy 19.1).

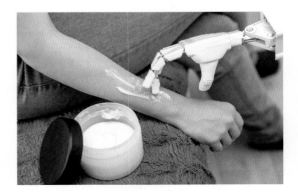

Research Fuels the Controversy 19.1

Kansei Robotic Use With the Elderly

The elderly population in Malaysia may increase to 15% from the country's current population by the year 2030, prompting health care researchers there to consider a future need for robot-assisted care with the aging population. Most robotic studies for the elderly, however, have been associated with Japanese culture. This study, using a *Personal Approach* research design, sought to investigate the feasibility of using robots for eldercare in Malaysia, focusing on possible emotional or learning benefits.

Source: Bidin, S. A. H., Lokmanb, A. M., Mohdc, W. A. R. W., & Tsuchiyad, T. (2017). Initial intervention study of Kansei robotic implementation for elderly. *Procedia Computer Science, 105*, 87–92.

Study Findings

Three elderly subjects from the Tanjung Malim Elderly Activity Centre (PAWE) participated in the study. Participants were interested in the use of robots as learning assistants but did not have any prior knowledge on robot learning. Participants found the use of the Kansei robots as learning and emotional support tools to be "interesting," "familiar," and "comfortable."

The researchers concluded that robotic interaction can provide an emotional benefit as well as learning opportunities for the elderly. They suggested this will be especially true if the technology is able to further embed the special values, perspectives, and emotions common to an elderly population.

Tarantola (2017) notes that in some difficult cases of depression, Paro could be the catalyst that helps people move on and get back to their healthy state. It is also another approach to use with other treatments for depression.

Many consumers and health care providers have expressed concern, however, about the lack of emotion in robots, suggesting that this is the element of human caregivers that can never be replaced. New technology, however, has resulted in a kind of robot intelligence known as "*kansei*," which means "emotion or feeling." *Kansei* robots use vision systems to monitor human expressions, gestures, and body language and voice sensors to pick up on intonation and individual words and sentences. When the *kansei* robot hears a word, it searches through its extensive database to match the results to emotional categories and then to generate an appropriate facial expression in response. In addition, *kansei* robots can sense human emotion through wearable sensors that monitor pulse rate and perspiration.

Similarly, a laboratory at Carnegie Mellon has designed a robot to work with therapists and people with autism (Bilton, 2013). The robot can develop a personality and blinks and giggles as people interact with it. Jim Osborn, a roboticist and executive director of the Robotics Institute's Quality of Life Technology Center at the university, noted that those who tested it loved it and hugged it and began to think of it as something more than a machine with a computer.

Indeed, Cynthia Breazeal, founder of the world's first social robot for the home called "Jibo," suggests that technology and humans can and should work hand in hand.

She argues that what is being created are robots that are really teammates and that these robots should complement the services that human professionals can provide (Fox, 2015). Jue (2017, para. 18) agrees, suggesting that "the train has already left the station," when it comes to consumer robots, and that the public will need to get acquainted with their new robot pals so that talking with any robot will just be second nature.

Discussion Point

To what degree can health care providers be replaced by technology? Can therapeutic "caring" be demonstrated by robots? Do you feel you could have a therapeutic conversation with a robot?

Sharkey and Sharkey (2012) suggest, however, that the increased use of robots in elder care raises a number of ethical concerns, including a potential reduction in the amount of human contact (opportunities for human social contact can be reduced); an increase in the feelings of objectification and loss of control (robots lack sensitivity to people's feelings and provide care at the convenience of caregivers); a loss of privacy; the loss of personal liberty; deception and infantilization (robots may restrict the behavior of humans); and a lack of clarity regarding the circumstances in which elderly people are allowed to control the robots (who is responsible if things go wrong?).

In addition, Jue (2017) notes that the halting speech and stiff movements seen in robots of the past, whether in movies, on television, and in real life, are now largely history. Huston (2017) agrees, noting that as technology continues to advance, robot caregivers have become increasingly life-like, and the ability to distinguish robot from human caregiver has become more difficult. Sharkey and Sharkey (2012) note that this physical embodiment may lead robots to be welcomed in the home and other locations (where for instance a surveillance camera would not be accepted) and their personable, or animal-like, appearance could encourage and mislead people into thinking that the robots are capable of more social understanding than is actually the case. Are the elderly and other vulnerable populations at risk of this deception? Can this population clearly differentiate between man and machine?

Discussion Point

Do mental health robots improve or further the problem of social isolation in the elderly and other vulnerable populations?

Susan Madlung, gerontologist and Clinical Educator for Regional Programs and Home Health Re-Design at Vancouver Coastal Health, argues that robot care may likely compound the issue of the social isolation of seniors (Tarantola, 2017). Indeed, she suggests that "Although robots might seem like a good response to the growing need for caregivers, I could see this as being quite detrimental to the emotional and psychosocial well-being of anyone, not just seniors," she continued. "Humans need humans" (Tarantola, 2017, para. 16).

Huston (2017) suggests then that one of the most significant challenges health care providers face in using technology is finding that balance between maximizing the benefits of technology and not devaluing the human element. Nurses need to make sure that the human element is not lost in the race to expand technology. Pols (2015) agrees, suggesting that nurses, patients, and ethicists have expressed concern that care through technology can become a cold and dehumanizing affair. This is certainly a potential concern with the use of robots as caregivers.

Robots as Couriers

Robots are also being used as robot couriers for mundane, repetitive jobs such as supply chain automation. Aethon Inc. has produced mobile robots called *TUGs* that can locate assets as well as transport them, including medications, supplies, equipment, and other goods that rely on scarce, valuable human resources for pushing carts (Aethon, 2018). The TUG, which has algorithms that determine if human intervention is needed, can haul up to 1,400 pounds and transport a variety of hospital carts. The hospital worker simply attaches a delivery to the cart, presses a button to select the destination, and pushes the "go" button. The TUG has been programmed to "remember" and navigate the layout of the facility. It automatically travels to its destination, announces that the delivery has arrived, and returns to its home base, where it waits on its charger for the next delivery. In addition, the TUG utilizes the hospital's existing Wi-Fi system to communicate with elevators, automatic doors, and fire alarms as well as the Aethon cloud command center that continuously monitors the TUG.

Biometrics

The health care environment continues to be rapidly transformed by new technology because of the need to provide confidentiality and security of patient data and to comply with the Health Insurance Portability and Accountability Act of 1996 (HIPAA). HIPAA calls for a tiered approach to data access in which staff members have access to only the information that they need to know to perform their jobs. New biometric technology ensures that such access being developed is both targeted and appropriate.

Biometrics is the science of identifying people through physical characteristics such as fingerprints, handprints, retinal scans, voice recognition, facial structure, and dynamic signatures. Fingerprint biometrics is still the most common type of biometrics in health care, primarily because of their ease of use, small size, and affordable price. Detection of facial geometry, however, is also beginning to make inroads. Facial geometry captures facial landmarks such as approach angles, eyebrow and mouth contours, skin texture analysis, and hairstyles, which can then be confirmed by facial recognition software.

Palm vein patterns are also being used as biometric identifiers. Using near-infrared light to capture each individual's unique palm vein pattern bypasses the need to have quality fingerprints. Right Patient (2018) notes that palm vein biometric patterns are difficult to forge, and because they exist inside of the body, it is practically impossible to recreate someone's biometric template. The palm vein recognition sensor needs the hand and blood flow to register an image. The use of palm veins as a biometric signature is expected to grow at a considerable pace from 2017 to 2025 owing to the growing need of securing confidential information and data in many organizations ("Trends in the Palm Vein," 2017).

Smart Cards and Smart Objects

Health care organizations are also increasingly integrating biometrics with "smart cards" to ensure that an individual presenting a secure ID credential really has the right to use that credential. *Smart cards* are credit card–sized devices with a chip, stored memory, and an operating system that records a patient's entire clinical history. The integration of biometrics and smart cards then can eliminate the need for multiple identification requirements.

Smart objects are everyday objects injected with easy-to-use software that give devices some degree of intelligence. For example, "smart hospital rooms" may include computer screens that pull up patient records and display diagnosis and treatment plans as well as vital signs, medications, and other personal information (Fareed, 2018). They can also provide caregivers with a real-time patient medical record and provide instant bedside access to the patient's electronic medical record. An advanced *Caregiver Alerting System* can let health care providers know if a confused patient is attempting to get out of bed or if vital signs suggest a change in patient condition. It can even prominently display patient risk indicators such as falls or isolation (Fareed, 2018).

In addition, hospitals are increasingly turning to *smart pumps* for intravenous (IV) therapy infusions. These smart pumps have safety software inside an advanced infusion therapy system that prevents IV medication errors by setting minimum and maximum dose limits, as well as preset limits that cannot be overridden at a clinician's discretion. Giuliano and Ruppel (2017) note that numerous examples in the literature attribute IV medication error reduction to the use of these smart pumps.

Still, end-user smart pump workarounds and IV-related medication errors are common. This is because health care providers become desensitized to false and repetitive alarms and they lower alarm volumes or simply turn off the alarms to decrease their alarm fatigue, placing patient safety at risk (Robert Wood Johnson Foundation, 2018c). As the primary end users of smart pumps, nurses need to be aware of potential safety issues and play an active role in improving the technology.

> **Consider This** Smart pumps cannot outsmart the provider who decides to override them.

Point-of-Care Testing

POCT, which has evolved into a multibillion dollar industry, is another technological advance that is bringing more timely decision making and treatment, which in turn improves bedside care and promotes more positive outcomes. The Washington State Clinical Laboratory defines POCT as at the point where patient care is given (Washington State Clinical Laboratory Advisory Council, 2017). In POCT, caregivers gather and test specimens near the patient or at the bedside using handheld analyzers, pulse oximeters, and blood glucose monitoring systems. Then, by networking via the Internet and downloading results to a central clinical lab, manual documentation of test results can be eliminated. This allows clinicians to recognize and begin treating life-threatening conditions in real time even when geographical distance is a barrier.

POCT also works for consumer use in the home. Patients can precisely monitor their laboratory values, submit them electronically to the lab, and then have results in minutes. POCT testing represents only a small portion of clinical laboratories' total testing volume, however, and evaluation challenges exist for all POCT programs in terms of accuracy, ease of use, quality control, and accurate data management. Indeed, delivering diagnostic tests at the bedside may be prone to errors because of a failure to follow procedures, inappropriate documentation, improper patient identification, and not performing required quality control tests. More pilot programs are needed to evaluate the use of POCT testing.

Bar Code Medication Administration

Bar coding has been developed to help caregivers ensure the right medication in the right dose is given to the right patient at the right time by the right route (the "*five rights*"). Bar coding works by requiring the medication giver to match, with a handheld scanner, his or her name tag, the bar code on the patient's identification band, and the medication to be given. When one of the five "rights" does not match, an alert is issued or the medication will not be dispensed from its storage system.

The *Leapfrog Group*, a conglomeration of non–health care Fortune 500 company leaders committed to modernizing the current health care system, has established standards that call for hospitals to implement a bar code medication administration (BCMA) system, linked to an electronic medication administration record, in 100% of hospital medical/surgical and intensive care units, to scan both patient and medication barcodes 95% of the time, and to have seven decision-support elements in place, as well as five best-practice processes and structures to prevent workarounds (The Leapfrog Group, 2017). Although 2016 results showed that nearly all reporting hospitals (97.8%) had a BCMA system connected to their electronic medication administration record in at least one inpatient unit, only 30% fully met the standard (The Leapfrog Group, 2017).

In addition, implementation of BCMA is not without problems. One recent study reported that nurses often develop workarounds that may undermine bar coding's safeguards. These workarounds typically occurred at the point of the human–machine interface and had significant potential to compromise patient safety (van der Veen, van den Bemt, Bijlsma, de Gier, & Taxis, 2017; Research Fuels the Controversy 19.2).

Computing and Communication

Computerized Physician/Provider Order Entry

CPOE is also a rapidly growing technology. Part of this growth has occurred because of its designation as one of three key patient safety initiatives by Leapfrog Group. In addition, the 1999 Institute of Medicine study, *To Err Is Human*, recommended the use of CPOE to address medical errors. CPOE is a clinical software application designed specifically for providers to write patient orders electronically rather than on paper. With CPOE, providers produce clearly typed orders, reducing medication errors based on inaccurate transcription. Because approximately 90% of medication errors occur during manual ordering and transcribing (handwriting and interpreting the prescription), the use of CPOE systems can help eliminate these types of errors (The Leapfrog Group, 2017).

CPOE also gives providers vital CDS via access to information tools that support a health care provider in decisions related to diagnosis, therapy, and care planning of individual patients. For example, physicians might access evidence-based medicine databases electronically for CDS when writing medication orders. If the provider has ordered a test or treatment that is contraindicated for a specific patient or condition, the CDS will inform that provider of the potential danger at the time the order is entered.

Translating CPOE into action has not, however, been without challenges. Although many health care organizations saw the value in CPOE technology, many did not consider it to be a necessity until government pressure (by law) to implement it began and reimbursement incentives were put into place. As of 2009, only 17% of hospitals in the United States had functional CPOE systems in place, which rose to 35% in 2012. As of 2017, CPOE was being fully used in 74% of U.S. hospitals (The Leapfrog Group, 2017).

There also may be cultural obstacles to CPOE; for example, a physician might prefer to write orders by hand instead of using a computer. This may be due to the normal resistance experienced with almost any change or it may reflect a reluctance to take on the increased cognitive workload associated with the use of CPOE. Physicians have also complained that the term "computerized provider order entry" had the potential to make them feel like data entry staff (Conklin, 2017).

Research Fuels the Controversy 19.2

Workarounds in Bar Code Medication Administration

The purpose of this prospective observational study was to assess the relationship between workarounds and medication administration errors in barcode-assisted medication administration (BCMA). Direct observation was used to collect data. The primary outcome measure was the proportion of medication administrations with one or more medication administration errors. A secondary outcome measure was the frequency and types of workarounds in medication administration.

Source: van der Veen, W., van den Bemt, P., Bijlsma, M., de Gier, H. J., & Taxis, K. (2017, April). Association between workarounds and medication administration errors in bar code-assisted medication administration: Protocol of a multicenter study. *JMIR Research Protocols, 6*(4), e74.

Study Findings

Researchers examined 5,793 medication administrations for 1,230 inpatients. Workarounds occurred in 66% of medication administrations and were associated with large numbers of medication administration errors. The most common procedural workarounds included not scanning at all (36%), not scanning patients because they did not wear a wristband (28%), incorrect medication scanning, multiple medication scanning, and ignoring alert signals (11%). Common types of medication administration errors were omissions (78%), administration of nonordered drugs (8.0%), and wrong doses given (6.0%).

The authors concluded that workarounds are associated with medication administration errors in hospitals using BCMA. In addition, they noted that BCMA needs more postimplementation evaluation if it is to achieve the intended benefits for medication safety.

In addition, cost is a factor. At Brigham and Women's Hospital, the cost of developing and implementing CPOE was approximately $1.9 million, with $500,000 maintenance costs per year since ("Leapfrog Fact Sheet," 2016). Installation of even "off-the-shelf" CPOE packages requires a significant amount of customization for each hospital and can be very expensive. Significant numbers of order sets must be created for CPOE to be put into place and revisions are ongoing as new evidence emerges about best practice. Providers also need and want some variance within the order sets. For example, providers want to store their preferences for medications, lab orders, and imaging orders in the EHR (Conklin, 2017). The EHR can then track deviations from the order set for review by clinical committees, which can use that information when order sets are updated. This approach allows for continuous learning that loops from the local level up to the system level and back again (Conklin, 2017).

Discussion Point

Should providers have a choice in whether to use CPOE when writing orders?

In addition, the requirements to fully meet Leapfrog's CPOE standards are stringent (Box 19.1). Still, institutional and clinician adoption of CPOE is crucial to helping caregivers to reduce medical errors and enhance patient safety, and health care institutions must commit the necessary human and financial resources to make this technological innovation a reality.

Clinical Decision Support and Artificial Intelligence

CDS is defined broadly as "a process for enhancing health-related decisions and actions with pertinent, organized clinical knowledge and patient information to improve health and healthcare delivery" (Healthcare Information and Management Systems Society, 2018, para. 2).

Like CPOE, CDS will likely be commonplace in the next decade, giving providers the promise for access at the point of care to cutting-edge research, best practices, and decision-making support to improve patient care.

> **Consider This**   Technology is never a substitute for clinical judgment or critical thinking. Technology is a tool—an adjunct to nurses' clinical skills—never a replacement.
> —Ann Scott Blouin, RN, PhD, FACHE, Executive Vice President of Customer Relations, The Joint Commission (RWJF, 2016a, p. 1)

In addition, AI will continue to gain ground as health care organizations begin to apply the technology to medical diagnoses and image recognition (Holman, 2018). Although the most common uses of AI in health care today are in natural language processing and robotic process automation, health care organizations are poised to do more with AI. Some are already using AI for CDS, population health, disease management, readmissions, and claims processing, but some experts believe that it will begin to provide value in areas such as cancer diagnostics, pathology, and image recognition in the near future (Holman, 2018).

Electronic Communication

Electronic communication technologies are also expanding at an exponential pace. Computers are increasingly a part of interdisciplinary team communication and care documentation in acute care hospitals, although futurists predict that computers will soon essentially be invisible, replaced with *smart objects*. Indeed, computerized charting is now the norm, with more institutions moving toward the use of *tablet personal computers*—flat-panel laptops that use a stylus pen or touch screen technology. In addition, *personal digital assistants* (PDAs; mobile, handheld devices including cell phones) give users access to text-based information

---

BOX 19.1   **Requirements for Full Compliance With Leapfrog's CPOE Standard**

In order to fully meet The Leapfrog Group's CPOE standard, hospitals must:
1. Ensure that physicians enter at least 75% of inpatient medication orders via a computer system that includes prescribing error prevention software; and
2. Demonstrate, via a test, that their inpatient CPOE system can alert physicians to at least 50% of common, serious prescribing errors (applies to adult hospital patients only.)

Source: Leapfrog fact sheet. (2016, April 1). *Computerized physician order entry.* Retrieved December 18, 2017, from http://www.leapfroggroup.org/sites/default/files/Files/CPOE%20Fact%20Sheet.pdf

and the latest computer and cellular applications. With institution-wide documentation systems, everyone uses the same documentation software, and the information is transferred to and retrieved from a central server via "hot synching" (putting the PDA into a cradle or connecting it via cable to the central server). In addition, the PDA can serve as a reference library, especially for drug information, and as a calculator for computing drug doses.

PDAs, however, are not cheap; in fact, the new iPhoneX can carry a hefty $1,000 price tag. In addition, PDAs can be lost or stolen, posing concerns about patient confidentiality. Finally, some health care providers feel uncomfortable using such technology in front of patients and some just feel uncomfortable with the technology itself. However, the quality and number of PDA applications continue to grow, as do their use.

Indeed, a report entitled *Point of Care Communications for Physicians 2014* revealed that physicians are universally (96%) using smartphones as their primary device to support clinical communications (HIT Consultant, 2018). Despite such universal smartphone adoption, the report found 70% of physicians believed hospital IT organizations were making inadequate investments to address physician mobile computing and communication requirements at point of care because of limited planned investments, poor mobile EHR tools, and inadequate mobile user support.

The use of *wireless local area networking* (WLAN) has also grown exponentially. WLAN uses a spread-spectrum radiofrequency to link two or more computers or devices without using wires. This allows caregivers to access, update, and transmit critical patient and treatment information despite moving between or being located at multiple sites of care. The area of outreach in the network is called the *basic service set*. Similarly, *Bluetooth* technology creates a small wireless network (called a *piconet*) between two pieces of hardware through short-range radio signals. This allows devices such as keyboards to link with personal computers and headsets to link with cell phones.

Electronic Health Records

Even health records have changed because of technology. The EHR is a digital record of a patient's health history that may be made up of records from many locations and/or sources, such as hospitals, providers, clinics, and public health agencies. For example, an EHR might include immunization status, allergies, patient demographics, lab test and radiology results, advanced directives, current medications taken, and current health care appointments. The EHR is available 24 hours a day, 7 days a week, and has built in safeguards to ensure patient health information confidentiality and security.

In January 2004, former President George Bush set a goal that most Americans would have an EHR by 2014. This goal was endorsed by former President Barack Obama and supported financially with $30 billion in stimulus funds to support hospital implementation over the next several years. It has not been easy, however, to make such system-wide changes. Cost, debates about ownership of data, and communication across computer systems have posed relentless challenges. Heavy investments are required upfront, with returns that occur only over time, if at all.

> ***Consider This*** The electronic record is not a single panacea for solving problems related to confidentiality or continuity of medical data access.

In addition, physicians have been especially slow to adopt EHRs. In a 2015 study, 83% of physicians expressed frustration using EHRs to support clinical communications because of poor interoperability, limited EHR messaging capabilities, and poor usability that made it difficult to find relevant clinical data (HIT Consultant, 2018). Similarly, a 2016 study found that poor usability and lack of desired functionality caused most physicians to be dissatisfied with their EHR technology (Heath, 2016). EHRs have also been shown to increase provider stress and reduce productivity because clinicians must often work longer hours to see the same number of patients (RWJF, 2016b).

In addition, the EHR may interfere with the patient–provider encounter, preventing quality information from being attained. Patients may feel less satisfied if providers focus on their computers instead of them as the face-to-face encounter may feel less personal. In addition, with the de-emphasis on the clinical narrative, the patient's medical record may become a series of "yes" or "no" data points (RWJF, 2016b).

> ***Consider This*** "As with any recordkeeping system, the value of an EHR is predicated on the amount and quality of information stored there, the way that information is organized, and the ease with which it can be retrieved, analyzed, and shared. EHRs represent a huge advance over paper records on all of these fronts, but they also place new demands on providers" (RWJF, 2016b, p. 3).

Virtual Care/Telehealth

Given declining reimbursement, health care provider shortages, and an increasing shift in care to outpatient settings, home care agencies are increasingly exploring technology-aided options that allow them to avoid the traditional 1:1 health care provider–patient ratio with face-to-face contact. Horner (2018) suggests that virtual care technology is increasingly applied to more use cases, more roles, more facilities, and more patient populations. For example, smaller and/or rural hospitals can use this type of technology to connect with specialists from other facilities and all patients can receive the care they need—whether it is in the form of virtual consults or a series of virtual visits—despite their geographical distance from their providers, related specialists, and traditional care settings (Horner, 2018).

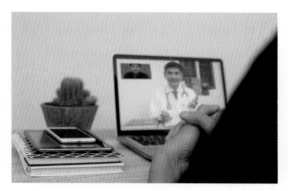

Telehealth, also called remote monitoring technology, telemedicine, telenursing, telecare, telehomecare, tele-management, e-health, and telephone care, is a form of virtual care, allowing health care providers to care for patients over a distance, using a combination of telecommunication and multimedia technologies. In more advanced telehealth, providers interact with patients through computer stations hooked up in the patient's home. These stations typically include a video monitor, a moveable color video camera, a speakerphone and microphone, and one or more medical peripherals for patient self-monitoring, such as blood pressure and pulse meter, stethoscope, pulse oximeter, scale, and glucometer. Patients record their heart rates, blood pressures, blood glucose levels, and other readings periodically and then transmit these data to a provider with a computer station like theirs. This gives the provider a real-time picture of the patient's health status. In less sophisticated telehealth programs, assessment, intervention, and evaluation occur by fax, by e-mail message, or simply by telephone.

For health care providers, telehealth has meant greater ubiquity—they can now practice across geographic boundaries and be directly involved in patient care, even when not directly on site with patients. It has also typically resulted in improved quality of care and lower costs and provided new strategies for dealing with the health disparities created by geographic location, age, and homebound status. For patients, telehealth has meant increased flexibility and, often, more personalized care.

Discussion Point

What, if anything, is "lost" when there is no face-to-face meeting between the health care provider and the patient? Can technology overcome this loss? What does technology offer that face-to-face visits do not?

Because telehealth continues to improve, performance indicators and appropriate measures of quality are evolving. More research also is needed to determine what telehealth system—or mix of telehealth and in-home visits—adds the most value both clinically and financially. Some individuals question what is lost when there is no face-to-face interaction between the patient and the care provider. A recent study by Tate, Antheunis, Kanters, Nieboer, and Gerritse (2017) suggests these concern, however, may be unfounded (Research Fuels the Controversy 19.3).

Desired patient outcomes for telehealth are a little better defined. They include patient satisfaction, increased involvement in health care decision making, reduced travel time and expense, increased time with health care providers, improved health care, improved quality of life, and increased medical record data for clinical decision making.

The Internet

The growth of the Internet as an information source for all types of information, including health, continues to grow exponentially. Just how significant is this impact? A May 2018 study suggested that Web MD has 80,000,000 unique monthly visitors, NIH has 55,000,000, and Yahoo Health has 50,500,000 (eBiz, 2018). Clearly, the scope of this use has changed the health care provider–patient relationship.

Historically, providers were recognized as the keepers of medical information. This allowed them to be the primary health care decision maker, often relegating patients to a somewhat passive and dependent role. The Internet, however, expanded the power and control of health information from providers alone to patients themselves. Indeed, the Internet, which is growing faster than any other medium in the world, has enormous potential to improve Americans' health by enhancing communications and improving access to information for care providers, patients, health plan

---

Research Fuels the Controversy 19.3

Quality of Web-Based Patient–Provider Contact

Despite the emergence of Web-based patient–provider contact, there is little evidence comparing the quality of Web-based doctor–patient interactions with face-to-face interactions. This study examined (1) the impact of a consultation medium on doctors' and patients' communicative behavior in terms of information exchange, interpersonal relationship building, and shared decision making and (2) the mediating role of doctors' and patients' communicative behavior on satisfaction with both types of consultation medium. Twelve medical interns and six simulated patients prepared four different written scenarios and were randomized to perform a total of 48 consultations. Effects of the consultations were measured by questionnaires that participants filled out directly after the consultation.

Source: Tates, K., Antheunis, M. L., Kanters, S., Nieboer, T. E., & Gerritse, M. B. (2017). The effect of screen-to-screen versus face-to-face consultation on doctor-patient communication: An experimental study with simulated patients. *Journal of Medical Internet Research*, *19*(12), e421.

Study Findings

The quality of doctor–patient communication, as indicated by information exchange, interpersonal relationship building, and shared decision making, did not differ significantly between Web-based and face-to-face consultations. Doctors and simulated patients were equally satisfied with both types of consultation medium, and no differences were found in the way participants perceived communicative behavior during these consultations. The findings suggest that concern about a negative impact of Web-based video consultation on the quality of patient–provider consultations may be unfounded.

---

administrators, public health officials, biomedical researchers, and other health professionals.

Indeed, thousands of health information Websites currently exist for consumers to explore in attempting to answer their health-related questions, and more are launched daily. The result is that patients have electronic access to medical information on virtually any topic, any time. This suggests that many consumers have at least the opportunity to be better informed about their health care problems and needs than in the past. In fact, this increased opportunity for consumers to access information has resulted in the creation of what is known as the *expert patient*—a patient who has the confidence, skills, information, and knowledge to participate in his or her health care.

Theoretically, expert patients are better informed and thus better able to be active participants in decision making. Although most providers appreciate well-informed patients who have demonstrated the initiative to learn more about their health care needs and problems, there are concerns regarding the accuracy and currency of information patients find on the Internet. In addition, many patients do not fully understand the information that is available to them, even when it is accurate. Some providers are concerned that patients will inappropriately self-diagnose, leading them to seek inappropriate treatment or no treatment at all. A smaller number of providers simply do not want to share decision-making power with patients. Students in health care programs must be taught not only to recognize patient expertise but also to actively encourage and support it.

Discussion Point

Empowering patients and involving them in their health care decision making is a socially encouraged value in health care today. Do you believe that most providers truly value and appreciate "expert patients?"

In addition, little research has been done to validate the currency or accuracy of the information on health care Internet sites. Krotoski (2011), citing a study or more than 12,000 people across 12 different countries, noted that more people than ever are using the web to find out more about an ailment before or instead of visiting the doctor. Alarmingly, only a quarter of the people surveyed checked the reliability of health information they found online by looking at the credibility of the source. In addition, Krotoski suggests that "a typical medical consultation follows this trajectory: 1) you discover a growth, 2) do a Google search, and 3) believe the first result that confirms your expectations" (para. 6). Krotoski concludes then that although the wealth of health information online has contributed to a more informed public, the expertise of the professional should not be undermined by the leveling power of the web.

Clearly, patients need to become experts at retrieving health care information and deciphering it to better empower themselves in health care decision making.

Genetics and Genomics

The National Human Genome Research Institute (2017) defines genomic medicine as "an emerging medical discipline that involves using genomic information about an individual as part of their clinical care (e.g., for diagnostic or therapeutic decision-making) and the health outcomes and policy implications of that clinical use" (para. 1). Ever since the Human Genome Project first began sequencing individual human genomes in 2001, we have learned much about how genetics influences both health and disease. In fact, the day will come soon when a medical checkup consists at least initially of a DNA readout and care will focus on preventing diseases patients are at risk of developing rather than treating illness.

Genetics and genomics will also help us to prevent or treat diseases now considered untreatable. For example, in August 2017, the U.S. Food and Drug Administration made the first gene therapy available in this country, ushering in a new approach to the treatment of cancer and other serious and life-threatening diseases (FDA News Release, 2017). Cellular therapy products include cellular immunotherapies, cancer vaccines, and other types of both autologous and allogeneic cells for certain therapeutic indications, including hematopoietic stem cells and adult and embryonic stem cells (U.S. Food and Drug Administration, 2018, para. 2). With human gene therapy, genetic material is introduced into a person's DNA to replace faulty or missing genetic material, bolstering the immune system to shut down the disease (U.S. Food and Drug Administration, 2018, para. 2). Because of these new cellular and gene therapy products, futurists suggest that cancer and heart disease deaths could diminish or disappear completely in the coming decade or two.

Organ transplants may no longer be needed because new organs can be grown from a patient's own tissue and because organs will be genetically matched to the patient, there will be far less chance of rejection. Stem cells will be used to generate replacement cartilage tissue to repair damaged joints, especially for osteoarthritis patients, and total knee and hip replacements may no longer be needed. Dentures will be replaced by stem cell therapies that grow natural teeth. In addition, biologic drugs are now available that can target molecular processes conventional drugs cannot, and they can treat a growing list of diseases including cancer, Lupus, Crohn's disease, rheumatoid arthritis, multiple sclerosis, kidney failure, asthma, and high cholesterol (Haydon, 2017).

Discussion Point

Do you believe that technology will someday eliminate "disease" as we know it today? If so, what are the implications in terms of life span and the prevalence of chronic disease?

Genetic testing has also created new opportunities for assessing genetic risk for disease so that preventive approaches to care can be taken. Direct-to-consumer companies such as 23andMe and Genos have proven particularly popular, with tens of thousands of people purchasing at-home testing kits every year (Pitts, 2017).

How common is genetic testing and how easy is it for a health care consumer to have it done? Provider orders are no longer necessary. In fact, genetic testing is now commonplace, with many commercial DNA sequencing companies charging as little as $300 to decode the human genome; and that figure could drop to $100 within the next 3 to 10 years (Herper, 2017). All the consumer must do is to send in a saliva sample and a form of payment. Results arrive in a few weeks to a few months. As a result, more than 500,000 human genomes had been sequenced as of 2017 (Herper, 2017), and global sales of genetic tests are expected to hit $10 billion within the coming decade (Pitts, 2017). In fact, Hansen (2017) suggests that more than a billion people worldwide will have their DNA mapped (and checked every year) by the year 2025. Hansen goes on to say that "if that trend continues, such sequencing eventually will become another standard lab test that doctors order as part of every patient checkup, making the promise of precision medicine a practical reality" (para. 3).

As patients gain access to information about their personal genetic sequencing, however, they are increasingly asking their health care providers to help them make informed decisions about what they should do or who they should see with that expertise. But some genetic tests have limited predictive value or may not be complete, leading patients and providers to consider making decisions with only some of the information they need. In addition, many ethical questions exist regarding whether relatives of someone with a positive predictive genetic test should or must be told about the results.

Consider This Genetic testing poses significant promise for precision medicine as well as significant risk for genetic discrimination.

In addition, Pitts (2017, para. 2) suggests that the significant growth in direct to consumer genetic testing "rests on a dangerous delusion: that genetic data is kept private. Most people assume this sensitive information simply sits in a secure database, protected from hacks and misuse." Pitts suggests this is far from the truth and that genetic testing companies cannot guarantee privacy. He also suggests that many are actively selling user data to outside parties.

Clearly, having genetic data can ultimately lead to better care and patient empowerment, but the ethical dilemmas associated with safeguarding such personal information and the potential emotional consequences of uncovering unknown medical data without the support of a primary care provider pose significant challenges for all consumers, as well as health care professionals.

IS TECHNOLOGY WORTH THE COST?

The rapid introduction of new technology is a leading cost driver in the U.S. health care system. Indeed, Clemens (2017) suggests that although technological advances in health care over the last several decades have been monumental and have served the industry well, new medical technology is responsible for 40% to 50% of annual cost increases. Indeed, many of the new biologic drugs such as T-VEC cost an average of $65,000 per patient—and that doesn't come close to topping the list of priciest biologic medications (Haydon, 2017). Indeed, the drug Brineura holds the top spot. It is a biweekly enzyme replacement therapy created to delay the loss of walking in individuals with a rare genetic disorder. Its price tag: $27,000 per injection, or more than $700,000 for a full year's treatment (Haydon, 2017). Clemens suggests we must ask why we spend so much on new technologies, knowing their significant potential to increase costs overall.

In addition, because access to technology is often dependent on a person's ability to pay for it, many health care disparities still exist in this regard. Dodds (2015) asks whether emerging technologies should be available only to those who can pay the additional cost. If so, patients who lack financial resources may not receive the same effective treatments that others can access for a range of serious conditions.

Huston (2017) agrees, noting that the reality is that emerging diagnostic and treatment technologies are expensive and thus may need to be used selectively. Decisions about who should have access to them and at what cost are at the heart of many ethical debates.

The Markkula Center for Applied Ethics (n.d.) echoes a similar concern in their assertion that the same technologies that offer hope for ever-increasing life expectancy (e.g., promising cancer treatments, surgical procedure and pharmacologic breakthroughs, and advanced genetic research)

are also leading to increased demands on the health care system from a growing population of senior citizens. "Ethicists and health professionals alike are now raising questions about when and from whom treatments should be withheld, as competition for the scarce medical resources of the health care system grows beyond the system's capacity to provide care for everyone. Already, some forms of rationing have been implemented, and more rationing of health care resources may be inevitable" (Markkula Center, n.d., para. 2).

Discussion Point

Should health care technology ever be rationed by age? By ability to pay? By perceived potential contributions to society at large?

In addition, some experts argue that technology is not only expensive (both initially and in terms of maintenance and technical support) but it needs constant upgrades, and the education needed to truly be competent in the use of all this technology is never ending.

In addition, not all health care providers embrace technology. This may simply represent a resistance to change, or it might be that health care provider input has not historically been used in technology acquisition decisions. In addition, it is possible that many health care providers have received inadequate orientation to the technology in place.

One must also remember that not all technology is worth the cost. Cost must always be weighed against possible benefits of the technology, effect on health care provider satisfaction, and projected utilization patterns. The bottom line is that health care providers and users alike must understand that technological advances come with an exorbitant price tag and we have not yet determined what makes technology worth the cost (Clemens, 2017).

Discussion Point

What makes new technology worth the cost? What criteria should be used in making these potentially value-based decisions (Huston, 2017)?

CONCLUSIONS

Emerging technologies offer great opportunities to improve the quality of patient care, but technology alone is not the answer. Indeed, "in recent years, the pace of technological change has outstripped the ability of many health care providers to fully reap the benefits or mitigate the challenges

BOX 19.2   **Pointers for Implementing Technology**

- Avoid being enticed by technology for its own sake—and be clear on the precise problem the new technology is designed to solve.
- Research the evidence related to new technologies and engage both experts and frontline users in preselection vetting.
- Make sure nurse leaders are represented on the technology and vendor selection committees and are involved in assessment and design implementation.
- Help establish evaluation criteria and an evaluation process for monitoring the introduction of major technology investments.
- Improve workflow as much as possible before implementation of a new technology, so that the new technology enhances workflow rather than impedes it.
- Take part in testing prototypes in real-life scenarios.
- Build in adequate educational resources to ensure a smooth transition.
- Remember that technology is an adjunct to care, not a replacement.

Source: Robert Wood Johnson Foundation. (2016d). *Boon or bane? Making sure technologies improve (not impede) nursing care.* Charting Nursing's Future. Issue No. 29. Retrieved May 30, 2018, from https://www.rwjf.org/content/dam/farm/reports/issue_briefs/2016/rwjf433148

that come with these advances" (RWJF, 2016a, para. 1). Regardless then of the system that is deployed, health care organizations must consider what technology can best be used in each individual setting and how it should be used. Some pointers to consider in implementing technology are shown in Box 19.2. In addition, successfully adopting and integrating new technology requires health care providers to understand that technology's limitations as well as its benefits.

> ***Consider This*** "We need to step back before we adopt new technology and have a conversation about how this will impact care. What do we lose by adding this technology? What will we gain? Nurses on the front lines of care 24/7 are the people to figure this out."
> —Carol Huston, as cited in RWJF, 2016d, p. 8.

In addition, debates about how best to merge the human element of care (caring) and emerging technology will undoubtedly continue. Historically, machines have been unable to demonstrate caring, although the development of new robotic devices is challenging this long-held belief.

Health care providers also need to overcome their "technophobia" because, clearly, care can be improved with the appropriate use of technology. But far too often, the response of health care providers has been to create "workarounds" to delay its adoption or, worse yet, mitigate any possible benefits it might bring. It is ironic that it is technology that would likely give nurses more time to do "nursing." Nurses must therefore keep the improvement of patient care first and foremost in their technology development agenda and embrace the use of technology as part of the skill set that will be expected of them in the 21st century.

For Additional Discussion

1. Is there a place for technology development in health care, even when it does not contribute to the improvement of patient outcomes? In other words, should the technology itself ever be the desired goal?

2. Are nursing schools adequately preparing students with the skill sets and competencies they will need to function successfully in a progressively more technological workplace?

3. How should organizations deal with "technophobic" health care workers? Should health care employers let employees decide what level of expertise they wish to acquire?

4. What safeguards are in place to ensure confidentiality of the EHR?

5. Do you believe confidentiality is greater with electronic or paper records?

6. What technology do you believe has the greatest potential to reduce health care worker shortages? Why?

7. What technologies currently in use would you predict to be obsolete in 10 years?

8. What barriers exist in health care environments that will impede the development of technology in years to come?

9. What safeguards do consumers have that the health information they find on the Internet is accurate and appropriate? If such safeguards are not in place, what could the consumer do to reduce their risk of inaccurate information?

References

Abate, C. (2016, August 10). *Is Davinci robotic surgery a revolution or a rip off?* Healthline. Retrieved May 30, 2018, from https://www.healthline.com/health-news/is-da-vinci-robotic-surgery-revolution-or-ripoff-021215#1

Aethon (2018). *Homepage.* Retrieved August 29, 2018 from https://aethon.com/why-aethon/

Andersen, L. R., & Rasmussen, S. (2015, February 12). *Tomorrow's technology will lead to sweeping changes in society—It must, for all our sakes.* The Conversation. Retrieved May 30, 2018, from http://theconversation.com/tomorrows-technology-will-lead-to-sweeping-changes-in-society-it-must-for-all-our-sakes-36023

Bidin, S. A. H., Lokmanb, A. M., Mohdc, W. A. R. W., & Tsuchiyad, T. (2017). Initial intervention study of Kansei robotic implementation for elderly. *Procedia Computer Science, 105,* 87–92.

Bilton, N. (2013, May 19). *Disruptions: Helper robots are steered, tentatively, to care for the aging.* The New York Times. Retrieved May 30, 2018, from http://bits.blogs.nytimes.com/2013/05/19/disruptions-helper-robots-are-steered-tentatively-to-elder-care/?_r=0

Clemens, M. (2017, October 26). *Technology and rising health care costs.* Forbes Community Voice. Retrieved May 30, 2018, from https://www.forbes.com/sites/forbestechcouncil/2017/10/26/technology-and-rising-health-care-costs/#33f926e4766b

Conklin, G. (2017, February 23). *Reframing CPOE to engage physicians.* Leadership+. Retrieved May 30, 2018, from http://www.hfma.org/Leadership/Share_Your_Story_Blog/2017/February/Reframing_CPOE_to_Engage_Physicians

Dodds, S. (2015, February 11). *3D printing raises ethical issues in medicine.* ABC Science. Retrieved May 30, 2018, from http://www.abc.net.au/science/articles/2015/02/11/4161675.htm

D'Onfro, J. (2018, May 30). *Technology companies could soon drive down health care costs, says Mary Meeker.* CNBC. Retrieved May 30, 2018, from https://www.cnbc.com/2018/05/30/mary-meeker-on-healthcare-consumerization-driving-down-costs.html

Do robots drive up prostate surgeries? (2011). FoxNews.com. Retrieved May 30, 2018, from http://www.foxnews.com/health/2011/07/20/do-robots-drive-up-prostate-surgeries

eBiz. (2018). *Top 15 most popular health websites | May 2018.* Retrieved December 23, 2017, from http://www.ebizmba.com/articles/health-websites

European Commission. (2015, April 24). *The walking robot set to help elderly people live an autonomous life.* Retrieved May 30, 2018, from http://www.euronews.com/2015/04/24/the-walking-robot-set-to-help-elderly-people-live-an-autonomous-life

Fareed, A. (2018, May 22). Building strategies for smart hospitals. Cerner. Retrieved August 29, 2018 from https://www.cerner.com/ae/en/blog/building-strategy-for-smart-hospitals

FDA News Release. (2017, August 30). *FDA approval brings first gene therapy to the United States.* Retrieved May 30, 2018, from https://www.fda.gov/NewsEvents/Newsroom/PressAnnouncements/ucm574058.htm

Fox, M. (2015, May 20). *Dramatic change for workforce ahead: Experts.* Retrieved May 30, 2018, from https://www.cnbc.com/2015/05/20/dramatic-change-for-workforce-ahead-experts.html

Freudenrich, C. (2018). *How biomechatronics works.* How Stuff Works. Retrieved May 30, 2018, from https://science.howstuffworks.com/biomechatronics.htm

Gabr, M. (n.d.). *Health ethics, equity and human dignity.* Retrieved May 30, 2018, from http://www.humiliationstudies.org/documents/GabrHealthEthics.pdf

Giuliano, K. K., & Ruppel, H. (2017). Are smart pumps smart enough? *Nursing, 47*(3), 64–66.

Hansen, D. (2017, December 23). *From DNA mapping to self-driving cars: 5 predictions for our digital future.* Forbes Brand Voice. Retrieved May 30, 2018, from https://www.forbes.com/sites/oracle/2016/10/12/from-dna-mapping-to-self-driving-cars-5-predictions-for-our-digital-future/#7e42e5737e76

Haydon, I. (2017, July 24). *Biologics: The drugs transforming medicine.* The Conversation. Retrieved May 30, 2018, from https://www.usnews.com/news/healthcare-of-tomorrow/articles/2017-07-25/biologics-the-drugs-that-are-trans-forming-medicine

Healthcare Information and Management Systems Society. (2018). *Clinical decision support.* Retrieved May 30, 2018, from http://www.himss.org/library/clinical-decision-support?navItemNumber=16563

Heath, S. (2016, October 11). *EHR vendors still seeing low physician satisfaction scores.* EHR Intelligence. Retrieved May 30, 2018, from https://ehrintelligence.com/news/ehr-vendors-still-seeing-low-physician-satisfaction-scores

Herper, M. (2017, January 9). *Illumina promises to sequence human genome for $100—But not quite yet.* Retrieved May 30, 2018, from https://www.forbes.com/sites/matthewherper/2017/01/09/illumina-promises-to-sequence-human-genome-for-100-but-not-quite-yet/#57c01ab0386d

HIT Consultant. (2018). *83% of physicians are resistant to use EHRs for clinical communications.* Retrieved December 18, 2017, from http://hitconsultant.net/2015/01/19/physicians-resistantehrs-clinical-communications

Holman, T. (2018, January 4). *Four healthcare technology trends to watch in 2018.* Tech Target Network. Retrieved May 30, 2018, from https://searchhealthit.techtarget.com/news/450432637/Four-healthcare-technology-trends-to-watch-in-2018

Horner, L. (2018, March 6). *How healthcare technology will change in 2018.* Becker's Healthcare. Retrieved May 30, 2018, from https://www.beckershospitalreview.com/healthcare-information-technology/how-healthcare-technology-will-change-in-2018.html

Huston, C. (2013, May 31). The impact of emerging technology on nursing care: Warp speed ahead. *The Online Journal of Issues in Nursing, 18*(2), Manuscript 1.

Huston, C. (2017). Technology in nursing: Emerging ethical dilemmas. In C. Robichaux (Ed.), *Ethical competence in nursing practice (2017)* (Chapter 11, pp. 253–273). New York, NY: Springer Publishing.

Jue, C. (2017, January 5). *CES 2017: As robots learn to become more human, are we more robotic?* NBC News. Retrieved May 30, 2018, from https://www.nbcnews.com/tech/tech-news/we-re-entering-age-friendly-robots-n703336

Kirkner, R. M. (2017, March 30). *Robot-assisted surgery: Twice the price.* ACS Surgery News. Retrieved May 30, 2018, from http://www.mdedge.com/acssurgerynews/article/134696/hernia/robot-assisted-surgery-twice-price

Kite-Powell, J. (2017, November 2). *New studies look at cost and benefits of robotic surgery.* Forbes. Retrieved May 30, 2018, from https://www.forbes.com/sites/jennifer-hicks/2017/11/02/new-studies-look-at-cost-and-benefits-of-robotic-surgery/#61a35a986d47

Krotoski, A. (2011, January 9). *What effect has the internet had on healthcare?* The Guardian. Retrieved May 30, 2018, from https://www.theguardian.com/technology/2011/jan/09/untangling-web-krotoski-health-nhs

Leapfrog fact sheet. Computerized physician order entry. (2016, April 1). Retrieved May 30, 2018, from http://www.leapfroggroup.org/sites/default/files/Files/CPOE%20Fact%20Sheet.pdf

Lee, J. (2014, April 19). *Surgical-robot costs put small hospitals in a bind.* Modern Healthcare. Retrieved May 30, 2018, from http://www.modernhealthcare.com/article/20140419/magazine/304199985

Markkula Center for Applied Ethics. (n.d.). *Unhealthy dilemmas.* Santa Clara University. Retrieved May 30, 2018, from http://www.scu.edu/ethics/publications/iie/v3n3/homepage.html

Matthews, K. (2017, September 1). *Robots and AI will take over these 3 medical niches first.* Singularity Hub. Retrieved May 30, 2018, from https://singularityhub.com/2017/09/01/robots-and-ai-will-take-over-these-3-medical-niches-first/#sm.0000134es1tcjgfpvttjjji7yqkwv

National Human Genome Research Institute. (2017, November 28). *What is genomic medicine?* Retrieved May 30, 2018, from https://www.genome.gov/27552451/what-is-genomic-medicine

Pitts, P. (2017, February 15). *The privacy delusions of genetic testing.* Retrieved May 30, 2018, from https://www.forbes.com/sites/realspin/2017/02/15/the-privacy-delusions-of-genetic-testing/#68979aad1bba

Pols, J. (2015). Towards an empirical ethics in care: Relations with technologies in health care. *Medicine, Health Care & Philosophy, 18*(1), 81–90. doi:10.1007/s11019-014-9582-9

Right Patient. (2018, January 11). *RightPatient® palm vein biometrics.* Retrieved May 30, 2018, from http://www.rightpa-tient.com/palm-vein-biometrics-patient-identification

Robert Wood Johnson Foundation. (2016a). *Boon or bane? Making sure technologies improve (not impede) nursing care.* Charting Nursing's Future. Issue No. 29. Retrieved May 30, 2018, from https://www.rwjf.org/content/dam/farm/reports/issue_briefs/2016/rwjf433148

Robert Wood Johnson Foundation. (2016b). *EHRs: Fundamentally changing the nature of care.* Charting Nursing's Future. Issue No. 29. Retrieved May 30, 2018, from https://www.rwjf.org/content/dam/farm/reports/issue_briefs/2016/rwjf433148

Robert Wood Johnson Foundation. (2016c). *Alarms: A classic case of unintended consequences.* Charting Nursing's Future. Issue No. 29. Retrieved May 30, 2018, from https://www.rwjf.org/content/dam/farm/reports/issue_briefs/2016/rwjf433148

Robert Wood Johnson Foundation. (2016d). *Nursing's role in guiding technological change.* Charting Nursing's Future. Issue No. 29. Retrieved May 30, 2018, from https://www.rwjf.org/content/dam/farm/reports/issue_briefs/2016/rwjf433148

Segre, L. (2018, May 1). *Cataract surgery cost.* All About Vision. Retrieved May 30, 2018, from http://www.allaboutvision.com/conditions/cataract-surgery-cost.htm

Sharkey, A., & Sharkey, N. (2012). *Granny and the robots: Ethical issues in robot care for the elderly.* University of Sheffield. Retrieved May 30, 2018, from http://staffwww.dcs.shef.ac.uk/people/A.Sharkey/sharkey-granny.pdf

Tarantola, A. (2017, August 29). *Robot caregivers are saving the elderly from lives of loneliness.* Engadget. Retrieved May 30, 2018, from https://www.engadget.com/2017/08/29/robot-caregivers-are-saving-the-elderly-from-lives-of-loneliness

Tates, K., Antheunis, M. L., Kanters, S., Nieboer, T. E., & Gerritse, M. B. (2017, December 20). The effect of screen-to-screen versus face-to-face consultation on doctor-patient communication: An experimental study with simulated patients. *Journal of Medical Internet Research, 19*(12), e421. Retrieved May 30, 2018, from https://www.jmir.org/2017/12/e421

The Leapfrog Group. (2017, April 27). *Latest report: First-ever data on bedside bar coding shows hospitals have the technology to safely administer medication, but fall short on using it effectively.* Retrieved May 30, 2018, from http://www.leapfroggroup.org/news-events/latest-report-first-ever-data-bedside-bar-coding-shows-hospitals-have-technology-safely

Trends in the palm vein biometrics market 2017 – 2025. (2017, September 21). Retrieved May 30, 2018, from https://www.lanews.org/trends-in-the-palm-vein-biometrics-market-2017-2025

Ulloa, J. G. (2018). *Applied biomechatronics using mathematical models.* Cambridge, MA: Academic Press.

U.S. Food and Drug Administration. (2018, February 2). *Cellular & gene therapy products.* Retrieved May 30, 2018, from https://www.fda.gov/biologicsbloodvaccines/cellulargenetherapyproducts

van der Veen, W., van den Bemt, P., Bijlsma, M., de Gier, H. J., & Taxis, K. (2017, April). Association between workarounds and medication administration errors in bar code-assisted medication administration: Protocol of a multicenter study. *JMIR Research Protocols, 6*(4), e74.

Wadhwa, V. (2014, April 15). *Laws and ethics can't keep pace with technology.* MIT Technology Review. Retrieved May 30, 2018, from http://www.technologyreview.com/view/526401/laws-and-ethics-cant-keep-pace-with-technology

Washington State Clinical Laboratory Advisory Council. (2017, July). *Point-of-care testing guidelines.* Retrieved May 30, 2018, from https://www.doh.wa.gov/portals/1/Documents/2700/POCT.pdf

Assuring Provider Competence Through Licensure, Continuing Education, and Certification

Carol J. Huston

LEARNING OBJECTIVES

The learner will be able to:

1. Differentiate between competence and continuing competence in a profession.

2. Identify stakeholders who would be affected by a movement to mandate continuing competence in nursing.

3. Identify driving and restraining forces to implementing mandatory reexamination as a prerequisite for license renewal in nursing.

4. Compare support for mandatory reexamination for license renewal in nursing with that of other health professions such as medicine and pharmacy.

5. Identify arguments for and against mandated continuing education for license renewal.

6. Compare continuing education requirements for nurses with those for other health care professionals.

7. Describe personal and professional benefits of professional certification.

8. Delineate the roles/responsibilities assumed by the American Board of Nursing Specialties as the accrediting body for nursing certification.

9. Identify the strengths and weaknesses of using professional certification as an indicator of entry-level competence in advanced practice nursing.

10. Describe how portfolios and self-assessment, as tools for reflective practice, can further the goal of professional competence.

11. Explore the roles and responsibilities of the individual, employers, the State Board of Nursing, and professional associations in assuring both the initial and the continued competence of health care practitioners.

12. Reflect on his or her beliefs regarding the need for and efficacy of mandating reexamination for licensure, continuing education, and certification for nurses to assure continuing competence.

INTRODUCTION

How can one determine whether a nurse is competent? Does licensure assure competence? Does clinical performance assure competence? Does competence require recency of clinical practice? Is it assured by professional certification? Would nurse residencies increase the competency of the new graduate nurse?

Unfortunately, in many states, a practitioner is determined to be competent when initially licensed and thereafter unless proven otherwise. Yet, clearly, passing a licensing examination and continuing to work as a clinician does not assure competence throughout a career. Competence requires continual updates to knowledge and practice, and this is difficult in a health care environment characterized by rapidly emerging new technologies, chaotic change, and perpetual clinical advancements based on new evidence.

For example, the Institute of Medicine (IOM, 2010) report *The Future of Nursing* suggests that nursing graduates now need competency in a variety of areas including continuous improvement of the quality and safety of health care systems, informatics, evidence-based practice, a knowledge of complex systems, skills and methods for leadership and management of continual improvement, and health policy knowledge, skills, and attitudes. One must at least question how many nurses currently in practice would be able to demonstrate competency in all of these areas.

In addition, new competencies must be integrated into nursing practice as new science emerges. For example, Watson Dillon and Mahoney (2015) note that population health will be a new competency for nurse executives patient care. The Quality, Safety, and Education for Nurses Institute (QSEN, 2018) suggests nurses now need competency for practice in patient-centered care, teamwork and collaboration, evidence-based practice, quality improvement, safety, and informatics. In addition, Calzone,

Jenkins, Culp, Caskey, and Badzek (2014) argue that genomics is another emerging competency. In their study of a 1-year genomics competency integration effort, the majority (89%) of nurses felt it was very or somewhat important to become more educated in the genetics of common diseases, but a competency deficit affecting all nurses regardless of academic preparation or role was observed. Thus, despite a recognized need to develop new clinical competencies, the workplace did not support or provide an environment that promoted such learning.

> *Consider This* "You can't be too qualified . . . technology and practice are always stretching new boundaries" ("Stepping Up Your Nursing Career," 2017, p. 7).

In 1995, the Task Force on Healthcare Workforce Regulations of the Pew Health Professions Commission recommended changing how health care professions, including nursing, were regulated and suggested that continued competence should be assured as a regulatory board function. The Citizens Advocacy Center, a public policy organization located in Washington, DC, concurred, as did the IOM (1999) in its report *To Err Is Human*, which included a recommendation for professional licensing bodies to assume the responsibility for determining licensees' competence and knowledge.

There is little disagreement that the knowledge health care professionals need must be current and appropriate to their area of practice and that their care should be competent at the minimum. The challenge lies, however, in determining how best to assure that competence and in determining who should be responsible for its oversight.

This chapter explores definitions of *competence,* giving particular attention to that of *continuing competence.* Licensure, periodic relicensure, continuing education (CE), and professional certification are examined as potential strategies for assuring provider competence. The chapter also discusses the limitations of each of these strategies for assessing both initial and continuing competence, as well as the difficulties inherent in standardizing continuing competence requirements in a health care system composed of varied stakeholders. Finally, the chapter concludes with an exploration of portfolio development and reflective practice: contemporary strategies that allow health care professionals to carry out a self-assessment of their practice and to develop a personal plan for maintaining competence.

DEFINING COMPETENCE

Competence in nursing can be defined in many ways. Dictionary.com (2018) defines competence as adequacy or the possession of required skill, knowledge, qualification, or capacity. As such, it is tied to experience and context. Hence, professional competence can be defined as the capacity to handle events and challenges effectively.

In 1999, the American Nurses Association (ANA) convened an expert panel that defined three types of competence in nursing: *continuing competence, professional nursing competence*, and *continuing professional nursing competence.* Special attention was given, however, to continuing competence because so many assumptions exist regarding the rights and responsibilities of consumers, individual nurses, and employers to see that such competence is present and promulgated. Indeed, it is continuing competence that is a primary focus of this chapter, given that initial licensure suggests that at least minimum competence levels were met at that time.

In 2007, the ANA released a draft position statement on competence and competency for public review and comment. The purpose of this position paper was to define *competence* ("performing successfully at an expected level") and *competency* ("an expected level of performance that results from an integration of knowledge, skills, abilities, and judgment within the context of current and projected professional directions"). Key excerpts from the final document released in 2008 and reaffirmed in 2014 are shown in Box 20.1.

Clearly, although there is some overlap among these definitions, there is still some lack of consensus around what competence is and how it should be measured. There also appears to be difficulty in relating the continuing competence of providers with the roles they are asked to assume in the clinical setting. For example, some nurses develop high levels of competence in specific areas of nursing practice as a result of work experience and specialization at the expense of staying current in other areas of practice. Yet employers, who espouse the support of continuing competence, often ask registered nurses (RNs) to provide care in areas of practice outside their area of expertise because staffing shortages encourage them to do so. In addition, many current competence assessments focus more on skills than they do on knowledge.

Consider This   Nurses are often asked to float to or work in areas where their competence may be in question because their license allows them to work in virtually any area of practice.

In addition, professional nursing organizations decline to implement continuing competence mandates because they fear membership repercussions. For example, the American Nurses Credentialing Center (ANCC) continues to offer certification examinations for RNs without

---

BOX 20.1   **Excerpts From the American Nurses Association (ANA) Draft Statement on Professional Role Competence (Approved March 28, 2008, and Reaffirmed November 12, 2014)**

The ANA supports the following principles in regard to competence in the nursing profession:
- The public has a right to expect nurses to demonstrate competence throughout their careers.
- Nurses are individually responsible and accountable for maintaining professional competence.
- The nursing profession must shape and guide any process assuring nurse competence.
- Regulatory bodies define minimal standards for regulation of practice to protect the public.
- Employers are responsible and accountable to provide an environment conducive to competent practice.
- Assurance of competence is the shared responsibility of the profession, individual nurses, professional organizations, credentialing and certification entities, regulatory agencies, employers, and other key stakeholders.

Source: American Nurses Association. (2014, November 12). *ANA position statement: Professional role competence.* Retrieved June 3, 2018, from https://www.nursingworld.org/practice-policy/nursing-excellence/official-position-statements

baccalaureate degrees, despite the recognition that such certification suggests advanced rather than basic practice.

The ANA advocates that states defer competence monitoring to the professional association, without governmental involvement in the process, partly because of concern about misconduct charges if state regulators are involved and partly because memberships and revenues are likely to increase if the association monitors competence. Clearly, then, stakeholders and politics continue to influence how continuing competence is defined, used, and promulgated.

The issue is also complicated by the fact that there are no national standards for defining, measuring, or requiring continuing competence in nursing. In addition, specialty nursing organizations, state nurses' associations, state boards of nursing, and professional nursing organizations have not reached a consensus about what continuing competence is and how to measure it, although there is little debate that it is needed. The reality is that given the multiplicity and variations of the definition of continuing competence and the number of stakeholders affected by its promulgation, identifying and mandating strategies that assure the continuing competence of health care providers will be very difficult.

Consider This There is no consensus about how to define or objectively measure competence in nursing practice.

PROFESSIONAL LICENSURE

Licensure can be defined as

the granting of permission by a competent authority (usually a government agency) to an organization or individual to engage in a practice or activity that would otherwise be illegal. Licensure is usually granted on the basis of education and examination rather than performance. It is usually permanent, but a periodic fee, demonstration of competence, or continuing education may be required. (The Free Dictionary by Farlex, 2003–2018, para. 1)

Most health care professionals must be licensed, and this license is assumed to provide at least some assurance that the practitioner was competent in his or her field at the time of initial licensure.

Licensure Processes in Nursing

One of the most important purposes of the National Council of State Boards of Nursing (NCSBN, 2018b) and its 59 state boards of nursing (1 in each of 50 states, 2 in 3 states, 1 in the District of Columbia, 1 in each of four U.S. territories, and 1 with both a Board of Nursing and a board for advanced practice nurses) is to protect the health, safety, and welfare of the public. This is done by having a regulatory role in the accreditation of nursing education programs, through licensure and by implementing and enforcing the Nurse Practice Act. In addition, the NCSBN has created and disseminated numerous nursing practice and regulation resources on nursing practice and education and maintains a database on nursing disciplinary actions taken across the nation.

It is the licensing examinations for RNs and licensed practical nurses/vocational nurses (LPNs/LVNs), however, that the NCSBN and its state boards of nursing are probably best known. The NCSBN has developed two licensure examinations to test the entry-level nursing competence of candidates for licensure as RNs and as LPNs/LVNs. These examinations, the National Council Licensure Examinations (NCLEX-RN and NCLEX-PN), are administered with the contractual assistance of a national test service (NCSBN, 2018c) and test-integrated nursing content. Passage of the NCLEX suggests that the individual has been deemed by the state to have met minimal competence standards for entry into practice; however, it may not reflect or measure the many higher-level competencies achieved in different types of education programs for nurses.

Despite this flaw, licensure by examination continues to be a highly regarded strategy for assuring competence levels of health care professionals such as nurses. Indeed, some professional organizations and regulatory bodies suggest that RNs should be required to repeat the NCLEX periodically or that nurses should be required to take examinations similar in scope to the NCLEX for license renewal.

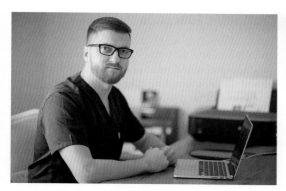

Efforts to implement mandatory reexamination as a prerequisite for license renewal in nursing, however, have met with minimal success. This is because there is little agreement about what such an examination should look like, how it would be administered, and how often it should be required. Nonetheless, multiple states have introduced legislation with varying approaches from retesting to requiring a provider to demonstrate competence in the workplace, but resistance is high, and there is little hope that periodic reexaminations to assess competence will be a part of nursing's immediate future.

In addition, the original *Nurse Licensure Compact* (NLC), with 25 participant states, allowed a nurse to have a license in one state and to practice in other states, as long as that nurse was subject to each state's practice laws and discipline (NCSBN, 2018a). That compact further reduced the likelihood that a nurse would require NCLEX reexamination during his or her career, despite crossing state lines where the initial nursing license was obtained.

The NLC was revised, however, in 2015, becoming the *enhanced NLC* (eNLC). Nurses with an original NLC multistate license were grandfathered into the eNLC but new applicants residing in the 29 states who have enacted eNLC legislation and the 9 states with pending legislation (as of January 25, 2018; Table 20.1) will need to meet 11 uniform licensure requirements (NCSBN, 2018a). The effective date for the eNLC is the sooner of the states enacting the eNLC or on December 31, 2018.

Licensure Processes in Medicine

In contrast to the NCLEX, U.S. medical licensure examinations are developed using a competence-based process that requires examinees to be cognizant of practice changes, the evidence required for practice, and the knowledge

TABLE 20.1	States That Have Enacted or Have Pending Legislation to Make the Enhanced Nurse Licensure Compact (eNLC) Effective

Enacted as of January 25, 2018

1. Arizona
2. Arkansas
3. Colorado
4. Delaware
5. Florida
6. Georgia
7. Idaho
8. Iowa
9. Kentucky
10. Maine
11. Maryland
12. Mississippi
13. Missouri
14. Montana
15. Nebraska
16. New Hampshire
17. New Mexico
18. North Carolina
19. North Dakota
20. Oklahoma
21. South Carolina
22. South Dakota
23. Tennessee
24. Texas
25. Utah
26. Virginia
27. West Virginia
28. Wisconsin
29. Wyoming

States With Pending eNLC Legislation as of January 25, 2018

1. Illinois
2. Louisiana
3. Massachusetts
4. Michigan
5. Minnesota
6. New Jersey
7. New York
8. Rhode Island
9. Vermont

Source: National Council State Boards of Nursing (2018a). Enhanced Nurse Licensure Compact (eNLC) Implemented Jan. 19, 2018. Retrieved August 30, 2018 from https://ncsbn.org/11945.htm

necessary to be competent into the future. In addition, to achieve full authority to practice independently, physicians are required to pass three licensure examinations

(U.S. Medical Licensing Examination, 1996–2018). Furthermore, a clinical skills examination was implemented in 2004.

In addition, although periodic reexamination was recommended in 1967 by the Bureau of Health Manpower of the U.S. Department of Health for licensure of physicians as of 1971, the decision regarding whether to do so has been left to the discretion of individual states. In most states, this is simply a matter of completing mandatory CE requirements and having no disciplinary actions filed against their license.

Licensure Processes in Pharmacy

Pharmacists have also been reluctant to embrace the IOM's *To Err Is Human* recommendation that periodic reexamination of key providers is critical to resolving health care quality problems, especially medical errors. Pharmacists take a licensing exam on graduation, known as the North American Pharmacist Licensure Examination (NAPLEX). The NAPLEX is a computer-adaptive examination that consists of 185 multiple-choice test questions. (Only 150 are used to tabulate the applicant's score. The remaining 35 are "trial balloon" questions under consideration for inclusion on future NAPLEX tests.) The NAPLEX is just one component of the licensure process and is used by the boards of pharmacy as part of their assessment of a candidate's competence to practice as a pharmacist (National Association of Boards of Pharmacy [NABP], 2018b).

In addition, 50 boards require a Multistate Pharmacy Jurisprudence Examination (MPJE), which combines federal- and state-specific questions to test the pharmacy jurisprudence knowledge of prospective pharmacists both for initial licensure and for license transfer (NABP, 2018a). The four boards that do not utilize the MPJE for their law examinations are Arkansas, California, Puerto Rico, and the Virgin Islands. The MPJE consists of 120 test questions. Reciprocity is then granted between states by an electronic licensure transfer program. At present, pharmacists are not required to retake the NAPLEX at any point for license renewal.

Discussion Point

Why are professional health care organizations reluctant to support reexamination as a means of assuring continuing competence? Who are the stakeholders involved?

What are some ramifications of adopting such a mandate?

CONTINUING EDUCATION

Instead of requiring health care providers to periodically repeat their initial licensure examinations, many professional associations and states have mandated CE for license renewal. This has been done in an attempt to promote continued competence and is less controversial than periodic reexamination for licensure.

CE in Nursing

A majority of the states in the United States have some kind of requirements for CE for professional nurse license renewal. These requirements typically vary from a few hours to 30 hours, every 2 years (Box 20.2). There is no requirement for CE for RNs in Arizona, Colorado, Connecticut, Georgia, Hawaii, Idaho, Illinois, Maine, Maryland, Mississippi, Missouri, Montana, New York, Oklahoma, South Dakota, Tennessee, Vermont, Virginia, Washington, and Wisconsin. Every other state has some sort of requirement for RNs ("Nursing CEU Requirements," 2017).

Some states—Colorado, for example—required CE at one time, but removed that requirement because it felt that CE did not guarantee competence. Similarly, Hawaii discontinued CE requirements for many professions, including nursing and physical therapy, because of the high costs of these courses to the individual practitioner, considerable costs to the state to administer the legislation, and the inability to demonstrate positive outcomes.

Discussion Point

Is the need for CE greater for one type of health care professional than another? When required, should the minimum number of mandated hours be the same for all health care professionals? If not, how many should be required for each health care specialty?

CE in Medicine

Sixty-two boards (46 states plus Guam, Puerto Rico, and the Virgin Islands) require some form of continuing medical education (CME) for relicensure of medical doctors (MDs) and for doctors of osteopathy (DOs), although the requirements frequently differ for the two groups (American College of Physicians, 2018; Medscape Education, 2016).

The number of required hours also varies dramatically by state. For example, Colorado, Indiana, Montana, and South Dakota require no CME hours for either MDs or DOs (Medscape Education, 2016). New York requires only

BOX 20.2   Sample State Continuing Education (CE) Requirements for Nurses

- *Arkansas:* 15 practice-focused contact hours every 2 years, or certification or recertification during the renewal period by a national certifying body or completion of 1 college credit hour course in nursing with a grade of C or better during licensure period (Arkansas Board of Registered Nursing, 2018).
- *California:* 30 hours every 2 years (California Board of Registered Nursing, 2018).
- *Florida:* 18 general hours of CE plus 2 hours on Medical Error, 2 hours on Florida laws and rules, 2 hours on Recognizing Impairment in the Workplace, and 1 hour of HIV/AIDS every 2 years (Florida Board of Registered Nursing, 2018).
- *Iowa:* 36 hours for a 3-year license (Iowa Board of Nursing, 2018).
- *Michigan:* Not less than 25 hours of CE, with at least 2 hours in pain and symptom management every 2 years. There is also a one time training in identifying victims of human trafficking beginning with the 2017 renewal cycle (Michigan Board of Nursing, 2018).
- *New Jersey:* 30 hours every 2 years (State of New Jersey, 2017).
- *New York:* 3 contact hours of infection control every 4 years and 2 contact hours of child abuse (one time; "New York Board of Nursing State CE Requirements," 2018).
- *North Dakota:* 12 contact hours every 2 years ("North Dakota Board of Nursing State CE Requirements," 2018).
- *Ohio:* 24 hours every 2 years (Ohio Board of Nursing, 2018).
- *Oregon:* One-time, 7-hour course on pain management. One hour must be a course to be provided by the Oregon Pain Management Commission. The remaining 6 hours can be from a choice of pain management topics. Once this requirement is fulfilled, there are no additional CE requirements for renewal ("Oregon Board of Nursing State CE Requirements," 2018).
- *Texas:* All nurses with an active Texas license are required to demonstrate continuing competency for relicensure. This includes 20 hours of CE every 2 years. In 2010, rules were changed to require contact hours to be in the nurse's area of practice (Texas Board of Nursing, 2015).

infection control and child abuse content. Illinois requires 150 hours every 3 years, whereas Wisconsin requires only 30 hours every 2 years, and Arkansas requires only 20 hours each year (Medscape Education, 2016). It should be noted, however, that some medical specialty societies, specialty boards, hospital medical staffs, the Joint Commission, and insurance groups require physicians to demonstrate CE, even if the state does not require this for relicensure.

In addition, some states have laws that direct the format of the CME. Required topics often include pain management, AIDS, and domestic violence. Other states require that physicians renewing their licenses must receive instruction on ethics and professional responsibility.

Furthermore, unlike nursing CE, which is typically monitored by the state boards of nursing, there is no central repository of CME. Instead, accredited CME providers are required to keep records of *CE credits* awarded to physicians who participate in their activities for 6 years, and physicians are responsible for maintaining a record of their CME credits from all sources.

CE in Other Health Care Professions

Almost all states require CE for pharmacists, and most require the CE be from approved sources such as the American Council on Pharmacy Education. Sometimes

carryover of hours or units is allowed, and sometimes the type is proscribed.

In addition, many states require acupuncturists, audiologists, and occupational therapists to have CE for license renewal. Physician assistants must log 100 hours of CME every 2 years and sit for recertification every 6 years to maintain their national certification (American Academy of Physician Assistants, n.d.).

> ### Discussion Point
>
> CE is mandated in most states for certified public accountants, optometrists, real estate brokers, nursing home administrators, and insurance brokers. Why are there fewer states mandating CE for health care professionals?
>
> What rationale can be given for why these occupations have a greater need for CE than health care professionals?

Does Requiring CE Ensure Competence?

The CE approach to continuing competence continues to be very controversial because there is limited research

Pros and Cons of Continuing Education (CE) Requirements for Nurses

Pros
- Demonstrates professionalism
- Reflects commitment to maintaining competence
- Directs attention to patient safety and a reduction in medical errors
- Motivates employers to support CE needs of RN employees
- Raises the standard for CE for all nurses
- Research supports the conclusion that CE positively affects nursing practice

Cons
- Seat time does not guarantee learning
- Difficult to agree on competence standards
- Administrative and monitoring costs
- Concerns about the cost, access, quality, and relevance of CE offerings
- Research is inconclusive about the benefits of mandatory CE over voluntary CE
- Difficult to measure outcomes of mandatory CE on patient care because of the many variables that influence patient outcomes, including the individual nurse, the choice of the CE program, the CE program itself, learning styles, professionalism, and accountability

Source: Taft, L., & Sparks, R. K. (2008). Mandatory continuing education for nurses. *Nursing Matters, 19*(3), 4.

demonstrating correlation among CE, continuing competence, and improved patient outcomes. In addition, many professional organizations have expressed concern about the quality of mandated CE courses and the lack of courses for experts and specialists. Likewise, there is no agreement on the optimal number of annual credits needed to ensure competence. Until consensus can be reached regarding how CE should be provided and how much is needed, and until research findings show an empirical link between CE and provider competence, it is difficult to tout CE as a valid and reliable measure of continuing competence. Taft and Sparks (2008) summarized the pros and cons of mandating CE for nurses (Box 20.3).

CERTIFICATION

The Accreditation Board for Specialty Nursing Certification suggests certification "is the formal recognition of the specialized knowledge, skills, and experience demonstrated by the achievement of standards identified by a nursing specialty to promote optimal health outcomes" (American Nurses Credentialing Center [ANCC], 2018b, para. 3). Certification does not, however, include a legal scope of practice. The ANCC suggested, however, that it does protect the public by enabling anyone to identify competent people more readily; aids the profession by encouraging and recognizing professional achievement; recognizes specialization; enhances professionalism; and, in some cases, serves as a criterion for financial reimbursement (ANCC, 2018b). Organizations offering specialty certifications for nurses include the ANCC, the American Association of Critical Care Nursing, the American Association of Nurse Anesthetists, The American College of Nurse Midwives, the Board of Certification for Emergency Nursing, and the Rehabilitation Nursing Certification Board.

Becoming Certified

To achieve professional certification, nurses must meet eligibility criteria that may include years and types of work experience, as well as minimum educational levels, active nursing licenses, and successful completion of a nationally administered examination. Certifications normally last 5 years.

The American Board of Nursing Specialties

In addition to the large numbers of certified nurses, there are many different types of nursing certification credentials, and certification programs often have very different standards. This makes it difficult for providers and consumers to determine the value of a particular nursing certification. For this reason, the American Board of Nursing Specialties (ABNS) was created in 1991 to bring about uniformity in nursing certification, advocate for consumer protection by establishing specialty nursing certification, and increase public awareness of the value of quality certification to health care (American Board of Nursing Specialties, 2016).

The ABNS is composed of nurse-certifying organizations from around the world. As the only accrediting body specifically for nursing certification, the Accreditation Council provides a peer-review process for accrediting nursing certification programs that demonstrate compliance with ABNS standards.

The American Nurses Credentialing Center

The ANA established the ANA Certification Program in 1973 to provide tangible recognition of professional achievement in a defined functional or clinical area of nursing. The ANCC, a subsidiary of the ANA, became its own corporation in 1991, and since then has certified more than a quarter million nurses and approximately 75,000 advanced practice nurses (ANCC, 2018b). The ANCC, as of 2018, offered 24 specialty certifications for RNs, nurse practitioners (NPs), and clinical nurse specialists (CNSs; ANCC, 2018a).

Certification and the Advanced Practice Nurse

Advanced practice nurses were the first nurses to use professional certification as a means of documenting advanced knowledge in practice. In 1946, the American Association of Nurse Anesthetists began certifying nurse anesthetists. The American College of Nurse Midwives soon followed. Most states now use certification as an indicator of entry-level competence in advanced practice nursing, which includes CNSs and NPs.

Even the NCSBN, which originally proposed second licensure for NPs, now recognizes the certification examination as the regulatory mechanism for advanced nursing practice. A master's degree is required to take the certification examinations for advanced practice nurses. Certification, then, in the case of the advanced practice nurse is not really voluntary; it is required to ensure public safety and enhance public health.

> ### Discussion Point
>
> The ANCC currently does not allow educational waivers for the CNS- or NP-certifying examination (all applicants must have at least a master's degree). Do you support this decision to not "grandfather" advanced practice nurses who completed their educations through certifying programs (no master's degree) and who are currently practicing in an advanced role? Why or why not?

The Effect of Professional Certification

A great deal of research has been completed in the past decade regarding the use of certification to ensure competence and its inherent value. Most of these studies suggest that certification does have an effect on both improved patient outcomes and the creation of a positive work environment (Box 20.4). For example, Boyle, Cramer, Potter, Gatua, and Stobinski (2014) examined the impact of specialty nursing certification on patient outcomes in surgical intensive care units and perioperative units and found lower rates of central line–associated

> **BOX 20.4**   **Personal Benefits of Professional Certification**
>
> - Provides a sense of accomplishment and achievement
> - Validation of specialty knowledge and competence to peers and patients
> - Increased credibility
> - Increased self-confidence
> - Promotes greater autonomy of practice
> - Provides for increased career opportunities and greater competitiveness in the job market
> - May result in salary incentives

bloodstream infections when nurses held specialty certification. In addition, Fitzpatrick, Campo, and Gacki-Smith (2014) found significant differences in perceived empowerment between emergency department staff nurses who held specialty certification and those who did not.

Creating Work Environments That Value Certification

It is middle- and top-level nurse managers who play the most significant role in creating work environments that value and reward certification. For example, nurse managers can grant tuition reimbursement or salary incentives to workers who seek certification. This is critical because significant barriers to nurses obtaining specialty certification are time and cost. Managers can also show their support for professional certification by giving employees paid time off to take the certification exam and by publicly recognizing employees who have achieved specialty certification.

Managers should also encourage certified nurses to promote their achievements by introducing themselves as certified nurses to patients and wearing their certification pins. In doing so, the certified nurse acts as a role model to other nurses considering specialty certification.

In addition, March 17, 2017 was designated by the AACN to celebrate certified nurses ("How Will You Celebrate Certified Nurses?" 2017). This Certified Nurses Day sought to publicly honor, recognize, and celebrate certified nurses in hospitals and health care facilities throughout the United States.

> ### Discussion Point
>
> Do most employers value professional certification? Do nurses value it?
>
> Does the general public value it? On what criteria do you base your answer?

REFLECTIVE PRACTICE

Reflective practice is defined by the NCBN (n.d.) as "a process for the assessment of one's own practice to identify and seek learning opportunities to promote continued competence" (para. 3). Inherent in the process is the evaluation and incorporation of this learning into one's practice. Such self-assessment is gaining popularity as a way to promote professional practice and maintain competence. Often this is done through the use of professional portfolios for competence assessment.

For example, North Carolina now requires RNs to use a reflective practice approach to carry out a self-assessment of her or his practice and develop a plan for maintaining competence (NCBN, n.d.). This assessment is individualized to the licensed nurse's area of practice. RNs seeking license renewal or reinstatement must attest to having completed the learning activities required for continuing competence and be prepared to submit evidence of completion if requested by the board on random audit (NCBN, n.d.).

Similarly, the Nurses Association of New Brunswick (NANB, 2018) developed a mandatory continuing competence program (CCP) for implementation in 2008 (again revised in 2013) that requires RNs to demonstrate on an annual basis how they have maintained their competence and enhanced their practice. The NANB argues that continuing competence is a necessary component of practice and the public interest is best served when nurses enhance their knowledge, skill, and judgment on an ongoing basis; and reflective practice, or the process of continually assessing one's practice to identify learning needs and opportunities for growth, is the key to continuing competence (NANB, 2018).

The three steps of the NANB mandatory CCP are as follows:

1. Self-assessment of nursing practice to determine learning needs
2. Development and implementation of a learning plan to meet the identified learning needs
3. Evaluation of the effect of learning activities

The College of Registered Nurses of British Columbia (CRNBC, 2018) also has a mandatory CCP in place. This program was created in 2000 in response to the Health Professions Act, which required the establishment and maintenance of a CCP to promote high practice standards among RNs.

> **Consider This** Competence is continually maintained and acquired through reflective practice, lifelong learning, and integration of learning into nursing practice (NANB, 2018).

Portfolios and Self-Assessment

Portfolio development is another strategy the individual RN can use to be reflective about his or her practice and/or to assess or demonstrate competence. The professional portfolio typically contains core components such as biographical information; educational background; certifications achieved; employment history; a resume; a competence record or checklist; personal and professional goals; professional development experiences, presentations, consultations, and publications; professional and community activities; honors and awards; and letters of thanks from patients, families, peers, organizations, and others.

Even nursing students can benefit from developing a *professional portfolio of learning* (PPL). Peddle, Jokwiro, Carter, and Young (2016) suggest that a PPL can support the assessment and development of nursing student's clinical competence by blending clinical, online, and class-based activities into one space for formative, summative, and personal assessment activities to support graduation and employment opportunities (Research Fuels the Controversy 20.1).

> **Consider This** All nurses should maintain a portfolio to reflect professional growth throughout their career.

WHO IS RESPONSIBLE FOR COMPETENCE ASSESSMENT IN NURSING?

Who, then, has the responsibility for competence assessment in nursing? Should it be the individual, the employer, the regulatory board, or the certifying agency? Is it a shared responsibility? If so, are these entities willing to work together to create an integrated and systematic approach to promoting continuing competence in nursing?

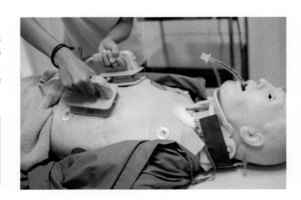

Research Fuels the Controversy 20.1

The Professional Portfolio of Learning

In 2013, the Professional Portfolio of Learning (PPL) was introduced in the Bachelor of Nursing at La Trobe University to support the assessment and development of nursing students' clinical competence. The aim of the PPL is to blend clinical, online, and class-based activities into one space for formative, summative, and personal assessment activities to support graduation and employment opportunities. The use of an action learning approach to design and implement the PPL allowed researchers to learn and improve/modify their approach as they progressed through each phase of the project.

Source: Peddle, M., Jokwiro, Y., Carter, M., & Young, T. (2016). A professional portfolio of learning for undergraduate nursing students. *Australian Nursing & Midwifery Journal, 24*(4), 40.

Study Findings

Following the pilot with first year students in 2014, review of the administrative, learning technology, business systems, clinical learning, and academic coordination elements of the PPL was modified in support of wider implementation across the curriculum.

   Benefits from the PPL included:

- Providing all students with a PPL to support professional development, life-long learning, and career transition from enrolment to graduation and beyond.
- Ability for students to review performance, identify strengths, and plan to address areas of weakness.
- Development of a far more comprehensive professional profile of the graduating student with supporting evidence.

- Improved rigor and administration of clinical appraisal systems and enhanced relationships with external partners.
- Real-time performance monitoring and timely opportunities to effectively manage student activity in clinical placement and identify students in need of support.
- Improved integration of theory and practice for teaching, learning, and assessment activities.
- The researchers concluded that the ultimate benefit for students from the PPL is the ability to record evidence of their development of competence as a RN.

Certainly, an individual responsibility for maintaining competence is suggested by the *ANA Code of Ethics for Nurses with Interpretive Statements* in its assertion that nurses are obligated to provide adequate and competent nursing care (American Nurses Association, 2015). State Nurse Practice Acts also hold nurses accountable for being reasonable and prudent in their practice. Both standards require the nurse to have at least some personal responsibility for continually assessing his or her professional competence through reflective practice.

> **Consider This**   The individual RN has a professional obligation to maintain competence.

The role of the professional association also lacks clarity. Although professional associations develop and promote standards, there is no oversight function of either initial or continuing competence.

Employers also play a role in assuring competence of employees by performing periodic performance appraisals and by carrying out the requirements of the accrediting bodies to ensure the ongoing competencies of employees. Yet employers are often among the first to argue that "a nurse is a nurse is a nurse" when it comes to meeting mandatory staffing or licensure requirements.

Regulatory boards, such as the state boards of nursing, regulate initial licensure, monitor compliance with requirements for license renewal, and take action when professional standards are breached. Yet, clearly, licensure and relicensure per se do not guarantee competence, particularly in a discipline as broad in scope and practice as nursing.

Finally, certifying organizations do help to identify those individuals who have expertise in a specific area of practice; however, knowledge expertise does not always translate into practice expertise. A lack of professional certification does not necessarily mean that the nurse lacks continuing competence. Recertification does not ensure continued expertise because recertification is usually a product of meeting CE requirements rather than reexamination.

CONCLUSIONS

The challenge in assuring competence in nursing is that nursing practice is dynamic, and thus best practice must be continually redefined as a result of new discoveries. Licensure, CE, and professional certification can ensure provider competence only if they reflect the latest thinking, research, and clinical practice needs. In addition, each of these three strategies is limited in its effectiveness as a competence assessment strategy.

Clearly, the NCLEX, as it currently exists, assures only minimum entry-level competence for professional nursing practice. Given that NCLEX content derives from a retrospective model and that technologic changes and the rate of knowledge acquisition are increasing exponentially in the 21st century, the knowledge base of the newly licensed nurse has a great likelihood of being dated even before examinations are scored. In addition, as long as a single NCLEX exists and there are multiple levels of educational entry into practice, the examination will continue to have to meet educational content directed at the lowest educational level of entry.

In addition, health care professionals, professional organizations, and regulatory bodies are reluctant to implement mandatory reexamination for licensure. One must at least question whether this is because of the fear that many providers would be unable to demonstrate the continuing competence necessary for relicensure.

CE has similar limitations for assuring provider competence. Some states do not require nurses to complete CE. Those that do demonstrate wide variation in how much CE is required, what content can be included, and how that CE can be provided. In addition, there is no guarantee that completing CE courses results in a change in the provider's knowledge level or practice or even that the content provided in the CE course is current and relevant.

Finally, professional certification does ensure that the nurse has some specialized area of knowledge and practice expertise. The reality, however, is that many nurses perform outside of the area of their certification expertise each and every day in their jobs, particularly if their area of specialty certification expertise is narrow. In addition, there are multiple certifying bodies and numerous types of certification. Determining the exact value of that certification in terms of improving patient care has not completely been ascertained.

How best to ensure provider competence cannot yet be answered. Efforts that address the need to do so are underway, but these efforts have not been coordinated or integrated by the professional associations, regulatory bodies, and stakeholders that are affected. In addition, most professional entities involved in ensuring continuing competence are reluctant to mandate interventions for fear of alienating stakeholders. Individual practitioners also seem reluctant to embrace reflective practice or to put thought and effort into creating portfolios that identify continuing competence in concrete and measurable ways. Until the focus rests solely on the need to protect patients and improve the quality of health care, mandated interventions for continuing competence are likely never to occur and provider competence will not be assured.

For Additional Discussion

1. Who should be responsible for the cost of ensuring provider competence—the provider, the employer, the clients that are served, or some other entity?

2. How likely is it that states, professional organizations, professional certifying organizations, and employers will be willing to agree on standardized measures for assessing professional competence?

3. Would most RNs support mandatory development of a continuing competence portfolio? Are most RNs actively engaged in reflective practice in an effort to assess their ongoing competence?

4. Why should the entry-level examination for nursing be broad and general in scope, whereas continuing competence is arguably demonstrated by professional certification in specialty areas?

5. Are cost and access deterrents to professional certification? If so, how can these barriers be overcome?

6. Do most nurses view CE coursework as a reliable and valid tool for increasing provider competence?

7. Should nurses be required to complete mandated CE hours in the area of nursing practice in which they work?

8. Are there core competencies all licensed nurses must achieve regardless of the setting in which they practice?

References

American Academy of Physician Assistants. (n.d.). *Information about PAs and the PA profession*. Linked In. Retrieved June 3, 2018, from https://www.slideshare.net/samueljack/information-about-pas-and-the-pa-profession

American Board of Nursing Specialties. (2016). *About us*. Retrieved June 3, 2018, from http://www.nursingcertification.org/about

American College of Physicians. (2018). *State continuing medical education requirements*. Retrieved June 3, 2018, from https://www.acponline.org/cme-moc/cme/state-continuing-medical-education-requirements

American Nurses Association. (2014, November 12). *ANA position statement: Professional role competence*. Retrieved June 3, 2018, from https://www.nursingworld.org/practice-policy/nursing-excellence/official-position-statements

American Nurses Association. (2015). *Code of ethics for nurses with interpretive statements*. Washington, DC: Author.

American Nurses Credentialing Center. (2018a). *Certification*. Retrieved June 3, 2018, from https://www.nursingworld.org/certification

American Nurses Credentialing Center. (2018b). *Why ANCC certification?* Retrieved June 3, 2018, from https://www.nursingworld.org/education-events/certified-nurses-day/overview/why-ancc-certification/

Arkansas Board of Registered Nursing. (2018). *Continuing education*. Retrieved June 3, 2018, from http://www.arsbn.org/continuing-education

Boyle, D. K., Cramer, E., Potter, C., Gatua, M. W., & Stobinski, J. X. (2014). The relationship between direct-care RN specialty certification and surgical patient outcomes. *AORN Journal, 100*(5), 511–528. doi:10.1016/j.aorn.2014.04.018

California Board of Registered Nursing. (2018). *Continuing education for license renewal*. Retrieved June 3, 2018, from http://www.rn.ca.gov/licensees/ce-renewal.shtml

Calzone, K. A., Jenkins, J., Culp, S., Caskey, S., & Badzek, L. (2014). Introducing a new competency into nursing practice. *Journal of Nursing Regulation, 5*(1), 40–47.

College of Registered Nurses of British Columbia. (2018). *Quality assurance for RNs and NPs*. Retrieved June 3, 2018, from https://www.crnbc.ca/PracticeSupport/QA/Pages/Default.aspx

Dictionary.com. (2018). *Competence* [Definition]. Retrieved June 3, 2018, from http://dictionary.reference.com/browse/competence

Fitzpatrick, J. J., Campo, T. M., & Gacki-Smith, J. (2014). Emergency care nurses: Certification, empowerment, and work-related variables. *Journal of Emergency Nursing, 40*(2), e37–e43. doi:10.1016/j.jen.2013.01.021

Florida Board of Registered Nursing. (2018). *Registered nurse (RN)*. Retrieved June 3, 2018, from http://floridasnursing.gov/renewals/registered-nurse-rn

How will you celebrate certified nurses? (2017). *AACN Bold Voices, 9*(1), 7.

Institute of Medicine. (2010, October). *The future of nursing: Leading change, advancing health*. Retrieved October 6, 2017, from http://thefutureofnursing.org/IOM-Report

Iowa Board of Nursing. (2018, January). *CE basic requirements*. Retrieved June 3, 2018, from https://nursing.iowa.gov/continuing-education/continuing-ed-licensees/ce-basic-requirements

Medscape Education. (2016, April). *State CME requirements*. Retrieved June 3, 2018, from http://www.medscape.org/public/staterequirements

Michigan Board of Nursing. Department of Licensing and Regulatory Affairs. (2018). *Nursing CE requirements*. Retrieved June 3, 2018, from http://www.michigan.gov/lara/0,4601,7-154-72600_72603_27529_27542---,00.html; https://www.michigan.gov/documents/lara/Continuing_Education_Information_for_Nurses_554819_7.pdf

National Association of Boards of Pharmacy. (2018a). *MPJE— Multistate Pharmacy Jurisprudence Examination. Frequently asked questions*. Retrieved June 3, 2018, from https://nabp.pharmacy/programs/mpje/faqs/#required

National Association of Boards of Pharmacy. (2018b). *NAPLEX: North American Pharmacist Licensure Examination*. Retrieved June 3, 2018, from https://nabp.pharmacy/programs/naplex

National Council State Boards of Nursing. (2018a). *Enhanced Nurse Licensure Compact (eNLC) implementation*. Retrieved June 3, 2018, from https://www.ncsbn.org/enhanced-nlc-implementation.htm

National Council State Boards of Nursing. (2018b). *Member boards*. Retrieved June 3, 2018, from https://www.ncsbn.org/member-boards.htm

National Council State Boards of Nursing. (2018c). *NCLEX and other exams*. Retrieved June 3, 2018, from https://www.ncsbn.org/nclex.htm

New York Board of Nursing State CE requirements. (2018). Retrieved June 3, 2018, from https://www.nurse.com/state-nurse-ce-requirements/new-york

North Carolina Board of Nursing. (n.d.). *Continuing competence—A reflective practice approach*. Retrieved June 3, 2018, from https://www.ncbon.com/myfiles/downloads/abcd.pdf

North Dakota Board of Nursing State CE requirements. (2018). Retrieved June 3, 2018, from https://www.nurse.com/state-nurse-ce-requirements/north-dakota

Nurses Association of New Brunswick. (2018). *Continuing competence program*. Retrieved June 3, 2018, from http://www.nanb.nb.ca/index.php/practice/ccp

Nursing CEU requirements. (2017, July 5). Career Trend. Retrieved June 3, 2018, from http://www.ehow.com/facts_4969045_continuing-education-does-nurse-need.html

Ohio Board of Nursing. (2018, May 15). *Education programs for nursing*. Retrieved June 3, 2018, from http://www.nursing.ohio.gov/Education.htm#ContinuingEd

Oregon Board of Nursing State CE requirements. (2018). Retrieved June 3, 2018, from https://www.nurse.com/state-nurse-ce-requirements/oregon

Peddle, M., Jokwiro, Y., Carter, M., & Young, T. (2016). A professional portfolio of learning for undergraduate nursing students. *Australian Nursing & Midwifery Journal, 24*(4), 40.

Quality, Safety, and Education for Nurses Institute. (2018). *Competencies.* Retrieved June 3, 2018, from http://qsen.org/competencies

State of New Jersey. New Jersey Division of Consumer Affairs. (2017). *New Jersey Board of Nursing. Continuing education FAQ.* Retrieved October 7, 2017, from http://www.njconsumeraffairs.gov/nur/Pages/Continuing-Education-FAQ.aspx

Stepping up your nursing career: Subspecialty certification. (2017). *AACN Bold Voices, 9*(5), 6–7.

Taft, L., & Sparks, R. K. (2008). Mandatory continuing education for nurses. *Nursing Matters, 19*(3), 4.

Texas Board of Nursing. (2015). *Education: Continuing nursing education and competency.* Retrieved June 3, 2018, from http://www.bon.texas.gov/education_continuing_education.asp

The Free Dictionary by Farlex. (2003–2018). *Licensure* [Definition]. Retrieved June 3, 2018, from http://medical-dictionary.thefreedictionary.com/licensure

U.S. Medical Licensing Examination. (1996–2018). *What is USMLE?* Retrieved June 3, 2018, from http://www.usmle.org

Watson Dillon, D. M., & Mahoney, M. A. (2015). Moving from patient care to population health: A new competency for the executive nurse leader. *Nurse Leader, 13*(1), 30–36. doi:10.1016/j.mnl.2014.11.002

Health Care Reform
The Dismantling of the Affordable Care Act
Carol J. Huston

CHAPTER OUTLINE

LEARNING OBJECTIVES

The learner will be able to:

1. Describe key elements contributing to health care costs in the United States and the impact of those costs on the federal budget.

2. Identify driving forces for health care reform in the United States.

3. Describe key components of the *Patient Protection and Affordable Care Act* (PPACA), more commonly known as the *Affordable Care Act* (ACA) or *Obamacare.*

4. Identify successes as well as flaws evident in the ACA, 6 years after its implementation.

5. Examine legislative efforts put forth in 2017 and 2018 to repeal and replace the ACA.

6. Consider what strategies Republican leaders in the 115th Congress might employ to further dismantle or eliminate the ACA.

7. Debate the degree to which partisanship will continue to be a factor in repealing and replacing the ACA.

8. Debate what Americans might be willing to pay or give up so that all Americans could have affordable, high-quality health care.

9. Consider what criteria are most important in a new health care reform bill.

INTRODUCTION

As we entered the second decade of the 21st century, 44 million people in the United States lacked any type of health insurance and an even greater number were under-insured. Of the millions of people who were too poor to afford health insurance, many did not qualify for Medic-aid. In addition, small businesses, in tough economic times, lacked the resources to provide health insurance benefits to all employees ("Health Care Reform Timeline," n.d.). All these factors suggested a need for health care reform that provided universal health care insurance coverage.

> **Consider This** As of 2016, the "typical family" paid about 35% of their income for health care (Moffit, 2016).

Yet, reform efforts to establish such coverage failed on six occasions over the last century, largely through oppo-sition of corporate stakeholders in the medical–industrial complex (Geyman, 2018). Indeed, comprehensive, system-atic efforts to reform a clearly broken health care system achieved no real momentum until late in the first decade of the 21st century. Even then, convergence on proposals for reform in the United States was very limited, so the rela-tively swift passage of the *Patient Protection and Affordable Care Act*, more commonly known as *the Affordable Care Act* (ACA) or *Obamacare*, came as a surprise to many. Over the first 6 years of its implementation, however, partisan efforts to revoke it were almost constant.

With the election of Donald Trump as President of the United States in November 2016, efforts to repeal and re-place the ACA became front and center. As of the writing of this chapter (mid-2018), there were more questions than answers about what health care reform will look like under the Trump administration. A politically contentious 2017 saw a clamor for the repeal of the ACA as well as a cry for more affordable health care without government mandates. The repeal for the individual mandate to purchase health insurance happened in late 2017 (the penalty for failing to maintain minimum essential health care insurance cover-age will be reduced to zero in January 2019), but formal replacement of a comprehensive health care reform act did not. As a result, as we entered 2018, millions of Americans still relied on ACA subsidies, health premiums were soar-ing, and provider choice was more limited than ever.

There was, however, momentum for reform. Health care was identified as the country's leading priority for Democrats (54%) and the second highest priority for Re-publicans (42%) at the close of 2017 (The Associated Press and NORC, 2014–2018). In addition, a recent poll by the Associated Press-NORC Center for Public Affairs Research found that nearly half of Americans, 18 years and older, wanted the government to address the issue of health care in the coming year, but few expressed confidence in the ability of the government to make progress (The Associated Press and NORC, 2014–2018).

Should desired health care reform be a remake of the ACA with less government subsidies, mandates, and regu-lation? Is there support for a single-payer, universal health care system? If so, what questions must be asked and what form should it take? Is an entirely new model of health care funding indicated, and if so, is the country prepared to make major shifts in cultural/value expectations about the "right" to health care regardless of ability to pay? To an-swer these questions, it may be helpful to first examine why health care reform itself is more necessary than ever.

WHY IS HEALTH CARE REFORM NECESSARY?

Costs Are Uncontrolled

Economics is a leading driver of health care reform in this country and the U.S. health care system is the most expen-sive in the world. In fact, the United States spent almost twice as much on health care, as a percentage of its economy, in 2016, as any other advanced industrialized countries—totaling $3.3 trillion, or 17.9% of gross domestic product (Frakt & Carroll, 2018). Much of this spending comes out of the coffers of the federal government (now the single largest insurer in this country), which subsidizes 43% of the health care for those over age 65 and those receiving Social Security disability through Medicare (Amadeo, 2018c). The federal government also heavily subsidizes health care for families below a certain income level through Medicaid. By 2030, it is estimated that payroll taxes will only cover 38% of Medicare costs, contributing significantly to the federal budget deficit (Amadeo, 2018c). Rising health care costs as well as increasing numbers in Medicare and Medicaid then threaten to consume the entire federal budget within sev-eral decades (Amadeo, 2018c).

In addition, for the past 40 years, real, per capita health care spending has grown at twice the rate of growth of real, per capita income, resulting in higher out-of-pocket health care costs for most American consumers (Goodman, 2015). As a result, medical bankruptcies have affected up to 2 million people in this country (Amadeo, 2018c).

> **Consider This** In a recent Gallup poll, Americans cited the high cost of care as their No. 1 financial concern (Allen, 2017).

Indeed, out-of-pocket health care costs borne directly by consumers rose 3.9% in 2016—the fastest rate of growth since 2007 (Johnson, 2017). Much of this increase came from the transfer of costs (increased deductibles and copayments) from insurance plans to consumers. "In 2016, 29 percent of people who received insurance through employers were enrolled in high-deductible plans, up from 20 percent in 2014. The size of the deductibles also increased over this time, a 12 percent increase in 2016 for individual plans, compared with a 7 percent increase in 2014" (Johnson, 2017, para. 1). Technological advances, prescription drugs, and the cost of medical equipment and supplies also contributed to cost increases.

In addition, health care costs are simply higher in the United States. Frakt and Carroll (2018) agree, noting that Americans don't consume significantly more health care than citizens in other industrialized countries; they're just paying more for that care. For example, the average cost of an MRI in the United States in 2015 was $1,119, compared to $811 in New Zealand (Mack, 2017). An MRI in Spain averaged $130. Similarly, the average cost of an appendectomy in the United States was $15,930, whereas it was $8,009 in the United Kingdom and only $3,814 in Australia (Mack, 2017). Similarly, pharmaceuticals cost far more in the United States because of government-protected "monopoly" rights for drug manufacturers.

Mack (2017) suggests the higher costs in the United States were borne from the historical fee-for-service reimbursement model whereby providers were rewarded for ordering more services rather than taking a more conservative approach. In addition, insurers, until the last couple of decades, simply paid what was billed, regardless of whether the cost was reasonable for the service provided.

> **Consider This** Fee-for-service reimbursement is like "going to an auto mechanic and agreeing to pay for whatever services he deems necessary, at whatever price he chooses, with no penalties to the provider if the service is poor."
> —Charles Hugh Smith (as cited in Mack, 2017, para. 15).

In addition, administrative costs account for 25% of total U.S. hospital spending, more than twice the percentage in Canada and the highest among eight nations studied in a 2015 Commonwealth Fund analysis (Mack, 2017). This inefficiency is only part of the wastes that are widely recognized as part of the U.S. health care system.

> **Consider This** The National Academy of Medicine has estimated the health care system wastes around $765 billion a year—about a quarter of what we spend (Allen, 2017).

Amadeo (2018c), however, suggests this cost difference is occurring because there is less price competition in U.S. health care than in other industries, and because most people don't pay cash for health care. When consumers don't pay for something out of pocket (because it is being paid by a third party), there are less incentives to care about overutilization or the cost itself, and there is no need to cost compare or shop for the most effective use of resources.

Access Is Unequal

There are also many access problems in the U.S. health care system that suggest a need for health care reform. Geographical access issues to health care providers create disparities for populations living in rural areas. Multiple studies have shown that rural residents are older, poorer, and have fewer physicians to care for them. This inequality is intensified as rural residents are less likely to have employer-provided health care coverage, and if they are poor, they often are not covered by Medicaid (Rural Health Information Hub, 2002–2018).

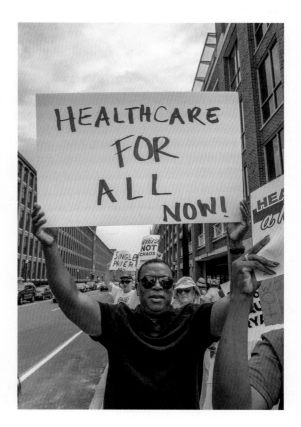

A lack of insurance also creates access barriers. Okoro et al. (2017) suggest that adults who lack health insurance coverage have coverage gaps and often skip or delay care because of limited personal finances. They also face increased risk for poor physical and mental health and premature mortality. In addition, with a limited number of primary care providers willing to take on patients without insurance, the uninsured are more likely to be diagnosed with diseases at later stages when treatment is more difficult and outcomes are poorer.

Unfortunately, this was the case in a study by Nguyen and Sommers (2016). In a telephone survey of U.S. citizens in three southern states, with family incomes below 138% of the federal poverty level (corresponds to the ACA's Medicaid eligibility guidelines), researchers found that low-income adults with Medicaid, private insurance, and Medicare reported significantly greater access and quality of care than uninsured adults, regardless of whether they had private or public insurance. Medicaid beneficiaries did report greater difficulty accessing specialists but less risk of high out-of-pocket spending than those with private insurance but for other outcomes, Medicaid and private coverage performed similarly.

It was the uninsured, however, who demonstrated the worst health outcomes. With limited access to primary and specialty care providers, the uninsured reported significant delays in needed care. They also reported having to skip medications because of cost and borrowing money or skipping paying to pay their medical costs (see Research Fuels the Controversy 21.1).

In addition, health insurance coverage has also been linked with increased access to clinical preventive services (CPS) and other medical services and, as a result, improvements in adult health (e.g., self-reported health and clinical depression), mortality, and financial security (Okoro et al., 2017). Adults who lack health insurance coverage or have inadequate coverage, gaps in coverage, or difficulties accessing or navigating the U.S. health care system often delay or forgo CPS and other needed medical care, leading to poor physical and mental health, premature mortality, increased health disparities, and increased financial risk, particularly among racial/ethnic minorities, persons with disabilities, and other vulnerable population groups (e.g., homeless persons, cancer survivors, or pregnant women; Okoro et al., 2017). Amadeo (2018c) notes that when people don't have health care insurance, preventive care becomes unaffordable, sending many people to the Emergency Department, raising costs even higher.

Research Fuels the Controversy 21.1

Access and Quality of Care by Insurance Type for Low-Income Adults

The objective of this study was to compare access to care and perceived health care quality for low-income adults with Medicaid versus other types of insurance coverage before the Affordable Care Act (ACA)'s coverage expansion in three southern states. Study data came from a telephone survey of U.S. citizens aged 19–64 years living in Arkansas, Kentucky, and Texas, with family incomes below 138% of the federal poverty level, corresponding to the ACA's Medicaid eligibility guidelines. The sample size was 2,765, divided evenly across the three states.

Source: Nguyen, K. H., & Sommers, B. D. (2016, August). Access and quality of care by insurance type for low-income adults before the Affordable Care Act. *American Journal of Public Health, 106*(8), 1409–1415. doi:10.2105/AJPH.2016.303156

Study Findings

Of privately insured respondents, 25% reported fair or poor health status, compared with 50% of Medicaid respondents and 54% of Medicare respondents. More than 80% of Medicaid and Medicare beneficiaries reported at least one chronic condition, compared with 54% to 57% among privately insured or uninsured respondents.

In the unadjusted models, Medicaid beneficiaries had more difficulty accessing primary and specialty care than those with private insurance and were more likely to use the Emergency Department because a doctor was unavailable. Their out-of-pocket costs, however, were lower than those with private insurance.

Uninsured individuals, however, consistently reported worse health care outcomes than those insured, regardless of whether the insurance was public or private. They were also at highest risk of not having a personal doctor for either primary care or specialty care. Uninsured individuals were also significantly more likely to report delaying care because of cost in the past 12 months, skipping medication doses because of cost, and borrowing money or skipping paying bills as a result of high medical costs compared with those with insurance. There were no significant differences for any of these outcomes between Medicaid beneficiaries and privately insured persons.

Quality Health Care Rankings Are Poor and Medical Errors Permeate the System

Quality concerns are another factor suggesting a need to reform the health care system. Despite having the most expensive health care system in the world, the United States ranks close to last in the quality of health care that it delivers, compared to all other developed nations ("Health Care Reform," 2016). A 2017 Commonwealth Fund think tank found the U.S. health care system fared especially badly on measures of affordability, access, health outcomes, and equality between the rich and poor (Khazan, 2017). The United States also had high rates of infant mortality and the highest rate of "mortality amenable to health care"—deaths that doctors and hospitals can prevent—and it experienced the smallest reduction in that measure in the past decade (Khazan, 2017).

Indeed, according to the Centers for Disease Control, the average life expectancy at birth in the United States fell by 0.1 years, to 78.6 years, in 2016, following a similar drop in 2015 (Blumenthal, 2018). This is the first time in 50 years that life expectancy has fallen for 2 years running. In 25 other developed countries, life expectancy in 2015 averaged 81.8 years. Blumenthal (2018) suggests it would be easy to place the blame for this drop entirely on the opioid epidemic, but suggests instead that it is an indictment of the American health care system.

In addition, medical errors are rampant in the U.S. health care system. Although the true number of medical errors is unknown (research suggests that less than 10% of medical errors are reported), recent studies have estimated medical errors may account for as many as 251,000 deaths annually in the United States, making medical errors the third leading cause of death (Anderson & Abrahamson, 2017; see Chapter 14). Indeed, error rates are significantly higher in the United States than in other developed countries such as Canada, Australia, New Zealand, Germany, and the United Kingdom.

Frances (2016) suggests that inexplicably, U.S. consumers tolerate these medical errors without public fear and rage, and as a result, no sustained or coordinated effort exists to identify the major sources of error and eliminate them. Health care reform must include greater attention to health care–acquired infections, clinical pharmacy, structured handoffs, diagnostic errors, and interoperable electronic health care records before the problem of errors will improve (Frances, 2016).

THE AFFORDABLE CARE ACT: SUCCESSES AND FAILURES

The ACA provided the first real hope for Americans of significant reductions in numbers of uninsured, greater access to coverage for those with preexisting conditions, and mandated health care insurance provision by employers (Marquis & Huston, 2017). *Bundled Payments, Accountable Care Organizations, Value-Based Purchasing,* and *Medical Homes* were critical strategies for the achievement of the ACA goals.

In addition, businesses with more than 50 employees were required to provide health insurance for their employees or pay a fine instead. Indeed, 46% more small businesses offered health care benefits in 2011 than in 2010 (Amadeo, 2018c). More insured small business employees meant fewer bankruptcies, better credit scores, and higher consumer demand. This allowed them to spend more, boosting economic growth. In fact, there were fewer bankruptcies in August 2011 than at the same time the previous year (Amadeo, 2018c).

In addition, the *individual mandate* clause of the ACA required individuals to buy insurance or pay a penalty at tax time, unless they qualified for a limited number of exemptions. The penalty for not having insurance for 2018 was $695 per adult or 2.5% of household income in excess of tax filing thresholds, whichever is higher (O'Brien, 2017). Several exemptions to this penalty, however, were implemented in early 2018 (see Table 21.1).

With the repeal of the individual insurance mandate, the incentive for people to purchase health care insurance goes away in 2019. The Congressional Budget Office estimates that repealing the individual mandate starting in 2019 will result in 4 million people losing coverage in 2019 and 13 million losing coverage in 2027 (O'Brien, 2017). Experts suggest the individual market will look very different if the penalty goes away. Many healthy people will voluntarily opt to go without coverage, and insurers could raise their premiums to cover the remaining, sicker population. These higher premiums would in turn cause more consumers to become priced out of the market.

Discussion Point

Should American citizens be required to have health insurance, just as they are required to have auto insurance?

New *Health Insurance Marketplaces,* also called *exchanges,* were created as part of the ACA for individuals without access to health insurance through work, for implementation in January 2014. Small businesses became eligible to buy affordable and qualified health benefit plans in this competitive insurance marketplace. Every health insurance plan in the marketplace offered comprehensive coverage and could be compared based on price, benefits, and quality, and tax credits were provided to lower the cost of insurance for individuals and families earning below certain levels (Marquis & Huston, 2017).

TABLE 21.1	**Congressional Efforts to Replace and Repeal the Affordable Care Act (ACA) in 2017**	
March–May 2017	*The American Health Care Act* (passed by the House on May 4, 2017, but failed in the Senate)	Provided a flat tax credit based on age, not income. This subsidy was not based on the cost of plans, so it would have raised costs for many. The Act also included a Patient and State Stability Fund that would help lower premiums by 20% after 2026. The Act would also have allowed states to waive several rules of the ACA under certain conditions. In the states that chose waiver rules, chronic disease sufferers would pay much higher rates. The Act also funded Medicare through a fixed block grant, and cut funding for Planned Parenthood and ACA taxes.
June–July 2017	*The Better Care Reconciliation Act* (put forth in the Senate but failed to pass)	Allowed states to decide whether to keep all 10 essential health benefits of the ACA. That would have allowed companies to charge more for those with preexisting conditions. The plan also penalized those who dropped their insurance then reapplied for coverage within 63 days. The plan also would have cut Medicaid spending starting in 2020 and reduced Obamacare tax credits and subsidies. The Act also allowed companies to charge seniors five times more than younger Americans, up from three times as much and stripped Medicaid and Title X reimbursement for Planned Parenthood health care services for a year. The Act also eliminated the tax on the individual insurance mandate and removed the tax on companies that don't provide health insurance. The bill also increased maximum allowable contributions to Health Savings Accounts.
July 2017	"Skinny Repeal" by the Senate (Senator John McCain, R-Ariz.,) cast the deciding vote against the "skinny bill." He disapproved of the process and urged a return to bipartisan lawmaking.	Would have repealed the ACA's mandate that individuals must buy insurance but didn't require companies to provide insurance benefits. It would have repealed the tax on medical device manufacturers as well and defunded Planned Parenthood, the Prevention and Public Health Fund, and the Community Health Center Fund.
September 2017	The Graham-Cassidy Bill (championed by Senators Lindsey Graham, R-S.C. and Bill Cassidy, R-La). On September 22, 2017, Senator McCain blocked the Graham-Cassidy bill. He said there wasn't enough information about how the bill would affect people because it was rushed through to meet Trump's deadline to repeal the ACA by the end of September 2017.	Would have converted Obamacare's federal Medicaid funding and insurance subsidies to state block grants. It left it up to the states to design their own health care programs with the funds, benefiting some states and disadvantaging others. The bill also would have allowed states to require that Medicaid recipients have a job unless they were seniors, children, disabled, or pregnant and cut off Medicaid funding by 2027. The bill also sought to eliminate the tax on those who don't buy insurance retroactive to 2016.
December 2017	*The Tax Cuts and Jobs Act* (passed by Congress and signed into law by President Trump in late December 2017)	The bill cut the corporate tax rate to 20% and changed individual tax brackets. It also made significant changes to the ACA, including elimination of the "individual mandate" to purchase health insurance. (O'Brien, 2017 notes that technically, the GOP tax bill didn't repeal the individual mandate; it simply reduced the penalty for going uncovered to zero. This, in practice, has the same result as eliminating the individual mandate altogether.)

TABLE 21.1   Congressional Efforts to Replace and Repeal the Affordable Care Act (ACA) in 2017 (*continued*)

February 2018	Expansion of Short-Term Health Plans	These regulations made it easier for consumers to obtain coverage through short-term health insurance plans—which didn't have to adhere to the ACA's consumer protections—by allowing insurers to sell policies that last just under a year.
April 2018	Broadening of the Individual Mandate Exemptions for 2018	The Trump administration announced that those who live in counties with no insurer or with only one choice could apply for a hardship exemption from the individual insurance mandate for 2018. In addition, prolife Americans who could only buy plans that covered abortion could also receive an exemption.
May 2018	President Trump revealed the *American Patients First Plan* to reduce drug prices	This plan reformed the rebates drug companies pay to pharmacy benefit managers (PBMs), who negotiate prices between drug manufacturers, pharmacies, and health insurance companies. The rebates create incentives for PBMs to suggest higher cost drugs. In addition, PBMs are allowed to charge insurers more than they're charging pharmacies. As a result, everyone pays different prices for drugs. To do this, Congress would have had to amend the act that established Medicare Part D because it prohibited Medicare from negotiating.

Source: Extracted from Amadeo (2018a, 2018b, 2018c); Luhby (2018a, 2018b).

In addition, all exchange plans were required to provide 10 essential health benefits (see Box 21.1).

What were the outcomes of the ACA? There were successes (Box 21.2) and well as failures (Box 21.3). Okoro et al. (2017) note that with the passage of ACA, approximately 20 million uninsured working-aged adults (aged 18–64 years) gained health insurance coverage. In addition, during 2013 to 2014, when many of the major coverage provisions of ACA went into effect (e.g., creation of the Health Insurance Marketplace, barring coverage exclusions for preexisting health conditions, expansion of Medicaid, establishment of tax credits, reductions in cost sharing, and other provisions to increase availability and affordability of coverage), the percentage of working-aged adults with health insurance increased by approximately 3% points.

Obama (2016) reported that because of the ACA, the uninsured rate in this country declined from 16.0% in 2010 to 9.1% in 2015 (a 43% decline), access to care improved, and health care payment systems were transformed (an estimated 30% of traditional Medicare payments began flowing through alternative payment models like bundled payments or accountable care organizations). In addition, reimbursement increasingly shifted from *volume* to *value*, reducing incentives for redundant and inappropriate care and increasing incentives for quality. The ACA also expanded Medicaid and CHIP to over 15 million men, women, and children who fell through the cracks in states that opt in ("Health Care Reform Timeline," n.d.).

Despite this progress, major opportunities to improve the health care system remained. The ACA itself was

> **BOX 21.1**
>
> **The 10 Essential Benefits Guaranteed by Insurance Plans in the Affordable Care Act Health Care Marketplace**
>
> 1. Ambulatory services (outpatient care)
> 2. Emergency services
> 3. Hospitalization
> 4. Maternity and newborn care
> 5. Mental health services and addiction treatment
> 6. Prescription drugs
> 7. Rehabilitative services and devices
> 8. Laboratory services
> 9. Preventive services (wellness visits including chronic disease management)
> 10. Pediatric care, including dental and vision
>
> *Source:* Health for California Insurance Center. (2018). *Essential health benefits*. Retrieved June 3, 2018, from https://www.healthforcalifornia.com/affordable-care-act/essential-health-benefits

BOX 21.2   Successes of the Affordable Care Act (ACA)

- Slowed the rise of health care costs (but didn't reduce costs)
- Required all insurance plans to cover 10 essential health benefits including treatment for mental health, addiction, and chronic diseases
- Protected people with preexisting conditions from predatory premiums or denials
- Eliminated lifetime and annual coverage limits (except for grandfathered plans)
- Allowed children to stay on their parents' health insurance plans up to age 26
- Required states to set up insurance exchanges or use the federal government's exchange
- Allowed those earning up to 400% of the poverty level to receive tax credits on their premiums
- Expanded Medicaid to 138% of the federal poverty level and provided this coverage to adults without children for the first time
- Eliminated the Medicare "doughnut hole" gap in coverage by 2020
- Required all qualified health insurance plans to provide free preventive and wellness visits without copays, deductibles, or coinsurance
- Required businesses with more than 50 employees to offer health insurance, although they received tax credits to help with the costs
- Encouraged 46% more small businesses to offer health care benefits in 2011 than in 2010. More insured small business employees meant fewer bankruptcies, better credit scores, and higher consumer demand. This allowed them to spend more, boosting economic growth. In fact, there were fewer bankruptcies in August 2011 than at the same time the previous year
- Altered the 80/20 rule provision so that 80% of premium dollars had to be spent on health care instead of administrative costs
- Lowered the budget deficit by $143 billion by 2022 (according to the Congressional Budget Office), by reducing government health care costs, raising taxes on some businesses and higher income families and shifting cost burdens to health care providers and pharmacy companies)

Source: Amadeo (2018a, 2018c); Anderson (2017); The Pros and Cons of the Affordable Care Act (2017); Federal Budget Bill to Delay ACA's Cadillac Tax & Suspend Two Other Taxes (2015); Kistler Tiffany Benefits (2015); Gold (2010); Bischoff (2012).

---

shrouded in confusion and misinformation, starting well before it was signed into law. This was due partly to partisan politics and partly to poor communication about the law to the public (Reisman, 2015). Indeed, Amadeo (2018a) notes that negative messages about Obamacare in the media outnumbered positive messages 15 to 1, and 3 years after it was approved, 54% of Americans opposed the Act.

Some of this discontent came about because of the broken promise that people who were satisfied with their previous coverage could remain on their plan. It quickly became apparent this would not be the case. Anderson (2017) notes that no one knows exactly how many people were kicked off their plans with the introduction of the ACA, but many of the estimates range into the double-digit millions. According to NBC News, 14 million people were kicked off their coverage because of the ACA, whereas the Washington Post reports a figure somewhere between 7 and 12 million (Anderson, 2017).

Consider This PolitiFact named the statement, "If you like your health care plan, you can keep it," the 2013 lie of the year (Anderson, 2017).

Other consumers found the rollout of the ACA and the marketplace confusing. They felt enrollment periods were too limited and the website was too complicated.

In addition, costs were often prohibitive, for both the government and consumers. The costs to implement the ACA increased about 5% each year (5.3% in 2014 and 5.8% in 2015; Amadeo, 2018b). In addition, despite implementation of the ACA, the cost of health care insurance continued

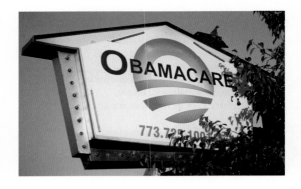

BOX 21.3   Failures of the Affordable Care Act (ACA)

- Consumers who were satisfied with their prior insurance plans and providers didn't necessarily get to keep them, a promise made to them when the ACA was introduced.
- Three to 5 million people lost their employment-based health insurance when businesses found it more cost-effective to pay the penalty and let their employees purchase insurance plans on the exchanges.
- Insurance companies cancelled many of the plans for the 30 million people who never had company plans and relied on private health insurance because their policies didn't cover the ACA's 10 essential benefits.
- Many insurance companies made their provider networks smaller to cut costs while implementing ACA requirements. This left customers with fewer providers that were "in-network."
- Increased coverage raised overall health care costs in the short term because many people received preventive care and testing for the first time. Since the end of 2013, health care premiums for the average family have increased by 140%.
- The ACA taxed those who didn't purchase insurance, but many avoided the tax through an ever-expanding list of exemptions.
- As of May 2011, more than 600,000 new young people became insured because of the ACA provision that children up to the age of 26 years could be covered by their parents' insurance. This resulted in record profits for the insurance companies for the first quarter of 2011, because the young, newly insured required fewer health services.
- Four million people chose to pay the tax rather than pay for coverage. The Congressional Budget Office estimated they paid $54 billion.
- In 2013, the ACA raised the income tax rate for 1 million individuals with incomes above $200,000. It also raised taxes for 4 million couples filing joint returns on incomes exceeding $250,000.
- Starting in 2013, medical device manufacturers and importers paid a 2.3% excise tax, although this tax was suspended for 2016–2018. Indoor tanning services paid a 10% excise tax.
- Starting in 2013, families could deduct medical expenses that exceeded 10% of income. Before, they could deduct any expenses that exceeded 7.5% of income.
- Pharmaceutical companies paid an extra $84.8 billion in fees between 2013 and 2023 to close the "doughnut hole" in Medicare Part D.
- In 2020, insurance companies were to be assessed a 40% excise tax on "Cadillac" health plans. These are plans with annual premiums exceeding $10,200 for individuals or $27,500 for families.

Source: Amadeo (2018a, 2018c); Anderson (2017); The Pros and Cons of the Affordable Care Act (2017); Federal Budget Bill to Delay ACA's Cadillac Tax & Suspend Two Other Taxes (2015); Kistler Tiffany Benefits (2015); Gold (2010); Bischoff (2012).

to be beyond reach for many Americans. Individuals found it difficult to find affordable plans in the Health Insurance Marketplace, often choosing lower cost plans with high deductibles or copayments, that ultimately they could not pay. In addition, choice was often limited in the Health Insurance Marketplace, existing coverage was disrupted, and bureaucracy created even more rules and regulations.

Of even greater concern was the staggering costs of the federal subsidies to insurers as well as what many perceived to be uneven allocation of their use. The bulk of the 8.8 million Americans who signed up for coverage via the federal health insurance exchanges in 2018 received subsidies ("Beyond Obamacare," 2018). "Heavy federal subsidies are designed to offset premium increases by insurers in the health care marketplace, or the health exchanges that individual states operate. As much as 80% of the Obamacare-insured population benefits from such subsidies" ("Beyond Obamacare," 2018, para. 5).

Consider This "As long as there are subsidies in place there will be people who will show up to claim them. That's sort of an iron law of economics."

—Mark Pauly, Professor, Health Care Management, Wharton

In addition, despite claims that the American public would come to like the ACA, more Americans opposed the law than favored it by 2016 (49.3% as compared to 39%; Moffit, 2016). Yet, many Americans openly espouse their view that care should be allocated equitably for the common good. Clearly, there is at least some conflict of values between justice and fairness, and the question about whether health care is a right or a privilege has not been fully answered. Stoltzfus Jost (2017, p. 13) agrees, noting that the ACA "really touched the live wire of political and ethical debates—it attempted to extend public support to low- and moderate-income people of working age who were not obviously among the worthy poor. It also extended government regulation of health insurance and specifically federal government regulation. It thereby came into conflict with a range of conservative values."

Consider This "For many Americans, opposition to the ACA was rightly rooted in their rejection of the tacit assumption underlying its centralized architecture: that Washington's political class possessed the wit and wisdom to restrain, guide, and direct this enormously complex and dynamic sector of the American economy and, in pursuit of that project, needed to exert greater control over their personal lives" (Moffit, 2016).

Discussion Point

Many Americans oppose some form of universal coverage because they view it as a form of social-ism. Do you foresee this public value changing anytime soon?

LEGISLATIVE EFFORTS TO REFORM A BROKEN HEALTH CARE SYSTEM

Multiple bills to repeal and replace the ACA were intro-duced into either the House or the Senate in 2017, although legislative consensus was not achieved (see Table 21.1). Al-though the bills were different in some respects, the com-mon theme was a reduction in mandates for individuals and businesses to buy or provide health insurance and a defunding of government subsidies for vulnerable popula-tions like the elderly and the poor.

The outcomes of these legislative efforts were highly partisan. Republicans tried to pass legislation to repeal por-tions of the ACA, and Democrats unanimously held the line in opposition. "But the Republicans failed not just because of uniform Democratic opposition but also, and primarily, because the range of political positions within the Repub-lican party in the Senate, and indeed in the House—from doctrinaire libertarians to practical moderates" (Stoltzfus Jost, 2017, p. 10).

In addition, virtually every stakeholder organization, in-cluding the American Medical Association, hospitals, State governors, insurance regulators, and Medicaid directors, weighed in to oppose repeal, and reliable Republican allies in

most efforts, such as the National Federation of Independent Business or the United States Chamber of Commerce, were largely silent, if not quietly opposed (Stoltzfus Jost, 2017).

Most believe that health care policy will remain at the fore-front as the 115th Congress enters its second session in 2018. The Republican Party has a narrow majority in the Senate and a more sizable one in the House of Representatives—but that is likely to change in November 2018 when all 435 House seats and 1/3 of the 100 seats in the Senate will be up for reelection. That essentially gives the Republican majority a 6-month win-dow for action ("Beyond Obamacare," 2018).

Mody and Blackwood (2018) suggest that Congress will continue its push to repeal the ACA in 2018, noting that although Republicans made strides in 2017, they did not fully deliver on their campaign trail promise to "repeal and replace" it. In addition, they suggest that Congress will consider legislation to stabilize the ACA individual market-place early in 2018 and push for entitlement reform. Indeed, Majority Whip Steve Scalise (R-La.) stated in early January 2018 that the repeal of Obamacare and entitlement reform were at the top of the agenda for House Republicans in 2018 (Weixel, Sullivan, & Hellmann, 2018). The legislation put forth by Sens. Lindsey Graham, R-S.C. and Bill Cassidy, R-La. in late 2017 (focused on providing block grants to states to give them new resources and greater regulatory flexibility to revive their individual and small group health insurance markets, rather than trying to adjust subsidy mechanisms) will likely provide some sort of foundation for new legislative efforts in 2018 (Mody & Blackwood, 2018).

The Medicaid program, which is projected to account for approximately $385 billion of federal spending in 2017, will be a prime target for reform in 2018 (Mody & Blackwood, 2018). The tax bill that President Trump signed into law in Decem-ber 2017 is projected to add $1 trillion to the federal deficit, making cuts to Medicaid an even more tempting target for some conservatives (Weixel et al., 2018). Mark Pauly, a Profes-sor at Wharton agrees, suggesting that entitlement programs such as Medicaid and Medicare will be targeted to make them look more market-like. For example, there could be attempts to rework Medicaid by including the addition of premiums for Medicaid beneficiaries, tightening standards for eligibility, and having some part of the Medicaid population purchasing coverage on exchanges ("Beyond Obamacare," 2018).

Consider This "Medicaid is front and center in any budg-et exercises, and now that deficits have increased, it puts Medicaid squarely in the bull's-eye." Joan Alker, Executive Director of the Georgetown University Center for Children and Families (as cited in Weixel et al., 2018, para. 16).

Tom Miller, a resident fellow at the conservative American Enterprise Institute think tank suggests, however, that "It might be time for Republicans to recalibrate, to think more in terms of containment, which is containing itself in terms of its future growth and spread, rather than some type of radical rollback" (Roubein, 2017, para. 3). "Supporters of the law, in contrast, feel as if the ACA has largely survived its first year in the face of a united GOP government committed to destroying it. They're hoping for a good election year that could bolster the health-care law's defenses going into 2019" (Roubein, 2017, para. 5).

Robert I. Field, professor of law and health care management at Drexel University and lecturer for Wharton, suggests, however, that the debate over U.S. health care reform and the future of the ACA could take a backseat in 2018 as the Trump administration faces other challenges such as keeping the government funded; dealing with the Children's Health Insurance Program (CHIP); and addressing the cost-sharing reductions (CSR) under the ACA ("Beyond Obamacare," 2018).

Pramuk (2018) agrees, suggesting that while Republican moves to overhaul Social Security, Medicare, or Medicaid appear unlikely—at least for 2018—Democrats are increasingly warning about the prospect because of the deficit concerns created by the 2017 tax plan. The GOP argues Democrats want to distract from the fact that they did not support the tax overhaul, the signature Republican achievement of Trump's first year in office.

PRESIDENT TRUMP'S INCREMENTAL DISMANTLING OF THE ACA

Despite the lack of legislation to fully "repeal and replace" the ACA, President Trump has been successful in undermining what is left of the ACA. The Trump administration's decision to cut the 2018 open-enrollment period to half that of the 2017 enrollment period, to cut advertising by 90%, to reduce navigator funding by 40%, to close the federal marketplace for maintenance several hours each week during open enrollment, and to bar regional office staff members from cooperating in enrollment efforts, portend his intent to dismantle the ACA (Stoltzfus Jost, 2017).

In addition, in October 2017, Trump issued an executive order endorsing approaches to siphoning off healthy individuals from the ACA market. He also cut off reimbursements to insurers to cover CSR that the ACA requires them to make for low-income individuals. These payments currently subsidize about 7 million consumers' copays and deductibles, as opposed to other subsidies that defray the costs of insurance premiums (Soffen & Uhrmacher, 2017).

Health insurance companies—lacking the information they needed to ensure their financial stability—are leaving the ACA's marketplaces ("The Pros and Cons of the Affordable Care Act," 2017). The companies that are staying then must hike their premiums because of uncertainty around losing CSR subsidies, the loss of which would destabilize the marketplace.

Trump also signed executive orders in October 2017, directing the Secretary of Labor to expand access to association health plans (Amadeo, 2018b). These are policies made available to trade groups, small businesses, and other associations that cross state lines. The order expands the types of groups that could form associations and prohibits them from refusing coverage or to charge more to those with preexisting conditions. In early January 2018, Trump proposed new rules to expand these association health plans as part of a broader effort to encourage the rise of cheaper coverage options that are exempt from certain Obamacare patient protections and benefit rules (Cancryn & Demko, 2018).

Trump also requested in October 2017 that the Labor Secretary ease restrictions on short-term health plans; allow employers to use pretax dollars for "health reimbursement arrangements"; to find ways to limit consolidation within the insurance and hospital industries; and to find additional means to increase competition and choice in health care (Amadeo, 2018b). All these new plans will negatively impact enrollment in the health care exchanges.

Trump also made cuts to the 340B Medicare drug discount program in 2017, a program designed to allow health care organizations to buy expensive drugs (commonly cancer therapies) at a discount and provide them to those who needed them but could not pay for them (Kalkanis & Trent, 2018). Trump questioned whether the drug savings were really being passed on for charity care, and proponents of the program suggested that although the program was long overdue for an update to add mechanisms for oversight and accountability, eliminating it was not the solution (Kalkanis & Trent, 2018).

The American Hospital Association, America's Essential Hospitals, and the Association of American Medical Colleges sued to block these rules from going into effect, but a judge dismissed the suit as premature in December 2017, suggesting the changes had not yet taken effect. Lobbyists and hospital groups also unsuccessfully pushed Congress to reverse the rule through a government funding bill (Weixel et al., 2018). In the end, the discontinuation of the 340B drug program will result in $1.6 billion in cuts to hospitals in 2018 (Weixel et al., 2018). Medicare will reimburse these expensive drugs at average sales price minus 22.5%, though reimbursement for other services were increased as an offset. For more than half of hospitals,.reductions in Medicare Part B drug revenue are estimated to be less than 5%, though about 6% of providers could see cuts exceeding 10% (Rosenquist & Boualam, 2018).

Discussion Point

Rosenquist and Boualam (2018) suggest the Trump Administration's cuts to 340B have pitted the pharmaceutical industry against 340B hospitals. How might this action still achieve the intended effect of helping safety-net hospitals serve poor and vulnerable populations?

Finally, in late December 2017, *The Tax Cuts and Jobs Act* was passed by Congress and signed into law by President Trump. The bill cut the corporate tax rate to 20% and changed individual tax brackets. It also made significant changes to the ACA, including elimination of the "individual mandate" to purchase health insurance as of 2019. It did not, however, impact the employer mandate or its related information reporting requirements. So even with the elimination of the individual mandate penalty, applicable large employers will still have to offer compliant plans or face tax penalties, and all coverage reporting requirements for employers, self-funded plans, and health insurance carriers will remain (President Trump Signs, 2018).

Cancryn and Demko (2017) note that state insurance regulators and Obamacare advocates have warned that new lax rules proposed by the Trump administration could open the door to a new wave of poorly regulated health plans that exclude coverage of key services required by the ACA, such as hospitalizations and prescription drugs. Larry Leavitt, Senior Vice President for Health Reform at the Kaiser Family Foundation, noted:

Any one of those steps in isolation wouldn't necessarily destabilize the markets, but the combination of all these actions is likely to make insurers very nervous. The ultimate risk is that more insurers decide that the market is too risky, and they exit, leaving counties with no options at all. (Cancryn & Demko, 2018, para. 8)

Discussion Point

Stoltzfus Jost (2017, p. 9) suggests that "we may be in a situation where the ACA cannot be repealed but will be left—or encouraged—to wither on the vine." Do you agree?

WHAT'S AHEAD?

As of mid-2018, it appears that some things will stay the same. Despite many insurers ending their participation in the ACA marketplaces because of uncertainties created by the Trump administration, every county nationwide will have an insurer in their ACA marketplace in 2018 (Soffen & Uhrmacher, 2017). Health care consumers will still be able to sign up on the federal exchange or their state marketplaces; get subsidies to help lower their premiums or reduce their deductibles and copays; and, if qualified, shop and compare coverage options (Luhby, 2017). It is of interest to note too that as of May 1, 2018, the uninsured rate remained basically flat at 9.1% despite all the efforts to reform the ACA in the prior 18 months (Sanger-Katz, 2018).

Many things, however, will change. Amadeo (2018b) suggests that if you are a young, healthy individual, health care reform under the Trump administration should mean lower costs and the elimination of the individual mandate penalty. Healthy individuals would also be eligible to purchase a short-term or association plan that would cost less but not guarantee them the unlimited annual or lifetime limits that the ACA did.

If you have a chronic illness, Amadeo (2018b) suggests your costs will rise because you'll have to rely on the ACA plans on the exchanges. As healthy customers leave those plans, the companies will raise prices to remain profitable, resulting in rising health care costs nationally. In May 2018, Maryland health insurers asked for an average 30% increase in premiums for that very reason (Amadeo, 2018b). Costs will skyrocket, however, for seniors who lose Medicaid coverage under newly proposed reform plans because many seniors need Medicaid to cover the out-of-pocket Medicare costs (Amadeo, 2018b).

In addition, fewer people will be enrolled in the health care exchanges in 2018, almost 3 million less than the 12.2 million who initially picked plans in 2017, but more than expected, given the shorter enrollment period for 2018 (Luhby, 2017; Mangan, 2017). In addition, about 5.8 million people enrolled in a marketplace were slated to lose at least one insurer in 2018 (Soffen & Uhrmacher, 2017). This will ultimately negatively impact health exchange enrollments as well.

In addition, premiums for the benchmark silver health exchange plan in 2018 will soar 37%, on average (Luhby, 2017). Increases will occur in the gold plan as well, although at a lower level. An analysis of health insurance costs by eHealth (2017) finds that these projected rate increases will make coverage unaffordable for 29% of individuals and 54% of families who bought their health insurance at eHealth during the 2017 open enrollment period.

CONCLUSIONS

With legislative failure to repeal the ACA in 2017, a stalemate is in place. "The Affordable Care Act remains in place as the law of the land, but the Trump administration seems committed to, at best, condemning the ACA to malign neglect and, at worst, actively undermining it at every opportunity. Although the ACA and most of the regulations and guidance for implementing it remain in place, the ACA will not operate on autopilot. It needs active support and guidance, with continual tinkering and adjustment" (Stoltzfus Jost, 2017, p. 9). Given the political stalemate, the time is right to reassess the deeper issues at stake and ponder the prospects for a considered compromise on health reform.

Anderson (2017, para. 12) agrees, noting that "the ACA is teetering on the edge of total collapse. It's not a matter of if, but when. Sticking with the status quo is no longer an option . . . and doing nothing would be catastrophic for the country." Anderson (2017) goes on to argue that there is no perfect solution, but an immediate major overhaul of the health care system is needed if we want to preserve the quality of health care Americans have come to expect. He notes that the ACA has a lot of great benefits, but the key is including these perks without bankrupting the country. He believes a more market-oriented solution is needed, one that allows individuals to choose what level of care is best for them, allows health care plans to freely move across state lines, and removes the individual mandate that forces every American to get coverage.

For Additional Discussion

1. Are current health care reform efforts being driven more by a political or health care agenda?

2. Can traditional market strategies (like competition) be used to increase efficiencies and control rising health care costs in the United States? Why or why not?

3. Did the ACA deliver on its promise to bring universal coverage to vulnerable populations without an increase in taxes or the deficit and with the ability to keep their current insurance plan if desired?

4. What strategies might induce more employers to offer health care insurance as a funded benefit? What keeps them from doing so?

5. Obama (2016) suggested that the ACA was likely the most important health care legislation enacted in the United States since the creation of Medicare and Medicaid in 1965. Do you agree or disagree?

6. Do current tax law and regulations discriminate against Americans who do not or cannot get health insurance as part of their employment?

7. Does expanding Medicaid eliminate the problem of American citizens "falling through the cracks" in terms of health care access?

8. What strategies will be needed to address the growing federal deficits related to government-subsidized health care (Medicare and Medicaid)?

9. Where do the major health care stakeholders stand on the repeal and replacement of the ACA?

10. How well informed were most Americans about the ACA at the time of its implementation? How much better informed were they 6 years later when efforts began to dismantle it?

11. What should the federal government's role be in assuring access to care for vulnerable populations?

12. Do Americans consider health care to be a right or a privilege?

References

Allen, M. (2017, December 28). *Want to cut health-care costs? Start with the obscene amount of waste.* Retrieved January 7, 2018, from http://healthcarereformarticles-philiphilipo .blogspot.com/2018/01/health-care-reform-articles-january-3.html

Amadeo, K. (2018a, May 10). *10 Obamacare pros and cons.* Retrieved January 11, 2018, from https://www.thebalance .com/obamacare-pros-and-cons-3306059

Amadeo, K. (2018b, May 14). *Donald Trump on health care. How Trump's health care policies will raise premium prices*

for you . Retrieved June 3, 2018, from https://www
.thebalance.com/how-could-trump-change-health-care-in-
america-4111422

Amadeo, K. (2018c, April 12). *Why reform health care.* The Balance. Retrieved June 3, 2018, from https://www.thebalance
.com/why-reform-health-care-3305749

Anderson, B. (2017, July 10). *Let's remember why health care
reform is needed.* Retrieved June 3, 2018, from https://www
.realclearpolitics.com/articles/2017/07/10/lets_remember_
why_healthcare_reform_is_needed_134418.html

Anderson, J. G., & Abrahamson, K. (2017). Your health care
may kill you: Medical errors. *Studies in Health Technology &
Informatics, 234,* 13–17. doi:10.3233/978-1-61499-742-9-13

Beyond Obamacare: What's ahead for U.S. health care in 2018.
(2018, January 5). Wharton, University of Pennsylvania.
Retrieved June 3, 2018, from http://knowledge.wharton
.upenn.edu/article/the-future-of-the-aca

Bischoff, B. (2012, June 28). *What Obamacare means for your
taxes.* Market Watch. Retrieved June 3, 2018, from https://
www.marketwatch.com/story/what-obamacare-may-mean-
for-taxes-1335896160486

Blumenthal, D. (2018, January 4). *Drop in U.S. life expectancy
is an 'indictment of the American health care system.'* STAT.
Retrieved June 3, 2018, from https://www.statnews
.com/2018/01/04/life-expectancy-us-health-care

Cancryn, A., & Demko, P. (2018, January 4). *Trump administration rolls out health plan rules that could weaken Obamacare.* Retrieved June 3, 2018, from https://www.politico
.com/story/2018/01/04/trump-administration-association-
health-plan-324021

eHealth. (2017). *Obamacare premiums will be officially unaffordable for many in 2018.* Retrieved June 3, 2018, from https://
resources.ehealthinsurance.com/affordable-care-act/obamac-
are-premiums-will-officially-unaffordable-many-2018

*Federal budget bill to delay ACA's Cadillac tax & suspend two
other taxes.* (2015, December 21). Horton. Retrieved June
3, 2018, from https://www.thehortongroup.com/resources/
federal-budget-bill-to-delay-acas-cadillac-tax-suspend-two-
other-taxes

Frakt, A., & Carroll, A. (2018, January 3). *Why the U.S. spends
so much more than other nations on health care.* Retrieved
June 3, 2018, from http://healthcarereformarticles-philiphilipo
.blogspot.com/2018/01/health-care-reform-articles-janu-
ary-3.html

Frances, A. (2016, September 27). *Medical errors should not be
our 3rd leading cause of death.* HuffPost. Retrieved June 3,
2018, from https://www.huffingtonpost.com/allen-frances/
medical-errors-should-not_b_12110648.html

Geyman, J. (2018, January). Crisis in U.S. health care: Corporate
power still blocks reform. *International Journal of Health
Services, 48*(1), 5–27. doi:10.1177/0020731417729654

Gold, J. (2010, March 18). *Cadillac' insurance plans explained.*
Kaiser Health News. Retrieved June 3, 2018, from https://
khn.org/news/cadillac-tax-explainer-update

Goodman, J. (2015, June 25). *Six problems with the ACA
that aren't going away.* Health Affairs. Retrieved June 3,

2018, from https://www.healthaffairs.org/do/10.1377/
hblog20150625.048781/full

Health care reform. The state of health care in America. (2016).
Healthcare Business and Technology. Retrieved June 3,
2018, from http://www.healthcarebusinesstech.com/health-
care-reform

Health care reform timeline. (n.d.). *Obama care facts.* Retrieved
June 3, 2018, from https://obamacarefacts.com/health-care-
reform-timeline

Johnson, C. (2017, December 6). *Out-of-pocket health spending
in 2016 increased at the fastest rate in a decade.* Retrieved
June 3, 2018, from http://healthcarereformarticles-philiph-
ilipo.blogspot.com/2018/01/health-care-reform-articles-
january-3.html

Kalkanis, S., & Trent, J. (2018, May 22). *For cancer patients,
Trump's drug pricing proposal falls short.* STAT. Retrieved
June 3, 2018, from https://www.statnews.com/2018/05/22/
cancer-patients-trump-drug-pricing-proposal

Khazan, O. (2017, July 14). *What's actually wrong with the U.S.
health system.* The Atlantic. Retrieved June 3, 2018, from
https://www.theatlantic.com/health/archive/2017/07/us-
worst-health-care-commonwealth-2017-report/533634

Kistler Tiffany Benefits. (2015, December 21). *IRS addresses
ACA rules for employer-provided health coverage.* Retrieved
June 3, 2018, from http://ktbenefits.com/2015/12/irs-
addresses-aca-rules-for-employer-provided-health-coverage

Luhby, T. (2017, November 1). *5 changes for Obamacare open
enrollment for 2018.* Retrieved June 3, 2018, from http://
money.cnn.com/2017/11/01/news/economy/obamacare-
open-enrollment-2018/index.html

Luhby, T. (2018a, February 20). *Americans will soon have
one more alternative to Obamacare, thanks to the Trump
administration.* CNN Money. Retrieved June 3, 2018, from
http://money.cnn.com/2018/02/20/news/economy/trump-
obamacare-short-term-health-insurance/index.html

Luhby, T. (2018b, April 9). *Trump administration offers two
more ways to escape Obamacare's penalty.* CNN Money.
Retrieved June 3, 2018, from http://money.cnn
.com/2018/04/09/news/economy/obamacare-penalty/index
.html

Mack, J. (2017, July 19). *7 Reasons U.S. health care is so expensive: Why do we pay more for less?* Michigan Live. Retrieved
June 3, 2018, from http://www.mlive.com/news/index
.ssf/2017/07/6_reasons_us_health_care_is_so.html

Mangan, D. (2017, December 21). *Obamacare enrollment blows
away expectations at nearly 9 million, despite short sign-up
window.* Retrieved June 3, 2018, from https://www.cnbc
.com/2017/12/21/government-reveals-final-obamacare-
enrollment-numbers-for-2017.html

Marquis, B., & Huston, C. (2017). *Leadership roles and management functions in nursing* (9th ed). Philadelphia, PA:
Wolters Kluwer.

Mody, P. R., & Blackwood, K. (2018, January 5). *5 Health
care policy issues to follow in 2018.* Retrieved June 3,
2018, from https://www.apks.com/en/perspectives/
publications/2018/01/5-health-care-policy-issues-

to-follow-in-2018?utm_source=Mondaq&utm_medium=syndication&utm_campaign=View-Original

Moffit, R. (2016, April 1). *Year six of the Affordable Care Act: Obamacare's mounting problems.* Retrieved June 3, 2018, from http://www.heritage.org/health-care-reform/report/year-six-the-affordable-care-act-obamacares-mounting-problems

Nguyen, K. H., & Sommers, B. D. (2016, August). Access and quality of care by insurance type for low-income adults before the Affordable Care Act. *American Journal of Public Health, 106*(8), 1409–1415. doi:10.2105/AJPH.2016.303156

O'Brien, E. (2017, December 2). *The Senate's tax bill eliminates the individual mandate for health insurance. Here's what you need to know.* Retrieved June 3, 2018, from http://time.com/money/5043622/gop-tax-reform-bill-individual-mandate

Obama, B. (2016, August 2). United States health care reform. Progress to date and next steps. *JAMA, 316*(5), 525–532. doi:10.1001/jama.2016.9797

Okoro, C. A., Guixiang, Z., Fox, J. B., Eke, P. I., Greenlund, K. J., & Town, M. (2017, February). Surveillance for health care access and health services use, adults aged 18-64 years—behavioral risk factor surveillance system, United States, 2014. *MMWR Surveillance Summaries, 66*(7), 1–41.

Pramuk, J. (2018, April 16). *It's not all about Trump: Democrats' midterm chances ride on health care and Social Security, too.* CNBC. Retrieved June 3, 2018, from https://www.cnbc.com/2018/04/16/not-just-trump-health-care-social-security-could-define-2018-midterm-elections.html

President Trump signs Tax Cuts and Job Act: Impact on health care and benefits. (2018, December 26). Kistler Tiffany Benefits. Retrieved June 3, 2018, from https://ktbenefits.com/2017/12/congress-passes-tax-reform-impact-on-health-care-and-benefits

Reisman, M. (2015, September). The Affordable Care Act, five years later: Policies, progress, and politics. *Pharmacy and Therapeutics, 40*(9), 575–578, 600.

Rosenquist, R., & Boualam, N. (2018, March 2). *The 340B program hits a crisis point.* Penn LDI. Retrieved June 3, 2018, from https://ldi.upenn.edu/healthpolicysense/340b-program-hits-crisis-point

Roubein, R. (2017, December 31). *GOP set to shift tactics on Obamacare in 2018.* Retrieved June 3, 2018, from http://thehill.com/policy/healthcare/366838-gop-set-to-shift-tactics-on-obamacare-in-2018

Rural Health Information Hub. (2002–2018). *Rural health disparities.* Retrieved June 3, 2018, from https://www.ruralhealthinfo.org/topics/rural-health-disparities

Sanger-Katz, M. (2018, May 22). *Despite attacks on Obamacare, the uninsured rate held steady last year.* Retrieved June 3, 2018, from https://www.nytimes.com/2018/05/22/upshot/despite-attacks-on-obamacare-the-uninsured-rate-held-steady-last-year.html?rref=collection%2Ftimestopic%2FHealth%20Care%20Reform&action=click&contentCollection=timestopics&region=stream&module=stream_unit&version=latest&contentPlacement=2&pgtype=collection

Soffen, K., & Uhrmacher, L. (2017, October 10). *Where the Obamacare exchanges lost insurers for 2018.* The Washington Post. Retrieved June 3, 2018, from https://www.washingtonpost.com/graphics/2017/national/obamacare-marketplace-insurers/?utm_term=.6496f32fc164

Stoltzfus Jost, T. (2017, November). The morality of health care reform: Liberal and conservative views and the space between them. *Hastings Center Report, 47*(6), 9–13. doi:10.1002/hast.774

The Associated Press and NORC. (2014–2018). *New year, same priorities: The public's agenda for 2018.* Retrieved June 3, 2018, from http://apnorc.org/projects/Pages/HTML%20Reports/new-year-same-priorities-the-publics-agenda-for-2018.aspx

The pros and cons of the Affordable Care Act. (2017, September 28). Health Markets. Retrieved June 3, 2018, from https://www.healthmarkets.com/resources/health-insurance/affordable-care-act-pros-and-cons

Weixel, N., Sullivan, P., & Hellmann, J. (2018, January 2). *Overnight health care: House GOP eyes entitlement reform, ObamaCare repeal in 2018 | Hospital groups dig in over discount drug program | Medicaid becomes GOP target.* The Hill. Retrieved June 3, 2018, from http://thehill.com/policy/healthcare/overnights/367114-overnight-health-care-house-gop-whip-entitlement-reform

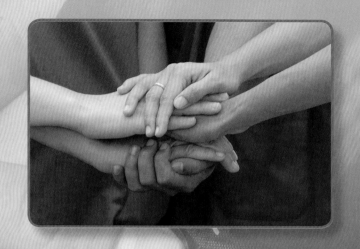

5

PROFESSIONAL POWER

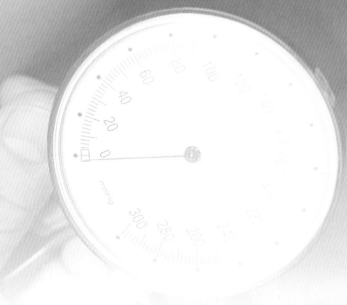

The Nursing Profession's Historic Struggle to Increase Its Power Base

Carol J. Huston

LEARNING OBJECTIVES

The learner will be able to:

1. Explore factors that historically led to nursing's limited power as a profession.

2. Examine characteristics of oppressed groups and analyze whether the nursing profession displays those characteristics.

3. Examine factors that led to the divergence of the nursing profession and feminism in the 1960s and

1970s and subsequently to their convergence in the mid-1980s as part of second-wave feminism.

4. Analyze the influence of gender on how many nurses view policy and politics, the willingness of nurses to work together collectively to achieve common goals, and the mentoring opportunities available to the profession's future leaders.

5. Identify driving forces in place to increase the nursing profession's power base.

6. Identify potential partners/external stakeholders/alliances that could strengthen the nursing profession's power in national and global policy arenas.

7. Identify nurses currently holding elected office in Congress and state legislatures, as well as the significant committees they serve on or positions they hold.

8. Identify issues currently being debated in the legislature that affect nursing and health care.

9. Explore individual, organizational, and professional responsibilities for succession planning to ensure that an adequate number of highly qualified nursing leaders exists in the future.

10. Reflect on whether the need to be politically competent should be internalized by nurses as a moral and professional obligation.

INTRODUCTION

Power is an elusive concept. The word *power* is derived from the Latin verb *potere*, meaning "to be able," thus, power may be appropriately defined as that which enables an individual or a group to accomplish goals. Power can also be defined as the capacity to act or the strength and potency to accomplish something (Marquis & Huston, 2017). Having power then gives an individual or a group the potential to change the attitudes and behaviors of others.

How individuals view power, however, varies greatly. Indeed, power may be feared, worshipped, or mistrusted, and it is frequently misunderstood (Marquis & Huston, 2017). Many women (and thus nurses) have historically demonstrated ambivalence toward the concept of power, and some have even eschewed the pursuit of power.

This likely occurred because some women have been socialized to view power negatively, believing that women do not inherently possess power (formal or informal) or authority. In addition, rather than feeling capable of achieving and managing power, some women feel that power manages them. These gender-based perceptions are changing, yet many women still need to learn how to use power as a tool for personal and professional success.

Similarly, the nursing profession has not historically been the powerful force it could have been in dealing with issues directly affecting health care and the profession itself. In a 2010 Gallup poll of more than 1,500 thought leaders from insurance, corporate, health services, government, and industry, as well as university faculty, the majority felt that nurses should have more influence in many areas of the health care system, including reducing medical errors, increasing the quality of care, promoting wellness, improving efficiency, and reducing costs (Robert Wood Johnson Foundation [RWJF], 2010). In addition, these thought leaders said that "nurses should have more influence than they do now on health policy, planning, and management. But when asked how much

influence various professions and groups are likely to have in health reform, opinion leaders put nurses behind government, insurance, and pharmaceutical executives, and many others—and they see real barriers to nursing leadership" (RWJF, 2010, para. 2).

Indeed, Nault and Kettering Sincox (2014) suggest that the idea of getting involved with legislation and legislators seems far removed from nursing practice and patient care for most nurses. But clearly, nursing can no longer afford to be reactive in the policy arena. The Institute of Medicine (National Academy of Science, 2011) suggests that "to be seen and accepted as leaders, nurses must see policy as something they can shape and develop rather than something that happens to them" (Lanier, 2017, p. 6). The general public has said it wants and expects nurses to be more involved in health care policy decision making, and both the American Nurses Association (ANA) Code of Ethics for Nurses and the Social Policy Statement recognize that influencing public policy is an essential professional expectation for registered nurses (RNs) in every practice setting (Lanier, 2017).

Unfortunately, though, nurses are often thought of as an apolitical group. As a result, nursing has all too often been reactive (rather than proactive) in the policy arena, addressing proposed legislation after its introduction rather than drafting or sponsoring legislation that reflects nursing's agenda. As a result, external forces have often controlled nursing.

These factors have contributed to the nursing profession having a relatively small power base in the political arena and some invisibility as a force in health care decision making. This chapter explores factors that have led to this relative powerlessness as a profession. Driving forces are identified, however, that are in place to increase nursing's professional power. The chapter concludes with an action plan to increase nursing's power base so that the profession is recognized as an increasingly significant force in health care decision making in the 21st century.

Discussion Point

Why is it that nurses, the largest group of health professionals, with perhaps the greatest firsthand knowledge of the health care problems faced by consumers, have not historically been an integral part of health care policy decision making?

FACTORS CONTRIBUTING TO POWERLESSNESS IN NURSING

Many factors have contributed to the nursing profession's relative powerlessness in health care policy setting. Six factors are discussed in this chapter (Box 22.1).

Oppression of Nurses as a Group

The attributes of oppression are unjust treatment, the denial of rights, and the dehumanizing of individuals. As such, it has been suggested that nurses and the nursing profession both work with oppressed groups and are themselves an oppressed group. Indeed, nursing was historically controlled by outside forces with greater prestige, power, and status. Generally, these forces were patriarchal and male dominated, such as medicine and hospital administration. For example, in the early 1900s, physicians attempted to exclude women from knowledge emerging from the basic sciences. Their refusal to let nurses use new instrumentation sustained women's subordination in nursing, although many nurses continually and actively sought greater scientific knowledge and techniques and incorporated these into their education.

Even at the start of this decade, some physicians openly suggested they should be the only health care professionals qualified to directly treat patients, even though many of the health care professions, including nurses, now hold advanced degrees including doctorates. Indeed, some physicians and their allies continue to push legislative efforts to restrict the right to use the title of "doctor," arguing that "nurses who want to be called doctors in a clinical environment should pay their dues and go to medical school" (O'Donnell, 2012, para. 7). One must question whether this elitism is more an effort to control money, power, and prestige than it is a concern about whether patients will be confused. Thus, the battle over the title "doctor" is likely a proxy for a larger struggle related to dominance and status.

In addition, some nurse practitioners work with physicians or within physician groups so that they can receive 100% insurance reimbursement for their services. This is called *incident to* billing and indicates that the physician is somehow involved with the care of the nurse practitioner's patients (Nursing Power, 2018). In many states in the United States, however, nurse practitioners have autonomous practice and do not require physician involvement or presence within their practice. In performing identical services, such as a primary care visit for yearly physical exam, the nurse practitioner typically receives only 75% to 85% compensation from Medicare, Medicaid, and private insurance companies. The Medicare Payment Advisory Commission (MedPAC) examined this payment disparity and determined that there was "no specific analytic foundation" for paying nurse practitioners less than physicians for the same services. This creates nurse practitioner invisibility and decreases nurse practitioner accountability for their own services (Nursing Power, 2018).

When a group is oppressed, it tends to have value confusion and low self-esteem. This occurs because the dominant groups identify their norms and values as the "right ones" and use their initial power to enforce them as the status quo.

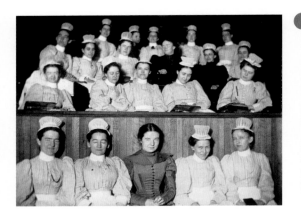

BOX 22.1   Factors Contributing to Powerlessness in Nursing

1. The oppression of nurses as a group
2. Nursing's failure to fully align with the feminist movement
3. Limited collective action by nurses
4. The socialization of women to view power and politics negatively
5. The inadequate recognition of nursing as an educated profession with evidence-based practice
6. The nursing profession's history of being reactive (rather than proactive) in national policy setting

Oppressed groups accept these norms, at least externally, to gain some power and control. For example, nursing's oppressors have not always held the same values as nursing (i.e., caring, nurturance, and advocacy). This has led to confusion for some nurses and even, at times, contempt for their own profession and what it represents.

> **Consider This** Badmouthing one's own profession may be a sign of oppression and values confusion.

Failure to Align Fully With the Feminist Movement

A second factor contributing to nursing's relative powerlessness is the profession's failure to align fully with the feminist movement. Although both nurses and women have improved their status in the last five decades, nursing has not kept pace with the progress women have made in other areas. This has occurred because, at least in part, nurses have not been fully engaged in the feminist movement.

This occurred for several reasons. One was that many feminists in the 1960s and 1970s were influenced by a more radical feminist perspective and, as a result, spoke out against women becoming nurses because it suggested that female nurses were in subordinate, caregiving roles. In addition, many nurses feared public identification with feminism.

The reality, however, is that nursing continues to be a profession composed of approximately 90% women, and this figure has changed only very slowly over time. This is noteworthy, given that there have been major gender shifts in virtually all of the other traditionally female-dominated professions (such as social workers, librarians, K-to-12 teachers) since the 1970s.

> ## Discussion Point
>
> Many nursing leaders in the early 1900s were political activists, actively involved in social issues such as women's suffrage and public health. At what point did nursing diverge from a sociopolitical agenda and why?

Although having female dominance in the profession may have some benefits, it also poses some liabilities. Indeed, some nursing leaders have suggested that nursing will never attain greater status and power until more men join the ranks (see Chapter 9). Others think that adding men to nursing's ranks is not the answer. Instead, nurses need to accept the responsibility for addressing the problems that have historically plagued the profession, and take whatever steps are necessary to proactively build a power base that does not depend on gender.

> **Consider This** Being a female professional in a male-dominated health care system brings to mind the "Ginger Rogers syndrome." Both Ginger Rogers and her dancing partner, Fred Astaire, were known as wonderful dancers, but Fred Astaire's name always came first, and he always received the greater recognition. In reality, "Ginger Rogers danced the same steps as Fred Astaire, but she did them backward and in high heels" (Wikiquote, 2017). So, who deserved the greater recognition?

In addition, recognition that assertive, independent nurses cannot exist if they have been socialized to be dependent women is growing. Similarly, it is improbable, if not impossible, for female nurses to implement expanded roles in advanced practice if they are unaware of or unwilling to recognize the social constraints imposed on them because they are women. Clearly, the battles between the AMA and advanced practice nurses about scope of practice, reimbursement, and the need for medical oversight are likely related as much to gender as they are to competition over patients (see Chapter 4). A reminder of this divide tore through social media recently when a male Florida anesthesiologist with ties to a major medical school posted demeaning and inflammatory comments about nurse practitioners (Kalensky, 2017, para. 3). He said:

> *Nurse practitioners are not, I repeat, not physicians. They lack the education, IQ and clinical experience. There is no depth of understanding. They are useful but only as minions.*

His comments were posted to Twitter, where many people reacted swiftly, calling for physicians to take a team-based approach and promote unity among health care professionals (Kalensky, 2017).

Sociologist Anne Bell suggests, however, that emerging trends in medicine and nursing may lead to a "flattening of the hierarchy" as women move into traditional male roles (Kalensky, 2017). Until then though, women will struggle to establish themselves as equals in health care professions.

Nurses need, then, to continue to examine the progress women have made in other professions and work with them inside and outside of nursing to strengthen power for women everywhere. This holds true for the men in nursing as well because the relative powerlessness of the profession transfers to them too, despite gender differences. Both male and female nurses must solve problems, work to advance the science of nursing, network to increase nursing's knowledge base and power, and provide mutual support.

Limited Collective Representation of Nurses

A third factor limiting the development of the nursing profession's power base is the inadequate collective representation of nurses by groups, such as collective bargaining agents and professional nursing organizations. As of 2014, only about 17% of the 3.1 million RNs in the United States belonged to collective bargaining units (Department for Professional Employees, 2018). Only about 5.5% of nurses (approximately 172,107) in 2014 belonged to the ANA, the nationally recognized professional organization for all RNs, whose mission is to advance and protect the profession (Union Facts, 2018). These relatively small membership numbers directly reflect the money that is available for lobbyists to represent nursing in the political arena. In contrast, the AMA has one of the most powerful lobbying organizations in the United States.

> **Consider This** Nurses must be represented in mass before they will be able to significantly affect the decisions that directly influence their profession.

There are many reasons for the small representation of nurses in the ANA. The dual and often conflicting role of the ANA as both a professional organization for nurses and a collective bargaining agent is certainly one reason (see Chapter 14). In addition, some nurses think that state nurses' associations have been burdened with the task of collective bargaining under the federation model of the ANA and that other programs have suffered as a result of funds being used for collective bargaining. Other nurses have expressed concerns about the cost of membership in the ANA or argued that the ANA is not responsive enough to the needs of the nurse at the bedside. Other nurses look at nursing as a job and not as a career and have little interest in professional issues outside of their immediate work environment.

Discussion Point

Do you belong to a professional nursing organization? Why or why not?
Do contemporary nursing leaders espouse this as a value? Is it encouraged in the workplace and in the academic world?

Whether these issues are valid is almost immaterial. As long as such a small percentage of nurses belong to the

ANA, the economic power of the ANA will be limited, as will its ability to significantly influence policy setting and legislation. Perhaps even more importantly, until nurses are willing to work together collectively in some form, they will be unlikely to increase either their personal or their professional power.

> **Consider This** At times, nurses have lacked pride in their collective groups and have viewed alignment with other nurses as alignment with other powerless persons, something that does little to advance an individual's professional power.

Unfortunately, at times, nurses in this country have not acted cohesively, whether at the local level, fighting for wage increases, or at the national level, attempting to influence health policy. Even the various professional nursing organizations to which nurses belong have not historically worked together cooperatively. The reality is that nurses continue to be widely divided on basic issues such as entry into practice, mandatory staffing ratios, and collective bargaining. Strategies to promote greater nurse unity are shown in Box 22.2.

BOX 22.2   **Strategies for Promoting Unity Within the Nursing Profession**

1. Nurses must respect each other's specialties and work toward enriching each other's job and work environments.
2. Nurses must acknowledge the different expertise that will help promote the quality care expected of them.
3. Nurses need to be self-aware regarding their behaviors that lead to disunity.
4. Nurses need to examine and learn from the nursing legacy that has negatively affected their behavior individually and collectively.
5. Accommodation of new vibrant views should be encouraged. This could be done through proper mentoring of the newly graduated nurses.
6. Collaboration among nursing organizations and working collectively would strengthen nursing.

Source: Thupayagale-Tshweneagae, G., & Dithole, K. (2007). Unity among nurses: An evasive concept. *Nursing Forum, 42*(3), 143–146.

> **Consider This** A metaphor for increasing nursing's power base through collective action would be a snowball. Individual snowflakes are fragile, but when they stick together, they become a powerful force.

Socialization of Women to View Power and Politics Negatively

A fourth factor contributing to powerlessness in the nursing profession has been the socialization of women (and thus the majority of nurses) to view power and politics negatively. Conscious efforts are changing this perception, however. For example, Taylor and Taylor (2017) reported that when nursing students participated in a theater-based workshop designed to increase student awareness of the micro-dynamics of power and the enactment of status in their day-to-day lives, they moved from seeing power as a generally bad thing, to a more neutral stance that power and status are at work in all of our interactions (Research Fuels the Controversy 22.1).

Politics is a part of life. It is also the art of using legitimate power wisely. Therefore, it requires clear decision making, assertiveness, accountability, and the willingness to express one's views (Marquis & Huston, 2017). It also requires being proactive rather than reactive and demands decisiveness.

Unfortunately, there is a persistent belief that political positioning is antithetical to quality nursing care. Perron (2013) suggests that nurses are not faced with choosing between caring for their patients and engaging with politics. Instead, she argues that the ethical merit of nursing care relies instead on positioning nurses squarely at the center-of-care activities, experiences, and functions. Nurses, then, become not a group that needs to be controlled and governed, but individuals who must care for themselves before they may care for anyone else.

The International Council of Nurses (ICN, 2014) and the World Health Organization agree, suggesting that nurses can and should be involved in policy development since they are uniquely positioned to provide crucial policy information. Furthermore, health policy often has a direct effect on nurses, and it is in their best interest to be engaged in its formulation. The ICN (2014) argues that a cultural shift must occur within the nursing profession to emphasize the importance of policy and nurses' role in setting and implementing it. In addition, a clear understanding of how policy affects nurses as well as how their unique knowledge regarding client care is crucial for policy development, must be embedded at the institutional level. This cultural shift must also occur in educational institutions where the integration of policy in practice must be emphasized in nursing classrooms and faculty must be given the proper support to develop and carry out policy research so that policy makers

---

Research Fuels the Controversy 22.1

Making Power Visible

An experiential, theater-based workshop was offered to undergraduate baccalaureate nursing students to increase their awareness of the micro-dynamics of power and the enactment of status in their day-to-day lives. This exercise allowed student participants to embody status and power and understand it in ways that they did not after simply completing assigned readings.

Source: Taylor, S. S., & Taylor, R. A. (2017). Making power visible: Doing theatre-based status work with nursing students. *Nurse Education in Practice, 26*, 1–5. doi:10.1016/j.nepr.2017.06.003

Study Findings

Participants' reflections, as shared in a single page reflective writing, showed two interesting trends. The first was that a relatively short workshop dramatically increased participants' awareness of power and status as ever present, including a substantial normative move from seeing power as being a generally bad thing that could be justified only in the interests of the organization's mission to a more neutral stance that power and status are at work in all of our interactions. The second trend that emerged was the tendency for participants to focus on agency-based explanations of power dynamics.

The researchers concluded that nurses can continue to ignore power and work around it, or they can recognize it and enact it appropriately and professionally. They argued that nurses must develop an awareness of their individual power, status, actions, intentions and values, and the assumptions they make about others, particularly those with less power or status. A lack of awareness and critical reflection contributes to the perpetuation of a powerless status quo.

and administrators can draw from the evidence base when developing policy.

> **Consider This** Changing nurses' view of both power and politics is perhaps the most significant key to proactive rather than reactive participation in policy setting.

Nurses, then, must perceive a need not only to be more knowledgeable about power, negotiation, and politics but also to be more involved in broad social and political issues. This requires becoming politically astute. Nurses need to understand what politics means, and they need to become experts in using politics to help nursing achieve both its professional goals and the needs of their clients.

Inadequate Recognition of Nursing as an Educated Profession With Evidence-Based Practice

A fifth factor contributing to the nursing profession's relative powerlessness is the inadequate recognition of nursing as a profession driven by research and the pursuit of higher education. Although nurses should value highly the caring, intuitive, nurturing part of nursing practice, the nursing profession has been negligent about equally emphasizing their extensive scientific knowledge base and the high level of critical thinking and analysis professional nurses use every day in their clinical practice.

Both the art and the science of nursing require highly developed skills and a well-developed knowledge base. The nurse of the 21st century has an extensive knowledge base in the sciences as well as in the arts. In addition, nurses must be expert critical thinkers, as they are required to continually look for and analyze subtle clues in their client data, make independent nursing diagnoses, and create plans of care. Constant assessment of and adjustment to the plan of care are almost always necessary, so nurses must be highly organized and know how to set priorities. In addition, nurses must have highly refined communication skills, well-developed psychomotor skills, and sophisticated leadership and management skills. This is the image nurses must promote to the public.

> ### Discussion Point
> If the public was asked to list five adjectives to describe nursing, what would they be? Would the art or the science of nursing be recognized more? Would nurses themselves use different adjectives?

The Nursing Profession's History of Being Reactive in National Policy Setting

The last factor discussed here as contributing to a relative lack of professional power in nursing is the profession's history of being reactive rather than proactive in national policy setting regarding nursing practice. *Reactive* means waiting until there is a problem and then trying to fix it. *Proactive* is more anticipatory; it means developing appropriate policy before action is taken or a problem occurs.

Unfortunately, the nursing profession has been far from proactive in shaping its own course or that of the health care system. In the 1990s, health care became big business. Managed care proliferated, and gatekeepers, not providers and consumers, began deciding who needed care and how much care was needed. Hospitals lost their place as the center of the health care universe as client care shifted from inpatient hospital stays to outpatient and ambulatory health care settings. Physicians lost much of their autonomy to practice medicine as they saw fit as insurers increasingly placed restrictions not only on which physicians, patients could see but also on what services the physician was authorized to prescribe.

Patients found themselves with limited choices of providers, longer wait times for care, more rules to follow, and more confusion about what would and would not be a covered expense. At the same time, RNs in record numbers, for the first time in history, were downsized, restructured, and often replaced by a cheaper counterpart to reduce costs.

Many nurses felt both overwhelmed and helpless with this degree of change. However, these changes did not happen overnight. Many of them were incremental and insidious, and the health care system changes occurred with little concerted effort by nurses to stop them.

Senge (1990) wrote about a brief parable in *The Fifth Discipline* that nurses should keep front and foremost when they think about the need to be proactive, even with incremental change. It is called "The parable of the boiled frog," and it goes like this:

If you place a frog in a pot of boiling water, it will immediately try to scramble out. But if you place the frog in room temperature water, and don't scare him, he'll stay put. Now, if the pot sits on a heat source, and if you gradually turn up the temperature, something very interesting happens. As the temperature rises from 70 to 80 degrees Fahrenheit, the frog will do nothing. In fact, he will show every sign of enjoying himself. As the temperature gradually increases, the frog will become groggier and groggier, until he is unable to crawl out of the pot. Though there is nothing restraining him, the frog will sit there and boil. He will boil to death, oblivious to what is happening to him.

Consider This Gradual but constant change may be even more dangerous than cataclysmic change because resistance is less organized.

DRIVING FORCES TO INCREASE NURSING'S POWER BASE

So what is the likelihood that the nursing profession will ever be a powerful force in health care decision making and the political arena? The answer is unclear, although the likelihood of this happening is increasing because of several driving forces in place. This chapter discusses six of these forces (Box 22.3).

The Timing Is Right. Consumers and Providers Want Change

Timing is everything. The political ferment regarding health care reform continues to escalate, and issues of cost and access are paramount in this country. For 2018, the United States was budgeted to spend US$1.57 trillion on health care, an amount equal to 22% of the gross domestic product (U.S. Government Spending, 2018). In fact, the United States spends more than any other industrialized country in the world (two to three times that of most industrialized countries). Yet its rankings in terms of life span, infant mortality, and teenage pregnancy are much lower than those of many countries that spend significantly less on health care.

The passage and implementation of the Affordable Care Act (ACA) only escalated public awareness and debate about flaws in publicly funded or subsidized health care in the United States. Furthermore, because of publications like *To Err Is Human*, consumers, health care providers, and legislators are more aware than ever of the shortcomings of the current health care system, and the clamor for action

has never been louder. Nickitas (2017, p. 54) agrees, noting that in today's political landscape, "nurses are hearing and experiencing the nation's anxieties over threats to health care access, insurance, rising prescription drug costs, and innovative efforts to improve the quality and value of health care." Clearly, the public wants a better health care system, and nurses want to be able to provide high-quality nursing care.

Both are powerful elements for change, and new nurses are entering the profession at a time when their energy and expertise will be more valued than ever. Nault and Kettering Sincox (2014) agree, suggesting that the present health care system is unreasonably costly with a myriad of access and patient safety issues. They argue that the creativity of nurses is needed to provide new solutions to problems and that it is time to individually and collectively determine what can be done to effectively influence the legislative process and policy development. The good news, then, is that the flaws of the health care system are no longer secret and nursing has the opportunity to use its expertise and influence to help create a better health care system for the future.

Size of the Nursing Profession and Diversity of Practice

The second driving force for increasing nursing's professional power base is the size of the profession and the diversity of nursing practice. Numbers are the lifeblood of politics. If nurses do not vote as a block, however, their political voice becomes diluted. The nursing profession's size, then, is perhaps its greatest asset, and its potential for a collective voting block should increasingly be recognized as a force to deal with.

Consider This Collective involvement of only a fraction of the nation's 3.1 million RNs in health care policy would produce a significant voting block.

BOX 22.3   **Driving Forces to Increase Nursing's Power Base**

1. The timing is right
2. The size of the nursing profession and the diversity of our practice
3. Nursing's referent power
4. Nursing's increasing knowledge base
5. Nursing's unique perspective
6. The desire for change among consumers and providers

Discussion Point

Have nurses ever made a concerted effort to vote collectively? What positions have professional organizations such as the ANA taken on recent election issues or candidates for office? Have endorsements by professional nursing organizations influenced how you vote?

Nursing's Referent Power

A third driving force for increasing the power of the profession is the referent power nurses hold. *Referent power* is the power one has when others identify with you or what you symbolize; therefore, you have their admiration or respect (Marquis & Huston, 2017). Nurses have a high degree of referent power because of the trust and credibility given to them by the public.

Lanier (2017, p. 7) notes that for more than 25 years, nurses have been recognized by the public as the most trustworthy of all professions. "When nurses speak, not only do people listen, but they also believe what is being said. Nurses are seen as selflessly looking after the needs of their patients rather than looking out for more selfish personal interests. In other words, they offer unbiased observations and suggestions that the public believes should be used extensively to shape policy decisions. The public believes nurses should be equal partners with physicians in efforts to address the many problems that challenge the health care system."

Nursing's Increasing Knowledge Base

A fourth driving force for increasing the power of the profession is nursing's increasing knowledge base. Indeed, the National Academy of Science (2011) in *The Future of Nursing: Focus on Education* notes that:

> Transforming the health care system to provide safe, quality, patient-centered, accessible, and affordable care will require a comprehensive rethinking of the roles of many health care professionals, nurses chief among them. To realize this vision, nursing education must be fundamentally improved both before and after nurses receive their licenses. (para. 1)

Fortunately, more nurses are being prepared at the master's and doctoral levels than ever before. Eileen Breslin, current President of the American Association of Colleges of Nursing, stated she "expects to see the momentum continue to build for advancing nursing education at all levels" since "employers are looking for highly skilled nurses able to translate the latest scientific evidence into practice" (Wood, 2015, para. 19). One of the greatest areas of growth will be in the number of Doctor of Nursing Practice students, with more than 15,000 students now pursuing a practice doctorate. Additionally, during the past decade, enrollment in PhD in nursing programs increased by 49% and is expected to further increase this year (Wood, 2015).

Furthermore, leadership, management, and political theory are increasingly a part of baccalaureate nursing education, although most nurses still do not hold baccalaureate degrees. These are learned skills, and, collectively, the nursing profession's knowledge of leadership, politics, negotiation, and finance is increasing. This can only increase the nursing profession's influence outside the field.

Nursing's Unique Perspective

A fifth driving force for increasing the nursing profession's power base is the unique philosophical perspective nursing brings to the health care arena. Nursing's perspective is unique as a result of its blending of art and science—a blending of "caring" and "curing," so to speak. The caring part of the nursing role is better known and better understood by the public. It is what historically has defined nursing. It is important that nurses not forget or underappreciate the unique values nursing represents because these are the values that make the profession different from all the others. These same values will make nursing irreplaceable in the current health care system.

The "science" part of nursing is less understood by the public. Nursing has an extensive scientific knowledge base, and the high level of critical thinking and analysis professional nurses use every day in their clinical practice is enormous. Nursing practice is increasingly becoming *evidence based*, meaning that nursing practice reflects what the literature says is *best practice*. That is, the practice of nursing is research based and scientifically driven (see Chapter 5). Unfortunately, consumers, legislators, and sometimes even other health care professionals fail to recognize this. Nursing then must do a better job of explaining and emphasizing both the art and the science of its practice. "Nurses are powerful because of the care they give, how they give it, and the relationships they have with patients" (Payne, 2016, p. 13).

ACTION PLAN FOR THE FUTURE

Based on these driving forces, an action plan can be created to increase the power of the nursing profession in the 21st century. This chapter identifies seven possible strategies to achieve this goal (Box 22.4).

Place More Nurses in Positions of Influence

The National Academy of Science (2011) suggested that for health care reform to work, nurses must be a part of decision-making processes in the health care system. This means placing nurses on advisory committees, commissions, and boards where policy decisions are made to advance health systems to improve patient care (National Academy of Science, 2011). Nault and Kettering Sincox (2014) agree, suggesting that since issues that can dramatically affect

BOX 22.4	**Action Plan for Increasing the Power of the Nursing Profession**

1. More nurses must be placed in positions of influence.
2. Recognize nursing's potential to make a difference.
3. Nurses must become better informed about all health care policy efforts.
4. Coalition building must occur within and outside of nursing.
5. More research must be done to strengthen evidence-based practice.
6. Nursing leaders must be supported.
7. Attention must be paid to mentoring future nurse leaders and leadership succession.

nursing practice can easily come through the legislative process, nurses must be at that table. Too much can go wrong if decision makers, who do not understand these changes, are left to make decisions without the input of those who provide professional care 24 hours a day, 365 days a year.

Training will be required, however, since many nurses lack basic skills in health care finance and policy. Indeed, a 2015 study suggested that increased orientation to liabilities and fiduciary duties were needed for nurses to be present and active on boards at all levels (Walton, Lake, Mullinix, Allen, & Mooney, 2015). Unfortunately, although nurses typically represent the greatest percentage of the workforce in hospitals, too few nurses serve on hospital boards or hold positions of significant power. A survey by the American Hospital Association (AHA) of over 1,000 hospitals in 2010 found that nurses made up only 6% of board members, whereas physicians held more than 20% of board seats (Walton et al., 2015).

For this reason, the Honor Society of Nursing, Sigma Theta Tau International (STTI, 2018) created a number of resources for nurses interested in gaining the skill set necessary to serve on the boards of health care institutions. One resource is a 2-year *Board Leadership Development* program that focuses on increasing knowledge and skills in the areas of strategic thinking and planning, fiduciary oversight, board and staff partnerships, and generative governance. Online educational resources are also available for nurses interested in learning how to be knowledgeable, contributing leaders on national and international not-for-profit boards.

In addition, the ANA, the American Academy of Nursing, and the American Nurses Foundation (ANF), the charitable and philanthropic arm of ANA, founded the *Nurses on Boards Coalition* (2018). This coalition is implementing a national strategy to bring nurses' valuable perspective to governing boards, as well as state-level and national commissions, with an interest in health. The goal is to put 10,000 nurses on boards by the year 2020.

Progress is being made. Beverly Malone, CEO of the National League for Nursing, predicts that in 2018, nurses will increasingly be taking seats at the table. "We will see more nurses on boards across the country—more than we've ever seen before in healthcare" (Stokowski, 2018, para. 2). Bob Dent, Senior Vice President, Chief Operating Officer, and Chief Nursing Officer, Midland Memorial Hospital, and President, American Organization of Nurse Executives (AONE), agrees, noting that "nurses at the point of service are continually stepping up in patient care settings and across other healthcare settings" (Stokowski, 2018, para. 3).

In addition, nurses must be placed in national positions that influence public policy. For example, a significant effort began in 2005 to establish an *Office of the National Nurse* in the United States, who would serve as an assistant to the surgeon general. A National Nursing Network Organization was formed, and legislation has repeatedly been introduced in Congress since 2006 to achieve this goal. Most recently, the *National Nurse Act of 2017* ("S.1106—115th Congress," 2018) was introduced (Congress.Gov, 2018). This bill would have designated the same individual serving as the Chief Nurse Officer of the Public Health Service as the National Nurse for Public Health. Thus, this bill elevated this nurse into a full-time leadership position to focus on the critical work needed to address national priorities of health promotion and disease prevention and to direct efforts at improving health literacy and decreasing health disparities in America. Proponents of the idea suggested that such a position would raise the profile of nursing and assist in a nationwide cultural shift to prevention and health promotion. Opponents suggested that this might not be the best way to effect change both within nursing and in the health care system. The bill was read twice and referred to the Committee on Health, Education, Labor, and Pensions in May 2017 (Congress.Gov, 2018).

Not all positions that influence public policy, however, occur at the national level. Indeed, few leaders burst on to the national scene directly. Instead, they assume leadership roles in entities such as medical centers, community hospitals, government agencies, and insurance companies.

Running for and holding elected office is, however, the ultimate in political activism and involvement. Only three nurses were serving in Congress as of mid-2018 (American Nurses Association, 2018). Many more nurses hold elected office in state legislatures.

In fact, nurses are uniquely qualified to hold public office because they have the greatest firsthand experience of problems faced by patients in the health care system, as well as an ability to translate the health care experience to the general public. As a result, more nurses must seek out this role. In addition, because the public respects and trusts nurses, nurses who choose to run for public office are often elected. The problem, then, is not that nurses are not being elected . . . the problem is that not enough nurses are running for office.

Recognize Nursing's Potential to Make a Difference

A second part of the action plan to increase the power of the nursing profession in the 21st century is to recognize the nursing professions' potential to make a real difference. It is critical that each nurse never lose sight of this potential. Payne (2016, p. 13) notes:

> One nurse working on a general med-surg unit cares for 6 patients 5 days a week, that's 30 patients a week. The nurse works 50 weeks a year, which equals 1500 patients a year. Say that nurse works in direct care for 30 years, that's 45,000 patients. And if they deal with 10 people that love each of those patients, that nurse could impact 450,000 people over the course of his or her career. Sure, you might have to adjust this for different units and shifts, more time off, or working less or more years, etc. either way it's a big number!

Consider This "Have you ever heard or said," "I am just a nurse...?" Perhaps something said in the face of a conflict or a problem? My response to that is, "No, especially a nurse. I am especially a nurse." (Payne, 2016, p. 13).

In addition, some legislators and employers have argued that "a nurse is a nurse is a nurse." This is wrong. Nurses can be whatever they want to be in nursing, and they can achieve that goal at whatever level of quality they choose. The bottom line, however, is that the profession will only be as smart, as motivated, and as directed as its weakest link. If the nursing profession is to be the powerful force it can be, it needs to be filled with bright, highly motivated people who want to make a difference in the lives of the clients with whom they work, as well as in the health care system itself.

Consider This Individuals may be born average, but staying average is a choice.

Become Better Informed About All Health Care Policy Efforts

The third step of the action plan is that nurses must become better informed about all health care policy efforts—especially those that influence their profession. This is difficult because no one can do this but nurses. This means grassroots knowledge building and involvement. O'Connor (2014) agrees, suggesting that the privileged intimacy the nursing role affords carries with it responsibilities beyond practice and professional responsibilities. It carries political responsibilities as well.

Consider This Nurses who do not understand the legislative process will not be able to influence the policy-making process.

One effort to increase the number of nurses who are well prepared to influence health policy at the local, state, and national levels was the launch of the American Nurses Advocacy Institute (ANAI) in 2009. ANAI fellows attend a 2+ day seminar in Washington, DC, to strengthen their competence in the political arena and participate in a year-long formal mentoring program. The institute covers content such as the advocacy process, criteria and methods for conducting political environment scans, effective strategies for creating and sustaining policy change, and coalition building ("RNs Hone Their Advocacy Skills," 2018).

Another program that helps nurses acquire the leadership skills to shape health care locally and nationally is the *Robert Wood Johnson Foundation Executive Nurse Fellows* program (RWJF, 2001–2018b). This 3-year program allows fellows to strengthen their leadership capacity and improve their abilities to lead teams and organizations in improving health and health care. The program targets leadership competencies focused on leading oneself, leading others, leading the organization, and leading in health care. In addition, RWJF launched the Future of Nursing Scholars program to develop the next generation of PhD-prepared nurse leaders who are committed to long-term careers that advance science and discovery, strengthen nursing education, and bring transformational change to nursing and health care (RWJF, 2001–2018a). The program advances the recommendation in IOM report, the *Future of Nursing: Leading Change, Advancing Health*, to double the number of nurses in the United States with doctoral degrees.

Not all nurses, however, need to or want to be this involved in politics and policy setting. Determining how directly or indirectly one should be involved is a personal decision. Certainly, being an informed voter should be considered a minimum expectation. O'Connor (2014) suggests that voting is an expression of respect for our freedom; conversely, not to vote is to disrespect our freedom, to take it for granted.

Fortunately, nurses are in the enviable position of having great credibility with legislators and the public. Nurses who choose to be directly involved in politics and policy setting can seek public office or become more involved in lobbying legislators about issues pertinent to health care and nursing. Such lobbying can be done either in person or by writing, and there are many good sources on how to do both. The legislator needs to understand why this is an issue that is critical not only to the nursing profession but also to his or her constituents. It is important, then, to create a need for the legislator to listen to what is being said.

Nurses can also give freely of their time and money to support nursing's position in the legislative arena. This can be done indirectly by contributing to professional associations such as the ANA, which have lobbyists in the legislative arena to protect nursing's interests, or by giving money directly to a political campaign. In this case, nurses should try to give early and to make as large a contribution as possible. It is the early and significant contributions that are remembered most.

Nurses interested in a more indirect contribution to policy development may work to influence and educate the public about nursing and the nursing agenda to reform health care. Either role is helpful—at least the nurse will have made a conscious decision to be involved.

Finally, nurses must also realize that part of the reason the profession has been invisible or portrayed inappropriately in the media is that nurses have not assumed the spokesperson roles they could have or should have for their profession. More nurses need to gain the skills needed to effectively interact with the media about nursing and health care. Other strategies for effecting change through political involvement are noted in Box 22.5.

BOX 22.5   **Political Activities to Effect Change**

1. Campaigning
   a. Know the issues associated with pending or potential legislation, and formulate a view related to that legislation.
   b. Organize a "call to action" by urging nursing health professionals to contact a legislator and identifying a legislator's position on an issue.
   c. Work for a political candidate.
   d. Attend political meetings.
   e. Make a campaign contribution.
   f. Provide links to a candidate's website.
2. Communicating
   a. Join organizations and assist in the development and wide dissemination of policy statements.
   b. Write letters to the editors of well-known lay newspapers and professional health care journals.
   c. Contact legislators.
   d. Present congressional testimony.
   e. Become a consultant to political candidates, help write their campaign message, and prepare policy briefings.
   f. Use social network media to get the message out to broader audiences.
   g. All television networks are required to provide free advertising space for public service announcements (PSAs). Volunteer to write the script for those PSAs.
3. Voting
   a. Register to vote and take the lead in organizing voter registration activities.
   b. Public universities are mandated to ensure that all college students are made aware of the process for registering to vote. Ensure that nursing students are aware of the process, and engage them in debating the issues.
   c. Promote the appointment of qualified nurses of key governmental positions.
4. Protesting
   a. Participate in a boycott.
   b. Support an action to strike.
   c. Organize a march.
   d. Oppose legislation.

Source: McNeal, G. J. (2011). Politicization: The power of influence. *ABNF Journal, 22*(3), 51–52.

Build Coalitions Inside and Outside of Nursing

The fourth step of the action plan to increase professional power in the 21st century is for the nursing profession to look within itself as well as beyond its organizations for coalition building. Belonging to professional nursing organizations is one way in which nurses can network for coalition building. Coalitions have been formed within nursing groups as well. The Tri-Council for Nursing is an alliance of four autonomous nursing organizations: the AACN, the ANA, the AONE, and the NLN. The Tri-Council focuses on leadership for education, practice, and research.

The Council for the Advancement of Nursing Science (CANS, 2016) is another example of coalition building among nursing groups. The Council is composed of representatives from the four major regional research societies, STTI, the American Academy of Nursing, the National Institute of Nursing Research, the Association of Women's Health, Obstetric and Neonatal Nurses; and the ANF.

Similarly, the National Federation for Specialty Nursing Organizations and the Nursing Organizations Liaison Forum, an entity of the ANA, merged in 2001 to become the Nursing Organizations Alliance, also known as The Alliance. The Alliance provides a forum for identification, education, and collaboration building on issues of common interest to advance the nursing profession (The Alliance, 2018).

> **Consider This** More collaboration among nursing organizations would increase the power of the nursing profession.

Discussion Point

All too frequently, the AMA and the ANA stand in opposition to each other in the legislative arena. Are there health care issues on which they could partner? Are there issues on which the ANA and the AHA could partner?

Nurses have not done as well, however, in building political coalitions with other health care professionals with similar challenges. Nor have they done well in building political coalitions with legislators. Most legislators have a great deal of respect for nurses but know little about their qualifications to speak with authority about the health care system. Nurses need to become experts at political networking, making tradeoffs, negotiating, and coalition building.

They also need to see the bigger picture of health care. This is not to say that nurses should lose sight of client needs but that they must do a better job of seeing the bigger picture and of building and strengthening alliances with others before they will be seen as powerful and capable.

Conduct More Research to Strengthen Evidence-Based Practice

Another critical strategy for increasing nursing's power base is to continue to develop and promote evidence-based practice in nursing. Great strides have been made in researching what it is that nurses do that makes a difference in patient outcomes (research on *nursing sensitive outcomes*), but more needs to be done. Nursing practice must reflect what research has identified as best practices, and a better understanding of the relationship between nursing practice and patient outcomes is still needed.

> **Consider This** Only relatively recently has research been able to prove that patients get better because of nurses and not in spite of them.

Building and sustaining evidence-based practice in nursing will require far greater numbers of master's and doctorally prepared nurse researchers, as well as entry into practice at an educational level similar to that of other professions. Social work, physical therapy, and occupational therapy all now have the master's or doctoral degree as the entry level into practice. Nursing cannot afford to continue debating whether a bachelor's degree is necessary as the minimum entry level into professional practice (see Chapter 1).

Support Nursing Leaders

Another part of the action plan to increase the profession's power is that nurses must support their nursing leaders and recognize the challenges they face as visionary change agents. Nurses have often viewed their leaders as rule breakers, and this has often occurred at a high personal cost to innovators.

In addition, nurses often resist change and new ideas from their leaders, and instead look to leaders in medicine and other health-related disciplines. Some of this occurs because of nurse leaders being discounted, at least in part, because of their female majority, and also in part to the low value placed on nursing expertise.

It is important to remember that, typically, it is not outsiders who divide nursing followers from nursing leaders. Instead, the division of nursing's strength often comes from within. Nursing leaders must be perceived as the

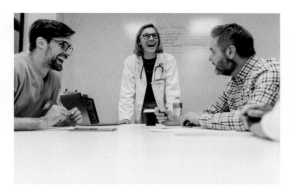

profession's best advocates. Differing viewpoints should be not only acknowledged but also encouraged. There is a proper arena for conflict and argument, but the outward force presented must be one of unity and direction.

Mentor Future Nurse Leaders, and Plan for Leadership Succession

Finally, and perhaps most important, before nursing can become a powerful profession, nurses must actively plan for leadership succession and care for younger members by providing mentoring opportunities. It is the future leaders who face the task of increasing nursing's power base in the 21st century.

Female-dominated professions have a history of exemplifying what is known as the *queen bee syndrome*. The queen bee is a woman who, after great personal struggle, becomes successful in her career. Her attitude, however, is that because she had to make it on her own with so little help, other novices should have to do the same. Thus, there has been inadequate empowering of young nurse leaders by older, more established nurse leaders. It is the young who hold not only the keys to the present but also the hope for the future. The nursing profession is responsible for ensuring leadership succession and is morally bound to do it with the brightest, most highly qualified individuals.

Discussion Point

Is the nursing profession proactive in planning its leadership succession, or is it a change that occurs by drift?

CONCLUSIONS

Although significant progress has been made, nursing, as a female-dominated profession, continues to face challenges in having a strong voice in health care policy. Nursing lobbyists in the nation's capital are influencing legislation on quality, access to care, patient and health worker safety, health care restructuring, reimbursement for advanced practice nurses, and funding for nursing education. Representatives of professional nursing organizations regularly attend and provide testimony at government agency meetings to be sure that the "nursing perspective" is heard on health policy issues.

Yet, clearly, nurses, as health care professionals, need to have greater input into and control over how the health care system evolves in this country. Nickitas (2017, p. 54) agrees, noting that

> *Nursing's value and voice matter in responding to the needs and demands of the populations they serve. As trusted listeners and communicators, nurses must express their values and use their voices to influence policy and decision-making processes. When nurses are more engaged (and better informed), they demand greater accountability around issues they care about. This can shape the quality of health care and, in turn, get to the core of when and how their values and voices can be effective.*

We need a health care system that will guarantee basic, affordable health care coverage for all citizens and in which all the members of the multidisciplinary health care team work together to create policy and provide care based on what is best for the patient. We also need a health care system that is accountable for its outcomes—that recognizes that individuality, autonomy, quality, and basic human dignity are essential components of health care services and that the bottom line is not always a number.

The nursing profession must be held accountable for being an integral force in shaping such a health care system. Indeed, nursing has a moral and professional obligation to do so. McNeal (2011) perhaps says it best:

> *For too long the discipline of nursing has quietly watched as other disciplines have slowly taken over many duties that were once only within the purview of the nursing profession. Pharmacy chains now conduct blood pressure screening and provide immunizations; retail stores have opened convenience clinics throughout the nation staffed by family nurse practitioners; and, social workers perform case management activities. At no other time in the history of this profession has the Office of the President recognized the value of nursing by creating ample provisions within the Healthcare Reform Act to facilitate nursing's ability to take the lead. This is our time, this is our moment. Let's not permit this time to pass us by. (p. 52)*

For Additional Discussion

1. Should the nursing profession target the recruitment of men into nursing in an effort to increase professional power?

2. What partners/external stakeholders should the nursing profession seek in terms of alliances or coalitions to strengthen its position in the policy arena?

3. What are the priority issues the nursing profession should identify in creating a proactive legislative agenda?

4. Will nursing ever be able to increase its power base if it does not increase its educational entry level to a level similar to that of other health care professions?

5. Do nursing schools provide enough content on politics, policy, and leadership for nurses to develop some degree of political competence? If not, what is missing?

6. Do most nurses internalize the need to be politically competent as a moral and professional obligation?

7. What legislative issues being debated have the greatest potential effect on nursing and health care?

References

American Nurses Association. (2018). *Nurses currently serving in congress.* Retrieved June 4, 2018, from http://www.nursing-world.org/MainMenuCategories/Policy-Advocacy/Federal/Nurses-in-Congress

Congress.Gov. (2018). *S.1106—National Nurse Act of 2017. 115th Congress (2017–2018).* Retrieved June 4, 2018, from https://www.congress.gov/bill/115th-congress/senate-bill/1106?q=%7B%22search%22%3A%5B%22sen.+merkley%22%5D%7D&r=1

Council for the Advancement of Nursing Science. (2016). *Homepage.* American Academy of Nursing. Retrieved June 4, 2018, from http://www.nursingscience.org/home

Department for Professional Employees, AFL-CIO. (2018). *Fact sheet 2015. Nursing: A profile of the profession.* Retrieved June 4, 2018, from http://dpeaflcio.org/wp-content/uploads/Nursing-2015.pdf

International Council of Nurses. (2014). Moving towards the greater involvement of nurses in policy development. *International Nursing Review, 61*(1), 1–2. doi:10.1111/inr.12092

Kalensky, J. (2017, November 3). *More than 'minions': Nurses deserve more respect from doctors.* STAT. Retrieved June 5, 2018, from https://www.statnews.com/2017/11/03/gender-gap-health-care-nurses

Lanier, J. (2017). Feel the power. *Ohio Nurses Review, 92*(2), 6–7.

Marquis, B., & Huston, C. (2017). *Leadership roles and management functions in nursing* (9th ed.). Philadelphia, PA: Wolters Kluwer.

McNeal, G. J. (2011). Politicization: The power of influence. *ABNF Journal, 22*(3), 51–52.

National Academy of Sciences (2011, Jan. 26). *The future of nursing: Focus on education.* Retrieved August 31,

2018 from http://www.nationalacademies.org/hmd/Reports/2010/The-Future-of-Nursing-Leading-Change-Advancing-Health/Report-Brief-Education.aspx

Nault, D. S., & Kettering Sincox, A. (2014). Nursing's voice in politics: The ongoing relationship between nurses and legislators. *Michigan Nurse, 87*(3), 17–21.

Nickitas, D. M. (2017, March). Speaking truth to power: Implications for nursing's values and voice. *Nursing Economic$, 35*(2), 54–95.

Nurses on Boards Coalition. (2018). *To improve the health of communities and the nation through the service of nurses on boards and other bodies.* Retrieved June 4, 2018, from https://www.nursesonboardscoalition.org

Nursing Power. (2018). *Invisibility, just another NP skill?* Posted by DrNurseSally on December 9, 2016. Retrieved November 25, 2017, from http://www.nursingpower.net/nursing-power/invisibility-just-another-np-skill

O'Connor, T. (2014). Wanted. Politically aware and involved nurses. *Kai Tiaki Nursing New Zealand, 20*(8), 24–25.

O'Donnell, M. (2012, April 23). *Why nurses should not be called doctor.* HealtheCareers Network. Retrieved June 4, 2018, from http://www.healthecareers.com/article/career/why-nurses-should-not-be-called-doctor

Payne, K. (2016, Summer). Especially a nurse: Find power in your practice. *Tennessee Nurse, 79*(2), 13.

Perron, A. (2013). Nursing as disobedient' practice: Care of the nurse's self, parrhesia, and the dismantling of a baseless paradox. *Nursing Philosophy, 14*(3), 154–167. doi:10.1111/nup.12015

RNs hone their advocacy skills through leadership program. (2018). The American Nurse. Retrieved June 4, 2018, from http://www.theamericannurse.org/2015/01/05/rns-hone-their-advocacy-skills-through-leadership-program

Robert Wood Johnson Foundation. (2001–2018a). *Future of nursing scholars.* Retrieved June 4, 2018, from https://www.rwjf.org/en/library/funding-opportunities/2017/future-of-nursing-scholars.html

Robert Wood Johnson Foundation. (2001–2018b). *Robert Wood Johnson Foundation executive nurse fellows.* Retrieved June 4, 2018, from https://www.rwjf.org/en/library/research/2011/05/robert-wood-johnson-foundation-executive-nurse-fellows.html

Robert Wood Johnson Foundation. (2010, January 20). *Nursing leadership from bedside to boardroom: Opinion leaders' perceptions.* Retrieved June 4, 2018, from https://cf.son.umaryland.edu/NRSG782/documents/RWJF-Gallup-Poll-January_2010.pdf

Senge, P. (1990). *The fifth discipline.* New York, NY: Doubleday/Currency.

Sigma Theta Tau International Honor Society of Nursing. (2018). *Board leadership institute.* Retrieved November 26, 2017, from http://www.nursingsociety.org/learn-grow/leadership-institute/board-leadership-institute-(bli)

Stokowski, L. A. (2018, January 22). *What will this year bring for nurses?* Medscape Nurses. Retrieved June 4, 2018, from https://www.medscape.com/viewarticle/891393

Taylor, S. S., & Taylor, R. A. (2017). Making power visible: Doing theatre-based status work with nursing students. *Nurse Education in Practice, 26,* 1–5. doi:10.1016/j.nepr.2017.06.003

The Alliance. (2018). *About us.* Retrieved June 4, 2018, from http://www.nursing-alliance.org/dnn/About-Us

Union Facts. (2018). *American Nurses Association (ANA).* Retrieved June 4, 2018, from https://www.unionfacts.com/union/American_Nurses_Association

U.S. Government Spending. (2018). *Total budgeted government spending expenditure GDP—CHARTS—Deficit debt.* Retrieved June 4, 2018, from http://www.usgovernmentspending.com

Walton, A., Lake, D., Mullinix, C., Allen, D., & Mooney, K. (2015, March–April). Enabling nurses to lead change: The orientation experiences of nurses to boards. *Nursing Outlook, 63*(2), 110–116. doi:10.1016/j.outlook.2014.12.015

Wikiquote. (2017, December 27). *Ginger Rogers.* Retrieved June 4, 2018, from https://en.wikiquote.org/wiki/Ginger_Rogers

Wood, D. (2015, January 12). *Top 10 things nurses can expect in 2015.* NurseZone.com. Retrieved June 4, 2018, from https://amsn.org/industry-career-news/top-10-things-nurses-can-expect-2015

Professional Identity and Image

Carol J. Huston

CHAPTER OUTLINE

LEARNING OBJECTIVES

The learner will be able to:

1. Explore the roots and prevalence of historical and contemporary nursing stereotypes, including nurse as angel of mercy, love interest (particularly to physicians), sex bombshell/naughty nurse, handmaiden to the physician, and battle-axe, as well as the stereotype of the male nurse as being gay, effeminate, or sexually predatory.

2. Identify common public portrayals or descriptions of nurses in terms of gender, dress, and role responsibilities.

3. Examine the role that organizations such as the *Center for Nursing Advocacy* and *Truth About Nursing* have assumed in addressing inaccurate or

negative portrayals of nursing in the media and the process they use to raise public and professional awareness of the issues surrounding nursing's public image.

4. Analyze the effect of inaccurate nursing stereotypes on the profession's ability to recruit the best and brightest students to nursing, as well as on the collective identity and self-esteem of all nurses.

5. Name well-known fictional nurse characters depicted in contemporary media (television and movies) and identify the nursing stereotypes they best represent.

6. Discuss the challenges inherent in attempting to change deeply ingrained stereotypes about nursing that are likely instilled very early in childhood.

7. Analyze how a lack of uniformity in dress and the way in which nurses introduce themselves to patients may contribute to the public's confusion about who is a nurse.

8. Explore the roles and responsibilities that individual nurses, employers, professional associations, and the media have, to ensure that nurses are portrayed accurately and positively to the public.

9. Identify image building strategies professional coalitions and corporations have used to promote recruitment and retention in nursing.

10. Reflect on the premise that every nurse controls the image of nursing.

11. Reflect on what image he or she would like the public to have of the nursing profession.

INTRODUCTION

An *image* can be defined as a reproduction or an imitation of something or as a mental picture or impression of something (Merriam Webster Online Dictionary, 2018). In other words, an image is often an unknown reality because it depends on the subjective perception of others. Perhaps that is why the public image of the nursing profession is at times, one-dimensional and inaccurate.

If asked to describe a nurse, most of the public would use such terms as *nice*, *hardworking*, or *caring*. They would also use the terms *ethical* and *honest*. There is little question that the public trusts and respects nurses. In fact, since they were added to the list in 1999, nurses have ranked number one on every Gallup poll on honesty and ethics except for 2001 ("Survey Says," 2018). Few people, however, would use the terms *highly educated*, *bright*, *powerful*, *professional*, or *independent thinker* to describe a nurse. Even fewer would call the nursing profession *prestigious*.

Clearly, public perceptions about the nursing profession are mixed and even contradictory at times. The public trusts and admires nurses, but this does not necessarily equate to respect or prestige. The reality is that much of the public does not understand what nurses really do.

Discussion Point

If the nursing profession is so well thought of, why are many of the brightest students encouraged to look at medicine rather than nursing? Why are there such significant differences in terms of occupational prestige and status between medicine and nursing?

Many people would, however, describe a nurse as a caring young woman, dressed in a white uniform dress, cap, and shoes, altruistically devoted to caring for the ill ("angel of mercy"), under the supervision of a physician. Common job functions would be identified as making beds, passing out pills, emptying bedpans, giving shots, and helping doctors. Some people, however, would allude, at least subtly, to a lustier image of sexy young females dressed in provocative attire and seeking sexual gratification from both patients and physicians. Still others might depict stern, aged "battle-axe" females thrusting hypodermic needles into recalcitrant patients and seemingly enjoying the discomfort they cause and the power that they hold.

What do these portrayals have in common? Almost nothing and yet everything. All are part of the convoluted, often conflicting stereotypical images of nurses. In addition, all these images demean the true nature and complexity of nursing, and most are based almost entirely in fiction. Yet these stereotypes are pervasive, and efforts to change them have yielded only limited progress. The result of this public image confusion is that old stereotypes of nurses as overbearing, brainless, sexually promiscuous, and incompetent women are perpetuated, as are images of nurses as caring, hardworking, altruistic, and selfless.

This image conflict is an enduring issue for nursing, and the profession's efforts to address the problem have been fragmented and largely unsuccessful. Indeed, many nurses believe nursing's image to be one of the most important and enduring issues they face as a profession. Waddington (2016) agrees, suggesting that nursing as a profession must build credibility by maintaining a modern image.

This chapter explores common historical and contemporary nursing stereotypes. The effect of these inaccurate stereotypes on recruitment into the profession and the collective self-esteem and identity of nurses is examined. In addition, strategies for improving the public image of nursing are presented, as are the challenges inherent in trying to change stereotypes that are ingrained in the profession's history and even in how nurses view themselves.

NURSING STEREOTYPES

Of the many nursing stereotypes, the most common ones are shown in Box 23.1: the nurse as an angel of mercy; the nurse as a love interest (particularly to physicians); the

BOX 23.1 **Common Nursing Stereotypes**

1. Angel of mercy
2. Love interest (particularly to physicians)
3. Sex bombshell/naughty nurse
4. Handmaiden to the physician
5. Battle-axe
6. Male nurses as homosexual, effeminate, or sexually predatory

nurse as a sex bombshell or "naughty nurse"; the nurse as a handmaiden to physicians; the nurse as a battle-axe; and the male nurse as homosexual, effeminate, or sexually predatory. All these stereotypes are profiled in this chapter. In addition, contemporary nursing images as depicted in movies and on television are profiled to better identify what images of nursing are before the public, especially the young people who represent the potential future nursing workforce.

Angel of Mercy

One of the oldest and most common nursing stereotypes is that of the nurse as an angel of mercy. Some individuals suggest that the image of the nurse as an angel with wings comes from the capes nurses historically wore as part of their uniforms. When most people think of nurses as angels of mercy, the image of Florence Nightingale bringing comfort to maimed soldiers during the Crimean War comes to mind. Clearly, Florence Nightingale's legacy of caring is beyond remarkable; however, few individuals outside of nursing would recognize Nightingale as a politically astute, assertive change agent who used her knowledge of epidemiology and statistics to document the effectiveness of nursing interventions. Both images should be equally important parts of her legacy.

The nurse "angel of mercy" stereotype continues to persist today, more than 100 years after Florence Nightingale's death. Indeed, a book published by Harlequin in 2008 titled *Single Dad, Nurse Bride* details the fictional life of an orthopedic doctor, Dr. Dane Hendricks, "who is every nurse's dream—handsome and a take charge kind of guy when it comes to medicine but also warm and humorous" (Amazon.com, 1996–2018b, para. 2). He is also wealthy. Rikki Johansen, "a conscientious nurse, taking to heart all the lessons she learned in nursing school, . . . always puts others before herself and as a result, she must drive a car that doesn't always start right away" (Amazon.com, 1996–2018b, para. 4). "When Dane's brother is diagnosed with cancer and Rikki turns out to be the only bone marrow match, there is never any doubt what her choice will be" (Amazon.com, 1996–2018b, para. 8).

The Center for Nursing Advocacy (2008–2018) has suggested that such images of the nurse as an "angel" or "saint" are generally unhelpful to the profession because they "fail to convey the college-level knowledge base, critical thinking skills, and hard work required to be a nurse. This image also suggests that nurses are supernatural beings who do not require decent working conditions, adequate staffing, or a significant role in health care decision-making or policy" (para. 1).

Some individuals argue that the angel of mercy stereotype is unconsciously promoted by nurses even today—in the Nightingale pledge, for instance (Box 23.2). When one looks closely at the pledge, which originated in 1893 but is still cited frequently in nursing graduation ceremonies, it speaks of nurses forgoing their personal wants and needs for the good of others. Being giving and caring in nature is a wonderful thing, but to suggest that it should be done to the extent of self-neglect is likely not the desired message.

It is important to remember, however, that being an angel of mercy is not all bad. It does encompass behaviors that many nurses typify, such as caring and dedication. Unfortunately, the angel of mercy image all too often also carries with it the idea that pay is never an issue and that suffering must

BOX 23.2 **The Nightingale Pledge**

I solemnly pledge myself before God and in the presence of this assembly, to pass my life in purity and to practice my profession faithfully. I will abstain from whatever is deleterious and mischievous and will not take or knowingly administer any harmful drug. I will do all in my power to maintain and elevate the standard of my profession and will hold in confidence all personal matters committed to my keeping and all family affairs coming to my knowledge in the practice of my calling. With loyalty will I endeavor to aid the physician, in his work, and devote myself to the welfare of those committed to my care.

Source: Florence Nightingale. (n.d.). *The "Nightingale Pledge."* Retrieved June 5, 2018, from http://www.countryjoe.com/nightingale/pledge.htm

be a part of the nurse's life if the role is to have value. This intrapersonal conflict between the values of altruism and pay befitting a professional is still experienced by many nurses.

Love Interest (Particularly to Physicians)

Another historical stereotype of nurses is that of a love interest, particularly to physicians. Doctor–nurse romance novels first appeared in the 1930s and 1940s, when becoming a nurse was one of the few career opportunities available to women. Nurses in these novels were generally cast as intelligent, strong women who felt fulfilled in their careers until they met the physician who would eventually become their husband. Then their career would end, and the nurses would live happily ever after, caring for their spouse and children.

With the women's rights movement of the 1970s, women's career opportunities expanded, and fewer books were devoted to women as nurses. In addition, readers' interest in medical romances dwindled. This is not to say that doctor–nurse romance novels do not still exist. They do, but the characters typically are different from what they were in decades past. The female character is now often a determined but compassionate physician or a charge nurse of a critical care unit in a large, urban medical center, who is beautiful. The male character, however, almost always continues to be a physician, coping with a tragedy in his past, who is "brilliant, tall, and muscular" and "with chiseled features, working in emergency medicine" ("Lovesick Doctors," 2007).

> *Consider This* Romantic relationships between nurses and doctors abound on recent television shows as well, such as Scrubs, House, Nurse Jackie, and Grey's Anatomy. It could be argued, however, that most of these relationships are not so much love interests as sexual liaisons.

Sex Bombshell/Naughty Nurse

Another common nursing stereotype is that of the nurse as a sex bombshell or "naughty nurse." Use of the word *naughty* probably is not powerful enough, however, given that the depiction of nurses in the sex and pornography industry is even more rampant than the general sexual stereotyping of nurses in the media. In fact, for at least 50 years, nurses have been portrayed as sex objects both on television and in the movies. Indeed, movies for at least six decades have been filled with images of nurses garbed in miniskirts, sleazy, low-cut tops, and high heels, who spend most of their time fulfilling sexual fantasies and virtually no time providing care to patients.

Nurses are even depicted as sex objects in television commercials. In 2003, Clairol Herbal Essences shampoo launched a commercial that showed a nurse abandoning her patient to wash her hair in his bathroom and then tossing her hair sensually at the patient as she left the room. Many nurses and nursing organizations condemned the unprofessional stereotype perpetuated in the ad and asked sponsor Procter & Gamble to discontinue it ("Procter & Gamble Pulls Offending Ad," 2003). Procter & Gamble did issue an apology to nurses and pull the ad, stating that the company "holds the nursing profession in the highest esteem" (p. 35).

> **Discussion Point**
> Do you think that the public truly believes that a nurse would abandon patient care duties to wash her hair in a patient's bathroom and then sensually shake her hair at the patient? If not, does the commercial still cause harm?

Another commercial sexualizing nurses was launched in September 2007 by Cadbury Schweppes Canada for Dentyne gum (Truth About Nursing, 2007). The Cadbury Schweppes ads showed female nurses being lured into bed with male patients the instant the male patients popped Dentyne into their mouths. The tag line for the commercial was "Get Fresh," and the message was that when hospitalized patients used Dentyne products, there would be an instant, erotic reaction from the "always available" bedside nurse.

More than 1,000 protest letters were sent from the website of the Registered Nurses Association of Ontario (RNAO) in response to the Cadbury Schweppes commercial (Truth About Nursing, 2007). Another 500 supporters from the Center for Nursing Advocacy wrote letters to top Cadbury Schweppes executives, leaving long messages explaining that such imagery reinforces a stereotype of workplace sexual availability that contributes to the global nursing crisis. Initially, the company responded that its ads were causing no harm. On October 6, 2007, however, the company told the Center and RNAO that it would pull the ads and consult nurses in creating future U.S. and Canadian ads that involved nurses.

Another recent example of the perpetuation of the naughty nurse stereotype became apparent when the *Heart Attack Grill*, a theme restaurant in Arizona, began dressing their waitresses in naughty nurse uniforms, which included micro miniskirts, fishnet stockings, and high heels. Because nurses are already a highly sexually fantasized profession, the Center for Nursing Advocacy asked the Heart Attack

Grill to reconsider their uniform choice when the restaurant opened in 2006. The Grill's owner, Jon Basso, who calls himself "Dr. Jon" and works in a medical lab coat, refused. In November 2011, a peaceful rally was held in front of the restaurant to protest the image of nursing being presented (Truth About Nursing, 2011a). Rally supporters argued that the Heart Attack Grill was reinforcing stereotypes that discouraged practicing and potential nurses (especially men), fostered sexual violence in the workplace, and contributed to a general atmosphere of disrespect that weakened nurses' claims to adequate resources.

In addition, the State Board of Nursing filed a complaint with the Arizona Attorney General's office that Basso was illegally using the term *nurse* in advertising for his restaurant (Arizona Statute A.R.S. 32–1636 states only someone who has a valid nursing license can use the title "nurse"). The Attorney General sent Basso a letter informing him that he was illegally using the word "nurse" at his restaurant and on his website. Basso's response was a refusal to remove the word "nurse" from his website, but he did agree to insert an asterisk next to every nurse

reference and to include a disclaimer that none of the women pictured on the website actually had any medical training or provide any real medical services (Truth About Nursing, 2011a).

More recently, in October 2014, Subway launched a television ad that used a naughty nurse costume, among others, to encourage U.S. customers to dine at the sandwich chain (Truth About Nursing, 2014a). In the ad, a young female office worker urged two colleagues not to eat burgers for lunch, but instead to emulate her Subway choices, because Halloween was coming and they had to "stay in shape for all the costumes!" She proceeded to demonstrate, donning a quick series of mostly naughty costumes that she helpfully labeled as "attractive nurse . . . spicy Red Riding Hood . . . Viking princess warrior . . . hot devil . . . sassy teacher . . . and foxy fullback!" "The nurse outfit wasn't the naughtiest ever, but it was a ridiculously short, flimsy dress" (Truth About Nursing, 2014a, para. 8).

And even more recently, a study by McAllister, Brien, & Piatti-Farnell (2018) of the Gothic imaging of nurses in popular culture found that the types of transgressive love nurses expressed to patients ranged from the obsessive and the pornographic to the monstrous. The authors concluded that this illuminates a hidden reality that nursing work is at once intimate and personal but also hidden, profane, repellent, horrifying, and feared. They also argued that it helps to explain phenomena—including nursing itself—which exists in the shadow of dominant and often stereotyped discourses.

Handmaiden to the Physician

Perhaps the most pervasive stereotype of nurses is that of handmaiden to physicians. In the handmaiden role, the nurse simply serves as an adoring backdrop to the omnipotent physician, demonstrating little, if any, independent thought or action. Certainly, this image is perhaps the most common image perpetuated on contemporary television and movie screens.

The image, however, is not new. This view of nurses as a handmaiden to physicians was reported in classic research by Philip and Beatrice Kalisch, in the 1970s, a time when nurses generally had no substantial role in television stories

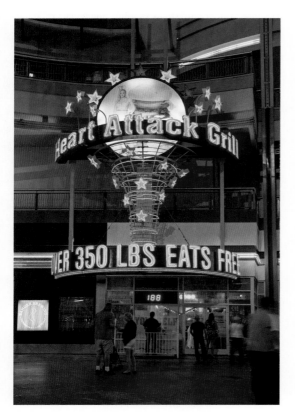

and were a part of the hospital background in programs that focused on physician characters. When nurses were the focus of a program, the storyline frequently involved the nurse's personal problems rather than his or her role as a nurse, and attributes such as obedience, permissiveness, conformity, flexibility, and serenity were emphasized.

Sometimes, though, even health care employers perpetuate this image, even if unintentionally. For example, in 2014, the Baylor Health Care System ran a television ad based on the idea that its employees were faithful "servants" (Truth About Nursing, 2014b). The one-minute ad featured many apparent nurses in clinical settings, intending to show them in a positive light. But many nurses objected to being presented as "servants." And the nurse scenes in the ad "emphasized what seem to be the most unskilled tasks with which nurses are associated, including hand-holding, mopping brows, wheeling gurneys, changing "hearts" and sheets, and picking things up off the floor" (para. 13). Meanwhile, apparent physicians in the ad acted as servants by doing research and cutting-edge surgeries and changing minds. Truth About Nursing suggested that "the servanthood theme may hold some appeal as a matter of spirituality or marketing, but it's dangerous to apply to a traditionally female profession that has struggled to overcome the notion that it simply serves physicians and to get respect for its advanced education and skills" (Truth About Nursing, 2014b, para. 13).

> **Consider This** Nursing care is frequently perceived by the public as simple and unskilled.

Many commercial representations of nurses also continue to represent the stereotype of nurse as a handmaiden. For example, in spring 2008, the Angela Moore jewelry catalog featured "Nurse Nancy" bracelets and necklaces. According to Truth About Nursing (2008), the jewelry was composed of four different types of balls; one ball featured a smiling, rosy-cheeked nurse in white uniform and cap giving a balloon to a girl; the second ball had a ladybug next to a stethoscope; the third ball featured a nurse's cap with a thermometer; and the fourth ball had a stuffed bear holding flowers next to a lollipop. The text in the catalog "asked readers to buy the Nurse Nancy jewelry to celebrate the ladies who give lollipops and band aids a whole new meaning" (Truth About Nursing, 2008, para. 1).

In response to letters of concern from nurses, the jewelry maker did agree to modify the description of the jewelry. According to Truth About Nursing (2008), however, what they changed it to was "Here's a special theme to celebrate the wonderful women who promote health and make us feel so much better. Talented, terrific and leaders to love!" (para. 3). Truth About Nursing (2008) suggested that "while this was probably an improvement over lollipops and band aids" (para. 4), it was still problematic in that it suggested that only women are nurses. In addition, they argued that "statements such as 'makes us feel so much better,' 'leaders to love,' and 'wonderful women' sound like adoration for someone's loving mom who makes them feel so much better by making them soup or tea" (Truth About Nursing, 2008, para. 5), not that nurses are highly trained health care professionals who use both science and art to make a difference in their patient's outcomes.

Even more distressing, however, was the February 24, 2017 suggestion of Nobel Prize winning economist Paul Krugman that nurses were one example of those who perform "menial work dealing with the physical world." When nursing advocacy groups urged Krugman to publicly apologize, he did so, explaining that nursing does deal with the physical work and have "manual" elements, but that it is not "menial" work. This type of uninformed stereotyping in influential media, is part of, however, what perpetuates the undervaluation of the profession (Truth About Nursing, 2017d).

Battle-Axe

Few stereotypes in nursing are as dark or demented, however, as that of the nurse as a battle-axe. The battle-axe stereotype often depicts an overbearing, unhappy, mean, senior nurse who intimidates both patients and staff. The movie *One Flew Over the Cuckoo's Nest* (1975) provides a perfect example of the battle-axe. Nurse Ratched, a nurse in a mental hospital, fits the description of a battle-axe in almost every way; craving power and control over others, and forcing her patients to obey her every whim or suffer the repercussions.

Nurse Diesel, in the movie *High Anxiety* (1978), was another stereotypical battle-axe nurse, with the addition of enormous prosthetic breasts. As an overbearing, evil-charge nurse, Nurse Diesel continually displayed a dark sneer and a love of domination. Annie Wilkes from the novel and movie *Misery* also gave new meaning to the sociopathic battle-axe nurse as she kidnapped, maimed, and held hostage a writer she admired and wanted to be close to. Similarly, the book *Doctors and Nurses* (Amazon.com, 1996–2018a) depicts Jen, a significantly obese nurse who partners (both sexually and career wise) with her married physician boss, to kill their patients. Jen's appetite for food, sex, and violence is whetted when her physician boyfriend happily scams patients and shrugs off lawsuit-worthy mistakes.

Battle-axe stereotypes of nurses have always existed; however, they seemed to hit their peak in the 1970s and

1980s. There are, however, still multiple images of battle-axe nurses available on the Internet and even contemporary television. Producer Ryan Murphy and Netflix announced plans in 2017 to revive the Nurse Ratched character from One Flew Over the Cuckoo's Nest for a two-season series on Netflix, starting in 2018 (Truth About Nursing, 2017b).

It is also of interest that the battle-axe counterpart of male physicians in medicine is viewed less negatively. For example, the television show *House* stars a drug-addicted, rule-breaking, rude, and crude male physician whose bad behavior is excused by his brilliance and ability to often cure patients when all hope is lost.

The Male Nurse: Gay, Effeminate, or Sexually Predatory

Female nurses are not the only ones who are stereotyped. Male nurse stereotypes are at least as prevalent as those for females, which only adds to the difficulty of recruiting men to the profession. For example, male nurses are frequently stereotyped as being homosexual (or at least effeminate). Indeed, a recent study (Goodier, 2013) reviewed one season of each of five American medical television dramas, including *Grey's Anatomy, Hawthorne, Mercy, Nurse Jackie,* and *Private Practice,* evaluating aspects of the episodes such as dialogue, costumes, casting, cinematography, and editing to compile a perspective on the ways that male nurses are characterized. Unfortunately, the shows tended to reinforce a stereotype of male nurses as men who are not traditionally masculine. The shows also reinforced images of the male nurse being mistaken for a doctor and the gay or emasculated male nurse. In addition, male nurses and midwives in the shows tended to suffer condescension from their colleagues and patients and were the object of comedy (Goodier, 2013).

Male nurses may also be stereotyped as being hypersexual and, as a result, the intent of their actions may be questioned as being either sexual in nature or, in some cases, even sexually predatory. Juliff, Russell, and Bulsara (2016) suggest this is especially the case in female intimate care where male nurses may feel vulnerable and uncomfortable about fulfilling role obligations. This makes it very difficult for male nurses to demonstrate the caring, therapeutic interactions that are such an important part of nursing. "One of the main responsibilities of a nurse is to show compassion to patients in their time of need, and men are quite capable of showing compassion as dedicated caregivers" ("Overcoming Gender Stereotypes," 2018, para. 1).

Consider This Many male nurses fear how their caring actions might be interpreted.

Another popular stereotype for male nurses is that they are nonachievers for going into nursing rather than more traditionally male occupations. This was certainly the case in the 2000 movie *Meet the Parents.* Unfortunately, despite the protestations of Greg Focker, the male registered nurse (RN) in the movie, that he loved nursing and became a nurse by choice, his future in-laws and other relatives constantly questioned his sexual orientation and manliness. They also clearly implied that Greg must have become a nurse because his test scores were not high enough for him to qualify for medical school.

Hodges et al. (2017) suggest that men face multiple gender-based barriers in nursing, including lack of history about men in nursing, lack of role models, role strain, gender discrimination, and isolation. In addition, finding and staying the path of nursing presents unique challenges for men.

Similarly, Sales Maurício and Fernando Marolan (2016) note that male nursing students often feel discriminated by society or even by the members of the profession. They suggest that "psychic suffering" occurs for male nursing students related to their gender and that social and political stereotypes as well as prejudices are significant issues for men in nursing. The researchers concluded that the psychic suffering of men in nursing needs to be further studied and that critical and proactive action are needed to emphasize masculinity as part of the profession.

Research by Wallen, Mor, and Devine (2014) concurs, suggesting that the extent to which male nurses perceive others respect nursing plays an integral role in determining their job satisfaction and affective commitment. Hospitals and other organizations can encourage perceived respect by offering interventions that cultivate feelings of increased occupational status among nurses, and male nurses in particular. Wallen et al. (2014) conclude that an apparent incompatibility exists between the expectations some people have for men, and the communal skills people think are necessary for such jobs. Their research suggests that how men in female-dominated jobs view their gender and professional identities—as compatible and overlapping, or conflicting and divided—affects their ability to navigate these different expectations.

How Ingrained Are Nursing Stereotypes?

Increasingly, researchers are concluding that inaccurate and negative stereotypes of nurses are not only well ingrained but also instilled early in life. Indeed, gender stereotyping about career opportunities begins at a very early age. By 3 years, most children already have firmly rooted gender-based ideas about the roles they can and should hold when they grow up.

The reality, then, is that by the end of middle school, most students report having their minds made up about desirable and undesirable careers. An unpublished study by Huston (Research Fuels the Controversy 23.1) suggested that basic beliefs and stereotypes about professions such as nursing may be ingrained at a far younger age, and that waiting until fifth, sixth, or even seventh grade to address inaccurate or negative images of nursing might be too late. Clearly, an early positive image for students is important if this is the population group the profession hopes will solve the current shortage.

Contemporary Nursing Stereotypes on Television

Television medical dramas currently provide the greatest number of visual images of nurses at work. There is little doubt, however, that television medical dramas build on traditional stereotypes of nurses, as well as suggest new ones. One of the best-known medical dramas in the past few decades, with strong nurse figures, was *ER* (1994–2009). This medical drama focused on the lives and events of the emergency department staff at County General Hospital in Chicago, a level I trauma center.

The character Carol Hathaway was perhaps the best-known nurse on *ER*. After surviving the September 1994 pilot episode in which, she tried to commit suicide, Hathaway became the charge nurse of the emergency department. She went on to have a sexual relationship with a physician and bore twins out of wedlock. Nurse Hathaway left the show in 1999—to join her physician love interest in another state.

Research Fuels the Controversy 23.1

Second-Graders' Image of Nurses

This unpublished study examined stereotypes held by 25 second-graders regarding "important" nursing roles and functions. In an effort to introduce students to nonhospital nursing roles, which students stated they already knew, a 30-minute slide show and discussion were held showing nurses actively engaged in less traditional nursing roles such as cardiac rehabilitation, primary care, flight nursing, education, management, and public health. In addition, nurse practitioners were introduced as primary care providers. Students were shown photos of nurses in all types of garb, except for white uniforms. Efforts were made to ensure ethnic and gender diversity in all presentation materials. At the conclusion of the presentation, students were asked to draw a picture of what they thought was the most exciting role that had been presented for nurses.

Source: Huston, C. (n.d.). Nursing stereotypes ingrained by second grade. Unpublished manuscript.

Study Findings

The caption on the first drawing was "the nurse is doing surgery on a real important disease." In the second, the nurse, with a red cross on her white uniform, was noted to be "rushing" into the hospital. In the third, the nurse, in her white starched cap, was making up a hospital bed. In the fourth drawing, the nurse was giving a hospitalized patient a backrub. In another, a dour nurse, as denoted by a capital N on her starched white cap with a red cross on it, was entering a hospital nursery. In the sixth, a patient in a bed was hooked up to an intravenous line, expressing pain. The smiling nurse was walking away from him.

In the seventh drawing, the nurse was helping the child in the hospital bed, and it included a caption that the "nurse is in a rush." In another drawing, nurses were scurrying to patients in their hospital beds. Rushing, for nurses, was a recurrent theme.

In the eighth drawing, the most exciting role for a nurse was noted as transporting a cot from room to room. Similarly, another student noted that the most important thing a nurse did was to transport people to the operating room, and yet another student noted that transporting patients in wheelchairs to their cars was the most important thing that nurses did.

Several drawings included stern nurses in white uniforms and caps and with red crosses on their chests making patients take medicine that tasted bad. Others depicted nurses working in nurseries or teaching mothers how to care for a crying baby. Another depicted a flight nurse taking an injured patient to the hospital, and yet another showed a nurse, in a white uniform with a red cross on her chest and wearing a cap, taking blood pressures.

All of the nurses in the drawings were female and white. The overwhelming majority wore white uniforms and caps and had red crosses on their chests. All but one drawing depicted nurses in hospital settings. Many associated the nurse with pain or an unpleasant experience. Despite the educational intervention, these second-graders already held deeply ingrained stereotypes about nursing and nursing roles, which were resistant to change. This suggests that if stereotypes are this difficult to modify in second-graders, the challenges in changing the image of nursing with the greater public will likely be very difficult.

Even with the departure of Nurse Hathaway, *ER* continued to provide probably the most influential portrayals of nurses on television. One of the highest-profile nurses remaining on the show was Abby Lockhart, an alcoholic, former obstetrical nurse from a family afflicted with bipolar disorder. She started on the show as a medical student, dropped out of medical school, worked as a nurse, and then became a doctor. Abby had sexual relationships with several doctors on the show and eventually married one of them.

In addition, Samantha Taggart, a nurse who joined the *ER* cast in 2003, was a tough, free-spirited, single mother of an emotionally troubled child, who almost immediately began a sexual relationship with one of the physicians. In her introductory scene, "Sam" (who had come to the hospital inquiring about employment) grabbed a syringe and leaped to sedate an unruly patient through a central vessel in his neck. This behavior earned her not only a job but also the respect of her soon-to-be coworkers.

One newer TV show to stir nurses to action, however, is *Grey's Anatomy* (2005–present). Physician characters on this show provide all the direct patient care as well as the emotional support of the patient and family. Indeed, in the 2017 lineup of its 15 regular characters, every single one was a surgeon (Truth About Nursing, 2017c). Nurses held only trivial roles. Even more distressing is the fact that one of the few visible nurses on the show gave sexually transmitted diseases to the male physicians. Truth About Nursing (2011b) notes that a few episodes in season 7 did feature a handsome male nurse (Eli), who "displayed a little skill and briefly stood up to the physicians, but by season's end, he was mainly a love interest for attending surgeon Miranda Bailey and no longer did any nursing work onscreen" (para. 8).

Similarly, nurses on NBC's show *The Night Shift* (2013–2017) "are mostly there to carry out physician commands. In general, the physicians run the ED, perform the complex life-saving procedures, and provide the patient advocacy and support. They also do some physician nursing, handling tasks that nurses are more likely to do in real life" (The Truth About Nursing, 2017a, para. 1). A similar invisibility of nursing characters exists on the new hit series *The Good Doctor* (2017–present).

One of the most alarming contemporary visualizations of a nurse on TV, however, was *Nurse Jackie* (2009–2015). The title character Jackie Peyton was a drug-addicted nurse who worked in the emergency ward at All Saints' Hospital in New York City. Jackie often made unethical and illegal decisions for the "good" of her patients, such as forging organ donor authorizations. In addition, although married, she often had sex with the pharmacist at the hospital in exchange for drugs. In season 2, her drug addiction led her to falsify an magnetic resonance imaging to get a phony prescription and to rip off a local drug dealer who embarked on revenge. Eventually, Jackie's addictions deepened to the point that she stole drugs from the oncology unit. When her theft was discovered, she was placed on probation by her employer, but a sympathetic colleague in the lab perpetuated her employment by discarding her next contaminated urine drug test. In addition, Jackie was a "world class liar," particularly about her addictions, and alienated almost everyone in her life (Truth About Nursing, 2015).

Perhaps what is most disturbing about Nurse Jackie is the attention this utterly dislikable nurse character received solely because of her independent and strong-willed thinking. The reality is that this was a drug-addicted nurse who had little regard for any codes of ethics or the patients she was charged to care for. Her primary mission in life and at work was to attain the drugs she needed to fuel an ever-increasing addiction, and this was often at the expense of patients. Unfortunately, "Jackie turned out to be arguably the strongest and the most skilled nurse ever depicted on serial U.S. television" (Campbell, 2013, para. 3).

Also disturbing was MTV's new reality show, *Scrubbing In*, which followed a group of 20-something travel nurses in Southern California (Campbell, 2013). Based on the trailer, in which these nurses were shown with a heavy focus on looking attractive, partying, and being "hell raisers," many nursing organizations launched campaigns to convince MTV Executives that the show should be cancelled for its unfair portrayal of nurses (most of these petitions occurred before the show had aired even one episode). Despite more than 30,000 letters of protest, the show aired as planned.

Finally, the May 20, 2014 segment of *Inside Amy Schumer* (Comedy Central), presented four female "RN" characters, in patterned scrubs embodying the unskilled physician handmaiden, the naughty nurse/physician gold-digger, the backwards female serf, and the petty, rule-bound battle-axe (Truth About Nursing, 2018). The first sketch indicated that the practical health advice that nurses deliver is in fact silly or dangerous, since it is delusional for nurses to think they may know more than physicians. The second sketch had the nurse proclaim that although the audience no doubt wanted to hear from physicians, it was going to have to "settle for the unsung heroes who do all the real work. The nurse went on to say that her statement was bogus, because nurses are as far from heroic hard workers as you can get. And the final segment indicated that nurses were helpless to address serious injuries they encountered outside the clinical setting" (Truth About Nursing, 2018).

Yet, there are some positive representations of nurses on contemporary television shows. Shows like *Chicago Med*, *Code Black*, *The Defenders*, and *Big Hero 6* offer glimpses of nursing skill, advocacy, and (more rarely) autonomy (Truth About

Nursing, 2017c). In *Code Black,* Latino "senior ER nurse" Jesse Sallander, greets each new class of physician interns by announcing possessively that he is their "mama" and that they are not "smarter than your mama because you have an MD." He also manages ED logistics, calls out vitals, describes symptoms, provides psychosocial care, and at times even suggests courses of action and diagnoses (Truth About Nursing, 2017c).

In addition, there are three notable nurse characters on *Chicago Med,* all African-American women. All three demonstrate some original thought and risk taking, although the show still spends as much time on their romantic lives and other personal issues as it does on their nursing skill (Truth About Nursing, 2017c). More positive contemporary representations of skilled professional nurses are needed on contemporary television.

The Image of Nursing on the Internet

The Internet is also filled with images of nurses, some accurate and some very stereotypical. A recent review of nurse images on Google found thousands of inappropriate images of nurses. Many were sexually suggestive, as well as demeaning. Some were in caricature, but many were of young women dressed in cleavage-baring uniforms and wearing fishnet stockings, high heels, and garter belts.

Even YouTube includes numerous stereotypical and distorted images. A 2012 study of the most viewed videos for "nurses" and "nursing" on YouTube suggested that nurses were depicted in three main ways—as a skilled knower and doer, as a sexual plaything, and as a witless incompetent (American Association for the Advancement of Science, 2018). The 10 most viewed videos reflected a variety of media, including promotional videos, advertising, excerpts from a TV situation comedy, and a cartoon. Some texts dramatized, caricatured, and parodied nurse–patient and interprofessional encounters. Four of the 10 clips, however, were posted by nurses and presented images of them as educated, smart, and technically skilled. They included nurses being interviewed, dancing, and performing a rap song, all of which portrayed nursing as a valuable and rewarding career. The nurses were shown as a distinct professional group working in busy clinical hospitals, where their knowledge and skills counted.

Finally, nurses should recognize that media stereotypes are not limited to nonprofessional sources. Even advertisements in medical and nursing journals often include stereotypical and demeaning nursing images, with frequent depictions of nurses as dependent, passive minor figures on the health care scene. If nurses are not depicted accurately in their own trade publications, how can they expect representation in other types of media to be better?

THE CENTER FOR NURSING ADVOCACY AND TRUTH ABOUT NURSING

Most nurses are upset about their depiction in contemporary media, but their efforts to respond to and change the situation have been fragmented. A more unified voice became possible with the creation of the Center for Nursing Advocacy in 2001. The center was created when Sandy Summers and seven other graduate nursing students at the Johns Hopkins University in Baltimore joined forces to address the media's disrespectful portrayal of nursing.

In 2009, the center was dissolved because of legal wrangling around record keeping and allegations of unpaid taxes. Sandy Summers then set up a new organization, called *Truth About Nursing,* a 501(c) (3) nonprofit organization that seeks to increase public understanding of the central, frontline role nurses play in modern health care, to promote more accurate, balanced, and frequent media portrayals of nurses, and increase the media's use of nurses as expert sources (Truth About Nursing, 2008–2018). "The Truth About Nursing's (2008–2018) ultimate goal is to foster growth in the size and diversity of the nursing profession at a time of critical shortage, strengthen nursing practice, teaching and research, and improve the health care system" (para. 1).

CONSEQUENCES OF INACCURATE OR NEGATIVE IMAGES

Inaccurate or negative public images of nursing have many consequences, particularly because these images influence the attitudes of patients, other health care providers, policy makers, and politicians. They even influence how nurses think about themselves.

A review of nursing image studies by Ten Hoeve, Jansen, and Roodbol (2014) noted that the self-concept of nurses and their professional identity are determined by many factors, including public image, work environment, work values, education, and culture. The researchers expressed concern that a lack of image clarity may negatively impact nurses' self-concept and the development of their professional identity and concluded that to improve their public image and to obtain a stronger position in health care organizations, nurses need to increase their visibility. This could be realized by ongoing education and a challenging work environment that encourages nurses to stand up for themselves.

Wood (2016) agrees, noting that professional socialization is the taking on of the identity, skills, and knowledge that are characteristic of a profession. The values and norms of the profession are also taken on and then embodied by individuals wishing to belong, so inaccurate or undesirable images negatively impact professional self-identity.

Inaccurate or negative images can also influence funding. When decision makers don't understand the value of nursing, they don't fund it. Nursing residencies in the United States receive almost no support compared with physician residency programs. Perhaps even more critical is that negative attitudes about nursing might discourage capable prospective nurses, who will instead choose another career that offers greater appeal in stature, status, and salary.

> **Consider This** Many nurses hold stereotypes about the profession to be true, just as the general public does.

Image Related Recruitment and Retention Challenges

As with other predominantly female professions, the literature suggests that many clients and their families undervalue nursing and do not understand what it is that nurses do that makes a difference in patient outcomes. Indeed, many nurses will honestly admit that they had little factual basis for what nursing would be like when they chose it as a profession. Instead, what drove them to become nurses were images that emphasized the caring, nurturing, and personal rewards associated with the profession.

Research by Price and McGillis Hall (2014) suggests that understanding how individuals come to know nursing as a career choice is of critical importance. Stereotypical imaging and messaging of the nursing profession shape nurses' expectations and perceptions of nursing as a career, which has implications for both recruitment and retention. Price and McGillis Hall conclude that strategies for future recruitment and socialization within the nursing and the health professions need to include contemporary and realistic imaging of both health professional roles and practice settings.

To recruit young people into the profession, the drug company Johnson & Johnson (J&J) began a series of television advertisements in 2002 as a part of its Campaign for Nursing's Future. Three new 30-second ads were released in 2005 and 2007, highlighting different aspects of nursing practice and promotion of diversity in nursing. New ads were released in 2011 and again several years later. Current ads are encompassing and include a website dedicated to promoting men in nursing, with career resources as related reading that emphasize challenges faced by minority male nurses as well as the pride engendered because of being a nurse (Johnson & Johnson, 2018).

CHANGING NURSING'S IMAGE IN THE PUBLIC EYE

Changing nursing's image in the public eye will not be easy. Nor will there be a silver bullet. Instead, multiple strategies are needed, including active interaction with the media and restriction of the term *nurse* to licensed nurses. In addition, nurses must increase their efforts to publicly praise and value nursing in addition to emphasizing how nursing uniquely contributes to patients achieving their desired health outcomes. Finally, nurses will need to become even more involved in the political processes that shape their profession.

Accomplishing this will take time and resources, including the time, energy, and funding of coalitions, foundations, and professional nursing organizations. Perhaps most important, it will take a concerted effort by individual nurses that will come only by first recognizing that there is a need to take action and then by doing what is necessary to achieve that goal. Carlson (2017, para. 16) notes that "Florence Nightingale was not a fading Victorian violet who avoided a fight. Rather, she was a disrupter, a change agent, a nurse who used her mind and heart to initiate change in the interest of the health and wellbeing of those she felt called to serve." Nurses today must view the call to change their public image in the same manner.

Indeed, global interest in changing nursing's image is increasing. In February 2018, The Duchess of Cambridge joined nurses and other health leaders across the world in launching a 3-year global campaign aimed at raising the profile and status of nursing ("Nursing Now Campaign," 2018). This *Nursing Now* campaign recognizes that nurses are at the heart of countries' efforts to provide health for all. The Duchess joined the World Health Organization's chief nursing officer, the president of the International Council of Nurses, health leaders, and nurses from countries around the world calling on governments, health professionals, and service users to value nurses and champion their leadership in providing the best quality of care ("Nursing Now Campaign," 2018).

Finding a Voice in the Press

One of the most important strategies needed to change nursing's image is to change the image of nursing in the mind of the image makers. That means proactively seeking positive and accurate media exposure of what nursing really is and what nurses really do. This job cannot be left to professional nursing organizations or to the image makers. Nursing's contributions need to be recognized and proclaimed. Unfortunately, many nurses feel ill prepared or lack the self-confidence to interact with the media. Knowing how to interact with the media is not intuitive for most nurses. Media training should always be provided to give nurses the skills and self-confidence to be effective in this role. Tips for interacting with the media are shown in Box 23.3.

> **Consider This** Far too few nurses are both willing and appropriately trained to interact with the media.

Instead of being fearful of the media, nurses should view media as an opportunity to expose the difficulties encountered in the profession as well as more accurate stories about what nurses do and the difference they make in the lives of the populations they serve. Nurses are uniquely qualified to speak with editors, reporters, and media producers on topics related to health care because they have a view from the frontlines and can localize national health care issues. Nurses are also well qualified to simplify medical terminology, explain the latest health care research, and identify current trends. Nurses, then, must be taught the basic skills necessary to self-confidently interact with the media. Nurses must also never pass up the opportunity to work with the media and should always view the media as playing a critical role in changing nursing's image.

BOX 23.3   **Tips for Interacting With the Media**

1. Be well informed about the topic.
2. Decide ahead of time what two to three key points you want to make and stay on track with the message.
3. Keep answers short, clear, and concise.
4. Stick to what you know and don't be pressured to answer questions you lack expertise in.
5. Talk in lay terms so that the public you want to reach understands your message.
6. Do not overestimate the reporter's expertise on the topic; be prepared to offer background information if necessary.
7. Remember that nothing is "off the record."
8. Be honest and friendly.
9. Respond immediately to media inquiries for interview since reporters are typically on short deadlines.
10. Be confident that you as a nurse are an expert on many issues consumers need and want to know.

> **Consider This** Nurses are experts in health care. Their invisibility in the media is likely a result of nurses lacking the basic skills and self-confidence to get involved, not that the media does not want to talk to nurses.

Reclaiming the Title of "Nurse"

Another strategy needed to improve the image of nursing is to ensure that use of the term *nurse* is limited to licensed nurses. The International Council of Nurses (ICN) reaffirmed in 2012 that the term "nurse" "should be protected by law and applied to and used only by those legally authorized to practice the full scope of nursing" (para. 1). In addition, all state boards of nursing have passed legislation restricting unlicensed personnel from using the title of "nurse." Unfortunately, on a regular basis, nursing aides and attendants either intentionally or unintentionally misrepresent themselves as nurses.

With the increased use of unlicensed assistive personnel and cross-training, a blurring of titles, roles, and responsibilities has occurred among RNs, licensed vocational nurses, and unlicensed support staff. Nametags increasingly recognized all staff as "care partners" or "associates," and some hospitals went so far as to prohibit the listing of RN on a name tag. At the same time, a loss of differentiated uniforms further adds to the public's confusion about who is truly caring for them. In addition, the media frequently perpetuates the inappropriate use of the term "nurse" by referring to all nurse's aides, volunteers who do health-related work, and medical assistants as "nurses."

In addition, RNs often contribute to the confusion by how they introduce themselves to patients. Nurses are often very casual when introducing themselves to patients, rarely identifying their specific role as the leader of the health care team. Nor do they explain how the roles of other members of the health care team differ. This may be due in part to typical female role socialization, which encourages women not to promote themselves, or it may be part of a team-building effort. Either way, patients end up confused about who the leader of the team is or how their roles differ.

Jacobs-Summers and Jacobs-Summers (2011) urge nurses to project a professional image in all interactions. They suggest that when nurses meet patients, they introduce themselves as a nurse and include their surname as professionals do. This introduction should not be perceived as cold or formal; instead it demonstrates respect and pride in the profession.

Jacobs-Summers and Jacobs-Summers (2011) also encourage "nursing out loud." "This means describing more of what you're thinking while you're providing care, consistent with patient confidentiality and sensitivity. If you do, then patients, families, physician colleagues and others will get a better sense of your education and skill" (Jacobs-Summers & Jacobs-Summers, 2011, para. 5).

Dressing as Professionals

Nurses in this country began shedding their white uniforms in the 1960s as part of the anti-conformist movement. As a result, the identity of the RN may be blurred. Whereas nursing caps and white starched uniforms were often impractical in caring for acutely ill patients, 30 years ago the public knew who the nurse was by the uniform he or she wore.

Today, many patients are unable to tell the members of the health care team apart, a problem that has become worse as the result of widespread adoption of scrubs as work uniforms. Advance Healthcare Network (2018) argues, however, that today's scrubs offer both comfort and convenience and allow nurses to look and feel good during a long shift. In addition, it argues that this evolution of the nurse uniform reflects society's view of the industry, as well as the increased roles and responsibilities nurses have.

Some nurse leaders have suggested, however, that a return to white uniforms would restore the public's perception of nursing's professionalism. Indeed, a study by Porr et al. (2014) noted that white pantsuit uniforms scored higher for professionalism than uniforms with small print, bold print, or solid color, and most patients preferred that their nurses dress in white. Even more compelling were the findings by Wocial, Sego, Rager, Laubersheimer, and Everett (2014) that for nurses to communicate assurance, patients perceive they must first be clean, well groomed, and understated in overall appearance.

Nurses themselves, however, are split on the issue of whether uniforms are essential to maintaining professionalism in nursing. They argue that comfort and uniformity of dress are equally important and that uniforms are not a requirement for professional trust and respect. Foster (2016) suggests, however, that it's not about whether nurses who conform to uniform policies can do their job better than those who do not. But patients and relatives of all ages expect professionals to appear in a certain way, and she considers it naive to believe that how broader society perceives a professional image or professionalism does not matter.

> **Consider This** Is it the white uniform that makes the professional, or is it the actions nurses take that define what a nurse is?

Positive Talk by Nurses About Nursing

Another strategy for improving the image of nursing is to change how nurses talk about nursing to others. Some nurses bad-mouth the profession and discourage young adults from considering nursing as a profession yet go on to bemoan the current nurse shortage. The effect of these comments by nurses on the public should not be underestimated in terms of their effect on the recruitment of young people into the profession.

The reality is that every nurse controls the image of nursing. Nursing, like any other profession, has strengths and weaknesses. It is important, however, that nurses enjoy their work, whatever it might be. Nurses should not stay in jobs that make them unhappy, because it demoralizes everyone around them. Whining and acting like a victim does little to improve the situation.

The bottom line is that nurses must be ambassadors for the profession and tell the public that nursing is an essential service with equal worth to other professions, that it can provide many services better than other health care disciplines, and that nursing is often more cost-effective than other disciplines. The public's demand for nursing likely rests on the demand nursing creates for itself in the public's eye.

Emphasizing the Uniqueness of Nursing

Another tactic nurses can use to improve nursing's image is not only to emphasize the profession's unique combination of "caring" and "curing" but also to underscore the depth and breadth of the scientific perspective that underlies its practice. Evidence-based practice and the application of best practice principles are an expectation for contemporary professional nursing practice. Nurses, then, must emphasize how clinical research and the use of current best evidence affect their decision making and the care they provide.

> **Consider This** "Competence and caring are interrelated" (Griffin-Stevens, 2018, para. 4).

In addition, newer research on nursing sensitivity and nursing outcomes is able to clarify what it is that nurses do that makes a difference in patient outcomes; there is increasing recognition that patients get better as a result of nursing interventions, not despite them. However, in many cases, the public knows very little about the research base that drives high-quality, evidence-based practice, and it is nurses who are in the best position to tell them about it.

Participating in the Political Arena

The political process can influence nearly everything nurses do and every problem they confront each day. In addition, public opinion is often based on inaccurate images, and nursing is no exception. Participating in the political arena, then, becomes a powerful strategy for changing the public's image of nursing.

The reality, however, is that although the nursing profession has some strong professional organizations, only a small percentage of nurses are members of national nursing organizations. This limits the profession's ability to be a force in the political arena. In addition, many nurses know little about the political process or feel too overwhelmed by the daily demands of their job to become involved in addressing larger professional issues in the political arena. Some nurses just assume that the best interests of the profession are being guarded by some unknown force out there. Legislators wonder whether inactivity means simply not caring or not having an opinion. The result is that nurses are inadequately represented in the political arena, and another opportunity for nurses to be represented as knowledgeable, active participants in the health care system is lost.

Because the underlying causes of the profession's political inactivity are numerous, just as the strategies needed to address this issue are complex, it is discussed only briefly here. Instead, a separate chapter has been dedicated to more fully discuss the issue (see Chapter 22).

CONCLUSIONS

Public identity and image have been a struggle for nurses for at least 200 years. From a sociological perspective, conflicting stereotypes of nursing have not served the nursing profession well, and a disconnect exists between reality and public image. The greater public clearly does not fully understand what professional nursing is all about, and the nursing profession has done an inadequate job of correcting long-standing, historically inaccurate stereotypes.

The responsibility for changing nursing's image lies squarely on the shoulders of those who claim nursing as their profession. Until nurses can agree on the desired collective image and are willing to do what is necessary to both tell and show the public what that image is, little will change. Damaging stereotypes are likely to continue to undermine public confidence in and respect for the professional nurse.

For Additional Discussion

1. Historically, images of physicians in the media have been more positive than those of nurses. Why? What factors have led to this difference?

2. Some nurses feel that no longer wearing white uniforms and caps has reduced the professionalism of nursing. Is how nurses dress an important part of public image? Would reverting to more traditional nursing attire improve nursing's public image?

3. Would you want your son or daughter to be a nurse? What have you told them about nursing that would either encourage them to enter the profession or discourage them from doing so?

4. Who are the best-known nurses currently depicted in the media (radio, television, movies) you access on a regular basis? Do their characters represent nursing stereotypes that have been discussed in this chapter?

5. What do you believe to be the greatest restraining forces that discourage nurses from interacting with the media? Is media training the answer?

6. The contributions of J&J to improve the image of nursing and increase recruitment into the nursing profession are unparalleled. Why would a corporation such as J&J be interested in this pursuit? Why did such an initiative not originate with a professional nursing organization?

7. Are nurses confused about what shared image they want the public to have of their profession?

References

Advance Healthcare Network. (2018, May). *From civil servant to classy surgeon: The evolution of nurse uniforms.* Retrieved June 5, 2018, from http://nursing.advanceweb .com/nurses-week-2018/?utm_source=hs_email&utm_ medium=email&utm_content=62769435&_ hsenc=p2ANqtz-8EvjLKyXXldmk6D0b_vOdvMFfOKhlK-2abIj0Frf7Ez0cVPvzGkAk13t_DpnHssexDtGP3VOz7s8Q-20QITLHho1Y-HnUw&_hsmi=62769435

Amazon.com. (1996–2018a). *Doctors and nurses: A novel (2006) (by L. Ellman).* Retrieved June 5, 2018, from http://www.amazon.com/dp/1596911026/?tag=reviewsofbooks1-20&link_code=as3&creative=373489&camp=211189

Amazon.com. (1996–2018b). *Single dad, nurse bride (2008) (by Lynn Marshall)* [Reader reviews]. Retrieved June 5, 2018, from http://www.amazon.com/Single-Nurse-Harlequin-Medical-Romance/dp/037319904X

American Association for the Advancement of Science. (2018). *Nurses need to counteract negative stereotypes of the profession in top YouTube hits (July 16, 2012).* EurekAlert. Retrieved November 29, 2017, from http://www.eurekalert .org/pub_releases/2012-07/w-nnt071612.php

Campbell, L. (2013, October 28). *Nursing stereotypes: The good, the bad and the ugly.* Vancouver, BC: Association of Registered Nurses of British Columbia. Retrieved June 5, 2018, from http://www.arnbc.ca/blog/nursing-stereotypes-the-good-the-bad-and-the-ugly

Carlson, K. (2017, June 7). *Nurses as disrupters and agents of change.* Retrieved June 5, 2018, from https://www.ausmed .com/articles/nurses-as-disrupters-agents-of-change

Center for Nursing Advocacy. (2008–2018). *Are nurses angels of mercy?* Retrieved June 5, 2018, from http://www.trutha-boutnursing.org/faq/nf/angels.html

Foster, S. (2016). Like it or not, the way we look matters. *British Journal of Nursing, 25*(16), 941.

Goodier, R. (2013). *TV may reinforce stereotypes about men in nursing.* Diversity Nursing Blog. Retrieved June 5, 2018, from http://blog.diversitynursing.com/blog/bid/152774/ TV-may-reinforce-stereotypes-about-men-in-nursing

Griffin-Stevens, D. (2018, May). Impacting the image of nursing. *Georgia Nursing, 78*(2), 14.

Hodges, E. A., Rowsey, P. J., Gray, T. F., Kneipp, S. M., Giscombe, C. W., Foster, B. B., . . . Kowlowitz, V. (2017). Bridging the gender divide: Facilitating the educational path for men in nursing. *Journal of Nursing Education, 56*(5), 295–299. doi:10.3928/01484834-20170421-08

International Council of Nurses. (2012). *Position statement: Protection of the title "nurse."* Retrieved June 5, 2018, from http://www.icn.ch/images/stories/documents/publications/ position_statements/B06_Protection_Title_Nurse.pdf

Jacobs-Summers, H., & Jacobs-Summers, S. (2011). *The image of nursing: It's in your hands.* Retrieved June 5, 2018, from http://www.nursingtimes.net/nursing-practice/clinical-specialisms/educators/the-image-of-nursing-its-in-your-hands/5024815.article

Johnson & Johnson. (2018). *Men in nursing.* Retrieved June 5, 2018, from http://www.discovernursing.com/men-in-nursing

Juliff, D., Russell, K., & Bulsara, C. (2016). Male or Nurse what comes first? Challenges men face on their journey to nurse registration. *Australian Journal of Advanced Nursing, 34*(2), 45–52.

Lovesick doctors and lovelorn nurses. (2007). Nurse Ratched's Place. Retrieved June 5, 2018, from http://nurse-ratcheds .blogspot.com/2007/11/lovesick-doctors-and-lovelorn-nurses.html

McAllister, M., Brien, D. L., & Piatti-Farnell, L. (2018). Tainted love: Gothic imaging of nurses in popular culture. *Journal of Advanced Nursing, 74*(2), 310–317. doi:10.1111/jan.13452

Merriam Webster Online Dictionary. (2018). *Image* [Definition]. Retrieved June 5, 2018, from http://www.merriam-webster.com/dictionary/image

Nursing now campaign launches. (2018, January). *Reflections on Nursing Leadership, 44*(1), 1–3.

Overcoming gender stereotypes: Why more men are becoming nurses. (2018, May 29). Retrieved June 5, 2018, from http://www.newdirectionsstaffing.com/2018/05/29/ overcoming-gender-stereotypes-why-more-men-are-becoming-nurses

Porr, C., Dawe, D., Lewis, N., Meadus, R. J., Snow, N., & Didham, P. (2014). Patient perception of contemporary nurse attire: A pilot study. *International Journal of Nursing Practice, 20*(2), 149–155. doi:10.1111/ijn.12160

Price, S. L., & McGillis Hall, L. (2014). The history of nurse imagery and the implications for recruitment: A discussion paper. *Journal of Advanced Nursing, 70*(7), 1502–1509. doi:10.1111/jan.12289

Procter & Gamble pulls offending ad. (2003). *Nursing, 33*(8), 35.

Sales Maurício, L. F., & Fernando Marcolan, J. (2016, December 2). The male being in psychic suffering in the nursing course. *Journal of Nursing UFPE/Revista De Enfermagem UFPE, 10*(Suppl. 6), 4845–4853.

Survey says: Nursing is the most ethical profession. (2018). StrategiesforNurseManagers.com. Retrieved June 5, 2018, http:// www.strategiesfornursemanagers.com/content/73908/5627 .cfm#

Ten Hoeve, Y., Jansen, G., & Roodbol, P. (2014). The nursing profession: Public image, self-concept and professional identity. A discussion paper. *Journal of Advanced Nursing, 70*(2), 295–309. doi:10.1111/jan.12177

Truth About Nursing. (2007). *Getting fresher.* Retrieved June 5, 2018, from http://www.truthaboutnursing.org/news/2007/ oct/06_dentyne.html

Truth About Nursing. (2008). *Let's "celebrate the ladies who give lollipops and band aids" with a Nurse Nancy bracelet!* Retrieved June 5, 2018, from http://www.truthaboutnursing.org/news/2008/mar/18_angela_moore.html

Truth About Nursing. (2008–2018). *Mission statement.* Retrieved June 5, 2018, from http://truthaboutnursing.org/ about_us/mission_statement.html

Truth About Nursing. (2011a). *November 2011 archives. Heart attack grill: Successful protest in Las Vegas November 12!* Retrieved June 5, 2018, from http://www.truthaboutnursing.org/archives/2011/oct_nov_dec.html#nov

Truth About Nursing. (2011b). *Understaffed: Fall 2011 TV review.* Retrieved June 5, 2018, from https://www.truthaboutnursing.org/news/2011/sep/fall_tv_preview.html

Truth About Nursing. (2014a). *All the costumes.* Retrieved June 5, 2018, from http://blog.truthaboutnursing.org/2014/10/all-the-costumes

Truth About Nursing. (2014b). *Servanthood: Is Baylor ad praising its nurses as "servants" a problem?* Retrieved June 5, 2018, from http://www.truthaboutnursing.org/news/2014/feb/baylor.html

Truth About Nursing. (2015). *Nurse Jackie episode reviews.* Retrieved June 5, 2018, from http://www.truthaboutnursing.org/media/tv/nurse_jackie.html

Truth About Nursing. (2017a). *No nurses. No care. The Night Shift's third season.* Retrieved June 5, 2018, from http://blog.truthaboutnursing.org/2017/10/night-shift-3

Truth About Nursing. (2017b). *Nurses vs. Netflix: Protests over Ryan Murphy's "Ratched."* Retrieved June 5, 2018, from http://blog.truthaboutnursing.org/2017/09/ratched-press-release

Truth About Nursing. (2017c). *The Defenders of San Fransokyo.* Retrieved June 5, 2018, from https://blog.truthaboutnursing.org/2017/09/fall-season-preview/#chicago-med

Truth About Nursing. (2017d). *Unskilled. Lowly. Servile.* Retrieved June 5, 2018, from http://blog.truthaboutnursing.org/2017/04/krugman

Truth About Nursing. (2018, May 23). *Inside Amy Schumer mocks nurses.* Retrieved June 5, 2018, from https://blog.truthaboutnursing.org/2018/05/amy-schumer

Waddington, A. (2016). Redrawing the nursing identity. *Canadian Nurse, 112*(7), 29.

Wallen, A. S., Mor, S., & Devine, B. A. (2014). It's about respect: Gender-professional identity integration affects male nurses' job attitudes. *Psychology of Men & Masculinity, 15*(3), 305–312. doi:10.1037/a0033714

Wocial, L. D., Sego, K., Rager, C., Laubersheimer, S., & Everett, L. Q. (2014). Image is more than a uniform: The promise of assurance. *The Journal of Nursing Administration, 44*(5), 298–302. doi:10.1097/NNA.0000000000000070

Wood, C. (2016). What do nurses do? Student reflections. *British Journal of Nursing, 25*(1), 40–44. doi:10.12968/bjon.2016.25.1.40

Nursing, Policy, and Politics
Understanding the Connection: Nurses' Role in the Policy Process

Sheila A. Burke, Donna M. Nickitas, and Jennifer Dine

CHAPTER OUTLINE

LEARNING OBJECTIVES

The learner will be able to:

1. Define the terms politics and policy and explore their relationship.

2. Differentiate among the problem stream, the political stream, and the policy stream in John Kingdon's three-stream model of policy development.

3. Explore the relationships among social inequity, health disparities, and access to health care.

4. Describe the role of research in assembling evidence to support policy change.

5. Identify nursing leaders who were pioneers in public policy, and describe their contributions in effecting social change.

6. Describe strategies and approaches that enhance the integration of health policy into nursing education and practice.

7. Identify roles that nurses may undertake to help shape policies that address the social determinants.

INTRODUCTION

This chapter examines the dynamic relationship between the nursing profession, policy, and politics from an underlying assumption that nursing is a public good. For years, society has expressed appreciation and approval that the profession fulfills a critical role to advance the nation's health and health care (Institute of Medicine [IOM], 2011; Riffkin, 2014). In 2016 the IOM was renamed the Health and Medicine Division of the National Academies of Science, Engineering, and Medicine.

Nurses have strong historical roots in advocacy and action which include identifying how to best distribute resources to individuals, families, and populations (Lewenson & Nickitas, 2016). In fact, these activities of advocacy and action toward obtaining and distributing resources align with Lasswell's (1936) classic definition of politics as activity that determines who gets what, when, and how. In addition, nurses work to create improvements in patient care; demanding increased access, and advancing health system changes that lead to better health and better health outcomes at lower costs. To conduct this work and achieve improved outcomes, nurses at all levels of the profession—education, practice, and research—are expected to understand and appreciate how they make crucial contributions to society (Kelly, Connor, Kun, & Salmon, 2008).

Nurses are also vital contributors to designing systems, which address emerging disease prevention, response, and management. They bring essential expertise and perspectives to health care teams to plan, implement, and evaluate response to emerging disease outbreaks and epidemics. The nursing profession also brings a unique perspective to care delivery models, which includes resources, infection prevention and control principles, and biopsychosocial human needs. This perspective makes nurses valuable assets as leaders and members of interprofessional health care, community, and legislative advocacy preparedness teams (Edmonson, McCarthy, Trent-Adams, McCain, & Marshall, 2017). The work of nurses in society to guide allocation and use of resources for the benefits of the populations can be viewed as the role of political agents.

An important way for nurses to assume leadership roles is through involvement in the policy-making process (IOM, 2011). Nurses have a specific accountability to participate in supporting a vision for health care that is affordable, accessible, and high quality (IOM, 2011). Because nurses are on the frontline of care delivery and have deep connections to patients, families, and communities, they are essential to ensuring that health care is consistently accessible, equitable, and of high quality. In addition, nurses are present at every level of the health care systems and can identify potential solutions to health issues and be instrumental in implementing effective solutions. To be influential in the development and adoption of intelligent health policy, it's vital that nursing professionals be prepared to use their professional knowledge and enter roles where they can influence policy makers or serve as policy makers. Nurses have both the capacity and expertise to influence health and public policy.

With the rapid pace of change in health care and the increasing complexity of health care and social policy issues, there are expanded opportunities for nurses to serve as leaders. It is important to recognize that though nurses are recognized as essential health providers and trusted professionals, they have not been seen as key players in influencing policy decisions related to health care access, delivery, and resources. Elevating nurses' participation in policy requires addressing this situation and taking steps to increase recognition of the roles nursing has in health and social policy issues.

> *Consider This* Professional nurses must work closely with Congress and other agencies in the governmental, private, and nonprofit sectors to advocate for nursing education, practice, and research to shape legislation, regulation, and standards of care impacting the profession.

For example, the Tri-Council is an alliance of four nursing organizations—the American Association of Colleges of Nursing (AACN), the American Nurses Association

(ANA), the American Organization of Nurse Executives (AONE), and the National League of Nursing (NLN)—each one has a focus on leadership for nursing education, practice, and research (Tri-Council for Nursing, 2015).

Each of the organizations is linked by common values and meets regularly to build consensus as well as provide stewardship within the profession. These organizations represent the voice of nursing and collectively speak to the diverse interests of the profession, including the nursing work environment, health care legislation and policy, quality of health care, nursing education, practice, research, and leadership throughout the health care delivery system. In 2017 the Tri-Council addressed the following policy positions:

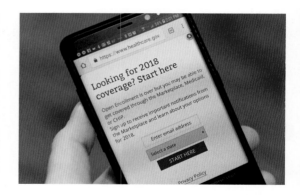

1. Increased awareness to incivility by issuing a resolution that spoke to the importance of advancing civility in nursing, within the profession and in the greater community. The resolution calls upon "all nurses to recognize nursing civility and take steps to systematically eliminate all acts of incivility in their professional practice, workplace environments, and in our communities."

2. Positioned authority and support toward advancing the role of Practitioner Nurses as a resource for improving health care by releasing a joint statement against the American Medical Association (AMA) Resolution, which has "call[ed] for the creation of a national strategy to oppose legislative efforts that grant independent practice to non-physician practitioners through model legislation and national and state level campaigns" ("American Nurses Association Responds," 2017, para. 1).

These initiatives reflect the breadth and scope of the Tri-Council's role in health care policy that involves, not only the nursing profession but also other professional groups to foster healthy, collaborative work environments that support all clinicians and the patients and communities they serve.

PATIENT PROTECTION AND THE AFFORDABLE CARE ACT

On March 23, 2010, President Obama signed H.R. 3590, the Patient Protection and Affordable Care Act (PPACA; hereafter called The Affordable Care Act). On March 30, 2010, the House and Senate both approved a package of fixes, H.R. 4872, the Health Care and Education Reconciliation Act of 2010.

The intention was that over the next decade health care reform activities contained in the Affordable Care Act (ACA) would result in new consumer protections, improved quality, and reduced costs. The ACA goals included increasing access to affordable care and holding insurance companies accountable to improve the consistency and scope of coverage. From 2010 to 2017 many changes to the ACA were proposed, and debates held about the degree to which its goals had been achieved. Though there were significant issues related to the implementation of the ACA, there were several important outcomes achieved regarding increasing the number of insured people and the extension or creation of coverage options for those with pre-existing conditions.

Following the 2016 change in the U.S. government administration, efforts to overhaul or eliminate the 2010 ACA accelerated. It appeared that several proposed changes would lead to reductions in the access to health care. Some of the proposed changes also seemed to be likely to result in increased costs for segments of the population.

Although decisions on the design and implementation of the health care policy had yet to be determined, the commitment of the nursing profession remained unchanged. "Nurses still have a responsibility to advocate for health care as a basic human right and access to an affordable package of essential health services" (Nickitas, 2011, p. 57).

Despite the changes in the health care systems, today's nursing workforce will be expected to address the myriad of health care challenges as noted listed below in Box 24.1.

Health care issues presenting complex challenges include:

- Opioid abuse and related deaths across the United States has increased at such a pace that it has been classified as an epidemic.

- Increasing incidence of suicides and depression, particularly in young adults and veterans.

BOX 24.1 **Key Features of the Affordable Care Act, by Year**

2010: A new Patient's Bill of Rights goes into effect, protecting consumers from the worst abuses of the insurance industry. Cost-free preventive services begin for many Americans.

2011: People with Medicare can get key preventive services for free, and also receive a 50% discount on brand-name drugs in the Medicare "donut hole."

2012: Accountable Care Organizations and other programs help doctors and health care providers work together to deliver better care.

2014: All Americans will have access to affordable health insurance options. The Marketplace allows individuals and small businesses to compare health plans on a level playing field. Middle- and low-income families will get tax credits that cover a significant portion of the cost of coverage, and the Medicaid program will be expanded to cover more low-income Americans. All together, these reforms mean that millions of people who were previously uninsured will gain coverage. Change in number covered between 2013 and 2016.

Source: Office of Disease Prevention and Health Promotion. Retrieved from http://health.gov

- Human trafficking as a social and health issue has been identified and nurses and other health professionals have key roles in implementing screening and intervention.

- Infectious diseases, including the unexpected spread of the Zika virus as well as global warming, have resulted in significant health issues with disproportionate impact on low and moderate resource countries.

- In 2015, the United States spent 17.8% of its gross domestic product on health care (Centers for Medicare & Medicaid Services, 2017) and rising costs impede utilization of preventive health initiatives.

Beyond being prepared with knowledge of health care systems and processes, it is essential for nurses to engage in policy development and be effective in working with other professions or stakeholders to support access to health care, cost management, and quality improvement initiatives.

NURSING AND POLICY

All aspects of the nursing profession are affected by policy issues, including safety and quality, health care standards, educational requirements, and nursing workforce conditions (which include adequate nurse-staffing, violence, and workplace incivility). Policy issues also encompass professional protections and requirements for nurses, including whistle-blowing, and the management of chemically impaired nurses. Nurses have been involved in shaping health care and public policy for over a century. For example, many early nursing leaders and activists, including Florence Nightingale, Lillian Wald, and Lavinia Dock, addressed the social issues of their times from the perspective of the nursing profession.

Nurses continue to this day to meet their social responsibility for initiating and supporting action to meet the changing health and social needs of the public (e.g., Research Fuels the Controversy 24.1).

It was professional advocacy and activism that created some of the earliest policy debates within nursing, including the requirements around the "training and education" of nurses. The 2011 IOM and the Robert Wood Johnson Foundation report, The *Future of Nursing, Leading Change, Advancing Health* (IOM, 2011), called for nurses to be better prepared with requisite competencies, such as leadership, health policy, system improvements, research, evidence-based practice, and collaboration, to deliver high-quality care, as well as competency in specific content areas including population and community health, and geriatrics.

The IOM (2011) report also represented a turning point for the nursing profession and called for nurses to achieve higher levels of education and training to ensure delivery of safe, patient-centered care across health care settings. The report recognized nurses are central to creating a genuinely effective U.S. health care system where all Americans will have access to high-quality and cost-effective care. The report defined four key recommendations:

- Nurses should practice to the full extent of their education and training.

- Nurses should achieve higher levels of education and training through an improved education system that promotes seamless academic progression.

- Nurses should be full partners, with physicians and other health care professionals, in redesigning health care in the United States.

- Effective workforce planning and policy making require better data collection and an improved infrastructure (IOM, 2011).

Research Fuels the Controversy 24.1

The Global Risks of Poor Physical and Mental Health in the Younger Populations

Many nurse researchers are identifying strategies that can significantly address the dramatic decrease in the health of the younger generations. For the first time in history the life expectancy for younger population is declining. The rates of obesity and obesity-related conditions, suicide, deaths by other forms of violence, and substance abuse are not only affecting life expectancy, these health issues are going to impact the costs of health care and the lifetime work productivity of the younger generations. Nurse researchers are identifying health-promotion and health-education strategies that incorporate early intervention and use of nonpharmacological treatments.

Source: Hart Abney B., Hovermale R., Lusk P., & Mazurek Melnyk B. (2018). Decreasing depression and anxiety in college youth using the creating opportunities for personal empowerment program (COPE). *Journal of the American Psychiatric Nurses Association.* doi:10.1177/1078390318779205.

Study Findings

Multiple nursing led studies in the United States and other countries are defining health education and treatment models that can reduce the risks associated with obesity, depression, and other mental health issues in the younger generation. For example, Dr. Bernadette Melnyk and colleagues developed the COPE (Creating Opportunities for Personal Empowerment) model for college students and obtained positive outcomes. COPE intervention included assessment and interventions that addressed depression, suicide risk, and anxiety in college students. There are other studies using the COPE model, which indicate the value of early implementation of evidence-based interventions. This is one example of how research provides policy opportunities for nursing. Through nurses engaging in policy development the value of programs such as COPE can be realized. Nurses can educate policy makers and work collaboratively with educational systems so that effective mental and physical health programs become part of the students' experience and can begin to affect the alarming trends toward reduced health quality in younger populations.

For nurses to practice to the fullest extent of their education and training, it requires that the nursing profession have both regulatory and legislative endorsement for entry into practice, licensure, and scope of practice activities. Since the 2011 IOM report, multiple statewide coalitions and strategic consortiums were launched and began working with state legislatures to adopt licensure laws that reflect new educational requirements for entry into practice and advanced practice parameters to ensure the protection of the public and remove barriers to practice.

One example was an initiative in Wisconsin, which was launched to address the projected nursing shortage in Wisconsin and across the nation. Multiple divisions of the University of Wisconsin (UW) nursing programs took part in a UW System Incentive Grant for economic and workforce development to address this problem. The Nurses for Wisconsin was awarded a 3.2-million-dollar grant with a goal to increase the number of baccalaureate registered nurses (RNs) by expanding the nursing education capacity within the UW System. The initiative was designed to accelerate the preparation of nursing faculty by increasing the number of nurses enrolled in doctor of nursing practice or nursing doctor of philosophy programs and offered pre- and postdoctoral fellowship awards and also included recruitment of faculty with a loan repayment program. In exchange for the financial support, fellows and faculty participants were required to make a 3-year commitment to teaching in a UW System nursing program (Adams et al., 2016).

Laws exist today that define the scope of nursing practice and licensure as distinctly separate from medicine and inclusive of responsibilities independent of medicine (National Council of State Boards of Nursing [NCSBN], 2015). The NCSBN is an independent, not-for-profit organization through which boards of nursing confer and develop approaches to address matters of common interest and concern that affect public health, safety, and welfare, including the development of nursing licensure examinations (https:// www.ncsbn.org/about.htm). NCSBN members include the boards of nursing in the 50 states, the District of Columbia, and four U.S. territories—American Samoa, Guam, Northern Mariana Islands, and the Virgin Islands.

To ensure the public continues to benefit from the care they receive, the NCSBN conducts innovative studies to evaluate safety and quality in nursing practice as well as in educational programs. For example, NCSBN conducted a landmark, national, multisite, longitudinal study of simulation use in prelicensure nursing programs throughout the country. This research study explored the role and outcomes of simulation in prelicensure clinical nursing education. "The study provided substantial evidence that substituting high-quality simulation experiences (for up to half of traditional clinical hours) produced comparable end-of-program educational outcomes and new graduates that were ready for clinical practice" (Hayden, Smiley, Alexander, Kardong-Edgren, & Jeffries, 2014, p. S3).

> **Consider This** Nursing's involvement in policy and politics has influenced state Nurse Practice Acts that regulate nursing practice for patient safety and public protection.

> **Consider This** The responsibilities of a licensed nurse include knowledge of, and adherence to, the laws and rules that govern nursing as outlined in the Nurse Practice Act and regulations. Review the nursing laws and rules by locating your state practice act and regulations at https://www.ncsbn.org/npa.htm.

Policy shapes and directs the environment in which nurses provide care and determines the scope of their responsibilities as well as the roles of other health providers and availability of resources. It is essential that nurses recognize how nursing science and high-quality research can support policy positions for which nurses are advocating and contribute to shaping public policy. This chapter traces nursing's involvement in policy activity and includes contemporary issues being debated today in the political arena such as health care restructuring. Because politics is part of every organization and a part of the government at every level, the chapter describes how becoming politically competent is essential for nurses to act on behalf of their profession and to influence the health care delivery systems where the patients and public will receive their care. Nurses can increase their influence in policy and make sure the contributions of nurses are visible through political advocacy and action (Lewenson & Nickitas, 2016).

The Future of Nursing: Campaign for Action is a national initiative of the American Association of Retired Persons (AARP) and the Robert Wood Johnson Foundation to implement the recommendations from the landmark 2011 IOM report. The Future of Nursing: Campaign for Action works with action coalitions in 50 states and the District of Columbia to implement the IOM's Future of Nursing recommendations and supports the role of nurses as essential partners in providing care and promoting health. The vision is to ensure that everyone in America can live a healthier life.

The campaign is coordinated by the Center to Champion Nursing in America, an initiative of AARP, the AARP

Foundation, and the Robert Wood Johnson Foundation. Since the 2011 report progress has been made in some areas. One initiative, the *Nurses on Boards Coalition* (NOBC), was developed in recognition that historically nurses have had a limited level of influence in the development of significant health care policies and in some cases where nurses have been active in policy development their contribution had not been widely recognized. The NOBC set a goal to have 10,000 nurses placed on boards and other influential bodies by 2020. This initiative was directly responding to the IOM report's recommendation that nurses attain a higher degree of influence through entering roles as decision makers on boards and commissions.

> **Consider This** Learn more about how the campaign is helping shape the future of health and health care by visiting the national Campaign for Action website and get connected at www.CampaignforAction.org.

DEFINING POLITICS AND POLICY

It is essential to describe and differentiate the terms policy and politics and to clarify the relationship between them. The word *policy* is Greek in origin and is linked to citizenship (Politics, n.d.). In government, policy involves the relationship of citizens to one another in public affairs (Aries, 2016) or defined as a government plan of action to solve a problem (Barbour & Wright, 2017). Government policy and programs often impact organizations and adjust the delivery of health care services to achieve certain outcomes, which have been identified as having value to the population. A broad definition describes policy as a set of standards that are intended to guide decisions and achieve certain outcomes. It often includes a statement of intent and is implemented as a procedure or protocol, for example, that all students must be vaccinated against measles, mumps, and rubella before admission into the school system.

Public policy is a term used that describes government actions. Policy is enacted through government systems, such as in the United States where the three branches of government are the legislative, executive, and judicial systems. These branches of government have the authoritative capacity to make decisions or influence the actions, behaviors, or choices of others. Each branch of government has a role in the formulation and regulation of health policy.

It is important for nurses to be connected to their elected representatives on Capitol Hill and be involved with governmental agencies as new laws are developed and enforced. Professional organizations such as the ANA have special departments such as the Department of Governmental

Affairs (GOVA) to amplify nurses' voices as policies are being created, fought for, and implemented. GOVA seeks to foster long-lasting relationships between nurses and their representatives so that nurses are positioned to influence governmental policy. Although policies are often reactive to societal and health issues, the foundation of nurses' policy work is toward creating an environment where health services are accessible, of high quality, and sustainable across diverse settings.

> ## Discussion Point
>
> How does health policy connect to how care and treatment are provided at the institutional level and the governmental level? What factors must be considered before policy development begins at both levels?

Governmental Policy

At the federal level, the U.S. Congress and the President make policy in three areas: *defense, domestic,* and *foreign.* Health-related policies can be found in all three areas. For example, health-related defense policies include the types of health care the military and their families will receive. Domestic policy refers to policies such as the enactment of the 2010 ACA, which originally was planned to be a comprehensive law aimed at protecting consumers, increasing access to care, promoting health, improving the health care delivery system, and controlling costs. Health-related issues are integrated into foreign policy as well. Congress decides whether to assist other nations in preventing HIV/AIDS, in providing family planning and nutrition assistance to developing countries, or responding to new health issues such as the 2016 Zika Virus outbreak, which impacted global, regional, and military health policies (Ai, Zhang, & Zhang, 2016).

By 2017, multiple global and national health issues that were causing significant strain on society (opioid crisis, suicide, etc.) created opportunities for nursing to significantly increase its participation in informing policy and advocating for effective strategies to address health issues that endangered existing and future generations.

For the overall good of the nation's health care system, "nurses must stay engaged to ensure appropriate attention and training occurs not only for themselves but also for all health care workers and hospitals" (Nickitas, 2014, p. 218). Nursing's voice and active participation in addressing these health and social issues are essential to shaping the quality and effectiveness of health care and public safety.

> ***Consider This*** Nurses serving in the military are affected by defense policy, nurses working to improve global health in developing countries are affected by foreign policy, and nurses working within the health care system anywhere in the United States are affected by the domestic policy. The President and the Congress decide on the allocations of tax dollars to be spent on defense, foreign aid, and domestic health care issues. When more money is spent to fund one policy initiative, less is available for others, unless taxes are increased.

Policies and Values

Policy involves the setting of goals and priorities by a society or an organization and the decisions about how and what resources should be used to achieve those goals. Thus, policies are often expressed as goals, programs, proposals, laws, and regulations that reflect the values and beliefs of those who develop the policies (Milstead, 2016). There are those occasions where policies may develop into moral dilemmas. This is because a policy relates to decisions about how to act toward others.

Policies developed by nurses have frequently demonstrated a commitment to the value of assisting people to care for themselves despite their illness or disability, and this belief has distinguished nursing from other professions (Research Fuels the Controversy 24.1). Caring, whether it is for families, for patients, or for the environment, is a value central to nursing. Watson (2008) suggests that to help the current health care system retain its most precious resource—competent, caring professional nurses—a new generation of health professionals must ensure care and healing for the public while learning about the value of serving others. For many years, caring had not been a value that received much attention from institutions and government policy makers. Nurses had some success at the state and federal levels moving such a policy agenda forward; however, results at a national policy level had been limited.

The importance of providing care within a context of caring with respect to person- and family-centered care has recently been receiving greater attention. Commonwealth fund research has shown that patient- and family-centered care that incorporates shared decision making can reap potential health care savings of $9 billion over 10 years. Accordingly, the National Quality Strategy seeks to ensure person- and family-centered care across the health care landscape and has outlined several goals to achieve this aim:

1. Improve patient, family, and caregiver experience of care related to quality, safety, and access to settings.

2. In partnership with patients, families, and caregivers—and using a shared decision-making process—develop culturally sensitive and understandable care plans.

3. Enable patients and their families and caregivers to navigate, coordinate, and manage their care appropriately and effectively (National Quality Forum, 2016).

Discussion Point

What values are reflected in state Nurse Practice Acts that address the scope of nursing practice for RNs and advanced practice nurses? Do these values promote or restrict nursing practice or nursing licensure, credentialing, and reimbursement for services?

Politics

Definitions of *politics* stem from the original Greek meaning, which referred to the government of the city-state; the actions of a government, politician, or political party; the process by which communities make decisions and govern; or the managing of a state or government. Politics involves power and influence for key decision making and requires significant investment in social capital. Politics is often defined as the process of who gets to decide how limited resources are allocated and distributed.

In government, politics is an activity that is central to developing the policy that protects the well-being of society. Therefore, nurses must understand how politics drives policy decisions and have the necessary skills and competencies to care for society, regardless of their institution or organizational affiliation. One way nurses can better understand politics is to first assess their political awareness and activity to express their participation in the political process (Box 24.2).

Consider This For nurses to realize their potential to successfully lead change, it is essential to understand the values and political issues at hand. Nurses who are effective advocates will

1. believe that they have the power and expertise to convince others of the need to change,
2. adapt themselves to handle the broader political value issues, and
3. learn to effectively mobilize their expert power and use strategic planning to influence key stakeholders for the needed change (Robertson & Middaugh, 2016).

Politics is a reality of all organized human activity; any group of two or more individuals has to establish how to make decisions that require common action and how to resolve conflicts. In fact, Kraft and Furlong (2010) suggest that politics involves how conflicts in society are identified and resolved in favor of one set of priorities or values over another. Because resources (money, time, and personnel) are limited or finite, choices must be made regarding their use. There is no perfect process for selecting optimum choices because whenever one valuable option is chosen, usually some other option must be left out. The challenge for policy analysts and political action is to understand how these choices are organized and which ones have the most influence and why.

For nurses to be effective advocates for others and to shape policy (and practice), it is necessary that they develop and practice political competence. This includes the ability to understand another's values and position and to use that insight to influence others to act. Nurses have expert knowledge in these practices because these practices are integral to the nursing process and are used to provide patient care.

BOX 24.2   Assessing Your Political Awareness and Activity

1. Are you a registered voter?
2. Are you affiliated with a political party (Republic, Democrat, or Independent)?
3. Did you vote in the last local or state primary election?
4. Did you vote in the most recent presidential election?
5. Did you vote in the last general election—local, state, and national?
6. Can you name your elected city, state, and national representatives?
7. Have you ever contacted any of these elected officials?
8. Have you ever lobbied your elected officials about a personal or professional issue that was important to you?
9. Are you actively monitoring the social media sites related to the policies you want to influence (not necessarily limited to the sites who support the policy as it may be very valuable to be aware of what opponents are doing to contest or dismantle policies you support)?

It is valuable for nurses to understand and appreciate how the nursing process approaches can be applied to the components of the political process. The skills that are integral to nursing practice provide a basis, which nurses can apply in the arena of political advocacy and action. To function in the area of policy at all levels requires competencies, which have not traditionally been adequately addressed in many nursing education programs. In 2017, the AACN launched an initiative and began a plan to increase the amount and depth of education related to preparing all nursing students to be prepared to fulfill their responsibilities in serving as leaders in advocating for and shaping health care (AACN). The *Faculty Policy Think Tank* (FPTT) initiative is focused on significantly improving nurses' preparation to impact policy through increasing this area of the educational experience.

Although the *AACN Essentials* describes the expectation for nurses' education at the baccalaureate, masters, and doctoral levels to address that practitioners will participate in policy and improvements to health care, the degree of curricular content and the approaches to teaching on the subject varied widely. The FPTT was created to inform and improve the state of health policy education in undergraduate and graduate nursing programs. The goal of the FPTT is to consider what steps lead to a generation of future practitioners who understand the elements that impact policy and have the appropriate competencies to bring nursing expertise and insight into the decision-making process and generate change.

CONCEPTUALIZING POLITICS AND POLICY DEVELOPMENT

Although there are many models for conceptualizing politics and policy development, Kingdon's streams of policy development (Sabatier, 1999) provide a broad and comprehensive framework for assessing policy development and a continuum for political engagement.

Kingdon's Three Streams of Policy Development

John Kingdon posited that three streams determine why some problems are chosen over others for policy development (Sabatier, 1999; Box 24.3). The three streams are the problem stream, the policy stream, and the political stream. These three streams often flow endlessly without converging, but when the streams come together, a window of opportunity opens to move an agenda, to legislate, or to regulate solutions to public problems.

The *problem stream* includes what are defined as problems, indicators of a problem, and the social construction of problems. It also includes how problems come to the

---

> **BOX 24.3**   **The Three Streams of John Kingdon's Streams**
>
> 1. **Problem:** embodies the process of problem recognition
> 2. **Policy:** embodies the formulation and refining of policy proposals as responses to problem recognition
> 3. **Politics:** considers the associated benefits and costs to subgroups of the population and the degree of external pressure the legislator feels to take action

attention of policy makers, such as in the form of causal stories or personal experiences. An example of such a problem is the current nursing faculty shortage. According to AACN's report on *2016–2017 Enrollment and Graduations in Baccalaureate and Graduate Programs in Nursing*, U.S. nursing schools turned away 64,067 qualified applicants from baccalaureate and graduate nursing programs in 2016 because of an insufficient number of faculty, clinical sites, classroom space, clinical preceptors, and budget constraints. Most nursing schools responding to the survey pointed to faculty shortages as a reason for not accepting all qualified applicants into baccalaureate programs. In October 2016, AACN released a report from its Special Survey on Vacant Faculty Positions. The survey achieved an 85.7% response rate from 821 nursing schools and reported a total of 1,567 faculty vacancies from schools with baccalaureate and graduate programs across the country. Besides the vacancies, schools also reported the need to create an additional 133 faculty positions to accommodate student demand. The data show a national nurse faculty vacancy rate of 7.9%. The majority of the vacancies (92.8%) were faculty positions requiring or preferring a doctoral degree.

Strategies to address the shortage have social relevance as the public's access to quality health care will be affected by a shortage of qualified nurses. Many statewide initiatives are underway to address both the shortage of RNs and nurse educators. For example, the UW announced the $3.2 million Nurses for Wisconsin initiative—funded through a UW System Economic Development Incentive Grant—to provide fellowships and loan forgiveness for future nurse faculty who agree to teach in the state after graduation. This program was launched in response to projections that Wisconsin could see a shortage of 20,000 nurses by 2035.

Kingdon's second stream is the *policy stream*. Ideas that are potential policy solutions are considered by their "technical feasibility and value acceptability" (Sabatier, 1999, p. 76). The reality is that policy makers are presented with many problems, and it is impossible to address all of them. Policy makers, then, are expected to set an agenda that reflects the values and issues on which to focus legislation or regulatory action. Because policy makers want to be successful (for their reelection and job security), most will avoid introducing legislative or regulatory proposals that are unlikely to pass and to be implemented.

For example, legislation introduced in the first session of the 113th Congress included the *Assault Weapons Ban of 2013* and the *Manchin-Toomey Amendment* to expand background checks on gun purchases. Both were defeated in the Senate on April 17, 2013. This legislation was defeated because Americans (and many special interest groups) advocated for the "right to bear arms" as protected by the Second Amendment of the U.S. Constitution. Since 2013 the increased incidence in mass shootings has caused national and international trauma and concern, with mass shootings in Las Vegas, Nevada (2017), Orlando, Florida (2016), Paris, France (2015), and Parkland, Florida (2018). At the same time nurses have continued to advocate for greater legislative action to reduce gun violence. For decades, ANA has called on Congress to enact sensible gun control–related legislation. In the wake of the Pulse shooting in Orlando in June 2016, ANA, representing the voices of more than 3.6 million RNs nationwide, renewed its call to action by urging lawmakers to immediately repeal restrictions prohibiting the CDC from studying gun violence.

Consider This "The time to unite and take action is now. Together we can halt the growing list of victims. We can stop the madness by forging solutions that address the myriad issues that promote cycles of violence. We must raise our voices to join with members of our communities and at every level of civil society in dialogue and action, to address the underlying issues that result in hate and motivate unspeakable acts of violence."
—ANA President Pamela Cipriano, PhD, RN, NEA-BC, FAAN

Consider This When support from the public, professional nursing, and consumer and hospital organizations came together to help fund the Nursing Education Act, it was because of the trust and value the public holds for the profession. In contrast, the ban on assault weapons met with opposition because of the change of national mood, the turnover of Congress and the White House to Republican rule, and opposition from the influential interest group, the National Rifle Association. This continues to be an issue where clear policy has not been established.

The significance of interest groups as part of the *political stream* cannot be overestimated. Throughout American history, political, ideological interest groups have shaped social change and policy decisions. Interest groups provide politicians with one of three resources essential for their success (i.e., reelection), including money, voter mobilization, and image. Image enhancement may be most significant for nurses regarding legislative interest. Having the support of nurses enhances a candidate's image. In 2017, nurses ranked as among the most highly trusted professions in public opinion polls for 16 consecutive years. The evidence supports the general public impression that the endorsement of nurses demonstrates a candidate's integrity.

Consider This Nurses continue to outrank other professions in Gallup's annual Honesty and Ethics survey. Eighty-one percent of Americans say nurses have "very high" or "high" honesty and ethical standards, a significantly greater percentage than for the next highest-rated professions, military officers, and pharmacists. Americans rate car salespeople, lobbyists, and members of Congress as having the lowest honesty and ethics, with the last two getting a majority of "low" or "very low" ratings (Gallup, 2014).

Nursing is a profession of more than 3.2 million members nationally. When divided by 435 congressional districts nationally, there are approximately 5,000 RNs per congressional district who can and have mobilized voters. The power of the "nursing numbers" converts to votes that can make the difference in electing officials who support and endorse nursing's core values and positions.

A strong political stream, however, is not enough. Convergence of the three streams is required. Nursing and the professional organizations that represent nursing (interest groups) in the legislature at the state and federal levels, then, have repeatedly worked to achieve this degree of stream convergence in public policy decisions related to health care. For example, the *Nurse–Family Partnership* (NFP) is a community-based program in which nurses work with first-time low-income mothers or vulnerable mothers from pregnancy until the child turns 2 years old. The NFP has been estimated to save $9,118 per child and as much as $26,298 as a return to society, for a net return savings of $17,180—cost–benefit ratio reported as 2.88. As health care delivery shifts from fee-for-service models of care to a value-based model, nurses are well positioned to use clinical and administrative data to measure nursing care, the quality of that care, and patient satisfaction from that care (Nickitas, 2014, p. 106). The NFP has effectively harnessed the value of clinical and financial data to illustrate how nurses are tackling important health problems and rigorously evaluating them.

> **Consider This** Nursing interest groups have seized upon the public's frustration with rising health care costs and promoted policies that emphasize the cost-effectiveness of advanced practice nurses (stream one—conditions, plus stream two—ideas/policies).

Analyzing Policy-Making and Professional Nursing

A more traditional approach to analyzing policy making uses a systems-based model that considers policy making in sequential stages. It is much like the nursing process: assess, plan, implement, evaluate, and assess again. In a policy system, a problem is identified and placed on the policy agenda; then developed, adopted, implemented, evaluated, and extended, modified, or terminated. The challenge of using a traditional systems model approach is that it fails to consider that the elected government's policy agenda rarely, if ever, reflect a consensus.

For example, leading up to and following the 2016 election cycle, the country became increasingly more divided along partisan lines, and significant differences were evident in the philosophical perspectives surrounding what role the government should have on health policy. Intense criticism of the ACA and its associated initiatives generated proposals from a variety of stakeholders. By the end of 2017, the newly proposed policies and the decisions regarding the distribution of resources led to an unsettled political environment. This situation created new opportunities for nurses, as individuals and as members of professional or other stakeholder organizations, to step forward and be active in bringing their expertise and influence to support the health care decisions that would provide quality, safety, and social justice.

In Kingdon's model, policy development, adoption and implementation, and politics are inextricably linked, and the political environment in which policy is formed is considered. Nursing has a responsibility to be a participant in all three of Kingdon's policy streams that create windows of opportunity to create and support policy that guarantees high-quality, patient-centered care.

> **Consider This** According to the IOM's definition, patient-centered care is "providing care that is respectful of and responsive to individual patient preferences, needs, and values and ensuring that patient values guide all clinical decisions" (IOM, 2011, p. 6).

It is a core responsibility of the nursing profession to elevate public awareness about the quality of care or lack of access to care. This includes addressing the social determinants of health. *Social determinants of health* include the issues of age, level of education, socioeconomic status, and access to health care. Through addressing these factors, there is a high capacity to improve the health of individuals and communities as well as reduce the costs of health care. To truly capture the inclusion of social and behavioral determinants of health data, nurses must lobby their legislators and others to ensure the social determinants of health are integrated into the policies and care delivery systems. These steps can yield significant benefits in increasing the quality and effectiveness of health care (Sigma Theta Tau International, 2017).

Professional nursing organizations and consumers collectively can develop ideas and propose policies to solve problems of health care access, health, and safety, or quality of care. Nursing professional organizations and interest groups like AARP can lobby and engage in political action to influence policy. In all of these examples, nursing is acting as an interest group. The unique thing about nursing as an interest group is that when nurses advocate for nurses and nursing, patients and the public get better care. Political action is a key part of interest group activity. Interest groups do more than support or oppose policies; they help to elect the policy makers by engaging in grassroots campaign activity and raising money for campaigns.

> ### Discussion Point
>
> Nursing has the potential to hold a significant leadership position in policy and politics. At the national level, the profession is represented by the ANA, the AACN, NLN, National Students Nurses Association, and many specialty organizations. What opportunities are available at the local, state, and national level for you to assume a leadership position?

POLICY MAKING AND POLITICS: THE KEY TO INVOLVEMENT

Nursing's potential to significantly shape health care and be active in policy making and politics requires participation. For changes in health care reform to be fully realized, nurses will need to see themselves as leaders in the process and engage with others, specifically stakeholders who are committed to health care quality who will share and support their goals. Political engagement can be viewed along a continuum that extends from no engagement to that of extreme activism, and each chooses when and how much political engagement along the continuum they want throughout their lives. For those who choose to enter the nursing profession, there is, however, an expectation that the nurse's professional role requires addressing policy as part of the care environment.

> *Consider This*   Political engagement is when individuals make things happen. From where you sit right now, identify three activities that you can make happen in school, in the community, and at home that can make a difference.

Political Advocacy

Nurses who make things happen fall into three categories: professionals, leaders, and political change agents. All three groups vote in every election and stay informed regarding issues affecting the health care system, and they speak out about working conditions and quality of care. They also participate in professional organizations, know who their local, state, and federal elected officials are, and communicate with them regarding issues of concern. Former ANA President, Karen Daley (2011) suggests there are a variety of ways that nurses can get involved and make a difference, including the following:

- Don't let policy happen "to you"—get involved in the policy committees at work and through state associations.

- Use your voice, experience, and expertise to help design and implement care environments and models. No one knows what patients want and need better than nurses do.

- Participate in workforce planning surveys and data-collection opportunities. Nurses must measure the value of what they do.

- Stay informed about and participate in the activities of a professional association. A few hours of volunteer time can make a big difference; remember there is strength in numbers.

- Embrace and act on the power of nursing expertise and wisdom.

Nursing Political Action Committees

In 1974, new laws were established allowing for contributions by *political action committees* (PACs). Those laws limited the amount an individual could contribute to a campaign and allowed groups to contribute up to $5,000 per election. Historically, nurses' political contributions continue to be outpaced in comparison to the contributions of physicians, nor do nurses' contributions approach the level of political contributions from the American Hospital Association (2014). ANA created the *Nurses Coalition for Action in Politics* (N-CAP; the precursor of the ANA-PAC) to establish political power through the endorsement of candidates and political contributions.

The proliferation of nursing specialty organizations and unions all claiming to represent "nursing" may have unintentionally limited the nursing profession's effectiveness in influencing elected officials because different nursing organizations bring different messages. Elected officials are unlikely to see how the goals of these organizations are related to each other. These officials tend to listen to those people they perceive as best positioned to help elect or reelect them, so whichever nursing organizations are most active in political campaigns through contributions and grassroots activity (usually only relevant in an official's first few elections because of the power of incumbency) are the organizations that will be heard.

It is essential for all nurses to be involved in the organizations that represent nurses, especially those with PACs, because of "money talks." Contributing to candidates that promote nursing's agenda to improve the quality of health care is important. The cost of campaigns has grown significantly, and it's a reality that it requires money to buy time in today's expanding media environment and conduct the social research that is now part of any elected official's career.

Nursing's future depends on nurses participating in activities that shape policy. Without significant participation, nurses risk having their presence and concerns unrepresented. Nurses can be active members of nursing organizations that take political action; they can take on active roles in a political party and attend political meetings, forums, and rallies; they can help register people to vote; they can contribute and raise money for causes and campaigns through PACs. The ANA-PAC evaluates the voting records of incumbent candidates campaigning for reelection, and the ANA state constituents develop relationships with candidates running for open seats.

Song (2011) states, "ANA does not use dues dollars to support candidates. Rather, ANA-PAC raises money through the voluntary donations from member nurses across the country. These nurses understand the importance of having a seat at the table when Congress is discussing nursing issues, such as appropriate staffing, home health, and safe patient handling. ANA-PAC donates to candidates who work to implement healthy public policy for our profession" (p. 15).

Discussion Point

Do all RNs benefit from the contributions and work for the members of the ANA who make monetary contributions to the ANA-PAC and help to elect "nurse-friendly" members of Congress? How would you go about determining the value of the contributions?

Nurses' professional work is linked to and affects policy in the workplace, though nurses often significantly underestimate how much of their work and the various practice settings are controlled by the government (policy). Across the country, nurses' capacity to influence policy will depend on having an increased awareness of how government policy decisions impact their practice and developing and applying skills where they can participate in influencing change. Achieving this level of increased awareness requires that nurses examine their values, use their voices, and take action. Nurses can no longer sit on the sidelines and say that government policy does not affect them. Health equity, access, and safe, affordable health care requires all nurses to become involved in public and health care policy.

To become engaged in civic participation will mean that nurses will have to balance the care of patients with the concerns of health care policy. Find an organization that speaks to your professional and core values. Then investigate the organization's legislative and policy agenda, learn what legislations impact nurses or nursing. There are several places where information about federal legislation can be located. These are listed in Table 24.1.

To become better informed about current issues affecting nursing and health care, consult additional websites of professional organizations. Other ways for nurses to learn about and increase their influence in politics and health care policy are shown in Box 24.4. These include becoming involved in electing candidates that nurses want to win. This requires that nurses learn about candidates and their agendas. When nurses support candidates that have a good chance of being elected or with a history of advocating for health care topics nurses support, there is greater opportunity to influence policy.

Nursing will benefit from managing its communication to avoid alienating elected officials involved with health care or social policies. One way to avoid eliciting negative responses from elected officials is for nursing (individually and as organizations) to present an evidence-based and objective approach to the issues, focusing on facts and not emotions. It is important for nurses to be aware that in elections where a candidate is an incumbent, the candidate will still need and value support. Activities nurses can undertake to support such a candidate include working with telephone or in-person outreach, fundraising, sending letters to the media, supporting the candidate in public forums, and either contributing funds personally or through engaging others to support the candidate.

Actions that nurses can take to increase their influence in the policy setting are also shown in Box 24.4.

TABLE 24.1 Federal Resources

Thomas website (http://thomas.loc.gov)
- Monitored by the Library of Congress
- Wealth of information available about the legislative process, including searches on bill status, public laws. House and Senate roll call votes, current activity in Congress.

Senate (www.senate.gov) and House (www.house.gov) websites
- Information about individual senators and representatives, committees, schedules, and search for legislation.
- Members of Congress can be contacted directly from each of these sites.

ANA Government Affairs website (http://www.nursingworld.org/MainMenuCategories/Policy-Advocacy)
- Contains legislation that has been identified as important to nurses and information about how nurses can contact their legislators to express concern and voice their opinion.

National League for Nursing website, the National League for Nursing's Public Policy Action Center (http://capwiz.com/nln/home).
- Social determinants of health include the issues of age, level of education, socioeconomic status, and access to health care. Through addressing these factors, there is a high capacity to improve the health of individuals and communities as well as reduce the costs of health care. To truly capture the inclusion of social and behavioral determinants of health data, nurses must lobby their legislators and others to ensure the social determinants of health are integrated into the policies and care delivery systems. Provides information about legislation affecting nursing and allows searches for elected officials using zip codes.

BOX 24.4   **Actions Nurses Can Take to Increase Their Influence in Politics and Policy**

To Influence Politics
* Be knowledgeable and get involved in campaigns (the earlier the better).
* Assist candidates in winning the endorsement of key organizations that you may be involved in, such as nursing organizations, parent–teacher organizations, and neighborhood organizations.

To Influence Policy
* Be a member of a nursing organization that influences policy at the local, state, and federal levels.
* Be informed. Subscribe to the social media sites for elected officials who have supported the policies you support and compare their involvement with that of your local representatives.
* Get to know your elected officials.
* Participate in the social media sites that your representatives and their staff monitor for feedback.
* Write letters presenting clear and concise information and a request for action on a specific area of policy (e.g., if there is pending legislation or a committee reviewing a particular policy, ask the official to support the position you have presented as benefitting the target population).
* Participate in the social media sites for the news. Write letters to the editor.
* Participate in coalitions of organizations, volunteering to participate in task forces, or to serve as an advocate in the community.

Consider This   Working together, speaking with one strong voice, nurses are a powerful political force. Consider the role social media has come to play in focusing public attention on health care issues. In 2017 an incident occurred where a nurse was assaulted by a law enforcement officer for protecting her patient's federally protected rights. The event was shared on social media and resulted in national attention and generated increased public awareness of the dangers faced by nurses. Many elected officials commented on the situation, and multiple national and local nursing organizations also used social media to address the issue ("American Nurses Association Calls for Action," 2017).

Shaping policy begins with a nurse selecting and learning about the policy issues that are personally and professionally important enough for that nurse to become an active participant in the policy activities. One way to become engaged is through joining or supporting professional nursing organizations or other relevant organizations that are aligned with professional goals and objectives. Professional membership organizations provide information, education, and opportunities to become active around key professional and societal issues. Most organizations, committees, and task forces provide opportunities for nurses to learn about organizational structure, function, and governance. In fact, all organizations have a legislative or PAC to address policy concerns or issues.

For years there have been resources for nurses and other members of society to access their legislative representatives. In general, local government representation is available through local offices and nearly all communities. All congressional offices have websites with directories and guidance on how to reach the legislators and their staff. The nurse interested in contacting a legislator, such as member of the state or national congress, can use the resources available to identify the staff members working with the legislator. Often the key step to accessing a legislator is to work through the legislator's staff.

Since 2010, the increased presence of social media and expanded avenues of nearly instantaneous communication seek help from their congressional representative's district office. The district Chief of Staff is often the only "policy person" in the district. The office in the Capitol deals with legislation and policy issues. Staff members are vital in getting access to a legislator, so the politically nurse must be polite and respectful ways reach out to these individuals.

Finally, nurses who want to influence policy should write their legislative representatives regarding health care issues (Box 24.5). Letters should arrive before any proposed legislation is heard in committee because crucial decisions on proposed legislation are made in committee. Bills that have a financial impact are listened to in a policy committee and a financial committee. Some bills are assigned to two or more committees. This is often a tactic used to defeat the bill before it comes to the floor. If your legislator is not on the committee, write to the Committee Chair at the committee office address. If you write to legislators who do not

BOX 24.5   Sample Lobbying Letter

[1]Lillian Wald, RN, BSN
Henry Street
New York, New York 00251
[2]The Honorable Harry Nemo
Member, U.S. House of Representatives
House Office Building
Washington DC, 20015
[3]RE: SUPPORT for HR 1435
[4]Dear Representative Nemo,
[5]I am a registered nurse, and I have worked in the area of home health care for over 5 years. In the past 2 years, more and more of the elderly patients I care for have had to be readmitted to the hospital shortly after being discharged from the hospital because they are not taking their prescribed medications.
[6]It will save costly hospitalizations to provide needed prescription drugs at affordable costs to seniors. Please support H.R. 1435 and please advise me of your current position on this bill.
Sincerely,
[7]Lillian Wald, RN, BSN

---

[1]Include your address.
[2]Use the proper form of address (most elected and appointed officials are addressed as "the Honorable").
[3]State what the letter is regarding.
[4]Use the office title in the salutation.
[5]State your credentials and experience/belief/position.
[6]Urge support/opposition, and ask for a response with the official's position.
[7]Sign letter.
(Please be sure when signing your name to include RN after your name.)

BOX 24.6   Letter to the Editor

Letter: When Doctors Humiliate Nurses
Published: May 14, 2015
Today, hospitals pride themselves on providing patient-centered care by a multidisciplinary team, a hallmark of their quality. When one team member bullies another, patient care suffers. As a nurse, I would not want my family member or my nursing student in a hospital where physicians demean and insult their nurse colleagues, thus hampering their ability to care. A culture and a climate of respect and dignity not only win the day but also ensure patient safety and quality care. It's time physicians learned that nurses are on their team, poised to manage complex critical decisions and care for their patients. Please no bullying—it hurts.
Donna M. Nickitas
Old Greenwich, Conn., May 8, 2015
The writer is a nursing professor at Hunter College, Hunter-Bellevue School of Nursing.

represent you (you do not reside in their district), however, they are unlikely to respond to your communications because you are not one of their constituents. It is generally more effective to send a copy of the letter with a brief cover letter to your legislator urging his or her support when the bill comes to the floor (if bills pass out of committee, they go to the "floor" or the entire house of the legislature). If your legislator supports your position on legislation, send a thank you note or post your gratitude to the legislator's website or social media site. Thank you notes tell legislators that you are watching what they are doing.

Finally, nurse political change agents are nurses who use their nursing expertise to lobby elected and appointed officials on issues of concern to the profession; write letters to the editors of professional journals and newspapers (Box 24.6 for an example of a Letter to the Editor, which was sent to the editor of the *The New York Times* and published).

The work of health and public policy cannot be done in isolation. Nurses must build and participate in coalitions, encourage the participation of other nurses, and mentor future leaders. Most importantly, nurses must use their political muscle to enact and implement policies that enhance access, affordable quality health care, including nursing care; seek appointments or assist other nurses and friends of nursing in securing appointments to governing boards in the public and private sectors; be active members of political parties; query candidates about their positions on health care and assist with fundraising for candidates that support nurses and nursing; seek elected and/or appointed office, and continue to identify themselves as an RN; work on staffs of elected/appointed officials; and extend their policy influence beyond the health system to the community and the globe.

NURSING LEADERS AS POLICY PIONEERS

Nursing has a long history of involvement in politics and policy development. There are numerous nursing leaders who served as pioneers in public policy formation in the early to mid-1900s. Only a few are presented here, as is the area of policy they were most noted for. Their stories are similar; all of them shared passion, courage, and perseverance. Also, they all shared commitment to collective strength. These same attributes are recognized in nursing policy activists today.

Lavinia Dock: Organizing Nurses for Social Awareness

At the 1904 ANA convention, Lavinia Dock, a founder of the ANA and the first to donate money to establish the American Journal of Nursing that same year, stated that it was essential that nurses exercise social awareness. As a result, delegates to the ANA convention that year considered social (policy) issues of the time, including child labor, women's suffrage, and sex education.

Lillian Wald: Public Health and Child Welfare

Lillian Wald, one of the founders of the ANA, exemplified involvement in social change, community leadership, and politics. She graduated from nursing school and entered Women's Medical College in New York to become a doctor. During her first year of medical school, she volunteered to teach hygiene to immigrant women attending a school program.

In 1893, she quit medical school with a classmate, Mary Brewster, and moved to New York's Lower East Side neighborhood to provide nursing care in the community. A friend and philanthropist, Jacob Schiff, and Solomon Loeb agreed to fund Wald and Brewster's purchase of a house to support their public health work. This house became the Henry Street Settlement and is considered the founding place for public health nursing.

Margaret Sanger: Birth Control

One of the many nurses whose training included experience at the Henry Street Settlement was Margaret Sanger (See Figure 24.1). Sanger witnessed maternal and infant mortality resulting from uncontrolled fertility in the neighborhoods of the Lower East Side of New York City. She cared for women suffering from self-induced abortions and was motivated to make birth control available to women.

She brought about policy change by first bringing the public and policy-makers' attention to a compelling issue: poverty-associated maternal and infant mortality. She also supported her agenda by leveraging the other relevant societal conditions, which included the women's movement and rights to controlling their pregnancies. Finally, policy change occurred with the legalization of birth control.

Martha Minerva Franklin: Segregation and Discrimination

Martha Minerva Franklin was another pioneering public policy nurse in the early 20th century. She founded

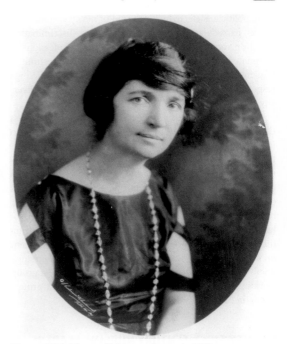

Figure 24.1 Photo of Margaret Sanger in 1922.

the National Association of Colored Graduate Nurses (NACGN) in 1908 with the fundraising assistance of Lillian Wald and Lavonia Dock, who mailed letters to more than 1,000 nurses ("ANA Hall of Fame: Martha Minerva Franklin," n.d.). The NACGN was formed because many states barred Black nurses from membership in state nurses' associations. Segregation, discrimination, and racism kept nursing education and hospitals separate.

The NACGN was instrumental, however, in political lobbying efforts to integrate Black nurses into the armed services during World War II. In 1951, the NACGN merged with the ANA (Flanagan, 1976). Today, the National Black Nurses Association exists as one of more than 70 national nursing organizations.

NURSES AND SOCIAL CHANGE

Historically, nursing leaders have participated in many efforts to bring about social change. Nurse leaders in the early 20th century were involved in passing socially focused legislation that outlawed child labor, supported the suffrage movement, and protected women abandoned by their husbands.

Nursing was also at the forefront of and lent integrity to the civil rights movement. As a result of the civil rights movement, poll taxes and literacy tests were made illegal.

Also, politicians elected with the aid of newly enfranchised Blacks passed laws intended to eliminate discrimination based on race. Nursing was one of the first professions to eliminate segregation. However, educational opportunities remain out of reach for many students of color, and nursing's responsibility to ensure that the profession reflects the diversity of those entrusted to its care still requires much work.

In 1974, the ANA set up a special account to help pass the Equal Rights Amendment to the Constitution and also joined a national boycott. The Amendment failed ratification by a sufficient number of states. The women's movement continued, and nursing and teaching were often used as examples of professions requiring a significant amount of knowledge and skill for which compensation fell far below male-dominated jobs requiring the same levels of knowledge and expertise, or "comparable worth." During the 1980s and beyond, nurses in a number of places went on strike to achieve wages of comparable worth. Nursing's involvement in the women's movement as its interest group working in coalition with other women's interest groups strengthened that movement.

TWENTY-FIRST-CENTURY NURSING LEADERS: NURSES SHAPING POLICY

Sylvia Trent-Adam, PhD, RN, FAAN

Deputy Surgeon General, as well as Chief Nurse Officer of the U.S. Public Health Service Commissioned Corps (USPHS), RADM Trent-Adams was appointed Acting Surgeon General in May 2017 to oversee the USPHS and is the leading spokesperson on public health in the federal government.

Patricia Brennan, PhD, RN, FACMI, FAAN

In August 2016, Dr. Brennan was appointed by National Institute of Health (NIH) to be the Director of the National Library of Medicine. As head of the world's most extensive medical library, she oversees all aspects of a vast collection used by scientists and health professionals around the world.

Patricia Grady, PhD, RN, FAAN

Dr. Grady has served as Director of NIH's National Institute of Nursing Research (NINR) since 1995. An internationally recognized researcher focused on stroke, she oversees an annual NINR budget of approximately $150 million that primarily funds the work of nurse scientists.

Bethany Hall-Long, PhD, RN, FAAN

In November 2016, Dr. Hall-Long was elected Lieutenant-Governor of the State of Delaware. She had previously served

14 years in the General Assembly, where she chaired the Senate Health and Social Services Committee. Dr. Hall-Long is also a professor at the University of Delaware School of Nursing.

> **Discussion Point**
> What can you do to help ensure nurses can use all their knowledge, skills, and experience to better help patients?

> *Consider This* The ANA was selected to testify at key hearings on national health insurance, amplifying nursing's voice on television to households throughout the country in advocating for comprehensive health coverage, including nursing care in all settings for all Americans.

CONCLUSIONS

What would Lillian Wald do about health care coverage for children and access to health care? What would Minerva Franklin do about racial health inequalities? What would Florence Nightingale do to elevate nursing in the policy debates? So the question for today is "What should nursing do to change the policies?"

At a time when the country is deeply divided along political party lines, the debates about health care insurance coverage and access have a profound impact on the citizens and residents of the United States regarding their health and well-being. Nurses must voice their concerns and speak to the public they serve. They are stakeholders in what happens within the delivery of health care (access, insurance coverage, cost, research), in the workplace (quality, staffing levels, safety, scope of practice, autonomy, working conditions), in the economy (unemployment's effect on mental and physical health and access to care), and in the social environment (addressing environmental-related illnesses and health crises related to social problems such as increased suicides, human trafficking, and opioid abuse).

Nurses can influence policies in the workplace and the community (both public and private). The bottom line is nurses must grasp their responsibility to be active participants and remain involved to address the nation's course of declining health by advocating for better health for all.

Pierce (2004) perhaps said it best:

> *As nurses, as voters, and as constituents, we must be a part of the solution. Our elected officials truly want to know what nurses think and it is our obligation as professionals and as citizens to let them know. Our patients and the American public trusts nurses and are counting on us to advocate on their behalf.* (p. 115)

For Additional Discussion

1. Are nongovernmental and governmental politics more alike than not? If not, how do they differ? If so, how are they alike?

2. Why do you believe nursing was the first profession to eliminate segregation?

3. What are the most significant nursing issues being debated in the policy arena?

4. With such limited membership in the ANA, will nurses ever have a political power base that is representative of the size of their voting block?

5. Why are so many nurses reluctant to become active in the political arena? What can be done to engage nurses in political work? The confidence? Do nurses perceive a lack of congruity between professional behavior and politics?

6. With the AMA typically being far better represented than the ANA in legislative lobbying, is nursing's risk of being dominated by medicine greater than ever?

7. How well informed are most legislators about contemporary health care and professional nursing issues?

8. What do you believe will be the next major policy issue affecting nursing to be debated in the political arena?

References

Adams, J. L., Lundeen, S., May, K. A., Smith, R. Wendt, E., & Young, L. K. (2016, July/August). Nurses for Wisconsin: A collaborative initiative to enhance the nurse educator workforce. *Journal of Professional Nursing, 32*(4). doi:10.1016/j.profnurs.2015.11.0

Ai, J. W., Zhang, Y., & Zhang, W. (2016). Zika virus outbreak: "a perfect storm." *Emerging Microbes & Infections, 5*(3), e21. doi:10.1038/emi.2016.42

American Hospital Association. (2014). *The value of membership in the American Hospital Association.* Retrieved from http://www.aha.org/about/membership/value.shtml

American Nurses Association calls for action in wake of police abuse of registered nurse. (2017, September 1). American Nurses Association. Retrieved January 2, 2017, from http://www.nursingworld.org/HomepageCategory/NursingInsider/NR-ANA-Calls-for-Action-Police-Abuse-Registered-Nurse-Utah-2017Sep1.html

American Nurses Association responds to Resolution 214 Amendment Presented by the American Medical Association. (2017, November 17). American Nurses Association. Retrieved January 2, 2017, from https://www.nursingworld.org/news/news-releases/2017-news-releases/american-nurses-association-responds-to-resolution-214-amendment-presented-by-the-american-medical-association/

ANA Hall of Fame Inductee: Martha Minerva Franklin. (n.d.). Retrieved from http://www.nursingworld.org/MarthaMinervaFranklin

Aries, N. (2016). To engage or not engage: Choices confronting nurses and other health professionals. In D. Nickitas, D. Middaugh, & N. Aries (Eds.), *Policy and politics for nurses and other health professionals* (pp. 16–33). Burlington, MA: Jones & Bartlett.

Barbour, C. and Wright. G. (2017). *Keeping the Republic: Power and Citizenship in American Politics* (8th ed). Thousand Oaks, CA: Sage.

Centers for Medicare & Medicaid Services. (2017). *National health accounts historical report.* Retrieved from https://www.cms.gov/Research-Statistics-Data-and-Systems/Statistics-Trends-and-Reports

Daley, K. (2011). Lessons in leadership. *American Nurse, 43*(3), 3.

Edmonson, C., McCarthy, C., Trent-Adams, S., McCain, C., & Marshall, J. (2017, January 31). Emerging global health issues: A nurse's role. *OJIN: The Online Journal of Issues in Nursing, 22*(1), Manuscript 2. doi:10.3912/OJIN.Vol-22No01Man02

Flanagan, L. (1976). *One strong voice.* Kansas City, MO: American Nurses Association.

Gallup. (2014). *Public rates nursing as most honest and ethical profession.* Retrieved from http://www.gallup.com/poll/9823/public-rates-nursing-most-honest-ethical-profession.aspx

Hayden, J. K., Smiley, R. A., Alexander, M., Kardong-Edgren, S., & Jeffries, P. R. (2014). The NCSBN National simulation study: A longitudinal, randomized, controlled study replacing clinical hours with simulation in prelicensure nursing education. *Journal of Nursing Regulation, 5*(2), S1–S44.

Institute of Medicine. (2011). *The future of nursing: Leading change, advancing health.* Washington, DC: National Academy of Sciences.

Kelly, M. A., Connor, A., Kun, K. E., & Salmon, M. E. (2008). Social responsibility: Conceptualization and embodiment in a school of nursing. *International Journal of Nursing Education Scholarship, 5*(1), Article 28.

Kraft, M., & Furlong, S. (2010). *Public policy-politics, analysis, and alternatives* (3rd ed.). Washington, DC: CQ Press.

Lasswell, H. (1936). *Politics: Who gets what, when, how.* New York: Meridian Books.

Lewenson, S. B., & Nickitas, D. M. (2016). Nursing's history of advocacy and action. In D. M. Nickitas, D. J. Middaugh, & N. Aries (Eds.), *Policy and politics for nurses and other health professionals* (2nd ed., pp. 3–13). Burlington, MA: Jones & Bartlett.

Milstead, J. (2016). *Health policy and politics: A nurse's guide* (4th ed.). Burlington, MA: Jones & Bartlett.

National Council of State Boards of Nursing. (2015). *About NCSBN.* Retrieved from https://www.ncsbn.org/about.htm

National Quality Forum. (2016). *Person- and family-centered care.* Retrieved from http://www.qualityforum.org/Topics/Person-_and_Family-Centered_Care.aspx

Nickitas, D. (2011). Cost and coverage in turbulent times. *Nursing Economic$, 29*(2), 57–58.

Nickitas, D. (2014). When nurses speak, will the nation listen. *Nursing Economic$, 32*(6), 218–282.

Pierce, K. M. (2004). Insights and reflections of a congressional nurse detailee. *Policy, Politics & Nursing Practice, 5*(2), 113–115.

Politics. (n.d.). In Online Dictionary of Social Sciences. Retrieved September 18, 2008, from http://bitbucket.icaap.org/dict.pl

Riffkin, R. (2014). *Americans rate nurses highest on honesty, ethical standards.* Retrieved from http://www.gallup.com/poll/180260/americans-rate-nurses-highest-honesty-ethical-standards.aspx

Robertson, R., & Middaugh, D. (2016). Conclusions: A policy toolkit for healthcare providers and activists. In D. Nickitas, D. Middaugh, & N. Aries (Eds.), *Policy and politics for nurses and other health professionals* (pp. 39–22). Sudbury, MA: Jones & Bartlett.

Sabatier, P. A. (Ed.). (1999). *Theories of the policy process.* Boulder, CO: Westview.

Sigma Theta Tau International. (2017). *Overcoming the health impact of social determinants.* Retrieved from http://www.sigmanursing.org/connect-engage/our-global-impact/gapfon; https://www.qualityforum.org/Overcoming_the_Health_Impact_of_Social_Determinants.aspx

Song, A. (2011). Defining ANA-PAC's role in the political process. *American Nurse, 43*(3), 15.

Tri-Council for Nursing. (2015). *Position statements.* Retrieved from http://tricouncilfornursing.org/Position-Statements.php

Tri-Council for Nursing. (2017). *A joint statement from the Tri-Council for Nursing: Increase access to care through APRN practice.* American Association of Colleges of Nursing | American Nurses Association American Organization of Nurse Executives | National League for Nursing. Retrieved from http://tricouncilfornursing.org/documents/Tri-Council-Joint-Statement-AMA-Resolution-2017.pdf

U.S. Department of Health and Human Services. (2010, March 23). *Key features of the Affordable Care Act by year.* Retrieved from http://www.hhs.gov/healthcare/facts/timeline/timeline-text.html

Watson, J. (2008). Social justice and human caring: A model of caring science as a hopeful paradigm for moral justice and humanity. *Creative Nursing, 14*(2), 54–61.

Professional Nursing Associations

Patricia E. Thompson and Cynthia Vlasich

CHAPTER OUTLINE

LEARNING OBJECTIVES

The learner will be able to:

1. Describe types of nursing associations and their value to members and the profession.

2. Explain the importance of nursing association missions.

3. Examine how nursing associations can strengthen their members' professional development across their careers.

4. Identify data an individual should access and review before selecting an association to join.

5. Identify challenges currently faced by nursing associations and possible solutions.

6. Explore the sustainability of nursing associations in the future.

INTRODUCTION

Nurses today have many choices in their careers. These include area and specialty in which they choose to practice, what work setting best suits them, how valuable unique certifications will be to them, and how they balance their careers with their lives, just to name a few. These choices can be relatively easy or quite hard to make, depending on the nurses' specific goals and career aspirations. Another choice nurses have is which professional associations they will join and, of those they join, how active they will be in each. Every association will have a unique mission and vision and offer different benefits to its members. The associations vary in focus from clinical specialty, academic development, scholarship, research, leadership, career advancement, to overall achievement. They also may vary in geographic scope, including local or state/provincial, national, and global.

Determining the associations that best meet the needs of each nurse is a personal decision and requires careful consideration, based on that nurse's individual career goals as well as expectations of association membership. However, it is critical for nurses to belong to and engage in professional associations, to enhance their own development, and to advance the profession.

TYPES OF NURSING ASSOCIATIONS

A nursing association is typically a not-for-profit entity that exists to serve and represent its members and meet the goals of the association based on its specific mission. Most are structured with an individual membership model; however, some organizations are association-membership based, such as the International Council of Nurses (ICN), which is a federation model. Other associations may be subsidiaries of a parent organization, such as the Association of Nurse Executives, which is a subsidiary of the American Hospital Association. Most associations, however, are autonomous.

One of the most important references for members of any association is that association's bylaws. An association's bylaws provide the governance structure through which that organization is led; incorporation laws within the country where the association is established provide the legal framework for the operation of the association.

Other key information about an association can frequently be found on that association's website, under the "About Us" or similarly labeled area. This information can help prospective members determine what type of nursing association it is, as well as the current initiatives, what is offered to members, and other resources that indicate

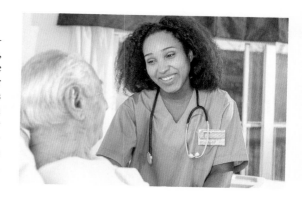

organizational priorities and where the organization invests its resources.

> **Consider This** Bylaws govern an association and provide a list of the association's purposes, but most members never review them.

Nursing associations are usually supported by a governing board of directors, elected officers, and paid and/or volunteer staff. These positions provide opportunities for members to serve in leadership roles on the board and network with stakeholders across the association. No matter how an association is structured, the main goal of every membership-based association should be to support its members and enable their success. Without members, associations would not exist. This goal, directly or indirectly, should be reflected in the association's mission, vision, and values, as well as in its programs, events, and services.

MISSION

Each nursing association has an identified mission that sets it apart from other organizations and addresses its main purpose for existence. The association may also have identified a vision and organizational values. The relationship between these is direct: the association mission is what the association does now, the association vision is what it hopes to become, and the association values are those specific beliefs that, with the mission and vision, guide the governing decisions of the association. The mission, vision, membership, and notable initiatives of three professional associations in nursing (American Nurses Association [ANA]; Sigma Theta Tau International [Sigma]; and the International Council of Nurses [ICN]) are compared in Boxes 25.1, 25.2, and 25.3.

BOX 25.1 **American Nurses Association**

About ANA

The American Nurses Association (ANA), part of the ANA Enterprise, represents registered nurses in the United States. ANA advances the profession by focusing on practice standards, positive work environments, nurse health, and issues affecting both nurses and the public.

Mission Statement

Nurses advancing our profession to improve health for all.

Members and Affiliates

The ANA represents the interests of the nation's 3.6 million registered nurses (RNs). Options for membership in the ANA include joint membership with constituent and state nurses associations, direct individual membership in the ANA, and through partnership specialty nursing and affiliate organization partnerships. For more information about the constituent and state nurses associations, ANA has an interactive association map.

Individual Members

ANA Only Membership (available in some states) and E-Membership are ways that individuals can become members of ANA directly. These members receive full member benefits at the national level, including the chance to influence decisions made at the national level that affect the practice of nursing and the health of our patients and our communities, but have no benefits at the state level. E-Members receive limited benefits and can access the members only section of NursingWorld.org.

Organizational Affiliates

ANA's affiliates are nursing organizations that belong to ANA as organizations. Working together, ANA and these organizational affiliates seek to share information and collaborate in finding solutions to concerns that face the nursing profession, across specialties. Affiliates are voting members in ANA's Membership Assembly.

Notable Initiative

Healthy Nurse, Healthy Nation

The Healthy Nurse, Healthy Nation™ Grand Challenge (HNHN GC) will:

• Engage nurses and partner organizations to take action in the areas of: "activity, sleep, nutrition, quality of life, and safety"
• Create a website to provide information and resources, motivate action, and connect nurses and other stakeholders.

ANA Enterprise Entities

American Academy of Nursing; http://www.aannet.org/
American Nurses Foundation; http://www.anfonline.org/
American Nurses Credentialing Center; http://www.nursecredentialing.org/

Sources: https://www.nursingworld.org/ana/; https://www.nursingworld.org/faqs/; http://www.healthynursehealthynation.org/en/about/about-the-hnhn-gc/

Meeting the Mission

To effectively support and engage their members, associations must first understand who their members are and why they choose to belong. This process begins with analyzing the organization's member demographics and needs. Age, level of education, place(s) of employment, range of financial income, areas of interest/specialty, certification(s), career goals, and motivation to join are examples of demographic data that an association may collect.

Associations should also collect data from potential members who have chosen not to join; determining why potential members chose not to join, and what their needs are, is important in reviewing association benefits. For example, a survey by Wiley Publishing (2014) indicated that 24% of potential members declined because of cost, 15% did not join because they were not asked, and 12% did not know what associations were available to join. Data such as these provide excellent opportunities for associations to learn and grow.

Associations must be in compliance with data collection rules, regulations, and policies, however, which limits the data they may collect. For example, the General Data Protection Regulation (GDPR) that went into effect in

BOX 25.2   **Sigma**

History

In 1922, six nurses founded the Honor Society of Nursing, Sigma Theta Tau International, now known as Sigma, at the Indiana University Training School for Nurses, which is now the Indiana University School of Nursing, in Indianapolis, Indiana, USA. The founders chose the name from the Greek words storgé, tharsos, and timé, meaning love, courage, and honor. Sigma became incorporated in 1985 as Sigma Theta Tau International Inc., a nonprofit organization with a 501(c)(3) tax status in the United States.

Mission

The mission of Sigma is advancing world health and celebrating nursing excellence in scholarship, leadership, and service.

Vision

Sigma's vision is to be the global organization of choice for nursing.

Membership

Sigma membership is by invitation to baccalaureate and graduate nursing students who demonstrate excellence in scholarship and to nurse leaders exhibiting exceptional achievements in nursing. Here are some additional facts about Sigma's membership:

* Sigma has more than 135,000 active members.
* Individual members live in more than 90 countries.
* More than 754 college and university campuses and three practice settings have a formal Sigma presence. Sigma has approximately 535 chapters located in 30 countries.
* Sigma communicates regularly with more than 100 nurse leaders who have expressed interest in establishing chapters globally, including those in Chile, China, Costa Rica, Denmark, Finland, India, Ireland, Israel, Germany, Jamaica, New Zealand, and Spain.

Notable Initiative

Sigma has convened a core panel of visionary global nurse leaders, the Global Advisory Panel on the Future of Nursing & Midwifery (GAPFON), to identify global health care issues, specifically noting those related to a voice and vision for nursing (Klopper & Hill, 2015). Additionally this panel is providing their thoughts on the current status of each of these issues and helping develop corresponding solutions that would effectively address them.

     Recognizing the need to actively involve key stakeholders from each global region and that the greatest opportunity to positively impact global health is multidisciplinary and intersectoral, the core panel has recommended expanding GAPFON to include engagement with a network of regional leaders across the world.

     Sigma officially released its 2014–2017 summary report on the GAPFON. Representing the culmination of 3 years of Sigma-led efforts, the report synthesizes data on global health care challenges and priority professional issues gathered at high-level meetings in each of the seven global regions. Sigma views the world's 19.3 million nurses and midwives as uniquely positioned to spearhead collaboration among health professionals from every discipline, and launched GAPFON to give nurses and midwives a unified voice and vision for the future to advance global health, while simultaneously strengthening professional roles.

Subsidiaries

Sigma Foundation for Nursing
The International Honor Society of Nursing Building Corporation
Sigma Marketplace

Source: Sigma Global Nursing Excellence. Retrieved from https://www.sigmanursing.org/why-sigma

2018 has bearing on many associations' ability to gather and utilize data.

     Existing data demonstrate that people join associations for multiple reasons, and those reasons differ between generational members (Myers, 2016). They may want to shape the future of the profession or enhance their careers. They may join to gain access to career support, association journals, continuing education opportunities, and other information that is available. They may believe in the association's mission and want to ensure it is achieved.

BOX 25.3 **International Council of Nurses**

About

The International Council of Nurses (ICN), founded in 1899, is a federation of more than 130 national nurse associations (NNAs). ICN focuses on quality care, health policy, evidence-based practice, professional workforce, and positive work environments.

ICN has strong collaborations and networks from the national to international levels. Examples include the World Health Organization, World Bank, and numerous nongovernmental organizations.

Mission

To represent nursing worldwide, advancing the profession and influencing health policy.

Vision (Strategic Intent)

"ICN's strategic intent is to enhance the health of individuals, populations, and societies by:
* championing the contribution and image of nurses worldwide
* advocating for nurses at all levels
* advancing the nursing profession
* influencing health, social, economic, and education policy."

ICN represents nurses globally in areas related to health, policy, and best practices. Population health and human rights are also a focus.

Membership

ICN is a federation ultimately representing millions of nurses globally. ICN works with these member associations related to the nursing profession. Individual membership in ICN is not available. Members of their national nurses association are part of ICN.

Notable Initiative

Girl Child Education Fund

The Girl Child Education Fund (GCEF) supports the primary and secondary schooling of girls under the age of 18 in developing countries whose nurse parent or parents have died. Your HYPERLINK "http://www.icn.ch/shop/en/donations/4-donation.html" donations to the GCEF support school fees, uniforms, shoes, and books. Donations to the GCEF can be made by credit card, bank transfer, or cheque.

Since the initiation of the program, over 350 girls have been enrolled in the GCEF. Currently 103 girls are being supported in Kenya, Swaziland, Uganda, and Zambia.

Foundations

Florence Nightingale International Foundation (FNIF)
The International Council of Nurses Foundation (ICNF)

Source: International Council of Nurses. *Who we are.* Retrieved from http://www.icn.ch/who-we-are/who-we-are; International Council of Nurses. *Members.* Retrieved from http://www.icn.ch/members/members; International Council of Nurses. *Girl child education fund.* Retrieved from http://www.icn.ch/what-we-do/girl-child-education-fund

Some join to enjoy the status of membership or because of the networking and mentoring available. Some join to celebrate and foster professional achievement, and some for the financial benefits of discounts and perks (Jacobs, 2014). Others join because of peer pressure or supervisor expectations.

Associations must leverage their strengths and determine what they provide that is unique for their members (Barnes & Nelson, 2014). Then, based on member assessments, associations must determine the scope and specific combination of services to offer, to meet their members' demands. They have a responsibility to determine member needs and appropriate

delivery modalities for programs and services. This allows current and potential members to make informed decisions on which association(s) will best meet their needs.

Today most associations have members across multiple age ranges and at different points in their careers. Because of generational issues in how people work and what they expect both from their workplace and from the associations they join, associations must provide support for members across generations, with differing career trajectories, with various levels of experience and motivations to join, for the association to meet its mission. Many organizations create a menu of benefit options to address the varied needs of their individual members. Additionally, given the geographic diversity of current and prospective members, as well as trends in virtual education and engagement, some professional associations offer virtual membership options to meet member needs.

Different interaction modalities are important to meet members' learning preferences and geographical locations. They include:

- Face-to-face programs and meetings
- Electronic mail, blogs, and communication boards
- Videoconferences, webinars, and other online options
- All forms of social media

Discussion Point

What strategies might be used to meet the needs of a geographically diverse membership?

For example, if association data indicate that a key motivator for membership is networking, then ensuring that rich opportunities to network one-on-one and with other members and member groups that have similar interests should become a priority. To be responsive, that association might create networking activities at events and through online communities and opportunities to collaborate on projects and programs that benefit not only the members involved with the actual work but also others in the profession.

CHOOSING TO BELONG

Nursing is a profession where association membership can provide great personal and professional value. Many of the nurse leaders in our profession today have not only become known within the field of nursing through their involvement in professional associations but also fine-honed their professional and leadership skills and created lifelong relationships with colleagues through such memberships.

According to the American Nurses Association Code of Ethics (2015, p. 35), "Individual nurses are represented by their professional associations and organizations. These groups give united voice to the profession. . . . Through its professional organizations, the nursing profession must reaffirm and strengthen nursing values and ideals so that when those values are challenged, adherence is steadfast and unwavering."

Benefits vary based on the mission of the association, but they are all important for professional growth across the members' career. Examples include:

- Educational programs providing continuing nursing education on topics related to association mission, with content focused on clinical practice, academic settings, leadership, scholarship, policy, and others.
- Association journals providing current knowledge and updates.
- Certification in specialty areas to demonstrate expertise and credibility.
- Networking to connect and collaborate with experts in your area of interest.
- Opportunities to identify mentors to assist the member with both short- and long-term goals related to career development.
- Content related to developing knowledge and skills to be a mentor.
- Awards and recognition such as research grants or travel stipends to present papers at conferences or public recognition for outstanding accomplishments.
- Discounts for goods or services, such as liability insurance, computers, or rental cars (Akans et al., 2013; Esmaeili, Deghan-Nayeri, & Negarandeh, 2013).

Discussion Point

Discuss how mentors/role models in professional associations might advance your professional development, providing specific examples.

We all balance personal and professional demands and need to carefully weigh opportunities and obligations to ensure we maintain the equilibrium needed for a healthy lifestyle and career. Association membership can assist with maintaining that personal/professional balance by providing the benefits listed above and many more—all in one place.

When considering which association(s) to join, it is important to review the benefits of the association based on a personal cost–benefit ratio. Each nurse must determine what they expect to gain from membership in any given association or a variety of associations, and in return, what they are willing to give in terms of membership dues and active engagement/participation. Individuals must be able to analyze and determine the value to them of both tangible and intangible benefits. Individuals should research various association options and analyze what each has to offer. In addition to culling through an association's website, they should call their membership offices to discuss the benefits of membership, and they should also speak with colleagues about what they recommend.

For example, if a membership association's annual dues are $100 and the benefits include free journal access, free continuing nursing education, and other tangible benefits, you can calculate a direct cost–benefit ratio based on the expense of these tangible items if purchased separately without the membership benefit. One must then determine and include the value of the intangible benefits, such as networking; the ability to meet and work with professional leaders within the association, to be mentored, to collaborate with others; and access to events or products. Based on that analysis, each individual can determine what the combined tangible and intangible cost–benefit ratio is, and thus the ultimate value, to them.

Many nursing colleagues choose to participate in two or more associations, gaining different value from each. Frequently this is a blend of associations with different missions, such as a unique specialty association combined with a more broadly focused national or global organization. Whether interests are focused at the local, state, provincial, national, regional, or global level, and whether they are specifically related to a specialty area or broader in nature, associations exist that can provide individuals with all those opportunities.

The benefits derived from professional association membership will be directly related to your level of involvement in the association. Many associations have a plethora of opportunities for their members, such as job opportunities and career advice, attending and networking at conferences and seminars, accessing professional journals and continuing education, daily or weekly news briefs/updates, and professional mentoring and networking. In addition, there are opportunities to serve on committees and boards that foster your leadership development and allow you to engage in policy and advocate for clients/patients. Taking advantage of all of the opportunities that are of interest to you will be critical to enjoying a full and valuable membership; engagement is key to realize the full benefits of an association. Association membership can provide a wonderfully well-rounded and rich professional experience and greatly enhance one's career.

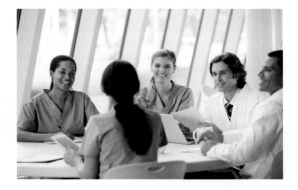

Discussion Point

Describe the factors important to you in deciding which nursing association(s) to join.

VALUE TO THE PROFESSION

Nursing associations exist to both support their members and address critical issues and challenges that face the profession and health care in general. Associations demonstrate support for their members and engage their members effectively through offering various professional education, networking, and mentoring opportunities. Many nursing associations, as a key part of their missions, also have a goal to improve health care, either directly or indirectly. This work may be quite broad or focused in specific educational or clinical practice areas, and may be local, regional, national, and/or global in scope.

Each organization's support of the profession should be mission specific and, depending on the organization, focus on one or more of the following:

- Policy, regulatory, and legislative support
  - Some associations exist to create, enact, and/or monitor compliance with professional practice laws and the standards created by various accrediting bodies. There are legal and voluntary standards that control the profession's work including licensure at all levels of nursing practice. Various accreditation bodies exist to support education, quality, and credentialing regarding practice.

- Developing practice standards
  - The mission of many organizations, including those with a specialty focus, is to develop and promote quality and evidence-based practice standards. These expected professional performance levels are often included or indicated in regulatory statements and used as a benchmark any time a legal question arises regarding professional performance.

- Creating positive work environments
  - Working conditions are often addressed by various accrediting bodies that relate to education and practice settings, as well as associations that may address this topic via research and dissemination of best practices. In addition, the missions of some organizations include collective bargaining, which is typically undertaken to support working conditions.

- Enhancing the profession
  - Professional associations are a voice for the profession to consumers and to policy makers. They maintain professional values and standards and support the profession through the opportunities they provide their members to grow and develop. Leadership opportunities to serve on boards, be involved on committees, and take action to move the organization and the profession forward in a positive way are often provided by professional associations.
  - Professional associations may also engage in or support conducting research related to professional enhancement in numerous ways, from support for practice standards, positive work environments, impact of performing to scope of practice, to identification of global professional issues and strategies to address them. For example, in 2017 Sigma (2017) published the *Global Advisory Panel on Nursing and Midwifery; Bridging the Gaps for Health* report that includes global priorities and strategies pertaining to all these areas.
  - Credentialing is another way organizations enhance the profession. It provides validity to knowledge and expertise for nurses in a particular area through assessment against established standards for that area.

Discussion Point

Explain why practice standards need to be evidence based.

Consider This Through maintaining professional values and standards, associations represent the profession to key stakeholders such as policy makers and the public.

Discussion Point

Some of the professional issues nursing associations address include scope of practice, quality and access to care, patient and nurse safety, and legislation that impacts practice. Select one of the above and explain the role of associations in addressing the issue. What other professional issues do nursing associations address?

PROFESSIONAL ASSOCIATION CHALLENGES

Professional associations are charged to remain relevant, valuable, and significant to all their members, at a time when membership crosses not only multiple generations but also multiple cultures. Whether a national, regional, or international organization, the reality is we are a global community with members from diverse cultures. Effectively recognizing and understanding a variety of norms, standards, and protocols, as well as meeting diverse cultural expectations is required for global success.

With the often-noted differences in Baby Boomers, Gen Xers, and Millennials, providing value and significance to all these generational members is a daunting challenge. Whether they value career success, personal time, or the ability to design a customized career life that suits their individuality ("Generational Differences Chart," 2015), each group has, in general, certain traits that, of course, do not hold true for all members of that generation. So what does this mean for associations? It means the association must be flexible in programming and approach and must offer a variety of options to provide value to different members.

As an association develops this menu of benefits, which may include programs, events, products, and services, each must be reviewed with keen attention to meeting the members' needs within both the mission and the resources of the organization.

Discussion Point

Discuss the challenges of meeting member needs across generations and options you feel would be effective for associations to reach such diverse membership.

In addition to generational diversity, today many associations are responding to an increasingly global community because of expansion into multiple countries and regions. This growth broadens the traditional local chapter model to encompass state, province, country, and global regional models. This global diversity not only impacts how the organization must grow but also brings additional complexity to meeting member needs, far beyond generational issues. Cultural diversity, combined with generational diversity, and the varying values that a rich cultural and generational membership mix provides, offers a unique opportunity and challenge for professional associations in meeting their members' needs.

Discussion Point

The practice of nursing differs greatly around the world. How do nursing associations bridge the chasm between diverse cultures, norms, and scopes of practice?

Associations must have strategic planning for global expansion, recognizing the implications for the organization and membership. Because organizations consider global growth, they must carefully scrutinize their organizational mission, vision for the future, intention, member demographics, and member demand, balanced against current and projected organizational resources, to ensure they are positioned not only to initiate global growth but also to achieve sustained, successful, and continued global expansion. Because associations design the best multiple strategy approach to reach their members, the strategy must include a variety of modalities to facilitate participation across the globe. Current and prospective members also need to consider the personal value they would find in being part of an association that is global in scope or one that is planning global expansion.

Discussion Point

What are the benefits and challenges to the association and to its members if a country-specific association decides to expand globally?

Members also value timely information about benefit opportunities, as well as how programs, events, products, and services are delivered. For example, an association may have an outstanding program; however, if it is not marketed effectively, and/or delivered in a manner that does not benefit the members, the program is of little value, and, indeed, can be detrimental if it leads to a disappointing experience for the members.

To that end, associations need to not only offer quality programs but also market them in such a way so that members recognize the value of the opportunities available for personal and professional growth. From a business construct, positioning the value of the association and its programs based on (1) features, (2) benefits, and (3) member value, customized to differing membership audiences may be a highly effective messaging strategy.

Communication with members must be fluid, flexible, and varied. For example, some members will prefer communication via phone calls and tangible mailings, whereas others communicate primarily via e-mail, text message, and social media. Being aware of their current member preferences regarding communications, communication trends in general, as well as specific guidance to meet legal limitations is vital for the success of any organization.

Discussion Point

How have you changed the way you communicate with colleagues, family, and friends over the past 3 years? How do you prefer to communicate now versus 3 years ago?

Another strategic decision for associations to make is where to focus their resources and how to prioritize what professional issues to address. There are many nursing and health care issues, and it is easy for the board of an association to enthusiastically slip into a mode of wanting to solve them all. However, it is critical that the association board of directors ensures all initiatives relate to the mission, so the association stays within its legal parameters. The focus should also support the association vision and uphold its values.

Discussion Point

Review missions of various professional nursing associations and determine which one(s) best meet your needs.

Consider This Nursing is the most trusted profession according to repeated Gallup poll results. And yet it is one of the least influential.

A major challenge faced by associations today is increasing their membership when current and potential members are careful in how they spend their money and time. Associations must develop strategies to demonstrate there is actual value in the dues a member pays and the time they volunteer. One strategy is to allow payment of dues over time. However, the most critical factor for members paying association dues is their ability to easily identify perceived personal value for their membership (Jacobs, 2014).

To address the demands of work, personal life, and other activities, associations need to help members recognize the many ways associations can help them, to improve their practice, save them time, increase their opportunities for advancement, and in many other ways. For example, easy access to mentors and networks can facilitate the members' ability to reach career goals more quickly. Members can connect with experts to assist with practice and educational, leadership, and scholarship goals (Esmaeili et al., 2013; Jacobs, 2014).

Engaging members can also be a challenge, but is essential for the success of an association. For example, ensuring members are offered opportunities to lead and govern the organization is critical for most associations whose board, committee work, and program content are accomplished through member volunteers. Special emphasis should be placed on engaging new members immediately and often, as well as engaging all members in activities and programs that are meaningful to them; these actions will in turn develop long-term loyalty. Providing a diverse variety of rich opportunities for member volunteers can be one of the most powerful strengths of an association. If these opportunities effectively address cultural, gender, generational, and geographic diversity, they can assist the association in providing value to membership through engagement, and this will lead the organization to success with positive outcomes for everyone.

SUSTAINABILITY

The association that is nimble, designed to respond quickly and efficiently to new opportunities, able to divest itself of ineffective programs, and provides diverse, meaningful, and impactful programs and opportunities for its members is best poised for long-term success.

Resilience

As with any organization, associations that thrive in a culture of change are best positioned to succeed. It is essential that organizations are flexible and able to adapt quickly for them to remain relevant. They must not only react to change, but must also be adept at predicting change. Nowhere is this more apparent than in professional associations. They must be responsive as well as responsible, be able to facilitate change, as well as assist their members in successfully navigating through a changing environment.

Knowledge Dissemination

Professional knowledge is vast and growing daily. Analyzing and sharing fresh and well-developed data in a way that is useful to members is a key value that organizations/associations provide and that members will continue to need in the future.

Leadership Development

Professional associations must have visionary leaders and highly competent staff to thrive. Associations also have a responsibility to help develop the next generation of nurse leaders both for the association and for the profession. They must create an environment to nurture and grow those nurse leaders. An association may barely survive or fully thrive depending on the knowledge and skill of its paid and volunteer leadership. Early identification, development, and mentoring of member and staff leaders, who bring expertise and loyalty to leadership positions within the association, are vital to both current success and long-term sustainability.

> **Consider This**   The IOM report on the Future of Nursing addresses the need for more nursing leaders now and in the future. Professional associations provide knowledge, skills, and opportunities to develop as leaders.

Collaboration

Although some associations feel a competitive model of work is beneficial, those organizations that have similar missions can benefit in great measure through collaboration with each other. Collaboration can provide a collective voice, a respectful diversity of opinion, experts, and expertise, and strengthen results while minimizing resource outlay.

> **Consider This**   Collaboration among nursing associations to address key nursing and health care issues conserves resources and strengthens the voice of the profession.

> ### Discussion Point
> Is interprofessional collaboration important for nursing associations in addressing health care issues? Why?

No one association is as powerful individually as all are collectively. With that, are associations the appropriate venue for sustaining nursing in the future? The answer is a resounding YES. The benefit of collaboration has proven to be powerful; it can change practice, establish standards, enact laws, sustain workplace settings in which nurses can best succeed, and support an environment in which our students and new graduates feel welcomed into the profession and are safe.

Resource Management

The key for sustainability in the future is an infrastructure that includes adequate human and financial resources. Associations need to engage and maintain their members and volunteer leaders, as well as hire expert staff. These are the people who provide the vision, accomplish the work, and maintain the relevance of the organization. Associations need to develop a multisource revenue base. Relying mainly on dues for revenue will not result in sustainability (Research Fuels the Controversy 25.1). Nondues revenue from programs, products, and services is often used as part of a multisource revenue strategy. However, other options need to be

Research Fuels the Controversy 25.1

Exploring Member Engagement

The focus of this research was to identify alignment and gaps between the reasons members state they engage with professional associations and why association staff believe members engage. In April 2016, an online survey was sent to 149 membership staff professionals and 1,030 active association members across generations from Millennials to Matures.

Source: Myers, A. (2016). *Member engagement study: Aligning organization strategy with what matters most to members.* Austin, TX: Abila.

Study Findings

Survey results demonstrated some similarities across generations for member engagement. A code of ethics and professional information rated as the highest benefits for Generation Xers, Boomers, and Matures. For Millennials opportunities for jobs was listed first with a code of ethics second.

Areas identified by members to maintain engagement were networking, professional development, and acquiring knowledge. Opportunities to volunteer were also important.

For organizational professionals, priority member engagement areas identified were attending conferences, ability to socialize, and acquiring information.

The article concludes with recommendations for association professionals to develop strategies to maintain and engage members across generations and their careers.

Conflict of Interest

This research was commissioned by Abila, a software company, with products for nonprofit associations. Abila paid Edge Research to conduct and analyze the online surveys for this study.

---

explored. Collaborating with other associations for programming events conserves resources, as well as increases networking opportunities for members and the reach of those programs. In addition, associations that are going to be viable in the future must have a strategy that includes building a reserve fund to access when unexpected situations occur.

Member Value

The association that not only meets member needs but surpasses member expectations, now and in the future, positions itself for long-term sustainability. And those associations that provide such value so that membership is seen as a necessity, not a choice, will flourish.

RESEARCH OPPORTUNITIES

The focus of professional associations is to meet the needs of members and the nursing profession. Although there are examples and some qualitative data available, there is limited evidence to document the outcomes of association work. Therefore, more research needs to be conducted in this area. Below are some ideas that can be developed into studies:

- Survey members in board-level association positions to determine what motivated them to become engaged members.

- What are the characteristics of associations that will thrive in the future?
- Analyze outcomes of associations with a policy focus.
- Survey association executive officers to assess the future of associations.
- Is there a relationship between association membership and nurses in leadership roles?
- Does leadership in student nurse associations translate into membership in professional associations after graduation?
- How can associations address the needs of an increasingly diverse membership?
- What effect will the large number of retiring baby boomers have on association viability?

CONCLUSIONS

Nursing associations seek to elevate the practice of nursing, with the ultimate goal of supporting their members and improving health care and health care outcomes. Every nurse can benefit personally and professionally from active membership in the organization(s) that best meet their needs. With visionary leadership and strong participation, associations advance our profession, locally, regionally, and globally.

For Additional Discussion

1. Determine the cost–benefit ratio for you to join a professional nursing association. Identify both the tangible and intangible benefits.

2. Explain how professional nursing associations enhance the nursing profession.

3. Discuss why effective marketing is key to a professional nursing association's success.

4. Explain how a professional nursing association should make decisions about which professional issues to address.

5. How can professional nursing associations help nursing become more influential?

6. How can collaboration benefit nursing associations and the profession?

7. How can professional nursing associations develop long-term loyalty from their members?

8. Identify key factors necessary for a professional nursing association to thrive.

9. "Resilience" is a popular term and is currently applied to many areas of health care. What does resilience really mean—in the broader framework of health care, as well as in your specific setting? Describe how a professional nursing association can develop and maintain resilience.

10. What professional nursing associations do you know most about? Least about?

11. If you could provide recommendations or advice to any professional nursing association on how best to recruit and retain members, what would those recommendations/that advice be?

12. As you analyze your career goals and direction, which professional nursing associations would be best for you to affiliate with and become a leader of?

13. If you were launching a new professional nursing association, what would its mission be?

14. Of the various types of diversity, for example, culture, gender, age, and socioeconomic status, which do you feel would be most challenging for a professional nursing association to effectively address?

References

Akans, M., Harrington, M., McCash, J., Childs, A., Gripentrog, J., Cole, S., … Fuehr, P. (2013). Cultivating future nurse leaders with student nurses associations. *Nursing for Women's Health, 17*(4), 343–346.

American Nurses Association. (2015). *Code of ethics for nurses with interpretive statements.* Silver Spring, MD: Author.

Barnes, J., & Nelson, J. (2014). *Exploring the future of membership.* ASAE Foundation Research Series, 1–18. Retrieved from https://www.asaecenter.org/publications/108025-exploring-the-future-of-membership-pdf

Esmaeili, M., Deghan-Nayeri, N., & Negarandeh, R. (2013). Factors impacting membership and non-membership in nursing associations: A qualitative study. *Nursing & Health Sciences, 15*(3), 265–272.

Generational differences chart. (2015, March 18). Retrieved from West Midland Family Center Website: http://www.wmfc.org/uploads/GenerationalDifferencesChart.pdf

Jacobs, S. (2014). *The art of membership: How to attract, retain, and cement member loyalty* (1st ed.). San Francisco, CA: Jossey-Bass.

Klopper, H. C., & Hill, M. (2015). Global Advisory Panel on the Future of Nursing (GAPFON) and global health. *Journal of Nursing Scholarship, 47*(1), 3–4.

Myers, A. (2016). *Member engagement study: Aligning organization strategy with what matters most to members.* Austin, TX: Abila.

Sigma Theta Tau International. (2017). *The Global Advisory Panel on the Future of Nursing & Midwifery (GAPFON®) Report.* Indianapolis, IN: Author. Retrieved from http://www.nursinglibrary.org/vhl/handle/10755/621599

Wiley Publishing. (2014). *Membership matters: Lessons from members and non-members* (pp. 1–8). Hoboken, NJ: Author.

Index

Note: Page numbers followed by *b*, *f* and *t* indicates boxes, figures and tables respectively.